AF818983

Exercise and Human Reproduction

Diana Vaamonde
Stefan S. du Plessis • Ashok Agarwal
Editors

Exercise and Human Reproduction

Induced Fertility Disorders and Possible Therapies

Springer

Editors
Diana Vaamonde, PhD
Department of Morphological Sciences
School of Medicine
University of Cordoba
International Network on Physical
Exercise and Fertility (INPEF)
Cordoba, Spain

Ashok Agarwal, PhD, HCLD (ABB), ELD (ACE)
American Center for Reproductive Medicine
Cleveland Clinic Foundation
Cleveland, OH, USA

Stefan S. du Plessis, MBA, PhD (Stell)
Division of Medical Physiology
Department of Biomedical Sciences
Stellenbosch University
Tygerberg, Cape Town, South Africa

ISBN 978-1-4939-3400-3 ISBN 978-1-4939-3402-7 (eBook)
DOI 10.1007/978-1-4939-3402-7
Springer New York Heidelberg Dordrecht London

Library of Congress Control Number: 2016932003

© Springer Science+Business Media New York 2016
This work is subject to copyright. All rights are reserved by the Publisher, whether the whole or part of the material is concerned, specifically the rights of translation, reprinting, reuse of illustrations, recitation, broadcasting, reproduction on microfilms or in any other physical way, and transmission or information storage and retrieval, electronic adaptation, computer software, or by similar or dissimilar methodology now known or hereafter developed.
The use of general descriptive names, registered names, trademarks, service marks, etc. in this publication does not imply, even in the absence of a specific statement, that such names are exempt from the relevant protective laws and regulations and therefore free for general use.
The publisher, the authors and the editors are safe to assume that the advice and information in this book are believed to be true and accurate at the date of publication. Neither the publisher nor the authors or the editors give a warranty, express or implied, with respect to the material contained herein or for any errors or omissions that may have been made.

Printed on acid-free paper

Springer Science+Business Media LLC New York is part of Springer Science+Business Media
(www.springer.com)

Foreword

When a female athlete asks you as her physician, or her science teacher, or her coach, or her pharmacist, or her trainer, a seemingly simple set of two questions, like:

"Can I continue to compete on my club soccer team and my husband on his while we are trying to get, and how will that affect our odds of getting pregnant?" and

"Will prenatal vitamins help for me or for him or for both so we do have a better chance of conceiving a healthy baby?"

You might probe with a few more questions, like how often and how intensely your patient and her partner practice and play. You would then think there would be an easy "Googleable source" to find answers. You had most likely be disappointed, until now. Yes, you would probably know that as the frequency and intensity of exercise increases, greater concern and major reactions might cause deleterious effects on somatic growth, pubertal development, and biological maturation. But you would almost certainly lack definitive answers. This book clarifies the questions to ask so that answers to these and many other key questions are clear, and does the most important part of knowing about any field, letting you know where the data are not available and/or are not definitive.

For example, the authors of Chap. 17 present the data clearly on the interactions between the various components of oral or transdermal contraception and factors influencing exercise performance. But the authors also state clearly where more data are needed to define specifically and with conclusiveness the impact of specific hormonal contraceptive use and exercise performance.

Yes, while sports and sex stories and videos are the most read and watched, it is rarer than seeing a 1947 Mercedes two seat convertible with a Spanish license plate on an American highway that practitioners of medicine or of coaching, or even trainers or participants have critical and well-informed conversations about how sex and sport performance relate to fertility and pregnancy outcomes. You want experts in the field to describe the current state of the art and the science, and that is what this book gives you.

Whether the most strenuous part of your day is shampooing your hair or galloping 1000 m repeats at dawn and at dusk, this book answers concerns that range from the effects of specific nutrition and meditation on pregnancy rates and outcomes of oral contraceptive and anabolic steroid use you should have for your own well-being, and for the practitioners ask casual or concentrated questions. No matter who you are (and whether you know definitively that "who" should be a "whom" or a "who"), your physical activities and nutritional patterns affect your sex hormones and physiology. And for those most at risk of disturbing their reproductive health—those who exercise the most, the least, or with abetting from steroids—mastering the distinctions between beneficial and harmful levels of activity and nutrient intake is critical.

Making sure you or your patients mechanics are primed for healthy baby making is simply one aspect, if a significant one, of exercise for both fitness and health (these are not the same, as the book differentiates). Bone health, nutrient availability, endocrine function, metabolism, mental well-being, and physical exercise intensity all interact—and the key knowledge about and parts of those complex interactions are described with enviable clarity in this book.

And by the way, for the practitioner or the coach, or player, it is indispensable in guiding answers about exercise and fertility in both men and women—if you would read the chapter on that very subject about chances of getting pregnant while competing in this book, you might know to ask a few more questions to help define your answers to the questions posed at the start of this foreword.

Whether you want just more information to advise your patients, or even your daughter, son, or yourself, or are a major researcher in the field, this book lets you know how to advise based on the current state of that area of this field. Yes, now there is a complete guide coupled with *Physiologic Reference Manual,* and you are reading from it. This book is unparalleled, unequalled, and indispensable for all touching others in any of the areas that affect the mix of sex and sport.

Chief Wellness Officer,
The Cleveland Clinic
Gorman Family Chair Holder and Chair of the
Wellness Institute at the Cleveland Clinic

Author of Four #1 NY Times Best Sellers, including *RealAge: Are You As Young As You Can Be?* and *YOU: The Owner's Manual.*

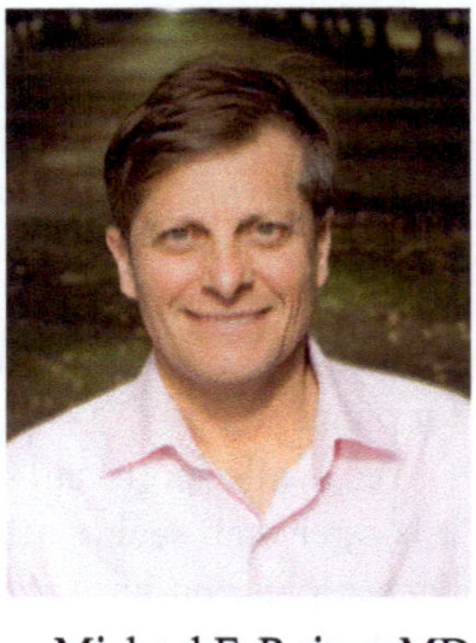

Michael F. Roizen MD

Preface

The etiologies of human reproductive disorders are fairly well known; yet, there are still many instances in which infertility is classified as idiopathic. This simply means that the cause behind the problem is unknown. There is growing evidence that physical exercise and sports practice may affect reproduction which may be the unknown factor in certain infertility cases.

With this first-of-a-kind textbook, we aim to provide a comprehensive review of the interaction between exercise and human reproduction, how exercise can have a positive or negative impact on male and female fertility with specific emphasis on the mechanisms that may lead to such effects. This textbook, which consists of 20 different yet interrelated themed topics, is intended to provide the reader with a meaningful and comprehensive review of the biological processes related to sports practice and how they interact with the reproductive function. The content covers the fundamental principles of human reproductive potential, sports physiology, the interaction between physical exercise and the endocrine and reproductive systems, associated nutritional aspects and possible strategies to avoid the potential harm of exercise on human reproduction. Each chapter was written by internationally recognized scientists and clinicians, making the text ideal for those seeking to increase their general knowledge in the field.

We trust that this book will have a broad and global appeal and be used not only as a reference for basic scientists, in the fields of sports medicine and reproductive medicine; but may also act as a guideline for physicians, physiologists, coaches, and professionals in the sports-human reproduction fields. Moreover, we anticipate that it may be an invaluable tool for multidisciplinary research teams since it brings together knowledge from a multitude of fields desiring that future research gaps and flaws will be diminished.

We want to thank all of the contributing authors for their inputs and are especially grateful to Michael D. Sova (developmental editor) and Kristopher Spring (executive editor) for their tireless efforts in reviewing and editing each manuscript. We would also like to acknowledge the University of Cordoba (Spain), the Division of Medical Physiology at Stellenbosch University (South Africa) and the American Center for Reproductive Medicine at the Cleveland Clinic (USA) for their institutional support. Finally, we want to express our gratitude toward our families for their support and patience in allowing us to complete this book.

Cordoba, Spain Diana Vaamonde

Tygerberg, Cape Town, South Africa Stefan S. du Plessis

Cleveland, OH, USA Ashok Agarwal

The original version of the book was revised.
An erratum can be found at DOI 10.1007/978-1-4939-3402-7_21

Contents

Contributors

Kathryn E. Ackerman, MD, MPH Division of Sports Medicine, Boston Children's Hospital, Sports Endocrine Research Lab, Neuroendocrine Unit, Massachusetts General Hospital Boston, Boston, MA, USA

Ashok Agarwal, PhD, HCLD (ABB), ELD (ACE) American Center for Reproductive Medicine, Cleveland Clinic Foundation, Cleveland, OH, USA

Carolina Algar-Santacruz, BSN Scientific Sport Association, Nutrir, Nutrición Médica y Ejercicio, Córdoba, Spain

Heather C. M. Allaway, MS Department of Kinesiology, Pennsylvania State University, University Park, PA, USA

Michelle Barrack, PhD, RD Department of Family and Consumer Sciences, California State University, Long Beach, CA, USA

Joao Sabino Cunha-Filho, MD, PhD Department of Obstetrics and Gynecology, Universidade Federal do Rio Grande do Sul, Porto Alegre, Brazil

Marzo Edir Da Silva-Grigoletto, PhD Department of Physical Education, Universidade Federal de Sergipe, Aracaju, SE, Brazil

Mary Jane De Souza, PhD Department of Kinesiology, Pennsylvania State University, University Park, PA, USA

Stefan S. du Plessis, MBA, PhD (Stell) Division of Medical Physiology, Department of Biomedical Sciences, Stellenbosch University, Cape Town, Tygerberg, South Africa

Maria de Lourdes Eguiguren, MD Department of Pediatric and Adolescent Medicine, Mayo Clinic, Rochester, MN, USA

Juan Marcelo Fernández, MSc, PhD Sport and Clinical Nutrition, Nutrition Group, Nutrir Medical Nutrition and Exercise Clinic, Andalusian Society of Sports Medicine (S.A.M.E.D.E.), Cordoba, Spain

Juan Manuel García-Manso, BS, MS, PhD Department of Physical Education, Universidad de Las Palmas de GranCanaria, Islas Canarias, Spain

Vanessa Krebs Genro, PhD Department of Obstetrics and Gynecology, Universidade Federal do Rio Grande do Sul, Porto Alegre, Rio Grand do Sul, Brazil

Neoklis A. Georgopoulos, MD, PhD Department of Obstetrics and Gynecology, Division of Reproductive Endocrinology, University of Patras, Medical School, University Hospital, Patras, Greece

Jenna C. Gibbs, PhD Department of Kinesiology, Pennsylvania State University, University Park, PA, USA

Anthony C. Hackney, PhD, DSc Department of Exercise & Sport Science, Department of Nutrition, University of North Carolina, Chapel Hill, NC, USA

Juan Ramón Heredia Elvar, MSc Department of Fitness and Health, International Institute for Exercise Science and Health, Alfàs del Pi, Spain

David R. Hooper, MA Department of Kinesiology, University of Connecticut, Storrs, CT, USA

Ignacio Jimena-Medina, MD, PhD Department of Morphological Sciences, School of Medicine, University of Cordoba, Cordoba, Spain

Luis Jiménez-Reina, MD, PhD Department of Morphological Sciences, School of Medicine, University of Cordoba, Cordoba, Spain

William J. Kraemer, PhD Department of Kinesiology, Physiology, Neurobiology, Medicine, University of Connecticut, Storrs, CT, USA

Thinus Frans Kruger, MBChB, MPharMed, MMed, MD, DSc Department of Obstetrics and Gynecology, Tygerberg Hospital, Stellenbosch University, Cape Town, Western Cape, South Africa

Michael I. Lambert, PhD Division of Exercise Science and Sports Medicine Department of Human Biology, University of Cape Town, Cape Town, Western Cape, South Africa

Amy R. Lane, BS, MA Department of Allied Health Sciences, University of North Carolina, Chapel Hill, NC, USA

Pieter Johann Maartens, BSc, HonBSc, MScMedSci Division of Medical Physiology, Faculty of Medicine and Health Sciences, Stellenbosch University, Cape Town, Tygerberg, South Africa

Rebecca J. Mallinson, PhD Department of Kinesiology, Pennsylvania State University, University Park, PA, USA

Roberto Matorras, MD, PhD Department of Obstetrics and Gynecology, Human Reproductive Unit, Cruces Hospital, Basque Country University, IVI Bilbao, Baracaldo, Vizcaya, Spain

Sarah J. Moss, PhD, MBA Physical activity, Sport and Recreation Research Focus Area, Faculty of Health Sciences, North-West University, Potchefstroom, South Africa

Sergio Oehninger, MD, PhD Department of Obstetrics and Gynecology, The Jones Institute for Reproductive Medicine/EVMS, Norfolk, VA, USA

Andries Fourie van Oort, MSc Physical activity, Sport and Recreation Research Focus Area, Faculty of Health Sciences, North-West University, Potchefstroom, South Africa

Jason Peng, BS Center for Reproductive Medicine, Cleveland Clinic Foundation, Cleveland, OH, USA

Juan Andrés Ramírez-González, MD, PhD Department of Morphology, Health Sciences Faculty, University of Las Palmas De Gran Canaria, Las Palmas De Gran Canaria, Spain

Nikolaos D. Roupas, MD, PhD Department of Obstetrics and Gynecology, Division of Reproductive Endocrinology, University of Patras, Medical School, University Hospital, Patras, Greece

Yves Schutz, PhD Department of Integrative Physiology, University of Fribourg, Fribourg, Switzerland

Alberto Da Costa Stein, PhD Department of Urology and Reproduction, Insemine Human Reproduction Center, Porto Alegre, Rio Grande do Sul, Brazil

R. James Swanson, BS, BSN, MS, HCLD, PhD Department of Biological Sciences, Old Dominion University, Norfolk, VA, USA

Diana Vaamonde, MS, PhD Department of Morphological Sciences, School of Medicine, University of Cordoba, International Network on Physical Exercise and Fertility (INPEF), Cordoba, Spain

Ricardo Vaamonde-Lemos, MD, PhD Department of Morphological Sciences, School of Medicine, University of Córdoba, Córdoba, Spain

Teresa Valverde Esteve, PhD Laboratorio de Investigación de Ciencias del Deporte, Universidad Católica de Valencia San Vicente Mártir, Valencia, Spain

Alex C. Varghese, PhD ASTRA Fertility Group, Mississauaga, Ontario, Canada

Mehis Viru, PhD Faculty of Exercise and Sport Sciences, University of Tartu, Tartu, Estonia

About the Authors

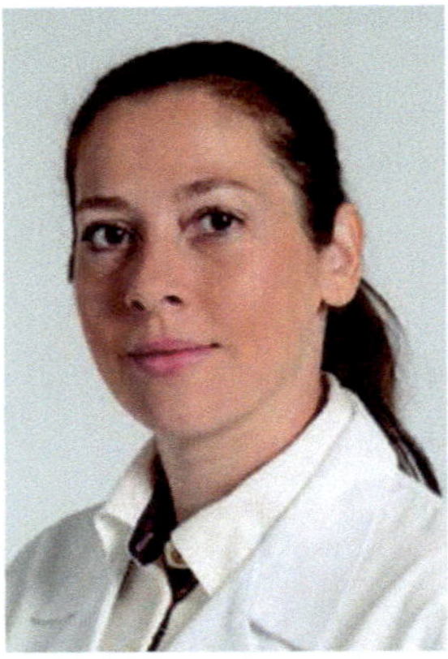

Diana Vaamonde MS, PhD (Diana Maria Vaamonde Martin) is a professor at School of Medicine of the University of Cordoba (Cordoba, Spain). Dr. Vaamonde currently leads a PhD research group in the area of physical exercise and fertility, with several ongoing doctoral theses.

She received her bachelors in biology from Washington and Lee University in 1998 and her masters in biology with emphasis on human reproduction from Old Dominion University/Jones Institute for reproductive medicine in 2004. She later completed a PhD program in physical activity and sport sciences at the University of Cordoba (Spain) where she brought together knowledge from the reproductive medicine and the sports medicine fields.

Her main expertise is in the area of male infertility and physical exercise. Most of her work has been on the effect of sports training, especially in elite athletes, on the male reproductive system. Her most recent work has included assessment of sperm DNA damage as a result of physical exercise as well as the use of antioxidant agents to revert exercise-associated damage in animal models. She has presented part of her work in prestigious international meetings (European Society for Human Reproduction and Embryology (ESHRE), American Society of Reproductive Medicine, European College of Sport Sciences). She has been invited as a speaker on the andrology pre-congress course of the ESHRE and embryology as well as a speaker for a plenary session on the topic of physical exercise and male reproduction for the ESHRE meeting of 2012. She serves as a reviewer for a number of journals including *Fertility and Sterility, Human Reproduction, Asian Journal of Andrology,* etc. and she is part of the Scientific Committee and Editorial Board for several journals (*Revista Andaluza de Medicina del Deporte, Histology Histopathology,* etc). She has also been the project leader for Gynemed (Germany) and embryologist and head of research at Reproductive Care Center (USA) as well as scientific consultant for FIV Marbella (Spain). She has recently created the International Network on Physical Exercise and Fertility (INPEF) along with Profs. Drs. Juan Manuel Garcia-Manso and Anthony C Hackney, who have extensively studied the effect of physical exercise on the endocrine system and fertility.

Dr. Vaamonde was funded by the Andalusian Government (Consejeria de Comercio, Turismo y Deporte) for studies on semen quality and endurance exercise.

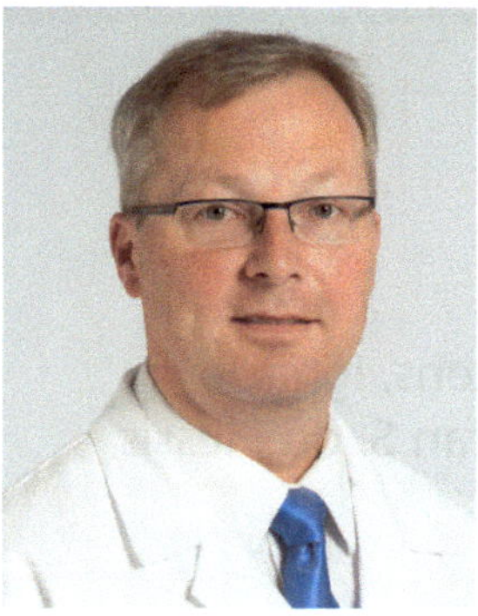

Stefan S. du Plessis MBA, PhD (Stell) is the head of Medical Physiology in the Faculty of Medicine and Health Sciences (Tygerberg) at Stellenbosch University (South Africa) where he is actively involved in undergraduate teaching and postgraduate training. He is also the head of the Stellenbosch University Reproductive Research Group (SURRG) and his research interests predominantly include male infertility and sperm function with the focus on factors that can influence it (e.g., lifestyle and noncommunicable diseases).

He graduated with a BSc (1989), BSc Hon (1990), MSc cum laude (1994), HonB, B&A (1997), MBA (1999), and PhD (2002) from Stellenbosch University and also received a certificate in human assisted reproduction from the CRM at the Cleveland Clinic (2014).

Till date Dr. Du Plessis has published 2 books, 57 peer-reviewed scientific articles, and more than 20 book chapters. He serves on the editorial board of three leading international journals; act as an ad hoc reviewer for various scientific journals and funding agencies, as well as moderator and examiner to several national and international universities.

He is regularly invited as a speaker, trainer, and mentor in semenology workshops; is an NRF rated researcher and has received numerous awards, the most notable of which include a Fulbright Research Scholarship (2015), Lasec Award for Excellence in Physiology Research (2013), and the Dr. Edmund Sabanegh Award for Excellence in Male Infertility Research (2012).

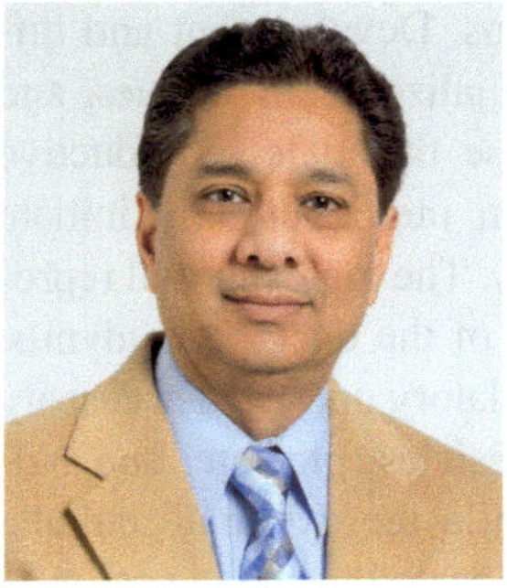

Ashok Agarwal PhD, HCLD (ABB), ELD (ACE) is a professor at Lerner College of Medicine, Case Western Reserve University and the head of the Andrology Center. He is the director of research at the American Center for Reproductive Medicine, Cleveland Clinic, USA. He has over 525 scientific papers and review articles in peer reviewed scientific journals. He has authored over 150 book chapters, and presented over 750 papers at both national and international scientific meetings. His current Hirsch index (h-index) is 97 on Google Scholar, 74 on Scopus, and 63 on Web of Science, while his citation count is 33,147 on Google Scholar. According to ResearchGate, Ashok has an RG score of 51.9 on 1516 publications. Ashok has served as an editor of over 26 medical text books/manuals related to male infertility, ART, fertility preservation, DNA damage, and antioxidants. He is the guest editor of four special journal issues. Ashok is a member or office bearer of several professional societies and he serves on the Editorial Board of a large number of journals in the area of reproductive medicine. Ashok is active in basic and clinical research and his laboratory has trained more than 500 basic scientists and clinical researchers from the USA and more than 50 countries. He has been invited as a guest speaker at important international meetings in over 25 countries, and is the program director of a unique and highly successful Summer Internship Course in Reproductive Medicine. In the past 8 years, over 180 pre-med and medical students from across the USA and overseas have graduated from this highly competitive program. His unique style of training and motivating young undergraduate and medical students into cutting edge original bench research and scientific writing of research articles for publication in medical journals has been recognized for the prestigious "Scholarship in Teaching Award" by the Case Western Reserve University School of Medicine every year since 2011. He serves on the editorial board of several key journals in human reproduction. His current research interests are identifying biological markers of oxidative stress, DNA damage and apoptosis using proteomic research tools and bioinformatics analysis as well as preserving fertility in patients with cancer. He is actively involved in laboratory and clinical studies assessing the efficacy of certain antioxidants in improving the male fertility.

Overview of the Male Reproductive System

1

Luis Jiménez-Reina, Pieter Johann Maartens, Ignacio Jimena-Medina, Ashok Agarwal and Stefan S. du Plessis

Abbreviations

HPG	Hypothalamic–pituitary–gonadal
SRY gene	Sex-determining region of the Y chromosome
ABP	Androgen-binding protein
GnRH	Gonadotropin-releasing hormone
FSH	Follicle-stimulating hormone
LH	Luteinizing hormone
DHT	Dihydrotestosterone
WHO	World Health Organization
PSA	Prostate-specific antigen

Introduction

Humans are sexually dimorphic; however, both male and female reproductive systems consist of different sets of structures, that is, gonads, internal genitalia, and external genitalia. This chapter will specifically focus on the male reproductive system and its functions. Development and differentiation of the specialized cells, tissues, and structures that comprise the male reproductive system already start in utero but only initiate function during puberty. The male internal reproductive organs consist of the ducts (epididymis, vas deferens, and ejaculatory duct) and accessory sex glands (seminal vesicles, prostate, and bulbourethral glands), while the external genitalia consists of the testes, located inside the scrotum as well as the penis. The testes are located inside the scrotum. Each of these structures is well vascularized and innervated and is controlled by an intricate interplay with the endocrine system which plays a very important role in the successful production and delivery of the male gametes. The testes have both exocrine and endocrine functions in the sense that they not only produce spermatozoa but also synthesize and secrete hormones. The process of spermatogenesis is furthermore highly regulated by the hypothalamic–pituitary–gonadal (HPG) axis. The most important reproductive processes are the following: initiation and maintenance of spermatogenesis, sperm transport, sperm maturation, semen production, sperm secretion, sexual response, and androgen production. The first part of this

L. Jiménez-Reina (✉)
Department of Morphological Sciences, School of Medicine, University of Cordoba, 14004 Cordoba, Spain
e-mail: cm1jirel@uco.es

P. J. Maartens
Division of Medical Physiology, Faculty of Medicine and Health Scineces, Stellenbosch University, Cape Town, Tygerberg, South Africa

I. Jimena-Medina
Department of Morphological Sciences, School of Medicine, University of Cordoba, Cordoba, Spain

A. Agarwal
American Center for Reproductive Medicine, Cleveland Clinic Foundation, Cleveland, OH, USA

S. S. du Plessis
Division of Medical Physiology, Department of Biomedical Sciences, Stellenbosch University, P.O. Box 19063, 7505 Tygerberg, Cape Town, South Africa
e-mail: ssdp@sun.ac.za

© Springer Science+Business Media New York 2016

D. Vaamonde et al. (eds.), *Exercise and Human Reproduction*, DOI 10.1007/978-1-4939-3402-7_1

chapter will emphasize the specific anatomy and histology of the male reproductive system, while the latter part will focus on the physiology and function of these structures.

Embryonic Development of the Male Reproductive System

Male reproductive development starts with gender determination. This occurs when the Y chromosome bearing spermatozoon fuses with the X chromosome bearing oocyte during the process of fertilization, creating a 46XY coded zygote. Thereafter, gonadal differentiation initiates as the foundation for testicular development. The bipotential gonads differentiate from the genital ridge which forms as a thickening of somatic cells on the inner surface of the mesonephros. Four structures are developed which later mature into the external genitalia: the genital tubercle, the urethral folds, the urethral groove, and the labioscrotal swellings. The sex-determining region of the Y chromosome (SRY gene) produces the SRY protein, which, in combination with other genes, promotes the development of the testis. After the gonadal differentiation process is completed, sexual differentiation starts. The testis develops steroidogenic cells, Sertoli cells, and cells responsible for completion of gonadal structural development from three bipotential cell lineages. The first fetal precursor cells are responsible for the formation of steroidogenic cells that are responsible for the secretion of sex hormones and subsequent onset of secondary sexual characteristics. The second cell lineage gives origin to Sertoli and mesenchymal cells. The Sertoli cells regulate the synthesis of the seminiferous tubules, while the mesenchymal cells differentiate into Leydig cells. Sertoli-cell and peritubular-cell secretions lead to the differentiation and migration of adult Leydig cells. The third cell lineage differentiates into the gonad structure. Development of the bipotential gonad is dependent on the anti-Mullerian hormone secreted by the Sertoli cells, with testosterone being secreted by interstitial cells and the insulin-like 3 hormone. The intermediate mesoderm is homologous for both male and female development and gives rise to the Wolffian ducts, Mullerian ducts, and the gonad precursors. During male development the Mullerian duct dissolves away, while the Wolffian duct gives rise to the epididymis, vas deferens, ductus deferens, ejaculatory duct, and the seminal vesicle. The development of the external male genitalia is dependent on dihydrotestosterone (DHT; secreted by Leydig cells) exposed to the fetus during the third trimester of pregnancy [1, 2].

The transfer of the testes from the genital ridge to the scrotum is a process of cardinal importance to sexual differentiation. Testosterone induces the relaxation of the cranial suspensory ligaments allowing the descent of the testes into the scrotum. The increased abdominal pressure due to the viscera growth and the elastic properties of the testes then cause the testes to be forced through the inguinal canal and into the scrotum. After the initial development of the essential male reproductive organs, the reproductive system lies dormant until puberty when the HPG axis becomes active and the process of spermatogenesis is initiated. The precursor cell development is of cardinal importance to spermatogenesis in the adult male. It is crucial that precursor cells proliferate unimpeded and give rise to an optimal amount of spermatogonia in later life [2, 3].

Anatomy and Histology of the Male Reproductive System

Testis

The two *testicles or* male gonads are responsible for spermatogenesis (the production of spermatozoa); simultaneously, they play a key role in the production of certain hormones, including testosterone, and can thus also be categorized as internal secretion glands (endocrine glands). The testes are housed within the *scrotum* (scrotal sac) below the penis, the left hanging a little lower than the right. The testis is oval shaped and slightly flat sided and has two smooth surfaces (internal and external), two poles (anterosuperior and posteroinferior), and two margins (anteroin-

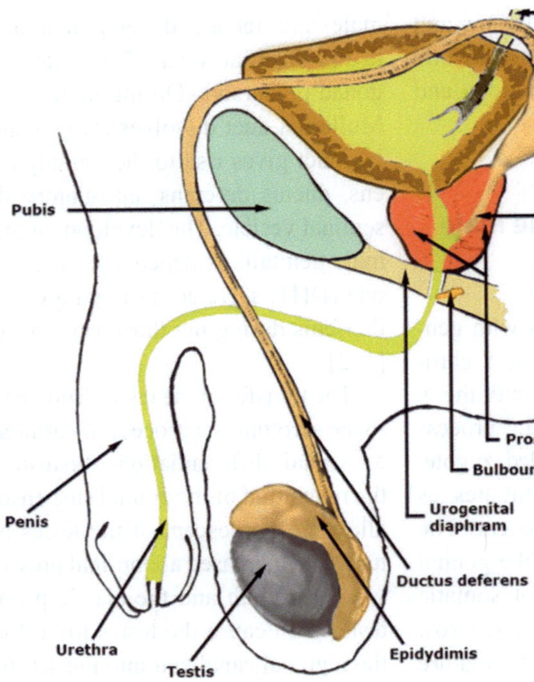

Fig. 1.1 Male genital system (scheme)

ferior and posterosuperior). It is covered by the *tunica vaginalis* (deriving from the peritoneum), which gives it its blue-white coloring. The adult testis is 40–50 mm long, 30 mm high, 25 mm wide, and weighs 16–20 g (Figs. 1.1 and 1.2).

The testis is surrounded by the *tunica albuginea,* a thick capsule of connective tissue and smooth muscle fibers. The innermost layer, known as the *tunica vasculosa,* is composed of loose connective tissue interspersed with numerous blood vessels. The tunica albuginea is thickest at the posterior margin, where it invaginates to form the *mediastinum testis*. The testis is secured to the scrotum by the *scrotal ligament*. Numerous connective-tissue septa arising from the mediastinum divide the testis into around 250 pyramid-shaped *lobules,* which are broad based at the surface of the capsule and become narrower as they converge to the mediastinum. Each lobule contains one to four highly-coiled *seminiferous tubules* (150–250 μm in diameter and 30–80 cm long). Towards the apex, straighter tubules known as *tubuli recti* connect the coiled tubules to the *rete testis* (rete of Haller) located in the mediastinum testis.

The *seminiferous tubules* are composed of a *seminiferous epithelium* lined by a *lamina propria* or peritubular tissue layer.

- *Lamina propria:* This layer is formed by connective tissue containing numerous fibroblasts and contractile myoid cells, whose rhythmic contraction facilitates the transport of spermatozoa.
- *Seminiferous epithelium:* This is a stratified epithelium composed of two main cell types: Sertoli cells and germ cells at different stages.

Sertoli cells are columnar cells that rest on the basement membrane and extend to the tubular lumen. They contain an oval nucleus, highly developed smooth endoplasmic reticulum, lysosomes, and Golgi complexes. Sertoli cells, which are bound to each other by tight junctions, have several functions:

- Promotion of nutrient exchange for germ cells
- Phagocytosis of degenerated germ cells and residual spermatid cytoplasm
- Production and secretion of testicular fluid

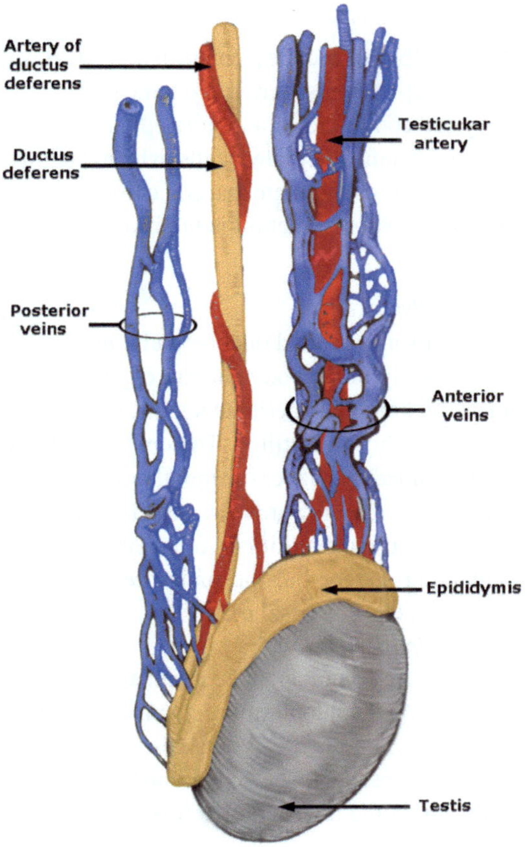

Fig. 1.2 Testis and epididymis (right lateral aspect)

- Production and secretion of *androgen-binding protein (ABP)* that binds specifically to the testosterone required for spermatogenesis
- Production and secretion of inhibin
- Regulation of germ cell movement in the epithelium, facilitating cell differentiation and the release of spermatozoa into the lumen
- Formation of the blood–testis barrier

Germ cells at various stages of maturity are found in the testis: *spermatogonia, spermatocytes, spermatids, and spermatozoa.*

- *Spermatogonia:*

These lie adjacent to the basement membrane of the tubular epithelium and are divided into two subtypes. *Type A* spermatogonia are stem cells which replicate and also divide by mitosis to produce *Type B* spermatogonia. The latter divide mitotically to produce primary spermatocytes. Due to incomplete cytokinesis during mitotic division, cells remain bound by cytoplasmic bridges during spermatogenesis.

- *Spermatocytes:*

Primary spermatocytes are the largest of the germ cells. They are formed in the *basal compartment* and migrate to the *adluminal compartment*. They are diploid cells which undergo meiosis I to produce secondary spermatocytes.

Secondary spermatocytes are haploid cells rarely seen under the microscope because they are present for only 8 h of the 64-day spermatogenic cycle. They divide by meiosis II to produce spermatids.

- *Spermatids:*

These are haploid cells found near the lumen of the seminiferous tubule. Rather than dividing, they undergo a process of differentiation to become spermatozoa.

- *Spermatozoa:*

These are fully mature haploid cells but are incapable of fertilization.

As referred to briefly above, the tight junctions between Sertoli cells form the histological basis of the blood–testis barrier, whose functions are to create a microenvironment for the correct development of spermatozoa and prevent contact between maturing (haploid) gametes and the immune system.

The barrier divides the tubule into two distinct sections:

1. Basal compartment: This compartment, which is in contact with the underlying connective vascular tissue, contains spermatogonia and primary spermatocytes.
2. Adluminal compartment: This compartment contains secondary spermatocytes, spermatids, and spermatozoa, and it is not in contact with underlying connective vascular tissue.

The final portion of the seminiferous tubules, containing a columnar epithelium composed entirely of Sertoli cells, opens into the rete testis, an anastomosing network of tubules lined by a cuboid epithelium, some of whose cells may contain flagella. Seminiferous tubules are separated from each other by peritubular interstitial tissue composed of loose connective tissue containing blood vessels, lymph vessels, nerves, and *Leydig cells (also referred to as interstitial cells).*

Leydig cells may occur singly or in clusters and are characterized by a euchromatic nucleus and eosinophilic cytoplasm. Their appearance is typical of steroid-secreting cells, that is, abundant smooth endoplasmic reticulum, lipid vacuoles, and numerous mitochondria with tubular cristae. These are testosterone-producing cells [4–7].

Sperm Ducts

A whole set of tubular structures are involved in transporting spermatozoa from their origin in the testis to the urethra, through which both semen and urine are removed. These structures, to be subsequently described, are the epididymis, ductus deferens, and ejaculatory ducts.

Epididymis

The *epididymis* is an elongated organ located over the posterosuperior border of the testis. It is roughly 50 mm in length and contains a highly coiled tube known as the *epididymal duct,* which is around 4 m long and 0.3 mm in diameter. The epididymis can be divided into three portions: the *head* or *caput* (wider upper portion), the *body* or *corpus* (middle portion), and the *tail* or *cauda* (lower portion), which continues into the ductus deferens. The head of the epididymis is attached to the testis by *efferent ducts* and fibrous tissue and the tail by fibrous tissue alone; the middle portion of the epididymis is not attached to the testis (Figs. 1.1 and 1.2). The visceral layer of the tunica vaginalis forms a recess between the testis and the body of the epididymis, known as the *sinus of the epididymis*. The functions of the epididymis include sperm storage, resorption of most of the testicular fluid produced in the seminiferous tubules, and secretion of the enzymes required for the maturation of spermatozoa.

As indicated previously, the two main structures of the epididymis are the *efferent ducts* and the *epididymal duct:*

- *Efferent ducts:*

Around 15–20 ductules connect the rete testis with the epididymis, across the tunica albuginea. They are composed of a simple epithelium containing columnar ciliated cells which facilitate the transport of spermatozoa, and cuboid non-ciliated cells whose function is to absorb testicular fluid.

- *Epididymal duct:*

This is a single, coiled duct around 4 m long, located mainly in the body and tail of the epididymis. It is here that spermatozoa acquire motility and the ability to fertilize. The epididymal duct is surrounded by a layer of smooth muscle which becomes thicker towards the tail. The lumen is lined by a pseudostratified columnar epithelium containing stereocilia; the major cell types are principal cells and basal cells.

Principal cells:

These are columnar and contain a basal nucleus, with rough endoplasmic reticulum and abundant Golgi complexes, lysosomes, and micropinocytotic vesicles. The apical surface contains long, nonmotile microvilli (stereocilia).

Basal cells:

These are stem cells which serve to renew the principal-cell population [4–7].

Ductus (Vas) Deferens

The *ductus (vas) deferens,* a duct around 40 cm long, is the continuation of the tail of the epididymis. It traverses the scrotal sac, the inguinal canal, the pelvic cavity below the peritoneum, and the rear lateral portion of the bladder, where it enlarges to form the *ampulla.* It is cylindrical in shape, with a diameter of around 2 mm and a caliber of 0.5 mm; this thick wall ensures great consistency.

The ductus deferens is divided into various anatomical portions: *scrotal, funicular, inguinal, iliac,* and *pelvic* (Fig. 1.1).

- *Scrotal portion:* Here, the ductus deferens ascends along the medial side of the epididymis, from which it is separated by the testicular veins.

- *Funicular portion:* From the anterior surface of the body of the epididymis, the ductus deferens continues upwards to the superficial inguinal ring. Here, it is accompanied by blood vessels supplying the testis and epididymis, nerves, pampiniform and *testicular* venous plexuses, lymph vessels, and a vestige of the peritoneum known as the *processus vaginalis*. All these structures are sheathed by the *external spermatic fascia* and together form the *spermatic cord* (Fig. 1.2).
- *Inguinal portion:* This portion of the ductus deferens traverses the inguinal canal to the superficial inguinal ring. At this stage it is accompanied not only by the elements forming the spermatic cord but also by the genitofemoral and ilioinguinal nerves and the cremasteric artery.
- *Iliac portion:* After passing through the deep inguinal ring, it enters the pelvic cavity (below the peritoneum) and moves downwards across the internal iliac vein and artery. Here, it separates from the other structures of the spermatic cord except for the artery of ductus deferens.
- *Pelvic portion:* Here, the ductus deferens runs first to the side and later to the rear of the bladder. From the side of the bladder, it is directed backwards (below and adhering to the peritoneum) towards the rearmost portion of the lateral border of the bladder, where it crosses in front of and above the ureter. Thereafter, it descends along the posterior wall of the bladder and then changes direction, moving downwards, forwards, and inwards until it reaches the base of the prostate. Over this last stretch, the ductus deferens becomes enlarged and tortuous, forming the ampulla, which is separated from the fundus of the bladder first by the peritoneum and later by the *rectovesical septum* or *retroprostatic fascia*.

The *mucosa* of the ductus deferens is lined by an epithelium similar to that of the epididymal duct, surrounded by a slender *lamina propria* of dense connective tissue. The star-shaped cross-sectional appearance of the lumen is due to a number of longitudinal folds. The thick *muscularis* of the ductus deferens is formed by inner and outer layers of longitudinal fibers and a middle layer of circular fibers. The longitudinal fibers shorten and widen the ductus deferens immediately prior to ejaculation, drawing in the content of the epididymis and expelling it towards the urethra. These muscle fibers receive abundant innervation from the sympathetic nervous system [4–7].

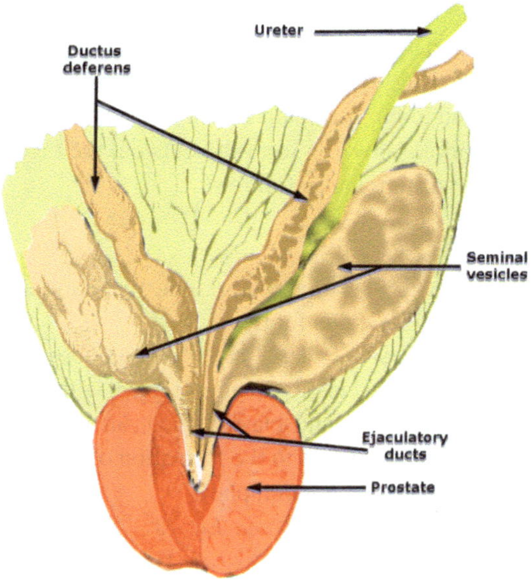

Fig. 1.3 Seminal vesicles, ejaculatory ducts, and prostate (posterior aspect)

Ejaculatory Ducts

The right and left *ejaculatory ducts,* tubes of around 25 mm in length, run from the terminal portion of the ampulla of the ductus deferens and the start of the seminal vesicles (Fig. 1.3), passing through the prostate and opening into the posterior portion of the prostatic urethra, to either side of the prostatic utricle, at the right and left *colliculi seminalis*. The ducts are lined by simple columnar epithelium and have no muscle layer [4–7].

Scrotum

The testes, epididymides, and a portion of the ductus deferens are sheathed in several layers of tissue which together form the *scrotum* or *scrotal sacs*. These sheaths derive from the abdominal wall, due to the descent of the testes from the abdomen into the scrotum. The two sacs are separated by a central septum (median raphe); the left sac hangs lower than the right and the two are attached to the perineum by the *scrotal pedicle*.

Working inwards from the outside, the layers of the scrotum are as follows:

- *Scrotal skin:* The scrotal skin is thin, dark, and shows numerous folds.
- *Tunica dartos:* This layer is composed of smooth muscle fibers interspersed with connective tissue and elastic fibers; at the midline, it contributes to the formation of the central septum (median raphe).
- *Subcutaneous cell tissue layer*.
- *External spermatic fascia:* This thin membrane is the scrotal prolongation of the lining of the abdominal external oblique muscle.
- *Cremaster muscle:* This muscle is formed by inner and outer layers of striated muscle, derived from the internal oblique and transverse abdominal muscles, which eventually insert into the internal spermatic fascia.
- *Internal spermatic fascia:* This layer, deriving from the abdominal *fascia transversalis,* extends downwards to line the spermatic cord, the epididymis, and the testis.
- *Tunica vaginalis:* This serosa, deriving from the peritoneum, lines the anterior and lateral surfaces of the testis but not the posterior surface. It comprises two layers: the *superficial or parietal lamina* and the *deep or visceral lamina* (which lines the tunica albuginea of the testis). Both are composed of mesothelial cells and submesothelial connective tissue. The interval between the visceral and parietal laminae is known as the *serous cavity of the scrotum* [4–7].

Accessory Sex Glands

Seminal Vesicles

These two oval structures (50 mm long, 10 mm wide, and 10 mm thick) are located behind the urinary bladder at either side of the ampulla of the ductus deferens and are separated from the *rectum* by the *rectovesical septum*. The end of each seminal vesicle joins the end of each *ampulla* to form the ejaculatory duct (Figs. 1.1 and 1.3). The seminal vesicle consists of a coiled, glandular tube around 15 cm in length, covered by fibrous tissue. It produces a yellowish, gelatinous secretion which accounts for 60–80 % of seminal fluid or semen. This secretion is particularly rich in fructose, citrate, amino acids, and prostaglandins.

Seminal vesicles do not store sperm. Contraction of the smooth muscle during ejaculation pushes this secretion into the urethra. The single tube, of which each vesicle is composed, comprises three concentric layers. The outermost layer of loose connective tissue surrounds two layers of smooth muscle tissue, a longitudinal outer layer, and a circular inner layer.

The innermost layer of the vesicle is a mucosa arranged into numerous folds, giving the lumen a highly irregular appearance. The mucosa comprises a *pseudostratified columnar epithelium* and a *lamina propria* of connective tissue. Epithelial cells are of two types: principal and basal. *Principal cells* are columnar, and their cytoplasm contains secretion vesicles, lipofuchsin granules, and lipid droplets, while *basal cells* are stem cells (progenitors of principal cells) [4–7].

Prostate

This is a chestnut-shaped gland and resembles an inverted cone, its apex pointing downwards. It is located beneath the urinary bladder (the base of the prostate is fused to the fundus of the bladder) and therefore surrounds the initial portion of the urethra. The vertical, transverse, and anteroposterior diameters are 25–30, 40, and 25 mm, respectively. It consists of anterior and posterior surfaces, two lateral surfaces (down-facing and out-facing), a base, and an apex (Figs. 1.1 and 1.3).

Although there are no clear divisions within the prostate, it is traditionally divided into four lobes:

- *Anterior portion* (in front of the urethra)
- *Posterior portion* (behind the urethra and between the ejaculatory ducts)
- *Right and left lateral lobes* (rest of the gland)

The anterior portion of the prostate, including the apex, is surrounded by fibers of the external sphincter muscle of the urethra and by fibrous laminae deriving from the periprostatic fascia of the pelvic floor. The posterior portion is lined by the *rectovesical septum* (the *Denonvilliers prostatoperitoneal* membrane or fascia); as indicated earlier, this posterior fascia also sheathes the ductus deferens and the seminal vesicles. Laterally, the prostate is surrounded by the prostatic fascia, which contains periprostatic venous plexuses. These fibrous fascia are attached in the anterior portion to the pubis, laterally to the elevator muscle of the anus and posteriorly to the sacrum. The prostate secretes a colorless fluid which makes up between 15 and 30 % of the volume of semen. This secretion contains acid phosphatase, citric acid for sperm nutrition, and fibrolysin for semen liquefaction. It should be noted that the prostate contains the prostatic urethra, the internal sphincter muscle of the urethra, the upper portion of the external sphincter muscle of the urethra, the ejaculatory ducts, and the prostatic utricle. The prostate is surrounded by a fibroelastic capsule containing bundles of smooth muscle fibers. It consists of 30–50 glands arranged in three concentric layers: an inner *mucosal* layer of glands surrounding the urethra, which is in fact invaginations of the urethral epithelium, an intermediate *submucosal* layer of tubuloalveolar glands, and a peripheral *principal* layer containing the main tubuloalveolar prostatic glands. The principal layer is the most susceptible to prostate cancer, while the mucosal and submucosal layers tend to be more affected by benign prostatic hyperplasia. The glandular parenchyma is surrounded by abundant connective tissue and bundles of smooth muscle fibers. During ejaculation, these muscles contract to expel the prostatic secretion into the urethra. The glandular mucosa is heavily folded, with a pseudostratified epithelium. It comprises *principal cells* containing numerous secretory granules and abundant acid phosphatase, and *basal cells* which are the precursors of principal cells. The alveoli of the prostatic glands often contain *corpora amylacea,* formed by precipitation of secretory material around cell fragments; over time, these may become calcified [4–7].

Bulbourethral Glands

These two lentil-sized glandular structures, also known as Cowper's glands, are located at the upper right and left of the urethral bulb, in the deep perineal pouch alongside the deep transverse perineal muscle. A duct, around 4 cm in length, arises from each gland to finish in the spongy urethra (Fig. 1.1). The glands produce a clear, viscous secretion which acts as a lubricant during sexual stimulation. They are surrounded by a capsule of connective tissue, with a simple epithelium comprising columnar mucus-secreting cells [4–7].

Penis

The penis is the male copulatory organ. It is located above the scrotum and in front of the symphysis pubis. The flaccid penis measures roughly 10 cm and is cylindrical in form, while the erect penis assumes the form of a triangular prism with rounded angles and measures around 16 cm (Fig. 1.1). Its anterior end is expanded in the form of an obtuse cone. This expansion, termed the *glans penis,* contains the external urethral orifice or *urinary meatus*. At the *neck* (the boundary between the glans and the body of the penis) the sheath of the penis folds in upon itself to form the *foreskin* or *prepuce*. The posterior portion of the penis, known as the *root,* is attached to the front of the symphysis pubis by the *suspensory ligament* and to the ischiopubic rami through the *corpora cavernosa penis*. The penis is formed by three blood-storing structures known *as erectile organs:* two dorsal tissue masses and one ventral tissue mass. The dorsal erectile organs, known as the *corpora cavernosa,* are capped by the glans. Behind, the corpora diverge, forming the *crura,* which attach to the ischiopubic rami, and terminate in a conical structure known as the *root of the penis*. The ventral erectile organ surrounding the urethra, termed the *corpus spongiosum,* is located in the lower longitudinal groove formed by the two corpora cavernosa. At its anterior end, the corpus spongiosum broadens out to form the *glans,* while the posterior end assumes a bulb shape to form the *bulb of corpus spongiosum*.

The integument of the penis is similar to that of the testis and comprises the following layers, working inwards from the outer layer:

- *Skin:* The skin is thin, mobile, and pigmented.
- *Dartos:* A layer of smooth muscle fibers underlying the skin.
- *Subcutaneous connective tissue:* It allows the skin to slide over the penis.
- *Deep fascia of the penis:* A layer of fibrous connective tissue covering the corpora cavernosa and the corpus spongiosum.

The skin surrounding the penis (dermis and epidermis) is very fine and contains small sebaceous glands. The hypodermis (superficial fascia) contains smooth muscle fibers but no adipose tissue, thus enabling the skin to slide freely over the underlying structures.

Inside the penis, the tunica albuginea is a layer of dense fibroelastic connective tissue surrounding the three erectile tissue masses. The erectile tissue is composed of highly irregular sinusoidal vascular structures, bounded by endothelium and surrounded by smooth muscle tissue. The corpora cavernosa are surrounded by a thick tunica albuginea, while that enveloping the corpus spongiosum is thinner [4–7].

Urethra

Although the urethra drains urine from the bladder and is thus part of the urinary apparatus, it is included here because it also carries semen out of the body.

The male urethra is divided into four portions, named after the location (Fig. 1.1):

- *Intramural:* This is the portion that traverses the bladder wall. It has a transitional epithelium *(urothelium)*.
- *Prostatic:* This portion, around 3 cm in length, crosses through the prostate gland, where it receives fluid from the seminal vesicles and the prostate (at the seminal colliculus). The epithelium is mostly transitional, although there are some areas of simple columnar epithelium.
- *Membranous:* This portion, measuring 1 cm in length, passes through the perineum. It is lined by a stratified columnar epithelium.
- *Spongy:* This portion, which is around 12 cm long, runs along the length of the penis, initially downwards and later forwards to the pubic symphysis; thereafter, it bends downwards in the flaccid penis or continues upwards in the erect penis. The distal portion has a pseudostratified columnar epithelium, while closer to the meatus the epithelium becomes squamous stratified.

The urethral lumen contains three dilations: the *prostatic sinus* (in the prostatic portion), the *intrabulbar fossa* (in the vicinity of the bulb of corpus spongiosum), and the *navicular fossa,* close to the *urinary meatus,* in which the urethra terminates [4–7].

Vessels and Nerves of the Male Reproductive System

Due to the importance of vascularization and innervation in the functioning of the male reproductive system, it is necessary to allude to the morphology and structure of these blood vessels, lymphatic vessels, and nerves.

Vascularization and Innervation of the Testis and Sperm Ducts

During embryonic development, the testis forms in the abdominal cavity, later descending into the scrotum. For that reason, the nerves and vessels of the testis originate or terminate in abdominal structures.

Arteries

- *Testicular artery* (Fig. 1.2): This is a branch of the abdominal aorta, which traverses the inguinal canal, where it forks to supply the epididymis *(epididymal artery)* and the testis; the latter then divides into two branches (internal and external), which give rise to the *interlobular arteries* of the testis.

- *Artery of ductus deferens* (Fig. 1.2): This is a branch of the superior vesical artery, which is in turn a branch of the internal iliac artery, alongside which the deferential artery runs throughout its course. It finally joins the epididymal branch of the testicular artery.
- *Cremasteric artery:* It is a branch of the inferior epigastric artery (which in turn arises from the external iliac artery). The cremasteric artery traverses the inguinal canal, where it supplies spermatic cord structures. It terminates in the tail of the epididymis, where it anastomoses with small arteries branching from the testicular artery and the epididymal artery.
- The *artery of ductus deferens,* the *prostatic branches of the inferior vesical artery,* the *inferior vesical artery,* and the *middle rectal (hemorrhoidal) artery* (all deriving from the internal iliac artery): These contribute to the vascularization of the seminal vesicles, the ampulla of ductus deferens, and the ejaculatory ducts.

Veins

- *Pampiniform plexus* (Fig. 1.2): This venous plexus, located in the anterior part of the spermatic cord, is a network of small veins originating in the testis and the anterior portion of the epididymis. Close to the *ductus deferens,* this plexus penetrates the abdomen and gives rise to the testicular veins. The right testicular vein empties into the inferior vena cava, while the left testicular vein drains into the left renal vein.

Some venous blood from the ductus deferens also drains into the pampiniform plexus.

- *Posterior spermatic plexus:* These are veins arising in the posterior half of the epididymis, which traverse the posterior portion of the spermatic cord and empty into the internal iliac vein system. Some venous blood from the ductus deferens also drains into the posterior spermatic plexus.
- *Prostatic, vesical, and seminal plexuses:* These are the networks in which the veins of the seminal vesicles and ejaculatory ducts terminate.

Lymph Vessels

The lymph vessels of the testis and epididymis terminate in the lumbar region, in lymph nodes close to the inferior pole of the right kidney and the anterior portion of the left renal vein. The lymph vessels of the ductus deferens and seminal vesicles lead to the external and internal iliac lymph nodes.

Nerves

The nerves of the testis and epididymis derive from the testicular plexus originating in the celiac plexus and from the deferential plexus originating in the inferior hypogastric plexus [4–7].

Vascularization and Innervation of the Scrotum

Arteries

- *Cremasteric artery:* As indicated earlier, this is a branch of the inferior epigastric artery. It supplies the cremaster muscle, the internal spermatic fascia, and the parietal lamina of testis.
- *Superficial arterial branches* of the *external pudendal arteries,* which derive from the femoral artery, and of the *perineal artery,* which arises from the internal pudendal artery.

Veins

- *Deep veins,* draining into the venous plexuses of the spermatic cord
- *Superficial veins,* draining into the external pudendal veins, which arise from the great saphenous vein

Lymph Vessels

The lymph vessels of the scrotum terminate in the internal inguinal lymph node groups.

Nerves

The scrotum is innervated by branches of the pudendal nerve, the perineal nerves, and genital branches of the ilioinguinal and genitofemoral nerves [4–7].

Vascularization and Innervation of the Prostate

Arteries

- *Prostatic branches of the inferior vesical artery* and the *middle rectal (hemorrhoidal) artery*

Veins

- *Prostatic veins:* These veins drain anteriorly and laterally into the *prostatic venous plexus,* and posteriorly into the *venous plexus of the seminal vesicles*. Blood from these two plexuses eventually empties into the internal iliac veins.

Lymph Vessels

The lymph vessels of the prostate terminate in the external iliac, internal iliac, lateral sacral, and internal pudendal lymph nodes.

Nerves

The nerves of the prostate arise in the inferior hypogastric plexus [4–7].

Vascularization and Innervation of the Penis

Arteries

- *Branches of the internal pudendal* and *perineal arteries,* located in the subcutaneous connective tissue layer, supply the integument and fibrous sheath of the penis.
- The *cavernosal arteries* (branches of the internal pudendal artery) supply the corpora cavernosa. Within the corpora, these branch off into numerous spirally arranged *helicine arteries.*
- The *arteries of bulb of penis, urethral arteries,* and *corpus spongiosum arteries* (all branches of the internal pudendal artery) supply the areas indicated by their name.
- The *dorsal arteries of the penis* (branches of the internal pudendal artery) flow from the dorsal aspect of the penis to the glans, passing through the corpora cavernosa and the corpus spongiosum.

Veins

- The *superficial dorsal vein of the penis,* located in the subcutaneous connective tissue layer, runs backwards to eventually drain into the left side of the great saphenous vein.
- The *deep dorsal vein of the penis,* located beneath the deep fascia and between the two dorsal arteries of the penis, arises through the merging of right and left venous plexuses in the neck region of the glans, formed by veins running from the glans. It is fed by lateral and superior venous branches from the corpora cavernosa and the corpus spongiosum and eventually drains into the prostatic venous plexus.

Lymph Vessels

- *Superficial lymph vessels* carry lymph from the integument and fibrous sheath of the penis to the inguinal lymph nodes.
- *Deep lymph vessels* carry lymph from the corpora cavernosa, corpus spongiosum, glans, and penile urethra. They run alongside the deep dorsal vein of the penis and terminate in the superficial and deep inguinal lymph nodes.

Nerves

- *Genital branch of the genitofemoral nerve.*
- *Dorsal nerve of the penis.*
- *Superficial branch of the perineal nerve.*
- The *cavernous nerves of the hypogastric plexus* provide vegetative innervation [4–7].

Physiology of the Male Reproductive System

Endocrine Regulation of the Male Reproductive System

The onset of puberty is associated with a rise in the cyclic secretion (peaking every 1.5 h) of the hypothalamic peptide hormone, gonadotropin-releasing hormone (GnRH). Factors that can stimulate GnRH production are leptin and noradrenalin, while substances such as dopamine, serotonin, prolactin and certain interleukins can inhibit GnRH production. GnRH is released into the hypothalamic–hypophyseal portal system binding to membrane receptors of specific cells (gonadotropic cells) in the anterior pituitary, thereby activating a protein kinase C-mediated pathway. This in turn stimulates the synthesis and secretion of the gonadotropins. These glycoprotein hormones are central in the regulation of normal growth, sexual development, and reproductive function and include follicle-stimulating hormone (FSH) and luteinizing hormone (LH). Both FSH and LH have similar α subunits but differ in their β subunit, which determines receptor-binding specificity. Low GnRH pulse frequency predominantly leads to FSH release, while higher GnRH frequencies are associated with preferential LH secretion [2, 3, 8, 9]. Once released from the anterior pituitary, they act on specific membrane receptors of their target tissue. LH is responsible for the stimulation of Leydig cells to produce mainly the steroidal hormone testosterone. FSH acts on Sertoli cells, which also have receptors for testosterone. The gonadotropins therefore initiate and support spermatogenesis. LH and FSH also promote the activation of ABP. The gonadal secretion of sex hormones also affects their own production by decreasing the release of GnRH, FSH, and LH in a negative-feedback manner. The gonads, furthermore, control the levels of FSH through testosterone secretion as well as by secreting a growth-factor-like peptide hormone, Inhibin B, from the Sertoli cells [10–14].

As previously mentioned, Leydig cells are responsible for the secretion of androgenic anabolic hormones. The primary androgen in the male reproductive system is testosterone, and its reduced form DHT binds to androgen receptors in Sertoli cells and modulates gene transcription. The endoplasmic reticulum and mitochondria of mature Leydig cells utilize cholesterol and acetate to produce testosterone. Testosterone and DHT are key to appropriate primary sexual characteristics of testicular development such as differentiation of male genitalia and pubertal growth in addition to initiating secondary sexual characteristics such as the characteristic male bodily and facial hair growth, body shape, muscular development, broadening of vocal chords, and development of libido. Testosterone is also a cardinal factor in the maintenance of spermatogenesis [15–17]. Maturation of the reproductive system is controlled by GnRH, the gonadotropins (LH and FSH), and the sex hormones. However, if thyroid hormone is not available in sufficient amounts, maturation of the reproductive system is delayed. Thyroid hormone cannot induce reproductive maturation and is thus regarded to have a permissive effect on reproductive maturation [18]. This system of combined hormonal interaction from various endocrine glands acting as a whole is referred to as the HPG axis and is illustrated in Fig. 1.4.

Spermatogenesis

Spermatogenesis is the process whereby the male gametes or spermatozoa are produced. Spermatogenesis is responsible for the production of haploid gametes from diploid spermatogonia and in so doing preserves the number of chromosomes in the offspring. This occurs in the seminiferous tubules of the testes through a complex and highly orchestrated process that initiates during puberty and continues throughout the rest of the male's lifetime. Spermatogenesis requires a combination of synchronized gene expression and cell division that takes place in the testes. Apart from the hormones necessary (FSH, LH, and testosterone), of fundamental importance to the normal occurrence of spermatogenesis are the Sertoli cells as they alter rates of spermatozoal production and produce factors essential to gamete development [19–22].

The whole process of spermatogenesis takes around 64–74 days during which mature spermatozoa (haploid cells) are produced from spermatogonia (diploid cells) and can be divided into three stages or phases (as seen in Fig. 1.5).

1. *Spermatocytogenesis:* This process includes division by mitosis and meiosis. Spermatogonia (diploid) divide in utero mitotically to

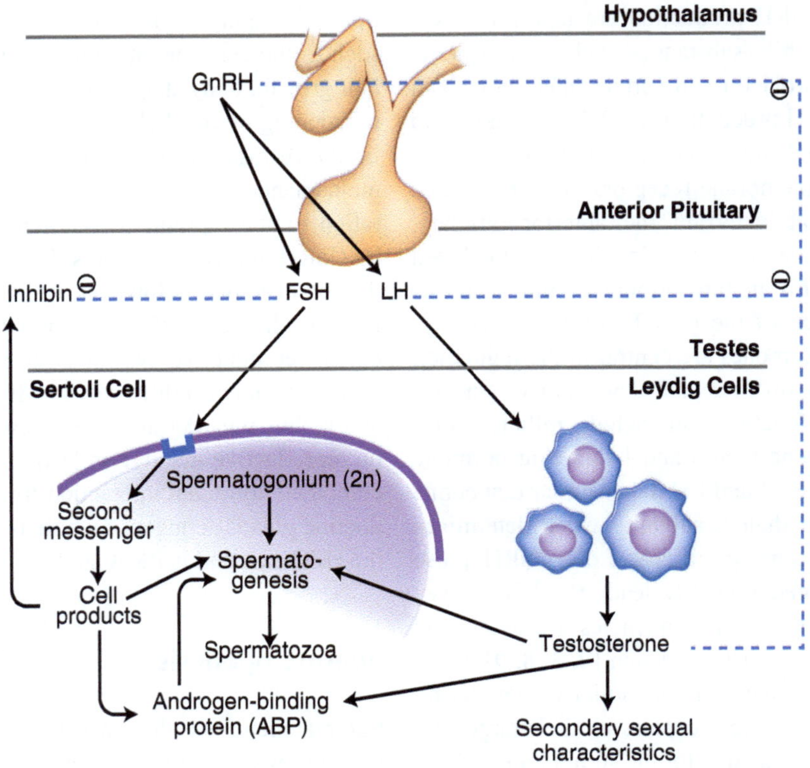

Fig. 1.4 Endocrine control and feedback of spermatogenesis and the hypothalamic–pituitary–gonadal axis *(HPG axis)*, follicle-stimulating hormone *(FSH)*, luteinizing hormone *(LH)*, androgen-binding protein *(ABP)*

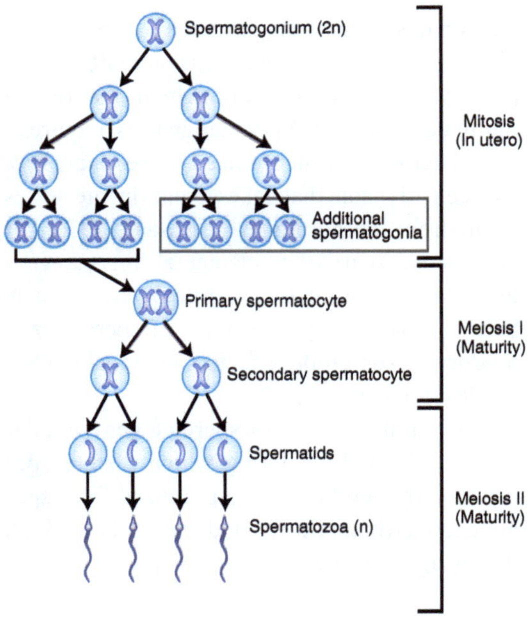

Fig. 1.5 Diagram representing three stages of spermatogenesis: mitosis, first meiotic division (meiosis I) and second meiotic division (meiosis II), and the development from diploid spermatogonia *(2n)* to haploid spermatozoa *(n)*

produce primary spermatocytes (diploid) and additional spermatogonia. After the onset of puberty, the first meiotic division takes place, and primary spermatocytes (which have replicated their DNA to two sets of chromosomes) give rise to secondary spermatocytes (diploid). During the second stage of meiosis, secondary spermatocytes (haploid) divide into spermatids (haploid). Sertoli cells nurture and support the developing spermatozoa throughout this process.

2. *Spermiogenesis:* This phase involves the differentiation of spermatids to produce spermatozoa (haploid). This process primarily entails maturation of the spermatozoon body and nuclear material. Maturation of the spermatozoon includes axoneme development via the thickening of the midpiece and microtubule congregation in addition to flagellum formation from one of the cell's centrioles. Nuclear maturation includes condensation of DNA and

packaging of the DNA, first with basic proteins and subsequently with protamines during spermatid elongation. The ensuing chromatin is not yet transcriptionally active. The chromatin is then enveloped by a Golgi apparatus which is then termed the acrosome. Testosterone is the main regulating factor with regards to spermatozoon maturation and results in the removal of excess organelles and cytoplasm, known as residual bodies, via phagocytosis by the neighboring Sertoli cells in the testicular tissue.

3. *Spermiation:* This is the process by which mature spermatids are released from the protective Sertoli cells into the lumen of the seminiferous tubule before their transition into the epididymis. Spermiation includes several steps including reorganization of the spermatid head and cytoplasm, disintegration of specialized adhesion structures, and the ultimate separation of the spermatid from the Sertoli cell. These processes take place at the apical edge of the seminiferous epithelium and take several days to complete. The newly matured and released spermatozoa are not yet motile and thus not yet able to penetrate the oocyte.

Due to the intricacy of the process, spermatogenesis is totally dependent on the existence of optimal conditions. It is extremely sensitive to changes in the external environment. Therefore, environmental and lifestyle insults that affect gonadal differentiation, Sertoli- or Leydig-cell proliferation, or spermatogenesis at any age could affect male reproductive development and thus lead to adverse reproductive pathologies such as oligozoospermia, asthenozoospermia, hypospadias, testicular cancer, and cryptorchidism [9–11, 20, 23].

Sperm Transport and Maturation

After production in the testes, immature spermatozoa are moved through the corpus and caput regions of the epididyma and are then stored in the proximal section of the cauda epididymis. The spermatozoa move a total of 6 m through the reproductive tract before leaving the urethra. The average transit time in the epididymis is estimated at 12 days. Sperm motion is driven by hydrostatic pressure that is created by the combination of fluids secreted by the seminiferous tubules and tubular peristalsis. Movement through the proximal epididymis is mediated by peripheral smooth muscle contractions, and movement through the epididymal head is mediated by contraction of the tunica albuginea. Fluidic rhythmic movements of the cilia, lining the walls of the ducts, and the cyclic contractions of contractile cells along the wall of the epididymal duct further propel seminal constituents. Epididymal duct contraction is believed to be regulated by cholinergic, adrenergic factors, and vasopressin [24–26].

Spermatozoa mature and acquire functional and motile characteristics during epididymal transit. These changes ensure that the sperm will be able to survive the female reproductive tract, capacitate, and fertilize the oocyte. Each epididymal section contains a unique gene expression profile of the epithelium that leads to specific and specialized secretion of proteins into the lumen. Maturational processes include changes in cell membrane, acrosome shape, and chromatin condensation and stabilization. Cell membrane changes primarily entail a reduction in cholesterol which leads to a downstream activation of kinases that promote capacitation. Chromatin condensation, structural changes to the acrosome and intracellular organelles, and migration of the cytoplasmic droplet, along the sperm tail, are all changes commonly observed during maturation. Lipids and proteins are also reorganized as signaling molecules in anticipation of fertilization. These changes are induced by the fluid milieu, secretions of the epithelium of the seminiferous tubules and epididymal lumen, which the cells are exposed to. This epididymal fluid contains many substances such as sodium, glutamate, albumin, bicarbonate, transferrin, immobulin, inositol, potassium, L-carnitine, sialic acid, lactate, metalloproteins, proenkephalin, taurine, clusterin

(SGP-2), glycerophosphorylcholine, and chloride. These substances are in part responsible for epididymal cell metabolism, activation of sperm motility, and regulation of fluid retention of sperm and epididymal cells [24, 25, 27–31].

Semen

Semen consists of cells suspended in fluid. Semen is generally observed to be a homogenous fluid opalescent to light greyish in color varying with difference in spermatozoal concentration. Semen coloration of reddish or yellow tints can be explained by red blood cells in the semen (hemospermia) or the influence of jaundice or drugs, respectively [32].

The bulk of the composition (99 %) is made up of the fluids secreted by the male reproductive accessory glands (i.e., the prostate, the seminal vesicles, and the bulbourethral glands). These secretions join spermatozoa secreted from the vas deferens, during ejaculation, to form a mixture called semen. It is commonly believed that the seminal plasma provides a nutritive and protective medium for the spermatozoa during their journey through the female reproductive tract. The main constituents of semen are listed below along with their functions:

- Water: fluid mechanism of transport for sperm.
- Buffers: protect sperm in acidic vaginal environment.
- Nutrients: fructose, carnitine, vitamin C, and citric acid provide nourishment for spermatozoa.
- Mucus: acts as lubricant for sexual intercourse.
- Spermatozoa: fertilization of oocyte.
- Enzymes: semen clotting in vagina and further liquefaction of clot. Prostate-specific antigen (PSA) is a glycoprotein enzyme encoded by the KLK3 gene produced by the prostate for semen liquefaction and dissolving of the cervical mucus for sperm penetration.
- Prostaglandins: stimulate smooth muscle contraction and transport through both reproductive tracts and improve sperm motility.
- Immunity particles: lysozyme, immunoglobulins, and leukocytes act as antibacterial agents and wash out the urethra; zinc acts as antioxidant.
- Other cells: genitourinary tract epithelial cells and immature germ cells [32–36].

The lower reference limits for semen parameters as described by the World Health Organization (WHO) are as follows: semen volume (ml) = 1.5; total sperm number (10^6 per ejaculate) = 39; sperm concentration (10^6 per ml) = 15; total motility (progressive + nonprogressive, %) = 40; vitality (live spermatozoa, %) = 58; sperm morphology (normal forms, %) 4, and pH = 7.2 [32].

Sexual Response

Erection and ejaculation are two key phases of the male sexual response that are of absolute necessity for copulation and fertilization to take place and are under the control of parasympathetic stimuli (tactile or psychological). Erection takes place through relaxation of the smooth muscle in the penile arteries, as a result of which the sinusoidal spaces become engorged with blood, the corpora become distended and compress the tunica albuginea, which in turn compresses the venous drainage system and traps blood within the penis (as seen in Fig. 1.6). The penile urethra does not close as the tunica albuginea of the corpus spongiosum is thinner and more extensible, thus allowing sperm to be transported during ejaculation. The movement of sperm out of the vas deferens and into the urethra where it encounters secretions from the accessory glands is known as emission. Ejaculation refers to the rapid muscular contractions that dispel semen from the urethra to the external environment outside of the body. Once parasympathetic stimulation ceases, the penis returns to its flaccid state [37–41].

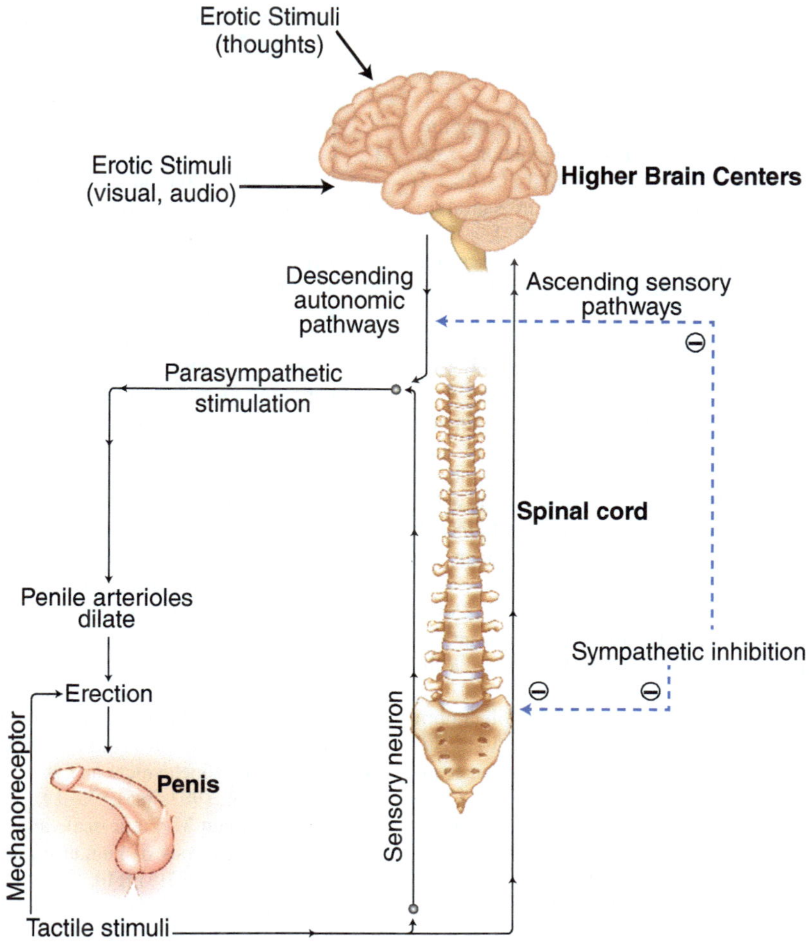

Fig. 1.6 Control, stimulation, and feedback pathways of the male sexual response

References

1. Lipshultz L, Sigman M. Office evaluation of the subfertile male. In: Howards S, Lipshultz L, Niederberger C, editors. Infertility in the male. Cambridge: Cambridge University Press; 2009. pp. 153–76.
2. Orth J, Jester W, Li L, Laslett A. Gonocyte–Sertoli cell interactions during development of the neonatal rodent testis. Curr Top Dev Biol. 2000;50:103.
3. Moffett D, Moffett S, Schauf C. Reproduction and its endocrine control. In: Moffett D, Moffett S, Schauf C, editors Human physiology: foundations & frontiers. Mosby Publishers; 1993. pp. 684–724.
4. Rouvière H, Delmas A. Anatomie humaine: descriptive, topographique et fonctionnelle. Tête et cou. vol. 1. Paris: Elsevier Masson; 2002.
5. Williams P, Bannister L, Berry M, Collins P, Dyson M, Dussek J, Ferguson M, Anatomy G. Tome II. 38ª edition. Churchill & Livingstone; 1995.
6. Kierszenbaum A. Histology and cell biology: an introduction to pathology. Philadelphia: Elsevier; 2007.
7. Ross M, Pawlina W. Histology: interactive atlas to accompany histology: a text and atlas; with correlated cell and molecular biology. Baltimore: Lippincott, Williams & Wilkins; 2007 (CD-ROM.).
8. Ferris H, Shupnik M. Mechanisms for pulsatile regulation of the gonadotropin subunit genes by GNRH1. Biol Reprod. 2006;74(6):993–8.
9. Silverman A, Livne I, Witkin J. The gonadotropin-releasing hormone (GnRH) neuronal systems: immunocytochemistry and in situ hybridization. In: Knobil E, Neill J, editors. The physiology of reproduction. 3rd ed. New York: Elsevier Academic Press; 2006. pp. 1683–710.
10. Rajalakshmi M, Sharma R, Pal P. Structure and physiology of mammalian testis. In: Kumar S, Tiwari R. Environmental and occupational exposures. Reproductive impairment. Delhi: Daya Publishing House; 2010. pp. 1–44.

11. França L, Ogawa T, Avarbock M, Brinster R, Russell L. Germ cell genotype controls cell cycle during spermatogenesis in the rat. Biol Reprod. 1998;59(6):1371–7.
12. Popa S, Clifton D, Steiner R. The role of kisspeptins and GPR54 in the neuroendocrine regulation of reproduction. Annu Rev Physiol. 2008;70:213–38.
13. Pinón R. Biology of human reproduction. Sausalito: University Science Books; 2002. pp. 171–2.
14. Filkenstein J, Whitcomb R, O'dea L, Longscope C, Schoenfeld D, Crowley W. Sex steroid control of gonadotropin secretion in the human male I. Effects of testosterone administration in normal and gonadotropin-releasing hormone deficient men. J Clin Endocrinol Metab. 1991;73(3):609–20.
15. Zimmermann S, Steding G, Emmen J, Brinkmann A, Nayernia K, Holstein A, Engel W, Adham I. Targeted disruption of the Insl3 gene causes bilateral cryptorchidism. Mol Endocrinol. 1999;13:681–91.
16. Calzolari E, Contiero M, Roncarati E, Mattiuz P, Volpato S. Aetiological factors in hypospadias. J Med Genet. 1986;23(4):333–7.
17. Svechnikov K, Landreh L, Weisser J, Izzo G, Colón E, Svechnikova I, Söder O. Origin, development and regulation of human Leydig Cells. Horm Res Paediatr. 2010;73(2):93–101.
18. Silverthorn D. Hormone interactions. In: Silverthorn D, Ober W, Garrison C, Silverthorn A, editors Human physiology: an integrated approach. San Francisco: Pearson; 2009. pp. 231–232.
19. Brink A, Lochner J. Infertility, obesity, cigarette smoke. In Brink A, Lochner J, editors. Pharos dictionary for the health sciences. Pharos dictionaries. Kaapstad: Pharos Woordeboeke; 2011. p. 359, 725, 869.
20. Mocarelli P, Gerthoux P, Patterson D, Milani S, Limonta G, Bertona M, et al. Dioxin exposure, from infancy through puberty, produces endocrine disruption and affects human semen quality. Environ Health Perspect. 2008;116(1):70–7.
21. Nef S, Parada L. Cryptorchidism in mice mutant for Insl3. Nat Genet. 1999;22:295–9.
22. Amann R. The male rabbit. IV. Quantitative testicular histology and comparisons between daily sperm production as determined histologically and daily sperm output. Fertil Steril. 1970;21:662–72.
23. O'Donnell L, Nicholls P, O'Bryan M, McLachlan R, Stanton P. Spermiation: the process of sperm release. Spermatogen. 2001;1(1):14.
24. Yamamoto M, Turner T. Epididymis, sperm maturation and capacitation. In: Lipshultz L, Howards S, editors. Infertility in the male. 2nd ed. St. Louis: Mosby Year Book; 1991. pp. 103–23.
25. Turner T. De Graaf's thread: the human epididymis. J Androl. 2008;29(3):237–50.
26. Clermont Y. Kinetics of spermatogenesis in mammals: seminiferous epithelium cycle and spermatogonial renewal. Physiol Rev. 1972;52(1):198–236.
27. Cornwall G. New insights of epididymal biology and function. Hum Reprod Update. 2009;15(2):213–27.
28. Hinton B, Lan Z, Rudolph D, Labus J, Lye R. Testicular regulation of epididymal gene expression. J Reprod Fertil Suppl. 1998;53:47–57.
29. Mortimer S. Essentials of sperm biology. In: Patton P, Battaglia D, editors. Office andrology. New Jersey: Humana Press; 2005. pp. 1–9.
30. Olson G, Nag Das S, Winfrey V. Structural differentiation of spermatozoa during post-testicular maturation. In: Robaire B, Hinton B, editors. The epididymis: from molecules to clinical practice. New York: Kluwer Academic; 2002. pp. 371–87.
31. Toshimori K. Biology of spermatozoa maturation: an overview with an introduction to this issue. Microsc Res Tech. 2003;61(1):1–6.
32. World Health Organization (editor). WHO laboratory manual for the examination and processing of human semen. 5th ed. Geneva: World Health Organization; 2010.
33. Owen D, Katz D. A review of the physical and chemical properties of human semen and the formulation of a semen simulant. J Androl. 2005;26(4):459–69.
34. Eliasson R. Biochemical analysis of human semen. Int J Androl. 1982;5(s5):109–19.
35. Pilch B, Mann M. Large-scale and high-confidence proteomic analysis of human seminal plasma. Genome Biol. 2006;7(5):R40.
36. Goldblatt M. Constituents of human seminal plasma. Biochem J. 1935;29(6):1346.
37. Weiss H. The physiology of human penile erection. Annals Int Med. 1972;76(5):793–9.
38. Holstege G, Georgiadis J, Paans A, Meiners L, van der Graaf F, Reinders A. Brain activation during human male ejaculation. J Neurosci. 2003;23(27):9185–93.
39. Bancroft J, Janssen E. The dual control model of male sexual response: a theoretical approach to centrally mediated erectile dysfunction. Neurosci Biobehav Rev. 2000;24(5):571–9.
40. Wespes E, Nogueira M, Herbaut A, Caufriez M, Schulman C. Role of the bulbocavernosus muscles on the mechanism of human erection. Eur Urol. 1989;18(1):45–8.
41. Wespes E, Schulman C. Study of human penile venous system and hypothesis on its behavior during erection. Urol. 1990;36(1):68–72.

Overview of the Female Reproductive System

2

Juan Andrés Ramírez-González, Ricardo Vaamonde-Lemos, Joao Sabino Cunha-Filho, Alex C. Varghese and R. James Swanson

Introduction

This chapter presents the most relevant and up-to-date aspects of the female reproductive system. The items directly involved are not many in number, consisting of the ovary, fallopian tubes, uterus, vagina, external genitalia, and breasts (the breast will not be discussed here). However, the reproductive system is coordinated with many other systems in the whole body for proper functioning. Our focus will be narrowly on the structures and function of the items listed as directly part of the female reproductive system with minimal inclusion of other ancillary systems. We present the gross anatomy first, then move to histological anatomy, and finish with physiology. A clear understanding of the female reproductive system necessitates understanding all three aspects. From a clinical aspect, we would also want to include biochemistry, pathophysiology, and pharmacology but many other excellent texts can be used if this broader picture is wanted.

Anatomy of the Female Reproductive System

The female genital system consists of internal organs (including ovaries, uterine tubes, uterus, and vagina—see Fig. 2.1a, b) and external organs (perineum and vulva—see Fig. 2.2).

This system is located deep within the pelvic cavity and consists essentially of two parts: a glandular body, the ovary, where the oocytes are formed and steroids synthesized, and an extended duct system, which successively takes on the names of uterine (fallopian) tube, uterus, and vagina. These tubes serve a dual purpose of providing a channel for ejaculated sperm to swim up into the peritoneal cavity and to bring either a fertilized or unfertilized egg down to the uterus and eventually out of the body at parturition or menses. The uterine tube is a simple duct that collects the oocyte on the ovarian surface and leads it to the uterus. The uterus is responsible for housing and feeding the fertilized egg during its development and, once it is mature, expelling the fetus

J. S. Cunha-Filho (✉)
Department of Obstetrics and Gynecology, Universidade Federal do Rio Grande do Sul, Av Nilo Peçanha, 2825/905, Porto Alegre 91330-001, Brazil
e-mail: sabino@insemine.com; sabino@via-rs.net

J. A. Ramírez-González
Department of Morphology, Health Sciences Faculty, University of Las Palmas De Gran Canaria, Las Palmas De Gran Canaria, Spain

R. Vaamonde-Lemos
Department of Morphological Sciences, School of Medicine, University of Córdoba, Córdoba, Spain

A. C. Varghese
ASTRA Fertility Group, Mississauaga, Ontario, Canada

R. J. Swanson
Department of Biological Sciences, Old Dominion University, Norfolk, VA, USA
e-mail: rjswanson@liberty.edu

© Springer Science+Business Media New York 2016

D. Vaamonde et al. (eds.), *Exercise and Human Reproduction*, DOI 10.1007/978-1-4939-3402-7_2

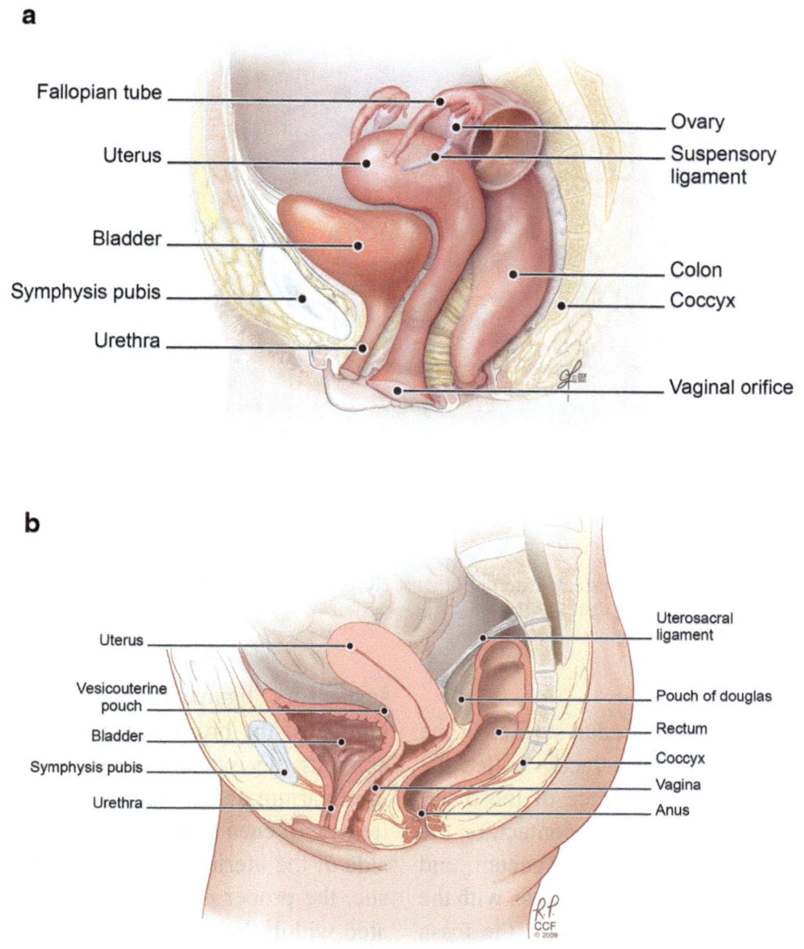

Fig. 2.1 **a, b** The female reproductive system: internal organs *(sagittal view)*. (Reprinted with permission, Cleveland Clinic Center for Medical Art & Photography © 2008–2015. All Rights Reserved)

outside the female body. The vagina gives way to the fetus and placenta during labor, but is also an organ of copulation, which receives the penis and semen during intercourse. The inferior vagina ends in the vulva, which is formed by a set of organs of varying nature (dermal and erectile tissues), connecting it external to the body.

An adnexal system is adjoined to the ovary, ducts, and vulva: This adnexa consists of various glands, developed around the lower end of the vagina and urethra, as well as muscles, membranes and fascia comprising the perineum.

Internal Organs

Ovary

The ovaries host oocytes and produce sex hormones. In the young woman, the ovary is an oval-shaped glandular body, pinkish white in color, measuring about 3–4 cm long, 1.5–2 cm wide, and 1–1.5 cm thick. Before puberty, the surface of the ovary is smooth and homogeneous: However, with age, repeated ovulations make it increasingly rough and irregular. The ovary has two surfaces, medial and lateral; two borders, mesovarian and free; and two extremities, uterine and tubal.

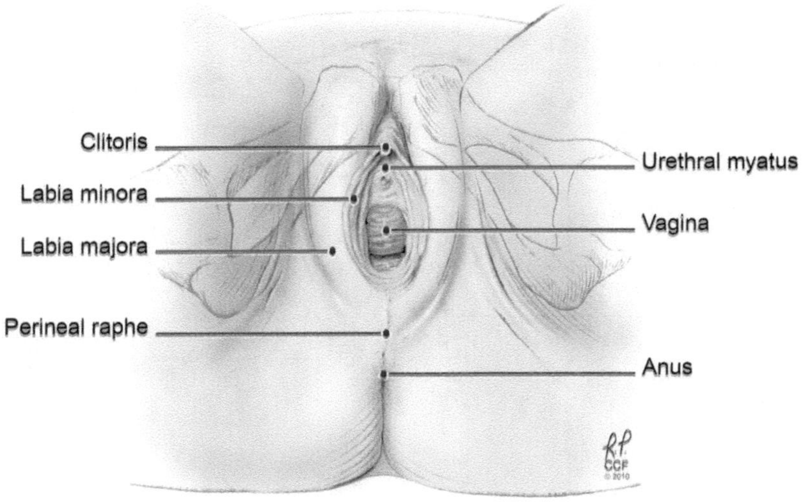

Fig. 2.2 The female reproductive system: external organs. (Reprinted with permission, Cleveland Clinic Center for Medical Art & Photography © 2008–2015. All Rights Reserved)

Relations

The ovary is located on the medial surface of the true (minor) pelvic wall, in a recess called the ovarian fossa. The medial surface of the ovary faces the pelvic cavity and it is in contact, on the right side, with the small intestine, cecum, and vermiform appendix and, on the left side, with the sigmoid colon. In nulliparous woman, the fossa is bounded by the broad ligament of the uterus, anteriorly; the external iliac vessels, superiorly; and the ureter and internal iliac vessels, with their uterine and umbilical branches, posteriorly. In multiparous woman, the ovary moves posteriorly, toward the infra-ovarian fossa, limited by the ureter and uterine vessels, superiorly; the border of the sacrum, posteromedially; and the superior edge of the piriformis muscle, inferiorly.

The anteroinferior border of the ovary presents the ovarian hilum and attaches to the posterior lamina of the broad ligament of the uterus by a peritoneal fold named mesovarium. The beginning of the uterine (fallopian) tube, fimbriated end, starts at the mesovarian border of the ovary, and lies along the superomedial border of the ovary, ending at the superolateral border of the uterus. The uterine entrance of the two fallopian tubes defines the inferior border of the uterine fundus (Fig. 2.3).

The lateral extremity of the ovary is attached to the lateral wall of the pelvis by the ovarian suspensory ligament, a fold of the posterior lamina of the broad ligament of the uterus that conveys the ovarian vessels and nerves to the mesovarium and ovarian hilum. The uterine extremity of each ovary is attached to the posterior side of the uterine horn by a band of fibrous tissue, the proper ovarian ligament, which is situated within the broad ligament and contains the ovarian branch of uterine artery.

Vascularization and Innervations

1. Arteries: The greatest part of the blood supply to the ovary comes from the ovarian arteries, direct branches of the abdominal aorta that arise at the L2–3 level. These arteries course inferiorly inside the suspensory ligament, along the posterior wall of the abdomen, running anterior to the psoas major muscle and ureter. The right artery also lies anterior to the inferior vena cava. Running superoanteriorly to the iliac crest, they cross anterior to the external iliac vessels and enter the broad ligaments to reach the ovarian flaps where they anastomose with the ovarian branches of the uterine arteries, the ovarian anastomotic arches. After sending branches to the ovary through the mesovarium, they continue medially to supply the uterine tubes.

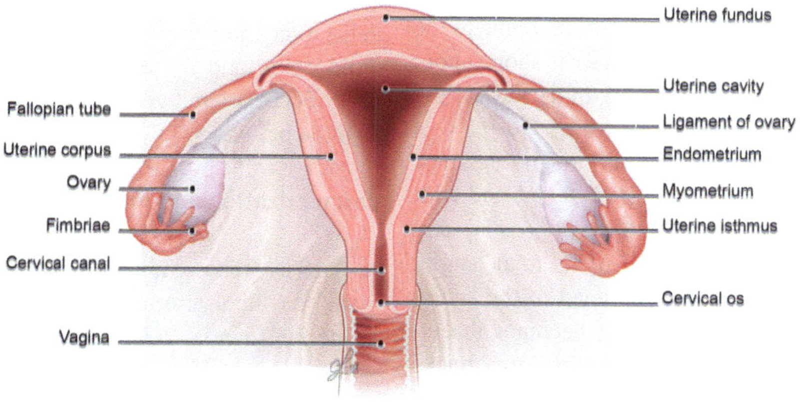

Fig. 2.3 The female reproductive system: internal organs *(coronal view)*. (Reprinted with permission, Cleveland Clinic Center for Medical Art & Photography © 2008–2015. All Rights Reserved)

2. Veins: The venous drainage of the ovary is through the ovarian veins, which leave the ovaries through the hila and form the pampiniform plexuses which surround the ovarian arteries. This plexus is situated in the thickness of the broad ligament and communicates with the uterine venous plexus, medially. Laterally, the plexus resolves in a single ovarian vein that follows the pathway of the ovarian artery and reaches the inferior caval vein, on the right, and the renal vein, on the left.
3. Lymphatics: The lymphatic vessels follow the ovarian artery and veins and join those from the uterine tube and fundus. They drain into aortic ganglia.
4. Nerves: The innervations of the ovary comes from the ovarian plexus, formed by fibers derived from the aortic and renal plexuses that descend along the ovarian vessels and contribute to the autonomic innervation of the ovary, uterine tube, and broad ligament of uterus. In addition, the ovary receives one or two branches from the lateral cervical nerve (branch of the inferior hypogastric plexus).

Fallopian Tube

Fertilization of the ovulated ovum may take place at the ovarian surface if sperm are in the rectouterine recess (pouch of Douglas) within the peritoneum at the time of ovulation, or in the fimbriated end of the fallopian tube. The fallopian tube subsequently transfers the zygote to the uterine cavity by ciliary and peristaltic action as estradiol increases.

The uterine tube is a muscular-membranous tubular-shaped structure that extends medially from the ovary to the uterine horn where it opens proximally into the uterine cavity through the myometrium and endometrium. The oviducts' distal end opens directly into the peritoneal cavity near the ovary; thus a direct communication exists between the peritoneal cavity and the body exterior coursing from the fallopian tube through the uterus and out the vagina.

The fallopian tube measures about 10 cm in length and 1 cm in diameter (isthmus). It stretches, posteriorly and laterally, in the direction of the pelvic wall, surrounding the corresponding ovary.

Topographically, the uterine tube can be divided into four parts: intrauterine, isthmus, ampulla, and infundibulum.

1. The intrauterine part, or intramural part, is the shortest (1 cm) and narrowest (1–2 mm) segment. It crosses the myometrium of the uterine horn and opens into the uterine cavity through the uterine ostium (its diameter is smaller than the abdominal ostium).

2. The isthmus is located immediately lateral to the uterus and connects the uterine tube to the horn of the uterus. The isthmus is short (about 2–3 cm), it narrows (2–3.5 mm) toward the uterus and has the thickest wall.
3. The ampulla begins laterally to the isthmus. The ampulla is the longest (7–8 cm) and widest part of the uterine tube (8–9 mm) and represents more than half of its total length. The ampulla curves at the level of the lateral extremity of the ovary as it becomes the infundibulum surrounding the ovary. Textbooks identify the ampulla as the normal place of fertilization, a theory not based on prospective, observable research, but rather a hypothesis needing confirmation. Normal fertilization could just as well take place in the infundibulum or in the peritoneal cavity.
4. The infundibulum, or ovarian part, is the distal (most lateral) end of the uterine tube. The infundibulum forms a funnel with the widest part directed laterally. The fimbriae are located on the peripheral edge and consist of 10–15 finger-like projections distributed around the surface of the ovary which are closely linked to the ovary by a variable fimbrio-ovarian ligament. The narrowest part of the infundibulum, directed medially, is the abdominal ostium, about 2–3 mm in diameter, which is the opening into the peritoneal cavity. After ovulation, the fimbriae "capture the oocyte" and lead it toward the abdominal hole in the uterine tube over approximately 3½ days. The inner surface of the uterine tube has numerous, intricate, mucous longitudinal folds that give it a labyrinthine aspect.

Except for the intramural portion, the uterine tube is covered by the peritoneum of the uterine broad ligament, the mesosalpinx, or mesentery of the tube, through which the vessels and nerves reach the oviduct.

Relations

The isthmus is posterior to the urinary bladder and the round ligament of uterus, anterior to the ligament of ovary, and inferior to the small intestine, greater omentum, and sigmoid colon. The ampulla and infundibulum are in close proximity to the ovary and share its relationships: left—sigmoid colon and mesocolon; right—inferior aspect of caecum and vermiform appendix when it is in the pelvis.

Vascularization and Innervation

1. Arteries: The oviduct receives arterial blood by the tubal arteries which branch from the uterine (medial 2/3) and ovarian (lateral 1/3) arteries reaching the uterine tube through the mesosalpinx, where they form the infra-tubarian anastomotic arch from which come numerous spiral arterioles that supply the wall of the tube.
2. Veins: The uterine tubes' venous drainage follows a reverse pathway to the arteries. They form arches and drain into the uterine (medially) and ovarian (laterally) veins.
3. Lymphatics: The lymphatic vessels of the fallopian tubes follow the same path as those coming from the uterine fundus, draining into the pelvic lymph nodes and from the ovary, ascending with the ovarian veins and draining into the aortic lymph nodes.
4. Nerves: Both, ovarian and uterine plexi share the innervation of the uterine tube. Sensory afferent fibers come from segments T11-L1.

Uterus

In the nonpregnant woman, the uterus is a hollow, muscular, thick-walled, inverted pear-shaped organ, where the fertilized oocyte develops. The nonpregnant uterus measures about 6.5–7.5 cm in length, 4.5–5.5 cm in width, and is about 2.5–3 cm thick. During pregnancy, it is greatly enlarged to accommodate the embryonic and fetal development. The uterus lies between the urinary bladder, anteriorly, and the rectum, posteriorly (Figs. 2.1a, b, 2.4a, b).

The uterus is made up of three parts: the fundus (superior to the fallopian tube entries), the body, and the cervix. The body and cervix are separated by a short isthmus.

The uterine body and fundus forms the superior two thirds of the uterus. Transversely expanded and ventro-dorsally flattened, the uterus

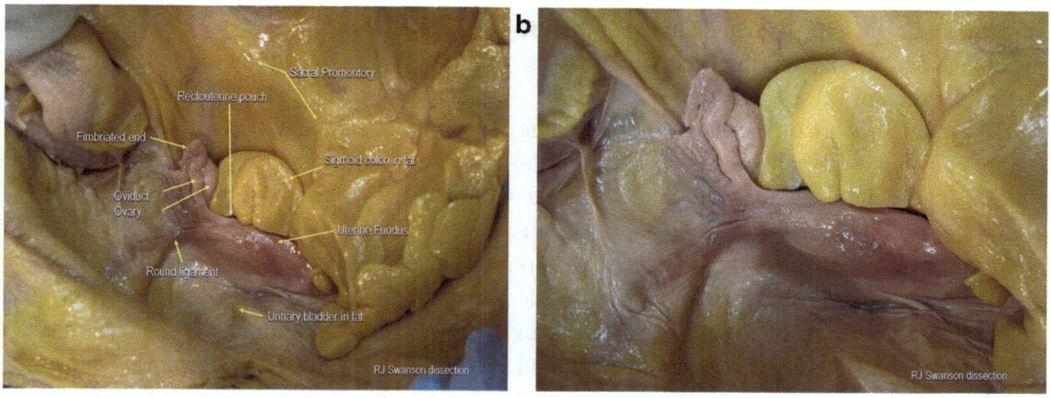

Fig. 2.4 **a** Uterine fundus, right oviduct and ovary in situ in 58-year-old cadaver abdomen *(labeled)*. **b** Uterine fundus, right oviduct and ovary in situ in 58-year-old cadaver abdomen *(close-up, unlabeled)*. (Courtesy of Dr. R. James Swanson)

shares its anterior surface with the urinary bladder (vesical surface) and its posterior surface with the rectum (intestinal surface). Both surfaces are convex.

The uterine fundus is superior to the uterine body and is the rounded part superior to the uterotubal union. The regions of the uterus where the fallopian tubes attach are the uterine horns. The proper ovarian ligament enters the uterine wall posterior and inferior to the fallopian tube insertion while the round ligament, a continuation of the proper ovarian ligament, leaves the uterine wall anterior and inferior to the fallopian tube to proceed into the internal inguinal ring, ending internally in the base of the labia majora.

The uterine cavity is triangular and flattened in the coronal plane presenting tubal angles, superiorly, and a cervical angle inferiorly. The cavity appears as a narrow slit in the sagittal plane.

The uterus is implanted in the superior aspect of the vaginal fornix. Two segments can be distinguished in the cervix, namely the vaginal and supravaginal portions. The supravaginal portion of the cervix is the uterine isthmus (approximately 1 cm in length), a narrow transition zone located between the body and the cervix. The isthmus is more evident in nulliparous than multiparous women. In this region the uterine cavity becomes significantly narrowed, forming the isthmic channel, and opening into the uterine cavity through the anatomical internal os.

The cavity of the cervix (cervical canal) is lined by longitudinal folds in which transversely oblique (palmate) folds converge. Superiorly the cervix continues into the isthmus and opens into the uterine cavity through the histological internal os. The inferior cervical aspect, the vaginal part, opens to the vaginal cavity through the external uterine os. This orifice is surrounded by the anterior and posterior cervical labia (Fig. 2.3).

The uterine wall consists of three layers from the lumen outward, that is, endometrium, myometrium, and perimetrium. The endometrium is a mucosal layer firmly attached to the myometrium which partially sloughs off during menstruation. The myometrium is a muscular layer which is 12–15 mm of smooth muscle in the nonpregnant state, but thickens considerably during pregnancy. The main branches of the blood vessels and nerves of the uterus are found in this layer. The perimetrium is the outer serosal layer of peritoneum resting on a thin layer of connective tissue (CT).

Pelvic Structure

An obtuse angle (100–120°) is formed between the cervix and the body of the uterus with the uterus tipped anteriorly, anteflexion (referred to as anteversion in relation to the vagina). The position of the uterus is maintained by dynamic factors, which include the muscles of the pelvic diaphragm and the urogenital part of the perineum, and by static factors, which include the pelvic ligaments and fascia, and the peritoneal folds of the pelvic region.

The main support of the uterus is the pelvic floor, formed by the pelvic diaphragm and reinforced superficially by the perineum. The pelvic viscera, vessels and nerves, surrounding the uterus, and the endopelvic visceral fascia that surrounds these structures support the uterus inside the pelvic cavity. The uterus is further fixed in place by a complex ligamentous system formed by the pubocervical, cardinal, uterosacral, and round ligaments which join the broad ligaments of uterus on either side. The pubocervical ligaments are equivalent to the puboprostatic ligaments in men. The cardinal ligaments expand from the supravaginal cervix and vaginal fornix to the lateral wall of the pelvis. They are situated at the base of the broad ligament, forming part of the parametrium (not lining the uterus but extending laterally from it in the cervical area). The uterosacral (rectouterine) ligaments extend from the lateral part of the uterine cervix and vaginal fornix to the pelvic surface of the sacrum. Located above to the levator ani muscle, they contribute to maintain the normal relation of the uterine cervix and the sacrum. The round ligaments of uterus (10–12 cm long) originate on the anterior surface of the uterine horn (near the uterotubal junction). They pass anteriorly between the layers of the broad ligament to pierce the internal inguinal ring and canal. These round ligaments leave the abdominal cavity and pass through the mons pubis to attach to the base of labia majora. They contribute to the maintenance of uterine anteversion.

The broad ligaments of uterus are folds of the peritoneum that extend between the borders of the uterus to the lateral walls and floor of the pelvis, contributing to the maintenance of the normal position of the uterus.

The fundus and the anterior and posterior surfaces of the body of the uterus are coated by the pelvic peritoneum. When they reach the uterine borders, the peritoneal laminae attach together and extend to the pelvic wall forming, on each side, the uterine broad ligament. Superiorly, the laminae of the broad ligament are continuous and surround the uterine tube, forming the mesosalpinx.

Relations

The pelvic floor and the complex system of attachments provide the uterus a relatively stable position inside the pelvis. Its central position gives the uterus anterior, posterior, and lateral relations with the surrounding organs.

1. Anterior: The anterior surface of the uterus rests on the posterior surface of the urinary bladder. The peritoneum that lines these two surfaces forms the vesicouterine pouch.
2. Posterior: The posterior surface of the uterus rests on the posterior surface of the rectum to form the rectouterine pouch. This peritoneal recess separates the uterus from the rectum and is usually occupied by the small intestine, the sigmoid colon, and a small amount of peritoneal fluid. This space is also where ejaculated sperm reside for up to 7 days after intercourse.
3. Lateral: The lateral surfaces of the uterus are attached to the broad ligament; mesometrium superiorly and parametrium inferiorly.

Vascularization and Innervation

1. Arteries: The arterial blood to the uterus comes from an anastomotic network of the uterine and vaginal arteries, branches of the internal iliac arteries, the ovarian arteries, and branches of the abdominal aorta. At the level of the uterine horn, the uterine artery is divided into several branches, including a tubal branch and an ovarian branch.

On its path, the uterine artery emits collateral branches downstream (vesicovaginal, cervical-vaginal, cervical, and ureteral), irrigating the uterine cervix, the superior part of the vagina, base of the urinary bladder, and terminal segment of the ureter.

2. Veins: The venous drainage of the uterus flows into the uterine venous plexuses that accompany the uterine arteries in their path through the mesometrium. Each plexus is drained mainly by the uterine veins (toward the internal iliac vein) and also by the ovarian

veins (toward the inferior vena cava on the right, and the renal vein on the left).

3. Lymphatics: The lymphatic vessels from the wall of the uterus form an abundant plexus located in the mesometrium and the parametrium. Drainage follows three main routes:
   a. The majority of the lymphatic vessels from the uterine fundus follows the ovarian vessels and drains into the aortic lymph nodes (a small part may follow the round ligament and drain into the external iliac or inguinal lymph nodes).
   b. Lymph vessels from the uterine body enter into the broad ligament and drain into the external iliac lymph nodes.
   c. Cervical lymphatic vessels follow the uterine artery and drain into the internal iliac and sacral ganglia.
4. Nerves: The uterine nerves come from the uterovaginal plexus and are grouped into two pedicles directed to the uterine body and cervical-isthmus, respectively. This plexus is located at the base of the broad ligament on each side of the cervix.

Vagina

The vagina is the lowest portion of the female genital tract. It receives the penis during intercourse and is the natural route for elimination of uterine secretions and the fetus and annexes during child birth.

The vagina is a fibromuscular tube 7–10 cm in length and 2.5–3 cm wide. Its inner surface is rough (vaginal rugae) with superior-to-inferior longitudinal folds called rough anterior and posterior columns. The anterior columns contain horizontal (medial to lateral) folds along the inferior 2 cm length.

The vagina stretches from the uterine cervix to the vestibule where it opens between the labia minora and majora. The vestibular end of the vagina is anterior to the cervix. The entire vagina is inferior to the uterus, posterior to the urinary bladder and urethra, and anterior to the rectum. It passes between the medial borders of the levator ani muscles to pierce the urogenital diaphragm in conjunction with the urethra. Both of these tubular structures are surrounded by sphincters that are derived from the levator ani muscle.

Relations

1. Anterior: The superior aspect of the anterior wall of the vagina is 1 cm shorter than the posterior aspect in their connection to the cervix. From mid-vagina inferiorly, it is related to the terminal segments of the ureters as they enter the inferior portion of the bladder at the trigone (bladder segment), and the upper part of urethra (urethral segment).
   The female urethra is only 3–4 cm long and opens in the vestibule, through the external urethral orifice. It has two sphincters. The internal urethral sphincter is smooth muscle, poorly vascularized, and sometimes so thin that it is discounted as a true sphincter. The external urethral sphincter is more robust skeletal muscle from the levator ani located in the perineum. These sphincters control the flow of urine.
2. Posterior: The posterior part of the vaginal fornix is covered by the peritoneum and comes in direct contact with the bottom of the rectouterine pouch (peritoneal segment). At this level, the vaginal wall allows entry into the pelvic cavity and a surgical approach to the abdominal and pelvic viscera (surgical transvaginal path). At the floor of the pelvis, the vagina is anterior to the perineal body, a central point of various ligamentous attachments which separates the vaginal os from the anal canal.
3. Inferior: The loose CT of the rectovaginal septum, which separates the back wall of the vagina from the rectum, provides vaginal palpation through the rectum.
4. Lateral: The superior vaginal fornix is in contact laterally with the base of the broad ligament of the uterus and the pelvic segment of the ureter. More inferiorly, the lateral vaginal walls come into contact with the edges of the levator ani muscles and, inferior to those pelvic diaphragm muscles, with the greater vestibular glands and bulbs of vestibule (perineal segment of vagina).

Vascularization and Innervation

1. Arteries: The vagina is supplied by the vaginal artery. This artery will either be a branch from the uterine artery or it will come directly from the internal iliac artery. Irrigation in the upper segment is directly from the uterine artery through its vesicovaginal and cervicovaginal branches. In addition, branches from the middle rectal artery usually reach the inferior segment of the posterior wall. From its origin, the vaginal artery descends toward the top of the vagina and anastomoses with branches from the opposite side and from the uterine and middle rectal arteries. This anastomosis forms a median longitudinal trunk known as the "azygos artery of the vagina." In addition to the vagina, the vaginal artery also participates in supplying the inferior urinary bladder, the bulbs of the vestibule and the contiguous portion of the rectum.
2. Veins: Each side of the vaginal veins form a plexus (submucosal and superficial), which communicates with the uterine, bladder, and rectal plexi, and are drained by the uterine, vaginal, and rectal medial veins (they terminate in the internal iliac veins).
3. Lymphatics: Lymphatic drainage from the vagina is abundant and shows a segmental distribution. The lymph vessels from the top accompany the uterine artery and drain into the internal iliac and obturator lymph nodes. The vessels of the middle part accompany the vaginal artery and drain into the internal iliac and gluteal lymph nodes. Lymphatics from the lowest part drain into the superficial inguinal and pararectal nodes.
4. Nerves: The nerves innervating the upper part of the vagina and cervix are autonomic and derive from the uterovaginal plexus. The inferior hypogastric plexus (sympathetic) and the pelvic splanchnic nerves (parasympathetic) are mainly vasomotor but also transmit mechanoreceptor impulses from muscle and adventitia. Nerves which innervate the inferior part of the vagina are somatic and reach the vagina via the pudendal nerve (sacral nerve roots).

External Organs

Perineum

The perineum is formed by the soft tissues inferior to the pelvic diaphragm ending with the skin. The external configuration of the perineum varies according to the position of the individual:

1. When standing, the perineum takes the form of a sagittal cleft between the proximal ends of both thighs. Narrow and hidden, this space broadens anteriorly to end at the pubic symphysis and broadens posteriorly to end at the coccyx.
2. In dorsal decubitus (gynecologic or lithotomy position), the perineum forms a rhomboid- or diamond-shaped area with an anteroposterior axis. The anterior vertex is the inferior symphysis pubis; the posterior vertex is the coccyx; the lateral vertices are the ischial tuberosities.

The diamond-shaped perineum has the urogenital diaphragm as its roof and the skin as its floor. In common language, the perineum is called a person's bottom. This area contains a significant amount of adipose tissue with nerves, vessels, erectile tissue, and a few very small muscles within it. From posterior to anterior, the three openings of anus, vagina, and urethra also pierce the perineum. For a more detailed treatment of the perineum, a number of excellent texts are cited in the bibliography.

Vulva

The vulva contains the external female genitalia and the urethral os (opening). The vulva's skin is ovoid shaped with an anteroposterior axis. Anteriorly, the vulva extends from the wall of the abdomen at the symphysis pubis, posteriorly to the anus. The lateral limits are the medial sides of the thighs at the genitofemoral folds.

When the thighs are abducted, the cleft opens exposing the mons pubis, the labia majora and minora, and the vestibule. The bulbs of vestibule and the clitoris, which are also part of the vulva, are located deep to the labial formations.

1. *Mons pubis:* The mons pubis is a rounded relief located anterior to the pubic symphysis and from which it extends inferiorly to the labia majora. The inguinal folds are its lateral boundaries. The mons pubis consists of a pad of fatty CT covered by skin. During puberty, thick hair begins to appear (pubarche), which acquires the typical triangular female distribution. Both fat and hair decrease after menopause.
2. *Labia majora:* The two labia majora are longitudinal skin folds, with adipose and fibrous tissue deposits, located infero-posteriorly to the mons pubis at each side of the pudendal cleft. They provide protection to the vestibule, where the urethra and vagina open. Although they are symmetrical, their size depends on fat content so they vary in size and distribution among women. They extend anteriorly from the mons pubis, posteriorly to the perineal raphe, about 2.5 cm from the anal orifice. The labia majora are joined superiorly to form the anterior (labial) commissure, a relatively thick arc that is continuous with the mons pubis. Inferiorly, a very thin and transverse skin fold, the posterior (labial) commissure, extends between the labia majora anterior to the anal orifice and perineal body.
3. *Labia minora:* The two labia minora are thin and delicate skin folds located medially between the labia majora and lateral to the vestibule. On each side, a labial sulcus separates the major from the minor labia. The labia minora surround the vestibular space on each side where the urethra and vagina exit. The anterior ends of the minor labia are divided into two expansions, one inferior and the other superior. The superior expansions meet with each other superoanterior to the clitoris forming a hood of skin named the prepuce or foreskin of the clitoris. The inferior expansions join with each other inferior to the clitoris and form the clitoral frenulum. Posteriorly in young women, the labia minora are linked by a small skin fold called the frenulum of the labia minora. The labia minora lack hair and fat and have abundant sebaceous and sweat glands opening onto their surfaces. The skin of the inner surface is very thin, presents the typical pink color of mucosa and contains many sensitive nerve endings, making it very sensible to direct mechanical stimulation.
4. *Vestibule:* The vestibule is the space located between the medial surfaces of the labia minora. When the vulva is closed, the vestibule is a virtual space and is reduced to a simple interlabial slit. However, when the vulva is open, it takes the shape of an oblong funnel. At the base or superior aspect of the funnel will be the opening for the urethra, paraurethral glands, vagina, and ducts of the greater and lesser vestibular glands.
   a. *The external urethral orifice* is situated 2–3 cm posterior to the clitoris and 1 cm anterior to the vaginal opening. Lateral to the vaginal os are the paired external orifices of the paraurethral gland ducts. The paraurethral glands are homologous to the male prostate.
   b. *The vaginal orifice* is posterior to the external orifice of the urethra. The size and appearance vary according to the condition of the hymen. The hymen is a thin fold of mucous membrane, skin, and fibroelastic tissue that attaches to the edge of the vaginal orifice. The hymen is usually perforated before menarche which allows unobstructed menstruation flow. Prior to intercourse or the use of tampons, the adult woman normally has a complete hymen with either a perforation or septum. After the first use of tampons or sexual intercourse, the hymen's torn remains form small tubers called hymenal caruncles.
   c. *The paired greater vestibular glands* are round or oval-shaped, 0.5–1 cm in diameter and located posterolateral to the vaginal orifice. The glandular duct is short, narrow, and emerges from the anterior part of the gland. The greater vestibular glands are homologues of the bulbourethral glands in the male and their secretion lubricate the vaginal vestibule during sexual intercourse.
   d. *The paired lesser vestibular glands* also lie in the vestibule and exit into the space

between the urethral and vaginal openings. They secrete mucus to moisten the labia minora and the vestibule.

5. *Erectile organs*: The bulbs of vestibule and the clitoris are erectile tissue located deep to the labial formations that surround the vulvar vestibule.
   a. *The paired bulbs of vestibule* are 3–3.5 cm long and 1.2–1.5 cm wide located on the side of the urethral and vaginal orifices, deep to the bulbospongiosus muscles. They are homologues to the singular bulb of the corpus spongiosum of the penis, but unlike the single structure in male anatomy, the bulbs of vestibule in the female are separated by the vestibule of the vagina. Their anterior ends are joined at the urethral orifice to form a commissure and they attach to the body of the clitoris through the intermediate venous plexus.
   b. *The clitoris* is 0.5–0.7 cm long and 0.6–0.8 cm wide, located deep to the prepuce and anterior labial commissure. When flaccid, the clitoris is hidden by the labia majora. The clitoris divides superolaterally into a pair of 3–3.5 cm long crura. Each crus of the clitoris is anchored to the ischiopubic ramus and covered by a thin ischiopubic muscle. The glans clitoris is the counterpart of the glans penis but does not contain the urethra, so it has no corpus spongiosum. The clitoris plays a fundamental role in female sexual arousal and enters erection through tactile stimulation, although it does not significantly lengthen.

Vascularization and Innervation of the Perineum and Vulva

1. Arteries: The rich arterial blood supply of the perineum comes from (1) the superficial and deep external pudendal arteries which branch from the femoral artery and are distributed under the anterior skin of the vulva over the mons pubis, and (2) the internal pudendal artery which branches from the internal iliac artery and is distributed to the posterior sector of the perineum and vulva to perfuse the labia, erectile organs, and vestibular glands.
2. Veins: The venous drainage of the mons pubis, foreskin of the clitoris, and the anterior part of the labia majora flows into the external pudendal veins to the great saphenous vein. Veins from the labia and clitoris are abundant, adopt the appearance of cavernous tissue and drain into the internal pudendal veins through their perineal branches.
3. Lymphatics: The vulva has an important network of lymphatic vessels that drain the lymph into the superficial and deep inguinal lymph nodes and into the internal iliac nodes.
4. Nerves: Sensory nerves of the anterior and lateral part of the vulva (mons pubis and anterior third of the labia) come from the genital branches of genitofemoral, ilioinguinal, and iliohypogastric nerves. Sensory supply to the rest of the vulva is by perineal branches of the pudendal nerve. The pudendal nerve (S2–S4) accompanies the internal pudendal artery along its length with perineal branches innervating the skin and deep perineal erectile tissues and muscles. In addition, the posterior femoral cutaneous nerve innervates the middle third of the labia majora.

Embryology and Histology of the Female Reproductive System

Histogenesis

The development of internal sexual organs, hormonally regulated according to the chromosomal sex of the embryo, follows a basic pattern. In both sexes, an "indistinct" stage in gonadal development can be observed in 4–20 mm embryos. This critical period encompasses most of the malformations and/or dysfunctions of reproductive organs. Genital ridges, made up of thickened mesodermal epithelium of the coelom in the mesonephric area (Fig. 2.5), give rise to the gonads. The basal membrane underlying such epithelium gets fragmented and the quick proliferation of the coelomic epithelium results in cellular cords immersed completely in the mesonephric

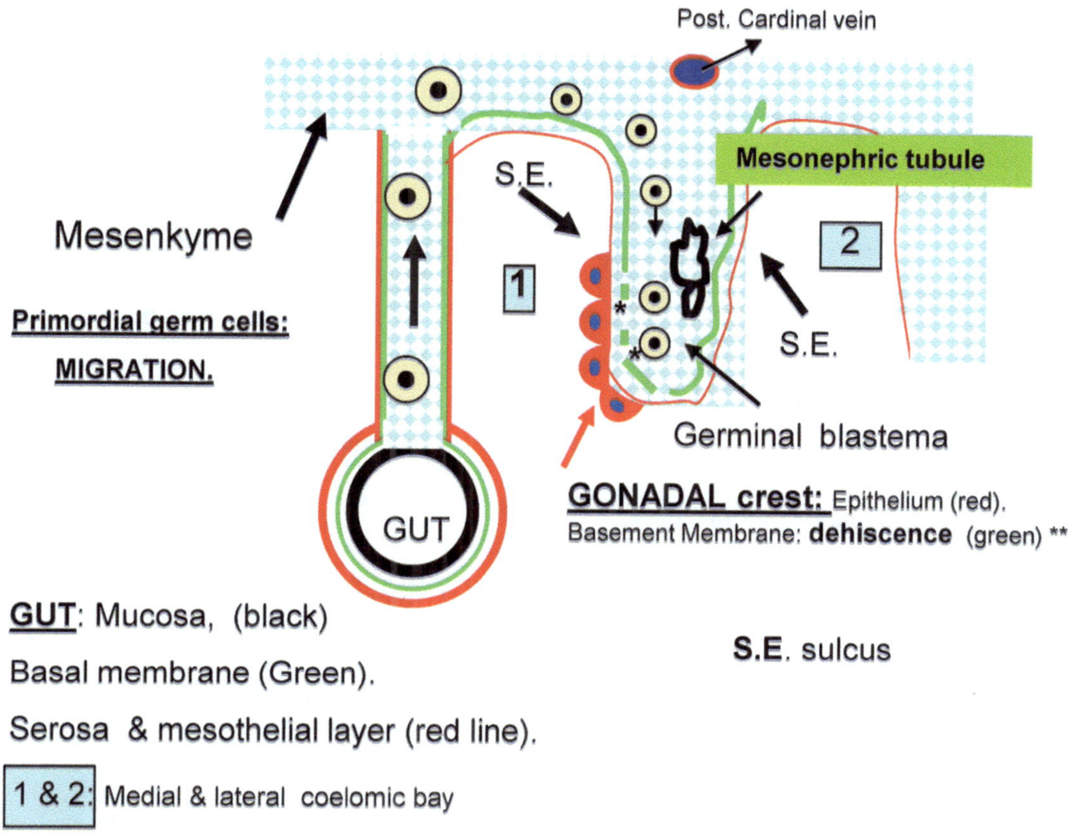

Fig. 2.5 Migration of primordial germ cells through the primitive gut to the gonadal ridge. (Courtesy of Ricardo Vaamonde-Lemos)

mesenchyme. At this point in development, a second type of cell appears, the primordial germ cells (PGCs; gonocytes).

These cells seem to originate in the dorsal wall of the yolk sac near the developing allantois, and are therefore of endodermal origin. The cells subsequently migrate to the posterior wall of the hindgut and midgut. At a later stage they migrate through the dorsal mesentery to the gonadal ridge [1]. Crests in the inner part of the mesonephros, having shorter caudo-cranial length, become more visible. In the XX female, the undifferentiated gonad will begin to differentiate into an ovary. The male mesonephric (Wolfian) ducts and testes will not begin to develop at week 7 due to the lack of testosterone and the female paramesonephric (Müllerian) ducts and ovary will begin to develop during week 11 of embryonic growth.

The adrenal gland develops suprainternally to the ipsilateral gonad, which explains the mixture of both tissues in some disorders.

The ovary develops its final structure at the end of the somitic period. The more central part of the mesenchyme turns into the medulla of ovary containing no PGCs. The cords fragment into small groups, each of which is completely separated and covered by a layer of cells of the mesodermal cords, giving rise to the "primordial follicle." Whether mesodermal cells also give rise to either "follicular cells" or "granulosa cells" remains unknown (Fig. 2.6). Nonetheless, mesonephric mesodermal cells are responsible for creating the secretory "interstitial" cells of the ovarian medulla [2].

In both genders, the Müllerian ducts (paramesonephric ducts) start to develop at the 10 mm

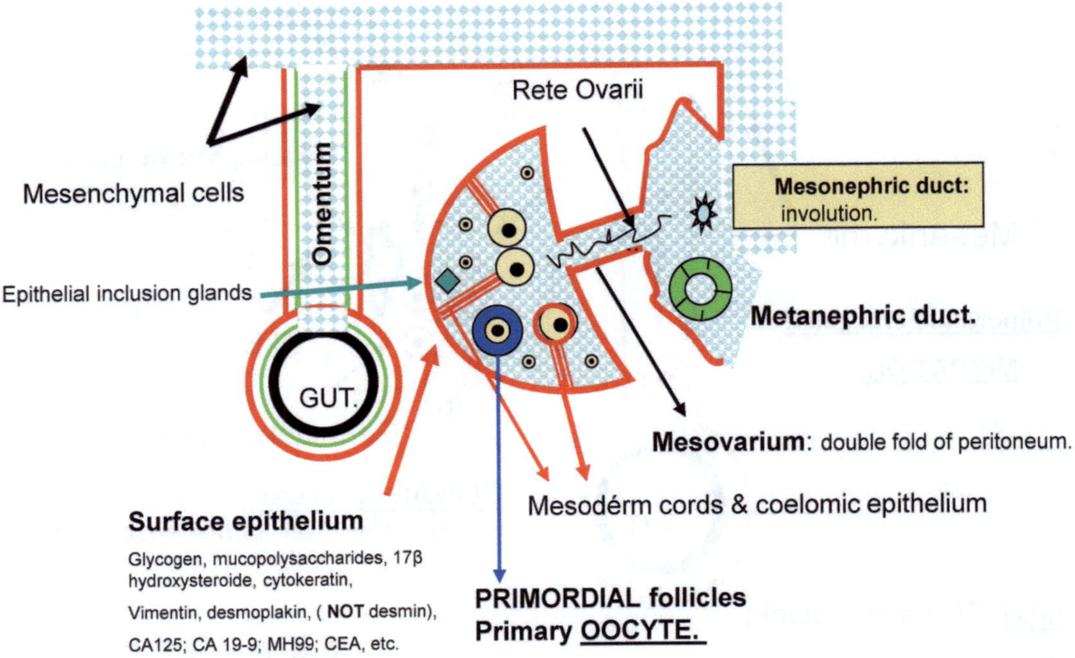

Fig. 2.6 Evolution of the primitive gonad into mature functioning ovary, with progressive differentiation and maturation of the different ovarian follicles as described in the text. (Courtesy of Ricardo Vaamonde-Lemos)

embryo stage, but in males, the Müllerian inhibiting hormone (MIH) produced by Sertoli cells arrests their development. In females, their cranial ends have a central lumen, the uterine orifice of the uterine tube, surrounded by fimbriae. The caudal ends form a thick solid structure which enters the mesenchyme, elongates cranio-caudally, while a lumen appears in its center. The caudal ends approach the embryonic median line, giving rise to the urorectal septum. This develops into the definitive "urogenital canal" and has a unique central cavity (except in cases of malformations, which are not uncommon), of which the more cranial two thirds develop into the uterine tubes. Its caudal part, which is also the largest and known as Müller's tubercle, gives rise to the fornix, body, and cervix of the uterus. The cervix enters the urogenital sinus differentiating into the vagina.

During the development of the mesoderm of both the ligamentous (mesosalpinx) and solid parts (uterus) of the Müllerian ducts, the Wolfian ducts persist. If the Wolfian ducts start to develop beyond their embryonic stage due to elevated testosterone, disorders can result. A neoplasm histogenesis can occur, of which the most common example is the hydatid of Morgagni. In the male, this is an appendix testis; in the female, it forms a paratubal cyst at the most cranial end of the ovary. These ducts can also develop abnormally at the level of the medulla of the ovary, forming the rete ovarii. In the male, MIH, mentioned above, and testosterone will inhibit the development of the Müllerian ducts through their paracrine effects.

Histology

Ovaries

A longitudinal section of a functional ovary shows a poorly delineated division into peripheral cortex and central medullary zones (Fig. 2.7). The medulla is rich in blood vessels and nerves and is thus mainly stroma while the cortex contains the follicles and is thus mainly parenchyma. From a histological and functional perspective,

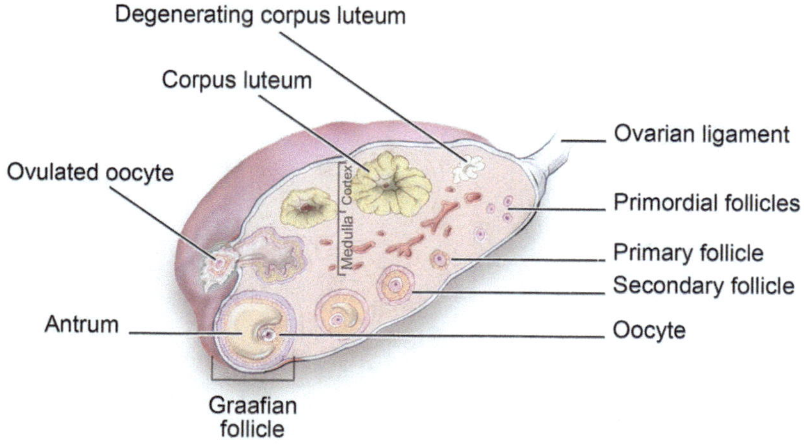

Fig. 2.7 The structure of the ovary. (Reprinted with permission, Cleveland Clinic Center for Medical Art & Photography © 2008–2015. All Rights Reserved)

the cortex is the most important part with the oocyte-containing follicles. Ovarian follicles are surrounded by cortical CT, which is cellular and has trophic functions.

The ovarian surface, except at the hilum, is covered by a simple flat epithelium, whose underlying CT is thickly condensed as the tunica albuginea (Fig. 2.8, #1).

The ovarian follicles are different sizes and have different cellular compositions according to their stage of maturation. Developed below the tunica albuginea during histogenesis, there are approximately 1–2.5 million follicles per ovary by the end of the fifth intrauterine month, and at birth only approximately 250,000–500,000 remain per ovary. Of these, in a normally cycling female, only about 260 in each ovary will reach complete maturity and release an ovum. This computation is approximate for a woman who has 40 years (10–50 years of age) of reproductively active ovaries ovulating every 28 days (13 times a year) with no pregnancies. Follicles do not ovulate during pregnancy and ovulation is also often reduced during nursing depending somewhat on frequency and genetics of the woman. The remaining follicles will undergo atresia (degeneration), which begins in the sixth month of intrauterine life resulting in the vast majority of ova being lost to this process.

Ovarian Follicles

There are two main types of follicles, namely primordial follicles (PF) and maturing follicles (MF). MFs can in turn be further divided into primary (PMF), secondary (SMF), and tertiary (TMF) or Graafian follicles.

PFs are in close proximity to each other under the tunica albuginea. Their number and development is not dependent on hormones. PFs are spherical, with a large eccentric nucleus (50 µm) and a small nucleolus. They also have a wide and acidophilic cytoplasm, which appears finely granular under the electron microscope (EM; Fig. 2.8, #4). Inside the cytoplasm are collections of Golgi cisternae, smooth endoplasmic reticulum (SER), mitochondria, lysosomes, and reticular membraniform structures (annulate lamellae). PFs are surrounded by a layer of squamous epithelial cells, follicular cells, which in turn are surrounded by the basement membrane that separates the follicle from the rest of the cortical parenchyma and stroma (Fig. 2.8, #2, 3).

PMFs develop from PFs after gonadotropin stimulation. The PFs undergoing a maturation process show changes in both oocyte and follicular (granulosa and theca) cells. The PFs become polyhedral or cuboidal and acquire several concentric layers. The oocyte begins increasing its volume from approximately 60 to 80 µm and the zona pellucida (ZP) develops between the

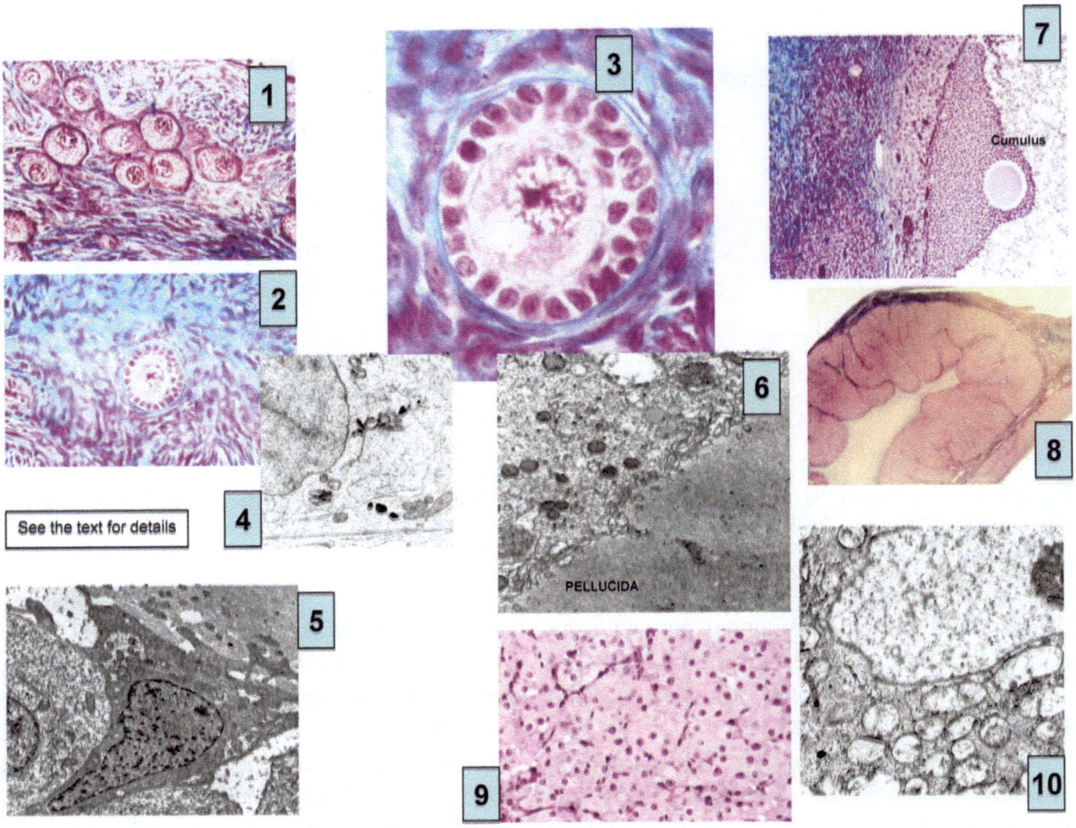

Fig. 2.8 Histology of the ovary. (Courtesy of Ricardo Vaamonde-Lemos)

oocyte and the follicular cells. The ZP is a highly refringent, homogeneous, acidophilic membrane rich in polysaccharides and three proteins (ZP 1, 2, and 3). An EM micrograph shows multiple digitiform and irregular elongations of the ovular cytoplasm (Fig. 2.8, #5, left upper side: granular ectoplasm of the oocyte; right upper side: ZP). The layer of cuboidal follicular cells is termed the granulosa layer. This stage shows increasing ribosomes, Golgi complex, mitochondria, microvesicles, lipids, liposomes, peroxisomes, and proteases. The vesicles are released during fertilization (cortical granule reaction; Fig. 2.8, #6).

During the maturation process of the ovarian follicles, the CT of the stroma, which is outside the basement membrane of the primary follicle, undergoes both morphological and functional differentiation to form two concentric layers called thecae. The inner layer is the theca interna, which is loose and vascular. Its cells have receptors for luteinizing hormone (LH) and follicle-stimulating hormone (FSH) and produce androgens as precursors of follicular estrogen. The blood vessels of the theca do not pierce the basement membrane to reach the layer of follicular cells except at the moment of ovulation and subsequent luteinization. The outer theca externa is less visible, more fibrous and dense, with dispersed smooth muscle cells, and it is gradually merged into the cortical stroma (Fig. 2.8, #7).

Follicular cells are multiplied in response to the action of FSH and insulin-like growth factor (IGF), giving rise to the SMFs. A cohort of 4–6 follicles increases their size and move toward the medulla. Gradually the vacuolated spaces (Call–Exner bodies), rich in hyaluronic acid and containing the follicular fluid, begin to appear among the follicular or granulosa cells of which there are two types: secretory and dense cells. The fluid-filled spaces increase in volume and coalesce to form the follicular antrum. The ZP of the oocyte is surrounded by follicular cells called the cumulus oophorus. Some of these cumulus oophorus cells form cylindrical spikes that have the appearance of a radiating crown around the zona called the corona radiata (Fig. 2.8, #7). Normally, as serum levels of FSH decrease, one of the follicles from the cohort will greatly upregulate its FSH receptors and outstrip the growth of the rest of the cohort and become the dominant follicle and the other follicles will become atretic. This dominant follicle will not grow to more than 10 mm (containing a 120 μm oocyte) until stimulated by LH. At the time of the LH surge, this dominant follicle will turn into the TMF or Graafian follicle and the abovementioned structures will reach their greatest development.

The LH surge will result in vasodilation and congestion of the blood vessels of the theca interna. Moreover, increasing LH will have three effects: (1) a sharp rise in antral progesterone (P_4), (2) the end of meiosis I with the appearance of the metaphase II oocyte, and (3) the rupture of the mature follicle (ovulation) with the release of the gamete ready to be fertilized. This rupture involves a hemorrhage that fills the antrum which has expelled the follicular fluid with the ovum.

Corpus Luteum

Due to the action of LH, cells from the ruptured empty follicle and the internal theca are converted into big polyhedral elements with a clear vacuolar cytoplasm called luteal cells which form the yellow body called the corpus luteum. These cells will secrete P_4 and estradiol (E_2), which increases ciliary action in the fallopian tubes (effect of E_2) to transport the zygote to the uterus, and induces and regulates the secretory phase of the endometrium (effect of P_4) in order to enable the implantation and early nutrition of the embryo. The corpus luteum ranges from 2 to 5 cm in diameter (Fig. 2.8, #8). Initially it has a center containing a blood clot which is quickly organized, fibrosed, and finally reabsorbed. It also has a wide peripheral undulating yellow band made up of "luteinized" granular cells (Fig. 2.8, #9; HE, 24x y; #10: MET 3500x). Inside these cells, there are typical mitochondria with tubular transversal crests and lipidic granules. Without implantation and pregnancy, the hormonal milieu changes, leading to decreasing LH secretion thereby causing endometrial shedding. Some subtle histological differences, not discussed in this chapter, occur, which distinguish those follicles having undergone atresia from those having undergone luteinization becoming corpora albicantia, if more than one follicle ovulates or corpus albicans (singular).

Uterine Tube

The uterine tubes or oviducts are funnel-shaped structures located on either side of the fundus of the uterus, each one reaching its ipsilateral ovary (Figs. 2.3, 2.9). They are 10 cm long and can be divided into four parts as already mentioned in the anatomy section: (1) intramural, (2) isthmus, (3) ampulla, and (4) infundibulum with fimbriae.

The entire tube has the same basic pattern from external surface to the lumen: (1) outer serous peritoneal layer with some CT; (2) muscular layer, with two divisions, (a) outer circularly oriented layer and (b) inner longitudinally oriented thinner layer; (3) mucous layer developing from a simple cylindrical epithelium with corresponding basement membrane and two types of cells. The number, appearance, and transition of these two cell types from one to the other vary depending on the cycle stage. One type of cell is ciliated, moving fluid and ovum/embryo toward the uterus and the other is secretory, producing a fluid rich in carbohydrates (uterine milk) for the early nutrition of the embryo. The fallopian mucosa is not smooth but has numerous longitudinal and transversal folds (Fig. 2.9) thereby creating a maze within the lumen of the tube (fimbriae). E_2 increases the length, number, and activity of the cilia, while P_4 increases the number and activity of the secretory cells, similar to what occurs in the endometrium. The function of the tubes is to transport, protect, and nourish the embryo during the first stages of its development. If embryo transport to the uterus does not progress, implantation might take place in the fallopian tube with an ectopic pregnancy developing. This event will lead to tubal rupture, acute abdominal pain, and emergency surgery.

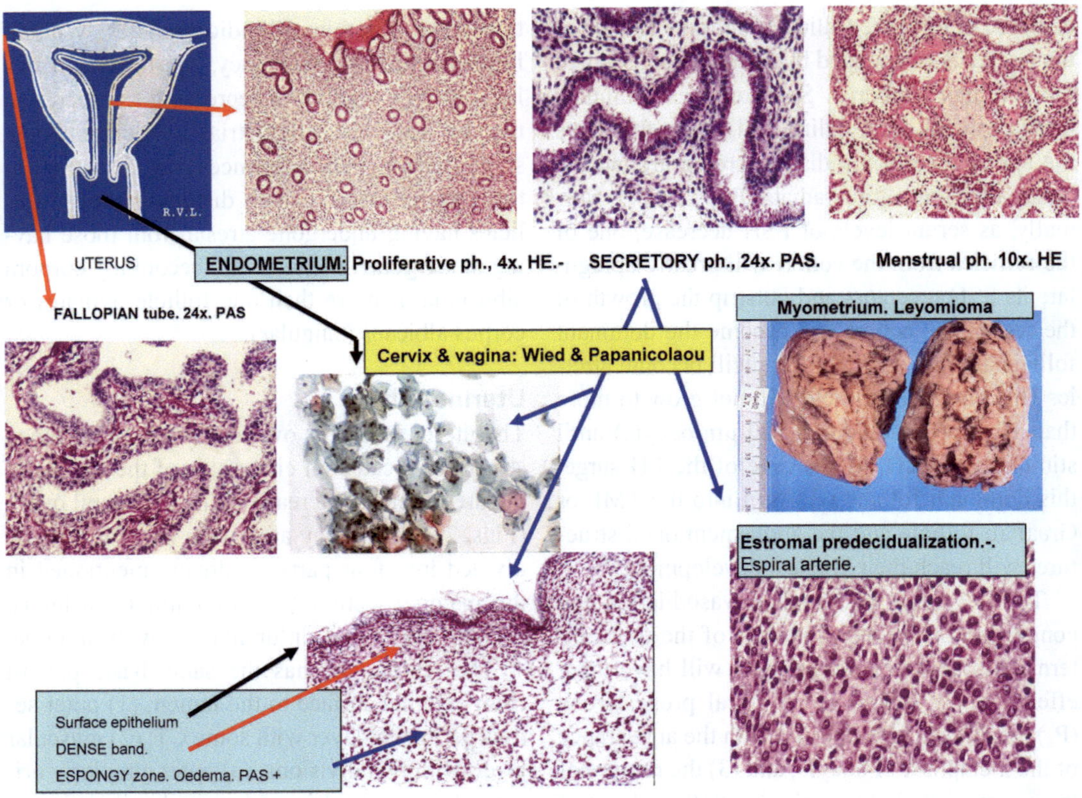

Fig. 2.9 Histology of the uterus. (Courtesy of Ricardo Vaamonde-Lemos)

Uterus

The uterus is a pear-shaped, single, central, thick muscular organ (Figs. 2.3, 2.9) that develops from the fusion of the Müllerian (paramesonephric) ducts. Divided into fornix, body, and cervix, the uterus protrudes into the vagina, as previously detailed in the anatomy section. The uterus has three histological layers: (1) the internal mucosal layer, endometrium; (2) the middle muscular layer, myometrium; and (3) the outer layer, perimetrium.

Endometrium

The endometrial mucous membrane is the most histologically complex part of the uterus. Mucous membranes are lined by a simple cylindrical secretory epithelium attached to a basal membrane lying on a chorion where the endometrial glands reside. These glands vary in size, morphology, and function depending on the stage of the menstrual cycle. Mobile cells (WBCs) are present, including the stromal granulocytes which produce relaxin. Immunohistochemical techniques show that these cells are hematolymphoid in origin and represent either a subpopulation of T lymphocytes or macrophages. Neutrophils are typically present in the normal menstrual and premenstrual endometrium. A rich vascular net displays the characteristic spiral arteries and autonomic nerves. The endometrium has a deep basal layer, *stratum basale,* adjacent to the myometrium, which is not shed during menstruation and serves for replenishing the functional layer, *stratum functionalis*. The basal layer is irrigated by straight arteries. The endometrial glands are simple, funnel shaped, and occasionally ramified, and their ducts are lined with epithelial cells that are secretory and can be cubic or cylindrical.

Myometrium

The myometrium is the thickest layer of the uterus and its contractions deliver the fetus. This is accomplished by its fibrillar bundles being longitudinally oriented both in the outer and inner muscular layer. The middle muscular layer is very vascular with arcuate arteries and the smooth muscle cells are circularly or spirally arranged. The smooth muscles of the uterus are highly dependent on E_2 stimulus and are thought to produce prostaglandins which are important, with oxytocin, in stimulating contraction at the time of delivery. The nuclei of myometrial cells are positive for E_2 and P_4 receptors (Fig. 2.10a, b).

Perimetrium

The perimetrium is a serosal layer covering the uterine body and fundus. This adventitia is continuous with the mesothelium in the area attached to the urinary bladder and rectum.

Uterine Cervix

The uterine cervix is the lower fibromuscular portion of the uterus at the point where it joins with the superior end of the vagina. A central lumen, the cervical canal, is lined by a cervical mucosa consisting of simple cylindrical mucus secreting epithelium. The lumen is invaginated, invested with ramified endocervical glands and retains some of these secretions as a defensive barrier or mucous plug. This plug is thicker during pregnancy, under the influence of P_4, and prevents pathogens from entering the uterine cavity. The plug becomes thinner during ovulation, enabling sperm to more easily enter the cervical lumen. The ectocervix, also called exocervix, is the part of the uterine cervix exposed at the superior aspect of the vagina with a speculum inserted. The ectocervix is lined with stratified squamous epithelium and subject to hormonal variations. These variations can be used for staging the female hormones in the reproductive cyclic (Papanicolaou staining test and cell cultures using the Wied or similar techniques, Fig. 2.8, #7). The characteristics of the ectocervix also allow screening for cervical cancer and detection of papillomavirus which can transform this epithelium into premalignant lesions. The area where endocervical and ectocervical epithelium join is the zone most susceptible to these pathological changes. The rest of the cervix consists of connective and smooth muscular tissue. As in the uterus, the stromal cells (both smooth muscle and myofibroblasts) are positive for E_2 and P_4 receptors which are also present in the ectocervical epithelium (Fig. 2.10c, d).

Vagina

The basic structure of the vagina is similar to other Müllerian duct-derived structures. The vagina has a muscular, funnel-shaped arrangement, which measures 10 cm in length and connects the vulva with the uterine cervix. The vaginal lumen is wide and its mucosa has folds, most of which are transverse on the anteroinferior aspect, lined by an epithelium similar to the ectocervix. The mucosa has the same kind of hormonal response as the cervix depending on the phase of the reproductive cycle. Cells in this epithelium, as in the skin, include Langerhans cells, which are antigen-presenting cells (APCs) for the numerous T lymphocytes (T cells) crossing the epithelial barrier, especially during the P_4 stage of the cycle. Estrogens stimulate the synthesis of glycogen which is subsequently converted by Döderlein's bacilli, into lactic acid, thus helping to regulate the acidic pH involved in the control of vaginal pathogens. In the chorion, there is a network of elastic and capillary fibers. The vagina has no glands; therefore, lubrication originates from the plasma transudate of the chorion blood vessels, the cervical mucus, and from the greater (Bartholin's) and lesser vestibular glands. An important fold in the most caudal portion of the vagina, which is only present in virgins, is the hymen. The muscular coat is poorly organized and differentiated in the external longitudinal and internal circular portions which, in the vaginal orifice (introitus), are combined with striated muscular fibers. The vaginal adventitia has no special features except for its rich venous network and important innervations.

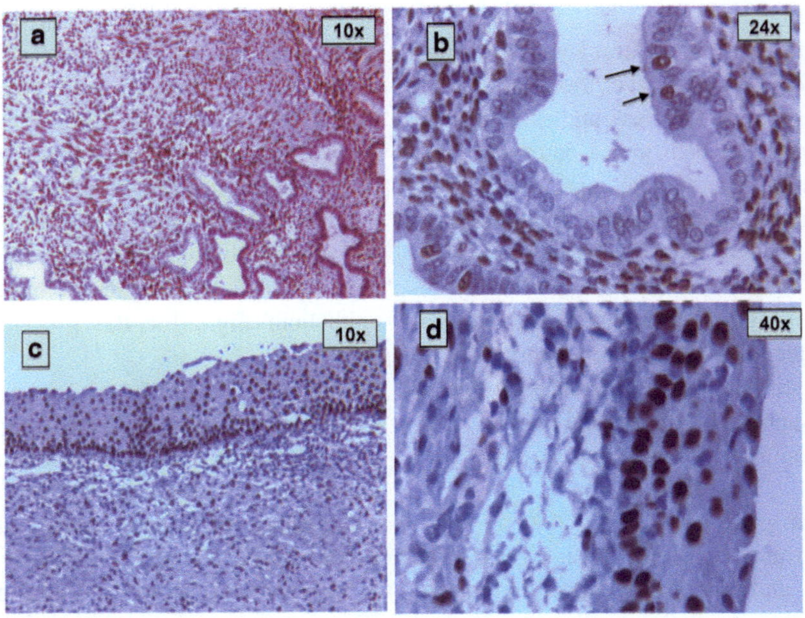

Fig. 2.10 Estrogen and progesterone receptors. **a, b** Uterus: smooth muscle. Endometrial glands—*arrows:* Nucleus (estrogen receptor) RE+. **c, d** Cervix: exocervical epithelium and cervical stroma. (Courtesy of Ricardo Vaamonde-Lemos)

Reproductive Physiology

Female Gametogenesis

Gametogenesis is the production of haploid sex cells or gametes known as oocytes and spermatozoa in humans. Each gamete carries one half of the genetic material from the male or female parent. Gametogenesis is divided into four phases: (1) extra-gonadal origin of PGCs; (2) proliferation of germ cells by mitosis; (3) meiosis; and (4) structural and functional maturation of the oocyte.

Primordial Germ Cells

Cells that are destined to become male or female germ cells can be identified during the fourth week of gestation within an extraembryonic membrane called the yolk sac. This sac contains precursor cells arising earlier in gestation during the phase of gastrulation and are known as PGCs. Most of the PGCs populate the region of the body wall at the level that will form the gonads. These precursor cells continue to multiply by mitosis during their migration and once these arrive in the presumptive gonad region, they stimulate cells of the adjacent coelomic epithelium to proliferate and form somatic support cells. Somatic support cells invest PGCs and give rise to tissues that will nourish and regulate development of maturing gametes. These support cells become the ovarian follicular cells in the female. PGCs undergo further mitotic divisions and give rise to female gametes (gametogenesis).

The PGCs differentiate into oogonia, and by the fifth month of fetal development all oogonia enter into meiosis, after which they are called primary oocytes. At this time, these primary oocytes will be housed in PF with squamous-shaped granulosa cells surrounding them. During the early phase of meiosis, all female germ cells enter a state of dormancy, and they remain in meiotic arrest (prophase of the first meiotic division) as primary oocytes until sexual maturity. Primary oocytes reach their maximum development at 20 weeks (5 months) of gestational age when 2–5 million total primary oocytes will have been created. However, at birth, this number will have been reduced by atresia to 0.5–1 million total oocytes.

At the onset of puberty, occurring at about 9–13 years of age, each month a few ovarian follicles (a cohort) resume development in response to the monthly surge of pituitary gonadotropic hormones. However, usually only one primary oocyte in the dominant follicle matures into a secondary oocyte and is ovulated in each individual ovarian cycle. This oocyte enters a second phase of meiotic arrest, metaphase II, and does not actually complete meiosis unless it is fertilized by the male gamete. These monthly cycles continue until the onset of menopause at approximately 50 years of age. The process of gametogenesis in the female is called oogenesis. On average, only one oocyte matures during each cycle, which occurs at approximately 28-day intervals. Therefore, the total number of oocytes to be ovulated in a female's lifetime is about 500.

As described previously, oogenesis already begins in early fetal life. Therefore, all oocytes to be ovulated by females are produced during fetal life. Many of them degenerate with time and at birth the ovaries contain only about 0.5–1 million total oocytes. However, two studies have challenged the belief that a finite number of oocytes are set around the time of birth in lower mammals. The renewal of ovarian follicles from germline stem cells (originating from bone marrow and peripheral blood) has recently been reported in the postnatal mouse ovary [3, 4].

Meiosis

Meiosis is the type of cell division that allows sexual reproduction since it reduces the number of chromosomes of the species to one half, making possible the combination of two gametes to form a new individual with the same number of chromosomes as each parent. Even though the timing of meiosis is distinct in the male and female, the basic chromosomal dynamics of the processes are the same in both sexes. Like all normal somatic cells, PGCs contain 23 pairs of chromosomes for a total of 46. One chromosome of each pair is obtained from the maternal gamete and the other from the paternal gamete. These chromosomes contain deoxyribonucleic acid (DNA), which encodes the molecular information required for development and functioning of the organism. Of the total complement of 46 chromosomes, 22 pairs consist of matching, homologous chromosomes called autosomes. The remaining two chromosomes are called sex chromosomes because they determine the sex of the individual and they are heterologous. The two sex chromosomes are designated X and Y. Individuals with one X chromosome and one Y chromosome (XY) are genetically male while individuals with two X chromosomes (XX) are genetically female. One of the X chromosomes in the female genome is randomly inactivated, leaving only one active X chromosome in each cell.

In females, the two meiotic cell divisions are dramatically unequal and yield a single, massive, haploid (one copy of chromosome) definitive oocyte and three minute, nonfunctional, haploid polar bodies. The first meiotic cell division produces a secondary oocyte and a first polar body in the female. DNA replication does not occur during the second meiotic division; thus, when these double-stranded chromosomes divide, they yield four haploid daughter cells (1N), one of which will be the oocyte plus three polar bodies.

In the female, the second meiotic division, like the first, is completely unequal, producing a large definitive oocyte and another tiny polar body. The first polar body may concurrently undergo a second meiotic division to produce a third polar body. In the female, the oocyte enters a second phase of meiotic arrest during the second meiotic metaphase (M-II) before replication of the centromeres. Meiosis does not resume unless spermatozoa fertilize the cell.

Functional Maturation of Oocytes

As described earlier, female germ cells undergo a series of mitotic divisions after they are invested by somatic support cells and then differentiate into oogonia. By 12 weeks of development, oogonia in the genital ridges enter the first meiotic prophase and then almost immediately become dormant. The nucleus of each of these dormant primary oocytes contains the partially condensed chromosomes and is referred to as a germinal vesicle. The swollen state of the germinal vesicle is thought to protect the oocyte's DNA during the long period, potentially decades, of meiotic arrest.

A single-layered, squamous capsule of epithelial follicular cells derived from the somatic support cells tightly encloses each primary oocyte. This capsule and its enclosed primary oocyte constitute a primordial follicle. By 5 months, the number of PF in the ovaries peaks at about 2–5 million total. The vast majority of these follicles subsequently degenerate by apoptosis, a process called atresia. During ovum maturation, there is a great increase in ribosomal RNA to handle the escalation of translation for protein synthesis required in the rapid cellular divisions that follow fertilization and thereby embryo development during the preimplantation period.

Abnormalities in meiosis may give rise to numerous chromosomal abnormalities. Nondisjunction is the usual mechanism by which abnormalities in chromosome number may occur.

Prior to a particular cycle, and independent of gonadotropin release by the pituitary, the follicular epithelium of a cohort of PF thickens, converting the single-layered follicular epithelium from squamous cells to cuboidal cells. These follicles are now called primary follicles. The follicular cells, called granulosal cells (the granulosum), and the oocyte jointly secrete a thin layer of acellular material, composed of only three glycoprotein, onto the surface of the oocyte. Although this layer, called the ZP, appears to form a complete physical barrier between the granulosum and the oocyte, it is actually penetrated by thin extensions of granulosal cells that are connected to the oolema by intercellular junctions known as gap junctions [5]. These extensions and their intercellular junctions remain intact until just before ovulation. They permit passage of amino acids, glucose, and metabolites for growth of the oocyte. The functions of the ZP include presentation of species-specific receptors to spermatozoa and induction of the acrosome reaction before fertilization. The granulosal cells secrete a Müllerian inhibiting hormone (MIH) that is responsible for the first meiotic arrest.

The granulosum of 5–12 of these primary follicles then proliferates to form a multilayered capsule of granulosal cells around the oocyte. The follicles are now called growing follicles. At this point, some of the growing follicles cease to develop and eventually become atretic, whereas in response to rising levels of FSH, a few continue to enlarge mainly by taking up fluid and developing a central fluid-filled cavity called the antrum. These follicles are called antral follicles. At the same time, the CT of the ovarian stroma surrounding each of these follicles differentiates into two layers, an inner layer called the theca interna and an outer layer called the theca externa. These two layers become vascularized, in contrast to the granulosum, which resides on its basement membrane and remains avascular, which is common to all epithelial membranes.

As E_2 synthesis increases from the growing follicles and produces a negative feedback on FSH production, FSH plasma concentration falls precipitously. One of the growing follicles now becomes dominant. This dominance is achieved by its increasing the insertion of FSH receptors into the membranes of the granulosal cells. Thus, the dominant follicle continues to enlarge by mitotic increase of granulosal cells and by producing more antral fluid. The remainder of the follicles recruited during the cycle undergo atresia since FSH is plummeting and the dominant follicle is binding all available FSH due to the increase in FSH receptors. The oocyte in the dominant follicle, surrounded by a small subset of granulosal cells called the cumulus oophorus, increasingly projects into the expanding antrum but remains connected to the layer of granulosal cells that line the antral cavity and underlie the basement membrane of the follicle. This multilayer of granulosum is called the membrana granulosa while the cumulus oophorus begins to send out radiating arms of granulosal cells that look like a crown. The large, swollen follicle is now called a mature vesicular follicle or mature Graafian follicle. The Graafian follicle is distended with protein-rich fluid and protrudes at the surface of the ovary like a blister. Rupture of the follicle occurs at ovulation, releasing the secondary oocyte through a raised area called the stigmata. At the time of ovulation, the second meiotic division is still not completed; the oocyte is still in the M-II phase. After ovulation, the secondary oocyte is surrounded by the cumulus oophorus and the corona radiata. The ability to mature, be fertilized, and finally to develop into a viable embryo is acquired gradually by the oocyte during progressive differentiation throughout folliculogenesis [6].

Menstrual Cycle

The reproductively functional time in the human female is characterized by the menstrual cycle. This cycle involves the uterine endometrium and the ovarian follicles. We will divide these two areas into ovarian and endometrial cycles. However, both occur in unison and in parallel and are highly coordinated through mutual interaction.

The Ovarian Cycle

In females, the normal reproductive years are characterized by monthly rhythmic changes in the rates of secretion of sex hormones and corresponding changes in the ovary. This rhythmic pattern observed in the ovaries is called the ovarian cycle. The ovarian cycle is most easily understood by describing it as an idealized 28-day cycle. In reality, the ovarian menstrual cycle has a range and varies from 21 to 35 days. In rare cases, some women cycle with an ovulation only once every few months or even once every few years. The ovarian cycle is driven by the dynamic changes in the concentrations of a few hormones. Gonadotropin-releasing hormone (GnRH), produced by the hypothalamus, stimulates the glandular cells of the anterior pituitary to synthesize and release LH and FSH. GnRH is released in a pulsatile manner, with peak concentrations at 60–90 min intervals. LH and FSH act on thecal and granulosa cells, inducing them to produce P_4, E_2, and some androgens. The thecal cells synthesize P_4 and androgens, whereas the granulosa cells synthesize E_2. The reason for the difference in the location of these steroid hormones is that the thecal cells lack the enzyme aromatase, which means that they cannot convert androgens to estrogens, and the granulosa cells lack the enzyme 17α-hydroxylase, which means that granulosa cells cannot convert P_4 to androgens. Also, the thecal cells only have LH receptors.

The ovarian cycle has two phases, follicular phase and luteal phase, which are separated by ovulation (Fig. 2.11).

The follicular phase is the period between the first day of menses and ovulation (usually the first 14 days of the ovarian cycle). At the beginning of the follicular phase, the developing cohort of follicles are stimulated by rising FSH to undergo rapid mitosis and start to produce steroid hormones. This rise in FSH occurs due to action potentials (APs) in the hypothalamus. A group of neurons in the hypothalamus produces microvolt APs that end on the GnRH-producing cells and is called a pulse generator. This pulsatile electrical activity stimulates the GnRH cells to synthesize and release GnRH in a pulsatile manner, which stimulates the anterior pituitary to release FSH and LH (first arrow for number 1, Fig. 2.11) Thus, the rise in FSH stimulates the granulosa cells and developing thecal cells to synthesize steroids and proteins and release increasing amounts of E_2 as seen with the second arrow from the FSH apex to the rising E_2 line (Fig. 2.11). Not shown on Fig. 2.11 is the release of the homodimer, inhibin A (also called activin), which can further increase the synthesis and release of FSH. Initially, the rising E_2 has a negative feedback effect on the pulse generator. GnRH release and consequently FSH and LH release thus begins to fall, giving rise to the atresia of all cohort follicles except for the dominant follicle (arrow 2, Fig. 2.11). As day 12 of the cycle approaches, E_2 blood serum levels reach a value of about 600 pg/mL (Fig. 2.11), and this very high E_2 level switches the negative feedback loop to a positive feedback loop on the pulse generator and thus produces a massive pulsatile surge in the FSH and LH gonadotropins from the anterior pituitary (arrow 3, Fig. 2.11). The high levels of E_2 are thought to stimulate the GnRH cells and gonadotropin cells to synthesize a second E_2 receptor protein into their cytosol that has positive feedback properties on mRNA transcription for GnRH, FSH, and LH. At about 18 h prior to ovulation, this LH surge stimulates the theca interna cells to synthesize and release large amounts of P_4 (arrow 4, Fig. 2.11). This rising P_4 initially has its major effect on the follicular cells

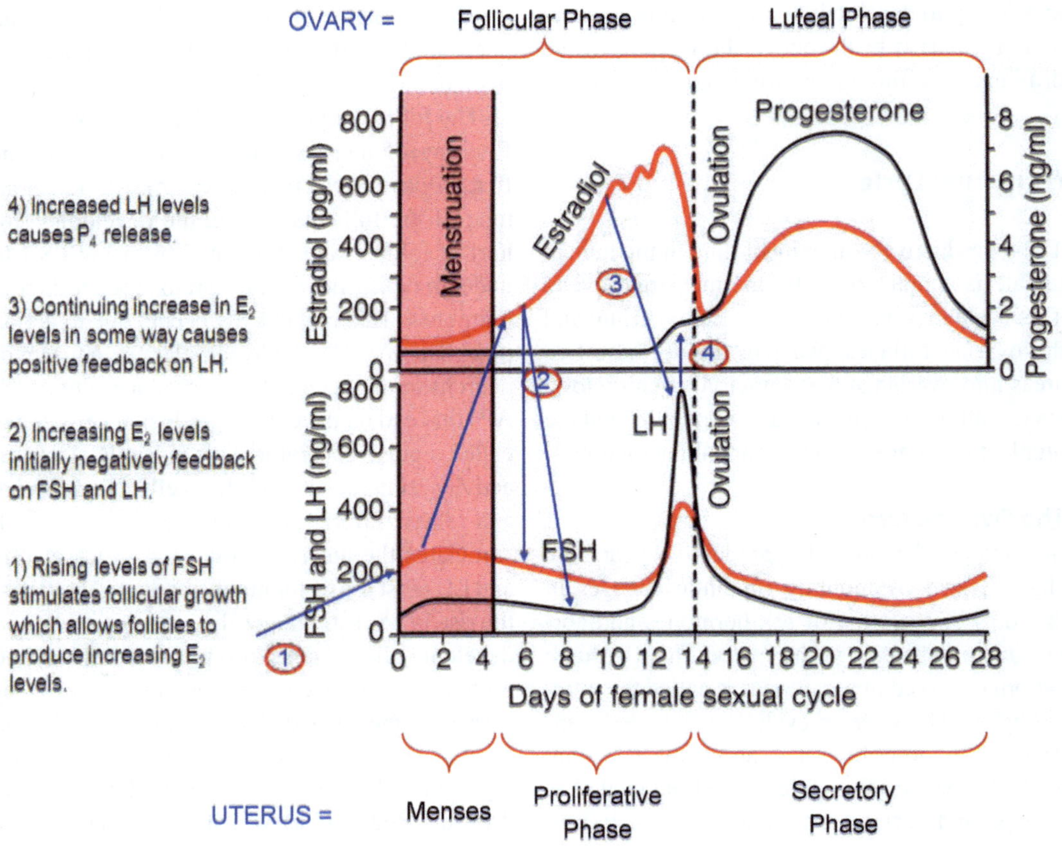

Fig. 2.11 Approximate plasma concentrations of gonadotropins and ovarian hormones during the female reproductive cycle. (Modified from [25] with permission from Elsevier)

causing the normal steroid-induced transcription of mRNA and resultant protein synthesis from both the theca interna and granulosum. Among the proteins produced are proteolytic enzymes that remove or degrade two items: (1) removal of the ovum maturation inhibiting (OMI) hormone, allowing the restart of oocyte meiosis from the germinal vesicle arrest stage to proceed to the M-II arrest stage; and (2) degrading the intracellular matrix of the follicular wall and the tunica albuginea at the ovarian surface. In addition, the level of antral proteins concomitantly increases so that there is a slight rise in colloid osmotic pressure within the follicular antrum. These three events produce a mature ovum ready to be fertilized and an expansion and rupture of the Graafian follicle allowing the release of this mature ovum (Fig. 2.7).

Ovulation marks the end of the follicular phase and the beginning of the luteal phase. The LH increase elicits luteinization, in other words, it causes the granulosa and the thecal cells in the remainder of the follicle to become a corpus luteum. During the early luteal phase, the corpus luteum synthesizes both P_4 and E_2. The P_4 and E_2 diffuse in and out of the cells throughout the body, but are retained by target cells and specifically bind to them with high affinity. Once bound to a P_4 or E_2 receptor in the cytosol, the receptor will undergo a conformational change allowing the receptor to move into the nucleus and bind with high affinity to chromatin and modulate transcription of target genes. Therefore, P_4 and E_2 by their modulation of genetic machinery of cells regulate many cellular activities through downstream production of effector molecules.

The corpus luteum is maintained by LH. Due to the high concentrations of P_4 and E_2, synthesis and release of FSH and LH are inhibited. FSH is further inhibited by inhibin B, a heterodimer with specific receptors in the anterior pituitary. During the late luteal phase, if an embryo is not produced and implanted, the low LH concentrations trigger luteolysis (luteal degeneration). This results in decreasing P_4 and E_2 levels, which in turn causes an increase in FSH and LH (Fig. 2.11), triggering a new cohort of follicles to develop for the succeeding cycle. The luteal phase lasts about 14 days and is the most consistent phase of the endometrial cycle.

Endometrial Cycle

The endometrium is crucial for embryo implantation and development and one of the most sensitive organs to ovarian steroid hormones. The composition of the functional endometrium is divided in two layers: (1) *stratum functionalis,* which is extremely responsive to steroids, and (2) the *stratum basale* (Fig. 2.12) [7].

During a normal and regular menstrual cycle, the first day of menstruation is considered day 1 of the menstrual cycle [8].

During the menstrual phase, the endometrium undergoes modifications mainly due to sex steroids (P_4 and E_2 action) [7, 9]. Both hormones act by binding to their corresponding receptors: Progesterone receptor A (PRA) (P_4 type A), Progesterone receptor B (PRB) (P_4 type B), and estrogen receptor ER (E_2) [7, 10, 11].

Estrogenic action is responsible for cellular proliferation and differentiation. E_2 causes the endometrial lining to thicken, transforming it into a proliferative pattern. Furthermore, E_2 acts in both the stroma and glands thereby causing elongation of the spiral arteries, and prepares, by an increase of P_4 receptors, the endometrial cells to be receptive to P_4 action [7, 12].

The secretory phase is defined as postovulation to onset of menstruation. After ovulation, the corpus luteum will produce and secrete a large amount of P_4 that causes the endometrium to secrete glycogen and mucus. In the mid-secretory phase (implantation window), the endometrium becomes decidualized and receptive to a fertilized embryo. This mid-secretory endometrium expresses several molecules, genes, and even some anatomical structures that are used for endometrial dating [13, 14]. In the late secretory phase, if pregnancy does not occur, there is a drop in P_4 and E_2 causing an immediate constriction of spiral arteries. Reduced blood flow leads to involution of the endometrium and, consequently, a bleeding breakdown [3, 4].

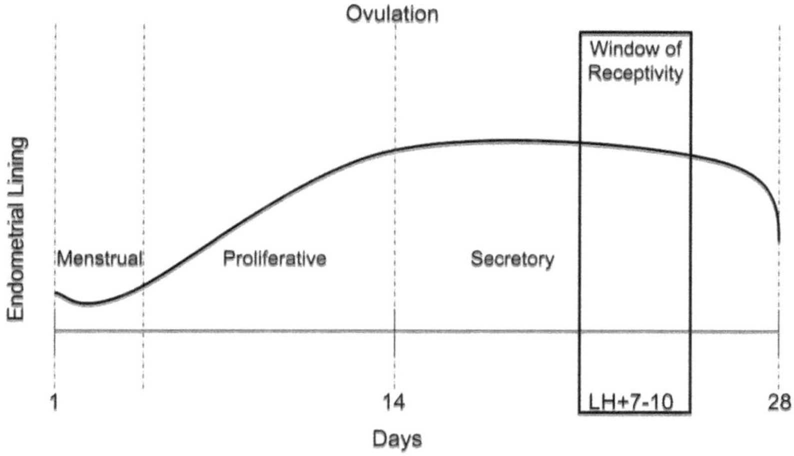

Fig. 2.12 Schematic representation of the endometrial cycle. This figure depicts the endometrium throughout the menstrual cycle. (Reprinted from [8] with permission from John Wiley & Sons)

Menopausal Transition

Menopausal transition was classified according to the Stages of Reproductive Aging Workshop (STRAW) [15].

A summary of STRAW classification table with some additional notes.

Summarizing the data gives the following picture of this period and the physiological implications of menopause during these years.

In the female's reproductive phase, the pubertal girl starts out with variable menses transitioning into regular monthly cycles. She will have normal GnRH, LH, FSH, AMH (anti-Müllerian hormone) and inhibin B levels, and between six and ten antral follicles with no vasomotor symptoms or urogenital atrophy. In the late period of the reproductive phase, the woman will begin to see subtle changes in the amount and length of the menstrual flow accompanied by lower hormone levels and there will be fewer antral follicles developing each month. No vasomotor symptoms or urogenital atrophy should be apparent during the late reproductive phase and pregnancy can occur with increased chances of birth defects that increase over time. This normally takes place between the age of 35 and 45 years but can be quite variable.

As a woman transitions into menopause, generally called perimenopause, the length of time between the first day of menses will be extended by at least 1 week (35-day cycles) and continue to increase over time to more than 60 days between cycles. Although less likely, some cycles can still produce ova and pregnancy can occur. This change will be accompanied by increasing levels of GnRH, LH and FSH, and continuing lower levels of AMH and inhibin B. In addition, vasomotor symptoms, sometimes called hot flashes, are likely to be experienced and are thought to be in response to spiking levels of P_4. The time for this transition can vary from less than a year up to about 3 years.

Finally, the woman will transition into the postmenopausal phase which will generally stabilize out to a constant state within 3–6 years. This time will be characterized by the highest GnRH and its responding gonadotropins (due to the nadir in negative feedback from steroids and inhibin) along with very low AMH and inhibin B. Vasomotor symptoms will peak early during this time and then eventually cease while increasing symptoms of urogenital atrophy reach their maximum for the remainder of the woman's life span.

Several cohort studies with a large number of subjects have been published so that comprehension and description of menopausal transition can be summarized as follows: (1) all stages have a vast variability in terms of duration and age of onset; (2) the decline of ovarian reserve starts 15 years before the complete cessation of menses (menopause) and is more pronounced after the age of 35; (3) clinically, one of the most important symptoms is the shortened follicular phase (and, consequently, the menstrual cycle length); and (4) the length of menopause is dependent on demographic characteristics of ethnicity, race, smoking, genetic background (family medical history), fat composition, and body mass index [15–21].

Menopausal transition starts physiologically when the inter-cycle FSH secretion increases and luteal P_4 decreases [22]. These events will decrease the follicular phase of the menstrual cycle. Consequently, older patients present with a shorter menstrual cycle interval [23, 24]. This observation occurs several years prior to the complete establishment of the post-climacteric stage (defined 12 months after the last menstrual period). Furthermore, anti-Müllerian hormone is a good marker of ovarian reserve but not an accurate marker for ovarian menopausal transition as a predictive test for the start-day of menopause.

Several investigators have defined some important demographic and social characteristics to better understand and predict pre- and post-climacteric events. Smoking habits are directly related to menopausal transition [20], while body mass index is associated only with hormonal markers (anti-Müllerian hormone and the number of antral follicles). Alcohol consumption as well as menarche age was also linked to menopausal transition [20].

Conclusion

The anatomical development of the female reproductive system involves a large and diverse number of structures. The primary gland begins as the undifferentiated gonad that develops into the ovary in the female and testis in the male. Except for the external genetalia, the remainder of the female reproductive system develops from a completely different set of tissues than the male structures. The orchestration of this interacting network of far-flung configurations that reside in brain, abdomen, pelvis, and perineum requires hundreds of specific enzymatic proteins to direct the construction and function of the system and requires thousands of specific structural proteins as the actual building blocks for the system. The complexity for the male is just as intricate as for the female. In this chapter, we have not even addressed the more difficult question of how these two very different male and female sexual systems developed in a synchronous way for the first male and first female of some reproductively competent species to actually mate for the first time and have all the parts fit together and function properly to produce a viable offspring. That topic will have to wait for another treatise.

The number of tissues, cell types, and molecules needed for the system to function properly are also multilayered and range from skeletal to smooth muscle, simple to pseudostratified to stratified epithelium, neurons and neuroendocrine cells, many types of CT cells and molecules, hormones, neurotransmitters, and the list could go on and on. The photographs as well as light and transmission electron micrographs of these different structures are fascinating and give an artistic perspective to the whole system at every level. The microscopic details that have been left to other publications will excite the interests of all interested in delving further into this amazing subject.

As described in the physiology section, the normal function of the cycling female reproductive system is even more remarkably complicated than the gross and microscopic structure of the organs and tissues involved. This complexity begins at the zygote stage where very specific genes must be turned on to start differentiation in the preimplantation embryo while at the same time the majority of mRNAs directing later stages of embryo, fetal, neonatal, toddler, pubertal, and adult development must be turned off. As the female develops in utero, the DNA-derived mRNA/protein units that were needed initially have to be inactivated with histones while inactivated genes have to become activated. This change would involve hundreds to even thousands of activating/inactivating steps every week for the embryo and fetus. In addition, the development must include the instructions for which cell type and what molecular synthesis is to go to the various endpoints in the body. The functional picture outlined in this brief overview barely scratches the surface of all the steps necessary for the female side of the reproductive unit (male and female together) to work normally to produce a viable *ex utero* person. One might be moved to ask how humans succeed in reproducing themselves at all. We have presented a concise summary of the anatomy and physiology of the normal female reproductive organization that should stimulate you to dig further into this topic and also give you an appreciation for the beautifully complex design of this very important system.

References

1. De Felici M. Origin, migration and proliferation of human primordial germ cells. In: Coticchio G, Albertini DF, De Santis L, editors. Oogenesis. London: Springer-Verlag; 2012.
2. Gillman J. The development of the gonads in man, with a consideration of the role of fetal endocrines and the histogenesis of ovarian tumors. Contrib Embryol Carnegie Inst. 1948;32:81–131.
3. Johnson J, Bagley J, Skaznik-Wikiel M, et al. Oocyte generation in adult mammalian ovaries by putative germ cells in bone marrow and peripheral blood. Cell. 2005;122(2):303–15. doi:10.1016/j.cell.2005.06.031. PMID 16051153.
4. Johnson J, Canning J, Kaneko T, Pru J, Tilly J. Germline stem cells and follicular renewal in the postnatal mammalian ovary. Nature. 2004;428(6979):145–50. doi:10.1038/nature02316. PMID 15014492.
5. Albertini D, Bromfield J. Soma–germline interactions in the ovary: an evolutionary perspective. In: Verlhac M-H, Villeneuve A, editors. Oogenesis: the universal process. Chichester: Wiley-Blackwell; 2010.

6. Guraya SS, editor. Cellular and molecular biology of human oogenesis, ovulation and early embryogenesis: fundamentals, biomedical and clinical implications in relation to infant disorders. New Delhi: New Age International Publishers; 2008.
7. Speroff LF, Fritz MA, editor. Clinical gynecologic endocrinology and infertility. Philadelphia: Lippincott Williams & Wilkins; 2005.
8. Hawkins SM, Matzuk MM. The menstrual cycle: basic biology. Ann N Y Acad Sci. 2008;1135:10–8.
9. Achache H, Revel A. Endometrial receptivity markers, the journey to successful embryo implantation. Hum Reprod Update. 2006;12(6):731–46.
10. de Ziegler D. Hormonal control of endometrial receptivity. Hum Reprod. 1995;10(1):4–7.
11. Beier HM, Beier-Hellwig K. Molecular and cellular aspects of endometrial receptivity. Hum Reprod Update. 1998;4(5):448–58.
12. Lessey BA. Endometrial receptivity and the window of implantation. Baillieres Best Pract Res Clin Obstet Gynaecol. 2000;14(5):775–88.
13. Lessey BA. Assessment of endometrial receptivity. Fertil Steril. 2011;96(3):522–9.
14. Revel A. Defective endometrial receptivity. Fertil Steril. 2012;97(5):1028–32.
15. Soules MR, et al. Executive summary: Stages of Reproductive Aging Workshop (STRAW). Climacteric. 2001;4(4):267–72.
16. Guthrie JR, et al. The menopausal transition: a 9-year prospective population-based study. The Melbourne Women's Midlife Health Project. Climacteric. 2004;7(4):375–89.
17. Burger HG, et al. The endocrinology of the menopausal transition: a cross-sectional study of a population-based sample. J Clin Endocrinol Metab. 1995;80(12):3537–45.
18. Burger HG, et al. A prospective longitudinal study of serum testosterone, dehydroepiandrosterone sulfate, and sex hormone-binding globulin levels through the menopause transition. J Clin Endocrinol Metab. 2000;85(8):2832–8.
19. Sowers MR, et al. Anti-Mullerian hormone and inhibin B in the definition of ovarian aging and the menopause transition. J Clin Endocrinol Metab. 2008;93(9):3478–83.
20. Sammel MD, et al. Factors that influence entry into stages of the menopausal transition. Menopause. 2009;16(6):1218–27.
21. Woods NF, et al. Is the menopausal transition stressful? Observations of perceived stress from the Seattle Midlife Women's Health Study. Menopause. 2009;16(1):90–7.
22. Sherman BM, West JH, Korenman SG. The menopausal transition: analysis of LH, FSH, estradiol, and progesterone concentrations during menstrual cycles of older women. J Clin Endocrinol Metab. 1976;42(4):629–36.
23. Klein NA, et al. Reproductive aging: accelerated ovarian follicular development associated with a monotropic follicle-stimulating hormone rise in normal older women. J Clin Endocrinol Metab. 1996;81(3):1038–45.
24. Klein NA, et al. Decreased inhibin B secretion is associated with the monotropic FSH rise in older, ovulatory women: a study of serum and follicular fluid levels of dimeric inhibin A and B in spontaneous menstrual cycles. J Clin Endocrinol Metab. 1996;81(7):2742–5.
25. Hall JE. Female physiology before pregnancy and female hormones. In: Hall JE, editor. Guyton and Hall textbook of medical physiology. 12th edn. Philadelphia: Saunders; 2011. p. 987–1000

Suggested Reading

26. Almog B, et al. Age-related normograms of serum antimüllerian hormone levels in a population of infertile women: a multicenter study. Fertil Steril. 2011;95(7):2359–63, 2363 e1.
27. Bouchet A, Cuilleret J. Anatomie topographique, descriptive et fonctionnelle. 2e edn. Villeurbanne cedex: Simep; 1982.
28. Burger H. The menopausal transition—endocrinology. J Sex Med. 2008;5(10):2266–73.
29. Chevrel JP, editor. Anatomie clinique. 1e edn. Hong Kong: Springer-Verlag France; 1994.
30. Cunha-Filho JS, et al. Physiopathological aspects of corpus luteum defect in infertile patients with mild/minimal endometriosis. J Assist Reprod Genet. 2003;20(3):117–21.
31. de Ziegler D, et al. The hormonal control of endometrial receptivity: estrogen (E2) and progesterone. J Reprod Immunol. 1998;39(1–2):149–66.
32. Drake RL, Vogl AW, Mitchell AWM. Gray, Anatomía para estudiantes. 2a edn. Barcelona: Elsevier-España; 2010.
33. Dauber W. Feneis. Nomenclatura Anatómica Ilustrada. 5a edn. Barcelona: Masson; 2006.
34. Federative Committee of Anatomical Terminology (FCAT), Sociedad Anatómica Española. Terminología Anatómica. 1a edn. Madrid: Editorial Médica Panamericana; 2001.
35. Gartner LP. Color textbook of histology. Philadelphia: W. B. Saunders Company; 1997.
36. Kamina P. Anatomie Gynecologique. 4e edn. Paris: Maloine Editeurs; 1984.
37. Moore KL, Dalley AF. Anatomía con orientación clínica. 5a edn. Madrid: Editorial Médica Panamericana; 2007.
38. Netter FH. Atlas de Anatomía Humana. 4a edn. Barcelona: Elsevier-Masson; 2007.
39. Orts-Llorca F. Anatomía Humana. 4a edn. Barcelona: Editorial Científico-Médica; 1972.
40. Paulsen F, Waschke J. Sobotta. Atlas de Anatomía Humana. 23a edn. Barcelona: Elsevier-España; 2012.
41. Pinkerton JH, et al. Development of the human ovary. A study using histochemical technics. Obstet Gynec. 1961;18:152–81.

42. Platzer W. Atlas de Anatomía con correlación clínica. 9a edn. Madrid: Editorial Médica Panamericana; 2008.
43. Rohen JW, Lütjen-Drecoll E, Yokochi EC. Atlas de Anatomía Humana. Estudio fotográfico del cuerpo humano. 6a edn. Barcelona: Elsevier; 2007.
44. Ross M, Romrell L, Kaye G. Histologia. 3a edn. Interamericana; 1998.
45. Schünke M, Schulte E, Schumacher U. Prometheus. Texto y atlas de Anatomía. 2a edn. Madrid: Editorial Médica Panamericana; 2010.
46. Sternberg SS. Histology for pathologists. Raven Press; 1992.
47. Testut J, Latarjet A. Anatomía Humana. 9a edn. Barcelona: Salvat Editores; 1982.
48. Williams PL. Anatomía de Gray. 38a edn. Madrid: Harcourt-Brace de España; 1998.

Overview of Fertilization, Gestation, and Parturition

3

Sergio Oehninger, R. James Swanson and Roberto Matorras

Introduction

An overview of fertilization, gestation, and parturition at the most basic level involves spermatozoa, ova, and a uterus. While many other anatomical areas of the body could be considered, we will concentrate on (1) fertilization, with emphasis on the sperm and its interaction with the egg's membrane (the zona pellucida, ZP) and cytoplasm; (2) oocytes and the preparatory steps to ovulation and fertilization; and (3) gestation of the embryo and fetus, and eventually, parturition of the neonate.

Overview of Fertilization: The Male and Female Gametes

The human spermatozoon contributes, at least, three components during fertilization: (1) the paternal haploid genome, (2) the signal to initiate metabolic activation of the oocyte, and (3) the centriole, which directs microtubule assembly leading to the formation of the mitotic spindles during the initial zygote development. Clinical evidence derived from the use of assisted reproductive technologies points to the fact that defective sperm contributions may extend beyond fertilization, highlighting the fact that early and late paternal effects may be determinants of abnormal development.

R. J. Swanson (✉)
Department of Biological Sciences, Old Dominion University, Norfolk, VA, USA
e-mail: rjswanson@liberty.edu

S. Oehninger
Department of Obstetrics and Gynecology, The Jones Institute for Reproductive Medicine/EVMS, Norfolk, VA, USA

R. Matorras
Department of Obstetrics and Gynecology, Human Reproductive Unit, Cruces Hospital, Basque Country University, IVI Bilbao, Baracaldo, Vizcaya, Spain

Sperm–Oocyte Interaction

In order to fertilize the egg, ejaculated spermatozoa must undergo capacitation, recognize and bind to the ZP, and undergo the acrosome reaction (AR) [1]. The most significant changes experienced by sperm during capacitation are plasma membrane changes, increase in certain intracellular messengers, and increased phosphorylation of a set of proteins by different kinases [2–4]. In the murine species, a well-characterized model of gamete interaction, tight gametes binding is probably achieved through interaction of the zona pellucida protein 3 (ZP3) and yet unidentified complementary sperm-binding protein(s) present in the plasma membrane. ZP3 triggers the AR followed by a secondary binding process involving the zona pellucida protein 2 (ZP2) and the inner acrosomal sperm membrane leading to zona penetration. Glycosylation appears mandatory for murine ZP3-ligand function. It has been demonstrated that O-glycosylation, and particu-

© Springer Science+Business Media New York 2016
D. Vaamonde et al. (eds.), *Exercise and Human Reproduction,* DOI 10.1007/978-1-4939-3402-7_3

larly terminal galactose residues of O-linked oligosaccharides, are essential for maintaining mouse gamete interaction. Others have provided evidence that the amino sugar N-acetylglucosamine (NAG) is the key terminal monosaccharide involved in sperm–zona interaction in the mouse. In contrast, AR-triggering activity of ZP3 seems to depend upon the integrity of the protein backbone [5–7].

For the past two decades, investigators have sought to identify an individual protein or carbohydrate side chain as the "sperm receptor." In earlier work performed in nonhuman models, diverse candidates were postulated as primary sperm receptors for ZP3: (i) a 95 kDa tyrosine-kinase [8], (ii) sp56 [9], (iii) trypsin-like protein [10], (iv) β1–4 galactosyltransferase [11], and (v) spermadhesins [12]. However, none of these molecules have been unequivocally established as an active receptor and physiological relevance of these candidates is still debated.

In more recent experiments performed in knockout mice with absence of either ZP2 or ZP3 expression, in the event that the ZP failed to assemble around growing oocytes, and females were infertile; on the other hand in the absence of ZP1 expression, a disorganized zona assembled around growing oocytes and females exhibited reduced fertility. These and other observations led to speculating a model for ZP structure in which ZP2 and ZP3 form long Z-filaments cross-linked by ZP1 [13].

The identity of the sperm-binding proteins remains a subject of active investigation and the most recent data indicate that many different proteins are likely involved. There has been recent progress in functionally characterizing other promising candidate proteins that interact with ZP3, including among others zonadhesin and polycystic kidney disease and receptor for egg jelly-related protein (PKDREJ) [14–17].

Previous reports suggested that murine ZP2 mediates secondary binding of spermatozoa and that cleavage of ZP2 by proteases released through cortical granule reaction causes zona "hardening" and thus prevents polyspermy. Using an elegant approach, an observed post-fertilization persistence of mouse sperm binding to "humanized" ZP was shown to correlate with uncleaved ZP2. These observations are consistent with a model for sperm binding in which the supramolecular structure of the ZP necessary for sperm binding is modulated by the cleavage status of ZP2 [18–21]. To test the alternative hypothesis that the protein sequence of murine ZP3 (mZP3) glycoproteins mediates sperm–egg binding, transgenic mice were created in which mZP3 was replaced with human ZP3 (huZP3). If initial gamete binding were protein mediated, such mice would bind human sperm. However, murine but not human sperm were found to bind to mouse eggs expressing huZP3 [18].

During fertilization, the acrosome-reacted spermatozoa fuse with the oolemma and the whole spermatozoon (with the exception of part of the sperm membrane, most of the outer acrosomal membrane and the acrosomal components) is incorporated into the oocyte [22]. The ZP binds to at least two different receptors in the sperm head plasma membrane. One is a G_i-coupled receptor that can activate phospholipase Cβ1 and regulates adenylyl cyclase to increase cyclic-AMP (cAMP) levels. The cAMP activates protein kinase A (PKA) to open a calcium channel in the outer acrosomal membrane, resulting in a relatively small rise in cytosolic Ca^{2+}. Calcium activates phospholipase Cγ, which is coupled to the second tyrosine kinase receptor. The products of phospholipase C (PLC) activity, diacylglycerol and inositol-3-phosphate (IP3), lead to activation of protein kinase C (PKC) and IP3 receptor, PKC opens a calcium channel in the membrane and IP3 activates the calcium channel in the outer acrosomal membrane leading to a higher increase in cytosol calcium, which results in membrane fusion and completion of the AR [23–25]. Results of recent studies indicate that components that are essential for intracellular membrane fusion in somatic cells, such as Rab3A, GTPase, and SNAREs, may be present in mammalian sperm and may also participate in membrane fusion during the AR [26].

Compelling evidence has now demonstrated that carbohydrate-binding proteins on the sperm surface mediate gamete recognition by binding with high affinity and specificity to complex glycoconjugates of the ZP [27–32]. A group of investigators has recently reported a series of studies that suggest that (i) the binding protein(s) on human spermatozoa recognize selectin ligands or molecules alike on the ZP to ensure recognition and attachment; and (ii) the human ZP expresses glycans structurally (and probably functionally) linked to natural killer (NK) cell inhibition [30, 32–36]. A new molecular model for human sperm–egg interaction has been proposed based on these observations [32, 35, 37–41].

In the human, native solubilized ZP triggers the AR. Cross et al. [42] were the first to report that treatment of human sperm in suspension with acid-disaggregated huZP (2–4 ZP/μl) increased the incidence of acrosome-reacted sperm. Lee [43] demonstrated that pertussis toxin treatment of human sperm inhibits the (solubilized) ZP-induced AR. In contrast, acrosomal exocytosis induced by the calcium ionophore A-23187 is not inhibited by pertussis toxin pretreatment. Studies by Franken et al. [44] showed a dose-dependent effect of solubilized human ZP on the AR in the range of 0.25–1 ZP/μl and also confirmed the involvement of G_i protein during ZP-induced AR of human sperm. Schuffner and colleagues [45] reported that: (i) acrosomal exocytosis of capacitated human sperm triggered by the homologous ZP is dependent on the activation of G_i proteins (pertussis toxin sensitive) and the presence of extracellular calcium; and (ii) progesterone and follicular fluid exert a priming effect on the ZP-induced AR. Recent studies have revealed that human ZP is made of four glycoproteins designated as human ZP1, ZP2, ZP3, and ZP4 [46, 47].

Sperm–Oocyte Fusion

Sperm–oocyte fusion is a cell–cell membrane fusion event. The inner and outer acrosomal membranes and the plasma membrane of the equatorial region remain intact after the completion of the AR and zona penetration [48, 49]. Acrosome-reacted sperm bind to and fuse with the egg plasma membrane at the postacrosomal region of the sperm; this region is capable of fusion only after acrosomal exocytosis has taken place [28]. Several candidate binding molecules have been reported.

Binding of sperm to the egg plasma membrane appears to be mediated by members of the cysteine-rich secretory protein family (CRISP1 and CRISP2), and a member of the A Disintegrin And Metalloproteinase (ADAM) family of transmembrane proteins on sperm, and the integrin alpha$_{vi}$ß$_1$ receptor on eggs [50]. Sperm binding to an egg integrin (ß1) is a prerequisite adhesion step for sperm–egg membrane fusion in mammalian fertilization [51]. The oocyte integrin is required for membrane fusion and its activity appears to be related to a sperm surface protein fertilin (termed PH-30) that was implicated in gamete fusion based on antibody inhibition studies. Although some ADAM proteins act to block or to promote protease activity, fertilin has no such roles [52].

P-selectin is expressed on the oolemma of human and hamster oocytes following sperm adhesion and is also detected on the equatorial region of acrosome-reacted human spermatozoa, suggesting that this selectin might be involved in gamete interaction [53]. In addition, epididymal protein DE or CRISP1 and testicular protein Tpx-1 also known as CRISP2, are cysteine-rich secretory proteins also apparently involved in gamete fusion through interaction with egg-binding sites [54]. Other candidates have been proposed, including equatorin and CD9 [55–57]. Inoue et al. [58] identified a mouse sperm fusion related antigen and showed that the antigen belongs to a novel immunoglobulin superfamily protein. The authors termed the gene Izumo and produced a gene-disrupted mouse line. Izumo2/2 mice were healthy but males were sterile. They produced normal-looking sperm that bound to and penetrated the ZP but were incapable of fusing with eggs. Human sperm also contain Izumo and addition of the antibody against human Izumo left the sperm unable to fuse with zona-free hamster eggs. However, glycosylation appears not to be essential for the function of Izumo [59]. The specific roles of all these molecules need to be further validated [60].

Oocyte Activation

The signaling mechanism utilized by the spermatozoa to initiate and perpetuate oocyte responses is unclear, and three theories have been proposed: (a) the fusion theory that suggests the presence of active calcium releasing components in the sperm head [61, 62]; (b) the receptor theory that proposes a receptor-mediated signal transduction localized on the oocyte plasma membrane [63]; and (c) the "calcium bomb" theory that proposes that upon fertilization Ca^{2+} enters the egg either from stores in the sperm itself or through channels in the sperm's plasma membrane [64].

A cytosolic sperm factor containing a protein called "oscillin," which is related to a prokaryote glucosamine phosphate deaminase and is located in the equatorial segment, appeared to be responsible for causing the calcium oscillations that trigger egg activation at fertilization in mammals [65]. However, experimental evidence has now shown that oscillin is not responsible for the mammalian sperm calcium oscillations [66].

Present evidence supports the concept that an IP3 receptor system is the main mediator of calcium oscillations in oocytes [67]. The soluble sperm factor that triggers calcium oscillations and egg activation in mammals is a novel form of PLC referred to as PLC zeta [67]. This triggering was demonstrated by injection into eggs of both c-RNA encoding for PLC zeta and recombinant PLC zeta [67, 68]. According to a present hypothesis, after fusion of the sperm and egg plasma membrane the sperm-derived PLC zeta protein diffuses into the egg cytoplasm giving as a result the hydrolysis of phosphatidylinositol 4, 5-bisphosphate (PIP2) from an unknown source to generate IP3 (inositol 1,4,5-trisphosphate) [69, 70].

The earliest visible indications of the transition of mammalian eggs, or egg activation, are cortical granule extrusion (CGE) by exocytosis and resumption of meiosis. Although these events are triggered by calcium oscillations the pathways leading to the intracellular calcium release are not completely understood. The Ca^{2+} transients stimulate the resumption of the cell cycle by decreasing the activity of both a M-phase promoting factor (MPF) and a cytostatic factor [71] and either the Ca^{2+} transients and/or PKC lead to CGE [72]. Therefore, the calcium transients and/or activation of PLC zeta lead to CGE by yet an undefined mechanism. Src family kinases (SFK) have been recently suggested as possible inducers of some aspects of egg activation, though a role for SFK upstream of calcium release remains plausible [73].

Recently, two sperm-borne proteins that induce formation of pronuclei in eggs have been described: (a) the truncated c-Kit tyrosine kinase (tr-kit), that activates the dormant egg by eliciting intracellular Ca^{2+} oscillations, which serve as a secondary messenger for downstream effectors of zygotic development [74, 75], and (b) the protein postacrosomal sheath WW domain binding protein (PAWP). PAWP exclusively resides in the postacrosomal sheath (PAS) of the sperm perinuclear theca (PT). Microinjection of recombinant PAWP or alkaline PT extract into metaphase II-arrested porcine, bovine, macaque, and *Xenopus* oocytes induced a high rate of pronuclear formation, which was prevented by co-injection of a competitive peptide derived from PAWP but not by co-injection of the point-mutated peptide. Intracytoplasmic sperm injection (ICSI) of porcine oocytes combined with co-injection of the competitive peptide or an anti-recombinant PAWP antiserum prevented pronuclear formation and arrested fertilization [76].

Pronuclear Interaction and Nuclear Fusion

In primates, the male pronucleus is tightly associated with the centrosome, which nucleates microtubules to form the sperm aster whose growth drives the centrosome and associated male pronucleus from the cell cortex towards the center of the oocyte. Structural abnormalities or incomplete junctioning of the centrosome have been identified as a novel form of infertility [77]. In contrast, the female pronucleus has neither associated centrosome nor microtubule nucleating activity. Nevertheless, the female pronucleus moves along microtubules from the cell cortex towards the centrosome located in the center of the sperm aster. The current model for the movement of the female pronucleus involves its translocation along the microtubule lattice using the minus-end directed motor dynein in a manner analogous to organelle motility [78–80].

Mammalian fertilization requires dynein and dynactin to mediate genomic union; dynein concentrates exclusively around the female pronucleus, whereas dynactin localizes around the pronuclei and associates with nucleoporins and vimentin, in addition to dynein [81, 82]. The findings that a sperm aster is required for dynein to localize to the female pronucleus and that the microtubules are necessary to retain dynein, but not dynactin, at theirs surface, suggest that nucleoporins, vimentin, and dynactin might associate upon pronuclear formation, and that subsequent sperm aster contact with the female pronuclear surface allows dynein to interact with these proteins [80–82].

Delivery of Sperm mRNA Transcripts into the Egg

New evidence has challenged the traditional view of the transcriptional dormancy of terminally differentiated spermatozoa. Several reports indicated the presence of mRNAs in ejaculated human spermatozoa [83, 84]. Hypothetically, these templates could be critically involved in late spermiogenesis, including a function to equilibrate imbalances in spermatozoal phenotypes brought about by meiotic recombination and segregation, but also they could be involved in early postfertilization events such as establishing imprints during the transition from maternal to embryonic genes. Others have instead proposed that mature spermatozoa are a repository of information regarding meiotic and postmeiotic gene expression in the human and are likely to contain transcripts for genes playing an essential role during spermiogenesis. The use of the whole ejaculate as a wholly noninvasive biopsy of the spermatid should therefore be evaluated [85]. The mRNAs accumulated in the sperm nucleus are possibly not residual nonfunctional materials but might be viewed as the male gametes contribution to early embryogenesis [86]. Thus, human spermatozoa could act not only as genome carriers but also as providers of specific transcripts necessary for zygote viability and development before activation of the embryonic genome [87].

Overview of Ovulation: The Female Gamete

Steps to Ovulation of a Mature Ovum

For a fertilizable ovum to be released from the ovarian follicle, several events must be completed in a carefully orchestrated sequence involving the ovum and the follicle: (1) The ovum must be stimulated to progress from the dictyate stage of the germinal vesicle and undergo the first meiotic division. This ovum, uninterrupted, will enter into the second meiotic division and arrest at the mature metaphase stage of meiosis two (MII-stage ovum). The MII ovum will remain at this stage until ovulated and fertilized. Immediately upon sperm–egg fusion, the ovum being fertilized will undergo the cortical reaction, sometimes referred to as the zona reaction, and will complete the second meiotic division, as outlined in the preceding section. (2) The follicular wall must thin and weaken in order for the stigma to form and rupture, allowing the ovum to be released. At the same time, the follicular volume must increase to gently pressure the thinning follicular wall to rupture for ovulation. This process is outlined in Hall [88] on the basis of unpublished research done in Dr. Harry Lipner's laboratory at Florida State University by one of the authors, Swanson.

FSH, LH, and Estradiol-17β

The well-known hormonal control of ovulation begins with the secretion of follicle stimulating hormone (FSH). As its name implies, this hormone stimulates a crop of primordial or primary follicles to begin developing. The follicular antral fluid contains proteins and proteoglycans, steroids, ions, and a liquid that is an ultrafiltrate of the capillaries outside the basement membrane which surrounds the granulosa cells (GC), ovum, and antrum. No blood vessels or neurons pass through the basement membrane into the granulosa layer, which is an epithelium. These cells must be fed by diffusion. The antral contents include (1) products of the GCs and (2) other substances which diffuse through both the basement membrane and the GCs. As a cohort of several follicles responds and begins to grow through the secondary, tertiary, and eventually mature or Graafian stages, one follicle will begin to insert more FSH receptors into the GC plasma membranes. This more aggressive follicle normally outstrips the other members of the cohort, becomes the dominant follicle, and results in the release of only one egg per menstrual cycle. The remaining cohort of follicles become atretic and form a microscopic scar called a cicatrix. Rarely in the natural cycle, multiple follicles, growing at the same rate simultaneously, result in multiple dominant follicles and produce multiple embryos and multiple births. With in vitro fertilization (IVF), multiple dominant follicles are induced via hormonal treatment (called superovulation), so that a large number of eggs can be collected for the assisted reproductive technology (ART). The ability to drive the system by ART superovulation, with its copious egg production, illustrates that the dominant follicle number is closely regulated by the woman's endogenous hormones in the natural (non-superovulated) menstrual cycle and results in only one egg normally being released. The one follicle outstripping the others to become the dominant follicle in a normal menstrual cycle contains the GCs that produce steroids. The main steroid at this stage (follicular phase) is estradiol-17β (E_2). Because E_2 has a negative feedback on the production of FSH and luteinizing hormone (LH), the level of the driving hormone for follicular development, FSH, decreases as the follicles grow and produce an ever increasing amount of E_2. Only the follicle that rapidly responds to the decreasing FSH levels by producing and inserting many FSH receptors on the GC membranes survives and continues to grow. This upregulation of receptors keeps the FSH level within those GCs at a sufficient level to maintain continued growth and division while the remaining cohort follicles become atretic.

As the dominant follicle continues to grow, E_2 blood levels continue to increase. At some point the E_2 reaches a value (approaching 1 nanomol/mL) that, by some as-yet-unknown mechanism, triggers a positive feedback release of both FSH and LH. Prior to this peak level of E_2 few if any LH receptors are present on the GC membranes. But at the same time, LH is stimulated to be released from the anterior pituitary, and the GCs synthesize and insert the necessary LH receptors into their plasma membranes. This LH rise triggers two events in the GCs: (1) the GCs change their steroid production from producing primarily E_2 to producing progesterone (P_4), and (2) the GCs begin undergoing a radical change in both structure and function to become corpora luteal cells. This morphological change produces the corpus luteum (CL), or "body of yellow," and the CL becomes a steroid factory eventually synthesizing large amounts of P_4 and E_2. The initial change from E_2 to P_4, which produces enough P_4 to cause antral levels to be very high (2–4 nanomol/mL), profoundly affects the GCs. All steroids function by passing through the cell membrane and bind to an intracellular receptor protein. This complex then couples to a very specific receptor on the DNA in the nucleus. This binding process allows P_4 to initiate transcription of a number of mRNA strands that are transported through nuclear pores to bind to ribosomes in the cytoplasm of the GCs. The proteins being translated from those mRNAs are enzymes that: (1) degrade the extracellular matrix, made up of collagen and several proteoglycans like chondroitin sulfate and polysaccharides like hyaluronate; (2) degrade the ovum maturation inhibitor (OMI) protein that keeps the egg arrested in the dictyate stage of development and allows it to develop to the MII stage; and (3) increase the colloid osmotic pressure in the follicular antrum by inserting proteins into this cavity. Figure 3.1 summarizes these hormonally interacting events with a graphic cartoon, based on data from Dr. Lipner's lab ([88], p. 988).

1. Rising levels of FSH stimulates follicular growth which allows follicles to produce increasing E_2 levels.

2. Increasing E_2 levels initially negatively feedback on FSH and LH.

3. Continuing increase in E_2 levels causes a positive feedback on LH.

4. Increased LH levels causes P_4 release thus initiating synthesis of new mRNA for enzymes to weaken the follicular wall, degrade OMI and increase colloid osmotic pressure in the follicular antrum.

(Text: RJ Swanson)

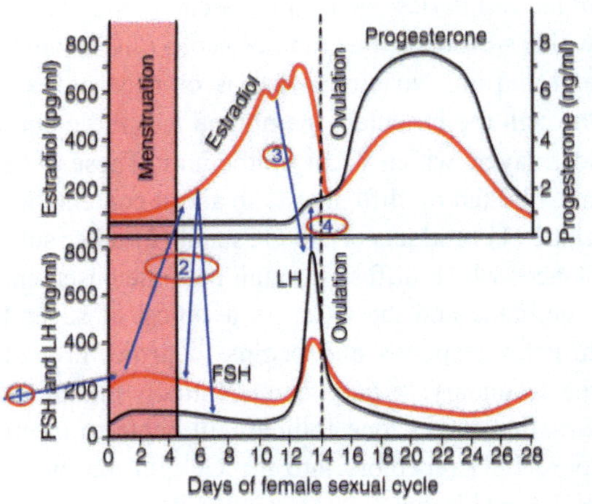

Fig. 3.1 Hormonal events of the menstrual cycle showing the direct ovulatory stimulus to be P_4. *FSH* follitropin, *LH* leuteotropin, *E2* estradiol-17β, P_4 progesterone. (Modified from [88, pp. 987–1000] with permission from Elsevier)

Progesterone and Ovulation of a Mature Ovum

The importance of progesterone for (1) creating a secretory endometrium that accepts the fertilized ovum and (2) maintaining pregnancy has been understood for many decades. The assessment of serum progesterone in normal pregnancy was accomplished from 1950 through 1970, while most of the assessment of pregnancy complications relating to progesterone was between 1963 and the early 1980s. The first use of progesterone as a contraceptive was reported by C. J. Andrews from Norfolk, Virginia, in 1936 [89]. However, the importance of progesterone in ovulation has not been conclusively confirmed in the literature, although this role has been implied over the past several decades. As seen in Fig. 3.1, the observation of high P_4 levels in the preovulatory follicle hinted at a role in ovulation but did not spark much interest in the research community. The importance of its role as the direct mediator of ovulation becomes evident when reading the effects of exercise on P_4 levels with a negative [90–95] or positive [96–97] effect on the menstrual cycle, which can be linked to the secondary effect of LH release from the anterior pituitary [98]. One author, in a review article [99], credits its ovulation induction exclusively to P_4 while rejecting any role of a positive feedback mechanism for E_2 on LH as the primary cause of ovulation. The mistake of failing to factor in this E_2 feedback mechanism has been addressed in hundreds of articles that clearly link rising E_2 as the primary stimulus for the LH surge, rising LH as the primary stimulus for P_4 secretion, and rising P_4 in the follicular antrum as the primary causal factor for ovulation. The effect of this P_4 production, while not initially great enough to give a large increase in blood serum levels, is seen later as the GCs become luteal cells. However, early P_4 production is clearly high enough to cause the GCs to produce the enzyme milieu to bring about the events necessary for ovulation to take place.

LH works through the second messenger system to initiate P_4 synthesis. LH and FSH are both potent stimulators of steroid synthesis and thus control E_2 and P_4. One major role of steroids is to bind to the nuclear receptors on DNA and transcribe mRNA molecules for protein transcription in the cytoplasm. Over the space of 5–10 h these proteins will produce the necessary thinning of the follicular wall, degrade the ovum maturation inhibitor (OMI), increase the antral colloid osmotic pressure, and begin the transition of GCs to luteal cells of the CL.

In Dr. Swanson's lab a total of 56 rabbits were mated with a buck to elicit ovulation in this coitus-induced ovulator species. The ovaries were then exposed with a flank incision and Graafian follicles were divided randomly into equal numbers of experimental anti-P_4 antiserum (a-P_{as}) or control normal rabbit serum (NRS) follicles to be injected with 2 µL of one or the other compounds. Rabbits ovulate predictably approximately 12 h after coitus. When injected with a-P_{as} within 4 h postcoitally, only 20 % of injected follicles ovulate and have entrapped MII ova in the antrum (Fig. 3.2a). When injected after 5 h postcoitally, there is no difference between a-P_{as} and normal rabbit serum (NRS) injected follicles; 80 % ovulation (Fig. 3.2b).

These results illustrate the driving force of P_4 in the ovulatory event (Fig. 3.3). This highlights the importance in recognizing the effects of strenuous exercise on the female reproductive cycle. Not only can perturbation of P_4 have a detrimental effect on embryo implantation and pregnancy maintenance, but low P_4 can negate the release of an egg on any cycle so that there would be no chance for fertilization. When the normal female reproductive cycle is clearly understood, a person can play a major controlling role in monitoring and managing her reproductive health in relation to exercise regimens, diet, and ingested recreational substances, all of which can improve or ravage the body with devastating effects on the reproductive system.

Beginning of Pregnancy

Human pregnancy starts with embryo implantation into the uterine wall at approximately day 6 or 7 postfertilization and is a very delicate mechanism that requires embryo–endometrium dialog. The time period during which implantation can occur (the implantation window) generally ranges from day 6 to day 10 post-ovulation (days 20–24 in a 28-day cycle). By day 10, the blastocyst has become totally encased within the endometrium and embryo development has started.

The Placenta

The human placenta is a highly specialized organ which plays a number of important roles, including embryonic/fetal nutrition and growth, endocrine function, and acting as a physical and immunological barrier. Furthermore, during gestation, the human fetus depends on the placenta for its pulmonary, hepatic, and renal functions.

Placental Barrier

During the early stages of pregnancy the placental barrier comprises four layers, namely the syncytiotrophoblast, the cytotrophoblast, connective tissue, and the endothelium of the capillary vessels, whereas at term only a hemo-monochorionic structure comprising the trophoblast and the fetal endothelium remains. Although the placental barrier separates fetal blood from maternal blood, this separation is not absolute, and a number of substances are able to either passively or actively cross the placental barrier.

Placental Transfer

The placenta plays a pivotal role in providing the fetus with the oxygen, water, and nutrients it needs while transporting the CO_2 and other metabolites resulting from fetal catabolism from the fetus to the mother. These different compounds cross the placenta by a number of mechanisms, including simple diffusion (gases, water, and the majority of electrolytes), facilitated diffusion (glucose and lactate), active transport (some cations, water-soluble vitamins, and amino acids), pinocytosis (lipoproteins and phospholipids), or by direct passage through a placental barrier's solution of continuity (for example red blood cells under both normal and abnormal conditions, such as placental abruption) [100].

The exchange of substances between the mother and the fetus depends on the characteristics of the exchange membrane, the hydrostatic or oncotic pressure on both sides of the membrane, the dynamics of placental maternal and

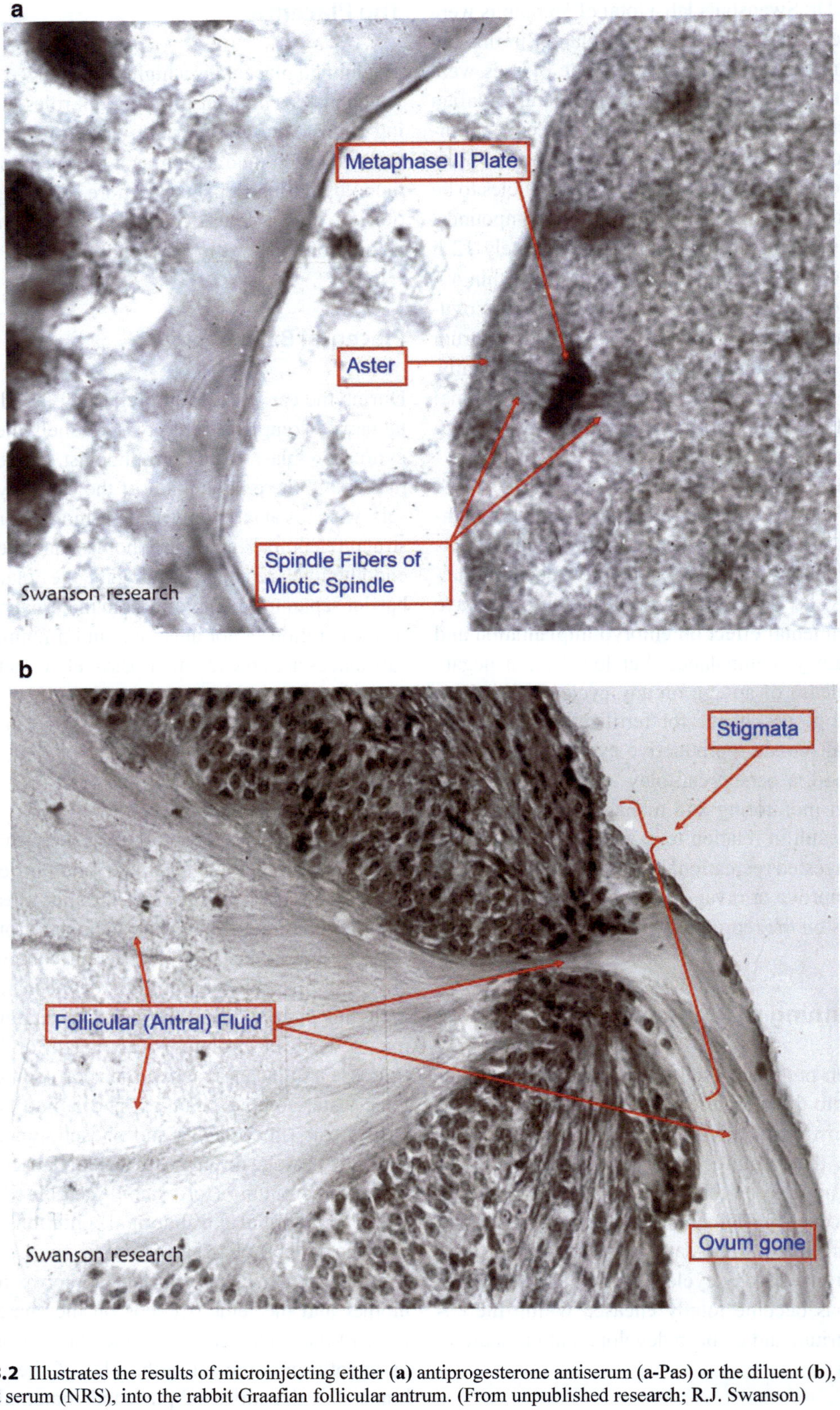

Fig. 3.2 Illustrates the results of microinjecting either (**a**) antiprogesterone antiserum (a-Pas) or the diluent (**b**), normal rabbit serum (NRS), into the rabbit Graafian follicular antrum. (From unpublished research; R.J. Swanson)

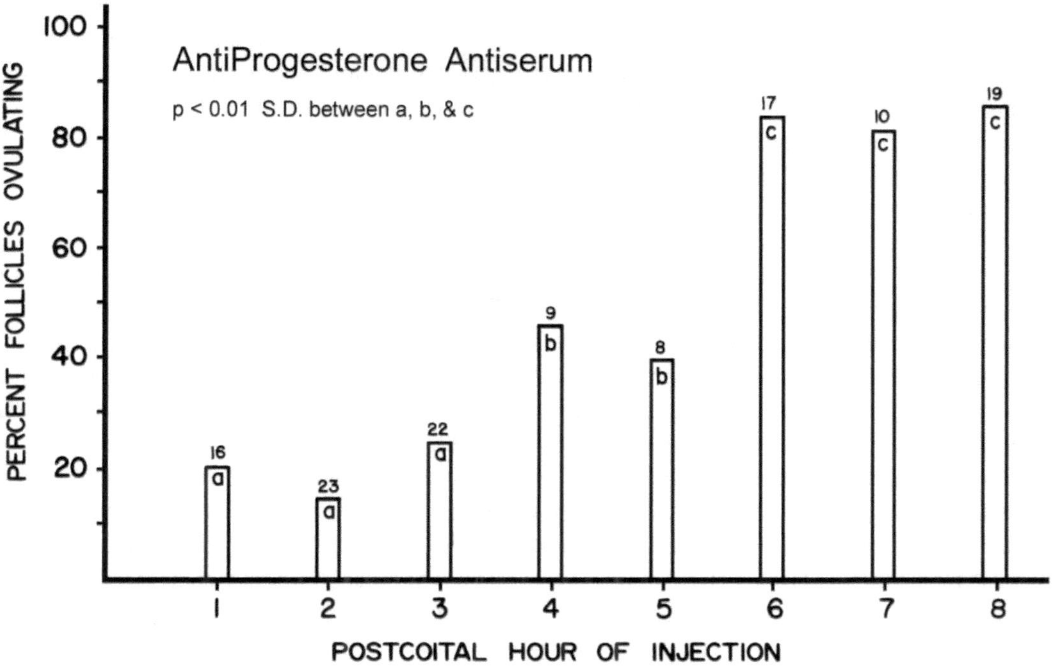

Fig. 3.3 Antiprogesterone antiserum injected into Graafian follicles 1–8 h postcoitally. Normal rabbit serum-injected follicles ovulated at 80 % for all hours of injection postcoitally. (From unpublished research; R.J. Swanson)

fetal circulation and its spatial configuration, the concentration of the different compounds on both sides of the placental membrane, and the placental metabolism [100].

Placental Respiration

Although the placenta is the first lung for the fetus, its respiratory efficiency is considerably lower than in the lung (1/5 per tissue weight unit). Both O_2 and CO_2 cross the placenta by simple diffusion, and the fact that the maternal blood reaching the intervillous space has a higher pO_2 than that in the villous capillaries results in a flow of O_2 to the fetal circulation. The direction of flow for CO_2 is the opposite since the pCO_2 is higher on the fetal side. Moreover, various unique characteristics of fetal blood favor O_2 uptake by the fetus: (a) higher hemoglobin concentration than in maternal blood, (b) the higher O_2 affinity of fetal hemoglobin, (c) the fact that O_2 transfer is facilitated by CO_2 transfer, (d) CO_2 transfer is 20 times quicker in the placenta and is facilitated by O_2 transfer [100].

Placental Endocrine Function

The placenta synthesizes a number of molecules, the function of many of which is still not well understood. These include:

1. Human chorionic gonadotropin (hCG)

This is a glucopeptidic hormone produced by the syncytiotrophoblast that comprises two subunits (α and β). The α unit is very similar to the α unit of LH, TSH, and FSH, whereas the β unit bears some resemblance to the β unit of LH, thus meaning that they share some of the same biological functions. Its main role is to maintain the CL during the first weeks of pregnancy. hCG levels are detectable soon after implantation and increase sharply up until the 10th week of gestation, at which point they begin to decrease.

2. Human placental lactogen (hPL)

This single-chain polypeptidic hormone is also produced by the syncytiotrophoblast and is very similar to the growth hormone (GH) produced by the anterior pituitary. hPL levels increase steadily throughout pregnancy, reaching a peak at the end of pregnancy, and correlate with placental weight. The biological role of this hormone is to guarantee the availability of glucose as an energetic substrate for the fetus. In the event of maternal fasting, the resulting hypoglycemia induces hPL production, which in turn triggers lipolysis in the mother, thereby increasing the level of free fatty acids, which cross the placenta and can be used as an energetic substrate. It also increases amino acid placental transfer by restricting protein use by the mother [100, 101].

3. Steroid hormones

The placenta produces huge amounts of progesterone and estrogens from precursors obtained from the mother. Progesterone is mainly synthesized from maternal cholesterol. However, since placental tissue lacks 17-hydroxylase activity, it is not able to synthesize estradiol or estrone from progesterone or pregnenolone. As a result, the aforementioned estrogens are synthesized from the dehydroepiandrosterone sulfate (DHEA-S) synthesized by the adrenal glands of both the mother and the fetus. Placental sulfatase reacts with DHEA-S to form DHEA, which is converted into androstenedione and testosterone, and subsequently into estrone and estradiol by placental aromatization.

The Amniotic Fluid

The embryo/fetus is immersed in the amniotic cavity, which is filled with amniotic fluid. The main functions of this fluid include protecting the fetus and the umbilical cord from external injury and the pressure resulting from uterine contractions, allowing the fetus to move freely (at least during the first part of pregnancy), which is necessary for normal fetal development, contributing to fetal thermoregulation, participating in fetal lung development, and, at labor, promoting cervical dilation. The mean volume of amniotic fluid at term is 800 mL, although this value can vary over a wide range (400–1200 mL).

The Fetus

Intrauterine life can be considered to comprise three stages: (a) the differentiation period (conception to week 12 of amenorrhea), during which organogenesis takes place, (b) the growth period (weeks 12–28), which is characterized by cell proliferation, and (c) the weight increase period (week 28 until the end of pregnancy), during which functional maturation of the organs occurs. The mean newborn weight at term is 3200 g (normal weight ranging from 2500 to 4000 g).

Fetal Circulation

Maternal/placental circulation begins once uterine spiral arteries penetrate the intervillous space. From that moment, these spiral arteries inject oxygenated blood into this space, where exchange with the chorionic plate occurs, and then this blood returns to the maternal circulation via the veins located in the placental septa [101]. Fetal blood reaches the placenta through two umbilical arteries that branch into the dividing villi.

Fetal oxygenation occurs via the placenta, which receives a significant proportion (close to 40 %) of cardiac output, whereas the lungs, which lack a respiratory function, receive only 8 %. Another peculiarity is that oxygenated and less oxygenated blood circulates through the same vessels in the fetal circulation. Oxygenated blood from the placenta reaches the abdominal wall of the fetus via the unique umbilical vein from where it penetrates into the liver. The majority of this blood passes to the inferior vena cava via the *ductus venosus,* with the remainder passing into the left hepatic lobule, which subsequently drains into the inferior vena cava via the left hepatic vein. The inferior vena cava contains two different blood flows, namely less oxygenated blood from the lower extremities and the abdomen (O_2 saturation 40 %) and more oxygenated blood from the ductus venosus (O_2 saturation 83 %) and the left hepatic vein (O_2 saturation 73 %). These two blood flows almost do not mix [100, 101].

Blood from the inferior vena cava flows into the left atrium very close to the interauricular communication, where a septum allows differential conduction of the flow, with oxygenated blood (from the *ductus venosus* and left hepatic vein) flowing to the left atrium and then on to the left ventricle and less oxygenated blood, together with blood from the superior vena cava, flowing directly to the right ventricle. The oxygenated blood leaving the left ventricle flows into the ascending aorta, from where it reaches the fetal encephalon. In contrast, the majority of the less oxygenated blood leaving the right ventricle flows into the descending aorta (via the *ductus arteriosus*), with a small proportion reaching pulmonary circulation. This means that whereas the fetal encephalon is only irrigated with more oxygenated blood, the lower part of the body receives a mix of oxygenated and less oxygenated blood.

Maternal Changes During Pregnancy

Pregnancy leads to a number of changes in almost every maternal organ and tissue. Although the majority of these changes are more evident at the end of pregnancy, many of them can also be detected in its earlier stages.

Gynecological Changes

Uterus

Perhaps the most remarkable of the local changes is the enlargement of the uterus, which increases progressively in size mainly due to the hypertrophia and hyperplasia of uterine smooth-muscle cells. At term, the uterus has a weight of 1100 g and a capacity of 5000 mL compared to its normal weight of around 70 g and capacity of 5 mL outside pregnancy. This increase in uterine size and weight is partially responsible for some of the compression-related effects on neighboring structures. Throughout pregnancy some irregular and painful contractions (known as Braxton-Hicks contractions) can occur, which are frequently misinterpreted as the beginning of labor at the end of pregnancy.

Cervix

Immediately after conception, the cervix is closed by a mucous plug, which forms a protective barrier against microorganism.

Ovaries

The CL enlarges during early pregnancy and remains active for 8–10 weeks, producing huge amounts of estrogens and progesterone.

Breasts

There is a remarkable increase in breast size as a consequence of adipose tissue hypertrophy, *acini* neoformation, and dilation of the lactiferous ducts during pregnancy. Breast vascularization also increases. Colostrum is produced from around week 12.

Systemic Changes

Cardiovascular Changes

A number of cardiovascular modifications, which are depicted in Table 3.1 [102], occur as a consequence of the need to irrigate a larger area (placenta, larger uterus, and breasts). Likewise, a number of symptoms and signs, such as asthenia, dyspnea, mild systolic murmurs, and peripheral edema, which outside pregnancy would suggest heart disease, can be completely normal during pregnancy [103]. Similarly, when the woman lies in the supine position, especially at the end of pregnancy, the enlarged uterus can obstruct blood flow to the inferior vena cava, thereby decreasing cardiac output, causing hypotension, and resulting in "supine hypotensive syndrome" or "aortocaval compression syndrome." This condition can affect fetal well-being and produce maternal lipothymy.

Table 3.1 Cardiovascular changes during pregnancy—Stages of labor and relationship between fetal descent and cervical dilation pattern

	Start (week)	Maximum (week)	Increase (%)
Blood volume	8	32–35	+40
Plasma volume	8	32	+50
Erythrocyte volume	8	40	+25
Cardiac output	10	24–32	+40
Heart rate	12	40	+22
Respiratory rate	8	40	+45
Oxygen consumption	14	40	+22
Blood pressure	1st trimester		−20
	3rd trimester		+40
Vascular resistance	8	22	−45

Venous varicosities are also common, especially in the legs, vulva, and rectum (hemorrhoids).

Hematological Changes

Pregnancy results in an increase in maternal erythropoiesis. However, the increase in plasma volume is higher than the increase in total erythrocyte volume, thus leading to a decrease in hematocrit values and resulting in the so-called "physiologic anemia of pregnancy" or "pseudoanemia of pregnancy." As a result, the cutoff for defining anemia in pregnancy is a hemoglobin level of 10.5 g/dL instead of the 12 g/dL used outside of pregnancy. A number of changes in the coagulation system, including a 50 % increase in fibrinogen values, an increase in clotting factors VII, VIII, IX, X, and XII, a decrease in factor XI, and a 50 % decrease in factor XIII, also occur [100, 101, 103].

Respiratory Changes

A number of changes occur in the respiratory function [104], all of which are aimed at obtaining a more efficient respiratory function in order to provide oxygen supply to the fetus (Fig. 3.4 [104]). One common finding during normal pregnancy is dyspnea, although its cause is not well established.

Nephro-Urological Changes

There is a 40 % increase in both renal blood flow and the glomerular filtration rate, and anatomical changes, such as an increase in renal size and urethral dilation, also occur.

Digestive Changes

The main digestive changes result from the relaxant effects of progesterone on the smooth muscle as well as the compressive effects of the gravid uterus on neighboring structures. The consequences include heartburn and esophageal reflux, risk of Mendelsohn's syndrome (chemical pneumonitis caused by aspiration of gastric contents), especially during general anesthesia, constipation, and hemorrhoids. The changes in liver function that occur result in alterations to the levels of many biochemical blood parameters (Table 3.2 [102]).

Musculoskeletal Changes

Lumbar lordosis develops progressively as a consequence of the increased weight in the anterior part of the body due to the enlarged uterus. Moreover, the feet of pregnant woman tend to be more widely separated than usual when standing.

Metabolic Changes

One of the most evident changes during pregnancy is the increase in maternal weight. Thus, the mean increase in maternal weight at the end of pregnancy is 11 kg, with 5.1 kg of this being due to the intrauterine contents (3.5 kg for the fetus, 1 kg the amniotic fluid, and 0.6 kg the placenta), 1.1 kg the uterus, 1.6 kg the blood, 0.5 kg the breasts, and the remainder to general storage. Nu-

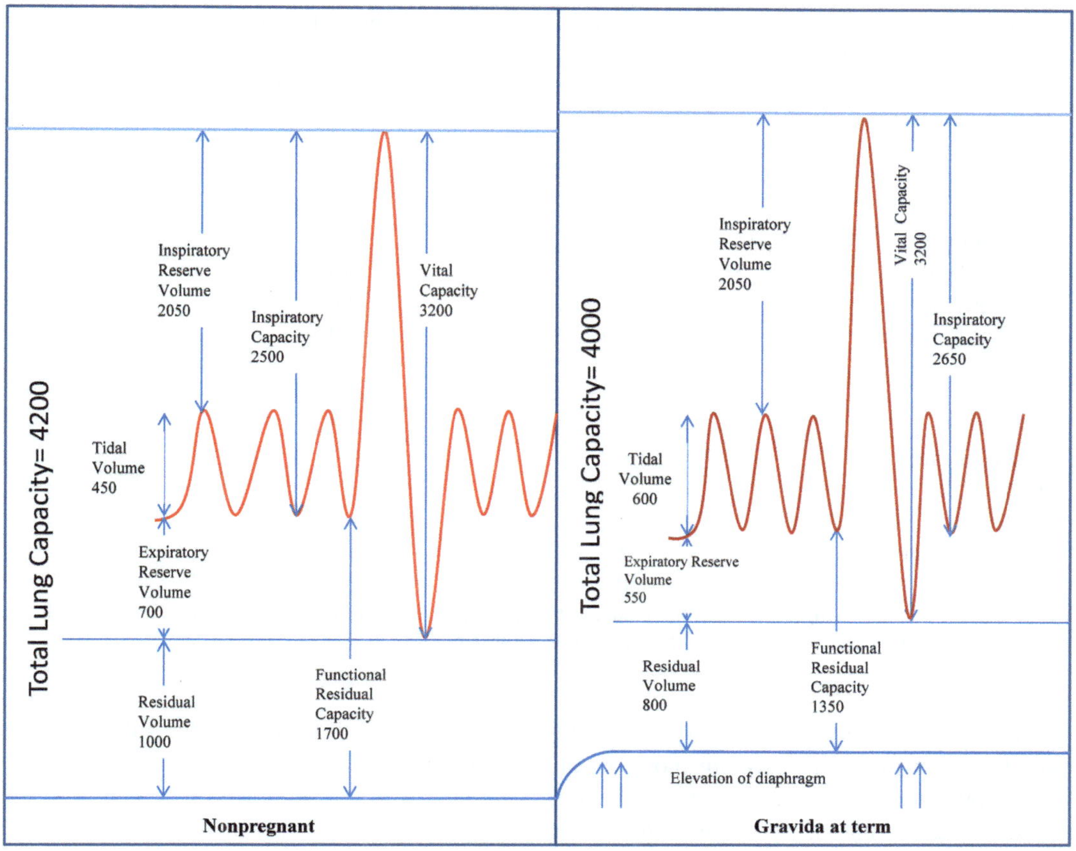

Fig. 3.4 Respiratory changes during pregnancy. (Based on data from Ref. [104])

tritional requirements increase during pregnancy up to an additional 20 % at term.

A remarkable volume of water is retained during pregnancy: 3.5 L for the fetus, amniotic fluid, and placenta, and a further 3 L for the increase in plasma volume, the increase in extracellular and extravascular water, and the water accumulated in the breasts and uterus.

The increased concentration of estrogens, progesterone, and especially hPL results in an increase in circulating insulin levels whose biological significance is to ensure a continual supply of glucose to the fetus. Pregnancy is a diabetes-enhancing condition and, as such, aggravates previously existing diabetes.

Labor

Term delivery in humans occurs at between 37 and 42 completed weeks. The mean gestational age is 280 days (40 weeks) after the last menstrual period if ovulation occurs 14 days after the onset of menstruation. Normal labor takes between 3 and 18 h.

The Elements of Labor

The Birth Canal

During delivery, the fetus must descend through the birth canal, which comprises a skeletal and a nonskeletal portion. The skeletal passageway of

Table 3.2 Effect of normal pregnancy on liver function tests—Stages of labor and relationship between fetal descent and cervical dilation pattern

Test	Effect	Trimester of maximum change
Alkaline phosphatase	2–4×	3rd
Cholesterol	2×	3rd
Fibrinogen	1.5×	2nd
Ceruloplasmin	↑	3rd
Transferrin	↑	3rd
Alpha-globulin	S ↑	3rd
Beta-globulin	S ↑	3rd
Lactate dehydrogenase	S ↑	3rd
GGT	S ↑	3rd
Bilirubin	N or S ↑	3rd
BSP	N or S ↑	3rd
Prothrombin time	=	=
SGOT	=	=
SGPT	=	=
Gamma globulin	N or S ↓	1st
Albumin	0.8×	2nd

N no change, *S* slight change, *GGT* gamma-glutamyl transpeptidase, *BSP* bromsulphthalein, *SGOT* serum glutamic oxaloacetic transaminase, *SGPT* serum glutamate pyruvate transaminase

labor is constituted by the pelvis which is composed of four bones: the sacrum, coccyx, and two innominate bones. Each innominate bone is formed by the fusion of the *ilium, ischium,* and *pubis*. The innominate bones are joined to the sacrum at the sacroiliac synchondroses and to one another at the symphysis pubis [101]. The nonskeletal portion comprises the uterine cervix, the vagina and its opening, the vulva, and the surrounding structures (rectum, bladder, and *levator ani* and perineal muscles). The birth canal follows an anterior curve rather than a straight line. Likewise, whereas the transversal diameter is larger than the anteroposterior diameter at the beginning of the birth canal, this situation is reversed at the end.

The Object of Labor (the Passenger)

During normal delivery, the fetus is in a longitudinal lie and in cephalic presentation. In this delivery, fetal presentation has an ovoid form, with the anteroposterior diameter being larger than the biparietal. In contrast, in the larger part of the remaining fetal body (the shoulders) the transversal diameter is much larger than the anteroposterior diameter.

The Power of Labor

The main power during labor is generated by the uterine contraction, which is helped by the voluntary pressure of abdominal muscles at the end of labor. Uterine contractions are produced by the uterine muscle, which is composed of smooth muscle fibers with some highly specific characteristics. During normal delivery, the contraction activity of the different muscle cells is synchronized, thus generating the normal uterine contraction. This type of contraction starts in the uterine fundus and progresses to the lower portions of the uterus, is more intense in the fundus, and ends later in the fundus. The characteristics of uterine contractions change throughout delivery, becoming more intense, more frequent, and lasting for longer as labor progresses. Thus, the contraction intensity is usually less than 30 mmHg at the beginning of labor, but more than 50 mmHg at the end. Although it is traditionally stated that uterine contractions become painful once their intensity exceeds 30 mmHg, there is great individual variability in this respect. As far as the duration is concerned, the length of the perceived contraction is 30–35 s at the beginning of labor and 60 s towards the end. However, the real length of contraction is considerably higher in both cases. On average, one uterine contraction occurs every 10 min at the onset of labor, with this value rising to three (or more) contractions every 10 min at the end [100–103].

Voluntary contraction of the diaphragm and of the muscles of the abdominal wall during the last part of the second period of labor increases the intra-abdominal pressure. This, together with uterine contractions, favors expulsion of the fetus once cervical dilation is complete.

Phases of Labor

Prodromal Labor

The mechanisms that trigger labor are complex and not yet fully understood. However, prior to the onset of labor there is an imprecise period, called prodromal labor, which is characterized by symptoms that include an increased uterine contraction frequency, descent of the uterine fundus, fixation of the fetal presentation, cervical plug expulsion, and changes to the cervix.

First Stage

The following phenomena occur during this stage: (1) cervical effacement (the length of the uterine cervix before starting labor is 3–4 cm, whereas when it is fully effaced it is paper-thin), (2) cervical dilation (from 0 to 3 cm at the onset of labor to 10 cm at the end), (3) an increase in the frequency and intensity of the uterine contractions, (4) rupture of the membranes, and (5) fetal descent.

According to Friedman [5], two different periods can be considered in the first stage of labor: the latent phase and the active phase, which usually starts at a dilation of 3–4 cm cervical dilation and is subdivided into the acceleration, maximum slope, and deceleration phases (Fig. 3.5 [102]).

Second Stage

The second stage starts at full dilation and ends with delivery of the infant. This stage lasts for a much shorter time than the first stage (average duration of 50 min in nullipara and 20 min in multipara). During this period the woman participates actively by "pushing" when she experiences (involuntary) contractions. Contractions are frequent and intense, similar to those at the end of the first period. Since fetal presentation is descended, uterine contraction forces the fetal head into the perineum, thus triggering the reflex abdominal push.

Mechanisms of Labor in the Second Stage The following processes take place during labor: (1) inlet into the birth canal, (2) passage through the birth canal (descent and engagement), and (3) exit from the birth canal. As a result, the fetal head experiences the following [100, 101]:

I. Engagement. In most cases, the vertex enters the pelvis with the sagittal suture lying in the transverse pelvic diameter, thus meaning that the maximal diameter of the head (anteroposterior) coincides with the maximal diameter of the pelvis inlet.
II. Descent.
III. Flexion. This allows the fetal head to adapt better to the birth canal, thereby presenting the smallest diameter.
IV. Internal rotation. This movement involves the head turning by 90° in such a manner that the occiput gradually moves toward the symphysis. The fetus has now descended and the presentation is in the pelvic outlet, with the widest fetal diameter (anteroposterior) coinciding with the widest diameter of the pelvic outlet (also anteroposterior). The fetal shoulders are located in the pelvic inlet, where their larger, transversal (bisacromial) diameter coincides with the widest diameter of the pelvic inlet (also transversal).
V. Extension and expulsion of the head: The change in direction of the birth canal causes the fetal head to tilt forwards so that its crown leads the way through the vagina.

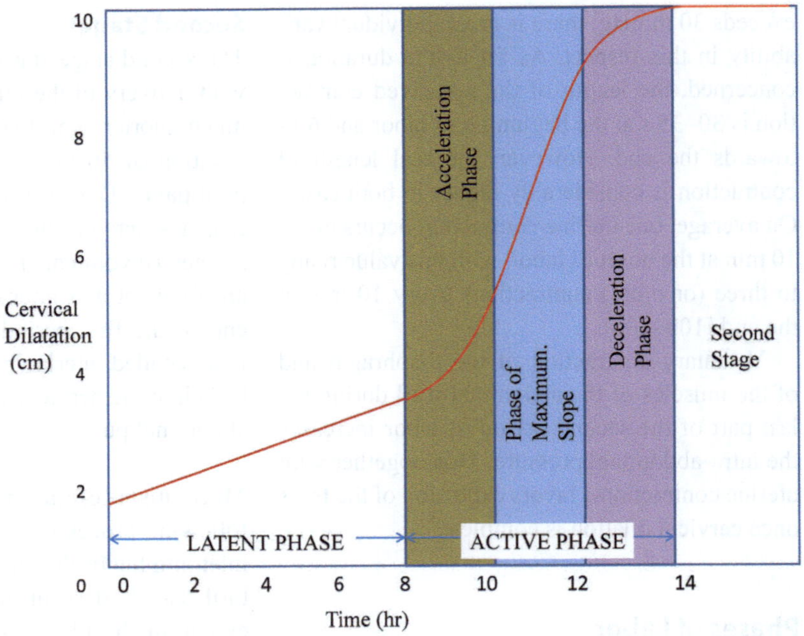

Fig. 3.5 Stages of labor and relationship between fetal descent and cervical dilation pattern. (Based on data from Ref. [102])

VI. External rotation (restitution) and delivery of the shoulders: The bisacromial diameter adopts the anteroposterior diameter of the pelvic outlet and the fetal head rotates again, placing itself in the same position as at engagement. The remaining fetal body is then easily expelled.

Although the aforementioned movements are sequential, they also overlap to a large extent. Furthermore, the fetal head may temporarily undergo a marked change in shape (becoming more elongated and decreasing its maximal diameters) as it descends through the birth canal (fetal head molding). At the same time, the pelvis increases its diameter due to distension of the sacroiliac synchondroses, especially the pubic symphysis, and backwards displacement of the coccyx.

Third Stage

The third stage of labor starts with the conclusion of fetal expulsion and ends with delivery of the placenta. The uterus contracts immediately after delivery of the fetus, thus decreasing its volume and causing the placental detachment. The resulting hematoma further increases placental detachment, which is followed by membrane detachment. A physiological hemorrhage (of up to 500 mL) occurs during delivery of the placenta and the membranes as a result of the highly vascularized area where the placenta was inserted into the uterus. This hemorrhage is effectively stopped by a number of mechanisms, the most important of which is the continuing uterine contraction. Due to the specific disposition of the uterine vessels and the uterine smooth fibers, this contraction strangles the uterine vessels, thereby preventing further hemorrhage. The other mechanisms involved include vascular contraction, clotting, and return of the blood previously retained in the uterus to general circulation [100, 101].

Conclusion

This chapter has presented an extremely complex set of events outlining some of what is currently understood about the sequential events in the roadmap to successful human reproduction. We must emphasize the phrase "currently understood" because within a few short years, the information in this chapter will be either confirmed, modified, or corrected. In addition, many more details about these processes will be discovered. As deeper understanding of the reproductive process is gained, we marvel at the miraculous design contained in the DNA blueprint that informs the events as a whole. Not only are structural proteins put in place and regulated by the enzymatic proteins for gamete-to-neonate construction, but all of the ancillary molecular machines for sequencing, organizing, and building the eventual human person are brought into play and then removed at precise intervals. With so many thousands of steps that are necessary to go right, we are amazed that we exist at all.

References

1. Amann R, Hammerstedt R. In vitro evaluation of sperm quality: an opinion. J Androl. 1993;14:397–06.
2. Storey B. Interactions between gametes leading to fertilization: the sperm's eye view. Reprod Fertil Dev. 1995;7:927–42.
3. Visconti E, Bailey L, Moore D, Pan D, Olds-Clarke P, Kopf G. Capacitation of mouse spermatozoa. I. Correlation between the capacitation state and protein tyrosine phosphorylation. Development. 1995;121:1129–37.
4. Baldi E, Luconi L, Bonaccorsi L, Krausz C, Forti G. Human sperm activation during capacitation and acrosome reaction: role of calcium, protein phosphorylation and lipid remodeling pathways. Front Biosci. 1996;1:d189–205.
5. Wassarman P. Mammalian fertilization: egg and sperm glycoproteins that support gamete adhesion. Am J Reprod Immunol. 1995;33:253–8.
6. Chapman R, Barratt L. The role of carbohydrate in sperm-ZP3 adhesion. Mol Hum Reprod. 1996;2:767–74.
7. Wassarman P. Mammalian fertilization: molecular aspect of gamete adhesion exocytosis, and fusion. Cell. 1999;96:175–83.
8. Leyton L, LeGuen P, Bunch D, Saling PM. Regulation of mouse gamete interaction by a sperm tyrosine kinase. Proc Natl Acad Sci U S A. 1992;89:11692–5.
9. Bookbinder H, Cheng A, Bleil D. Tissue- and species-specific expression of sp56, a mouse sperm fertilization protein. Science. 1995;269:86–9.
10. Boettger-Tong L, Aarons J, Biegler E, George B, Poirier R. Binding of a murine proteinase inhibitor to the acrosome region of human sperm head. Mol Reprod Dev. 1993;36:346–53.
11. Shur BD. Glycobiology. The beginning of a sweet tale. Curr Biol. 1994;4:996–9.
12. Gao Z, Garbers DL. Species diversity in the structure of zonadhesin, a sperm-specific membrane protein containing multiple cell adhesion molecule-like domains. J Biol Chem. 1998;273:3415–21.
13. Wassarman P, Jovine L, Litscher ES. Mouse zona pellucida genes and glycoproteins. Cytogenet Genome Res. 2004;105:228–34.
14. Bi M, Hickox R, Winfrey P, Olson E, Hardy M. Processing, localization and binding activity of zonadhesin suggest a function in sperm adhesion to the zona pellucida during exocytosis of the acrosome. Biochem J. 2003;375:477–88.
15. Sutton A, Jungnickel K, Ward J, Harris C, Florman M. Functional characterization of PKDREJ, a male germ cell-restricted polycystin. J Cel Physiol. 2006;209:493–500.
16. Turner M, Hoekstra E. Reproductive protein evolution within and between species: ZP3 sequence variation. Peromyscus Mol Ecol. 2008;17:2616–28.
17. van Gestel A, Brewis A, Ashton R, Brouwers F, Gadella M. Multiple proteins present in purified porcine sperm apical plasma membranes interact with the zona pellucida of the oocyte. Mol Hum Reprod. 2007;13:445–54.
18. Rankin L, Tong B, Castle E, Lee E, Gore-Langton R, et al. Human ZP3 restores fertility in Zp3 null mice without affecting order-specific sperm binding. Development. 1998;125:2415–24.
19. Rankin L, Coleman S, Epifano O, Hoodbhoy T, Turner G, Castle E, Lee E, et al. Fertility and taxon-specific sperm binding persist after replacement of mouse 'sperm receptors' with human homologs. Dev Cell. 2003;5:33–43.
20. Castle E, Dean J. Manipulating the genome to study reproduction. Mice with 'humanized' zonae pellucidae. Hum Reprod. 1999;14:1927–39.
21. Hoodbhoy T, Dean J. Insights into the molecular basis of sperm-egg recognition in mammals. Reproduction. 2004;127:417–22.
22. Yanagimachi R. Intracytoplasmic sperm injection experiments using the mouse as a model. Hum Reprod. 1998;13:87–98.
23. Breitbar H. Role and regulation of intracellular calcium in acrosomal exocytosis. J Reprod Inmunol. 2002;53:151–9.
24. Florman M, Tombes M, First L, Babcock F. An adhesion-associated agonist from the zona pellucida activates G protein-promoted elevations of internal Ca^{2+} and pH that mediate mammalian sperm acrosomal exocytosis. Dev Biol. 1989;135:133–46.
25. Florman M, Corron E, Kim D, Babcock F. Activation of voltage-dependent calcium channels of mammalian sperm is required for zona pellucida-induced acrosomal exocytosis. Dev Biol. 1992;152:304–14.
26. Yunes R, Michaut M, Tomes C, Mayorga LS. Rab3A triggers the acrosome reaction in permeabilized human spermatozoa. Biol Reprod. 2000;62:1084–9.
27. Fraser R, Ahuja K. Metabolic and surface events in fertilization. Gamete Res. 1988;20:491–519.

28. Yanagimachi R. Mammalian fertilization. In: Knobil E, Neill JD, editors. *The physiology of reproduction*. 3rd ed. New York: Raven Press, Ltd.; 1994. pp. 189–317.
29. Miller J, Macek B, Shur D. Complementarity between sperm surface beta -1,4-galactosyltransferase and egg-coat ZP3 mediates sperm-egg binding. Nature. 1992;357:589–93.
30. Clark F, Oehninger S, Patankar S, Koistinen R, Dell A, Morris R, et al. A role for glycoconjugates in human development: the human feto-embryonic defence system hypothesis. Hum Reprod. 1996;11:467–73.
31. Clark F, Dell A, Morris R, Patankar M, Oehninger S, Seppälä M. Viewing AIDS from a glycobiological perspective: potential linkages to the human feto-embryonic defence system hypothesis. Mol Hum Reprod. 1997;3:5–13 (Review).
32. Oehninger S. Molecular basis of human sperm-zona pellucida interaction. Cells Tissues Organs. 2001;168:58–64.
33. Patankar S, Ozgur K, Oehninger S, Dell A, Morris H, et al. Expression of glycans linked to natural killer cell inhibition on the human zona pellucida. Mol Hum Reprod. 1997;3:501–5.
34. Oehninger S. Normal fertilization. In: Shafie M EI, Sousa M, Windt M-L, Kruger TF, editors. An atlas of the ultrastructure of human oocytes. A guide for assisted reproduction. London: Partheon Publishing Group; 2000. pp. 23–35.
35. Oehninger S. Biochemical and functional characterization of the human zona pellucida. Reprod Biomed Online. 2003;7:641–8.
36. Ozgur K, Patankar MS, Oehninger S, Clark GF. Direct evidence for the involvement of carbohydrate sequences in human sperm-zona pellucida binding. Mol Hum Reprod. 1998;4:318–24.
37. Seppala M, Taylor N, Koistinen H, Koistinen R, Milgrom E. Glycodelin: a major lipocalin protein of the reproductive axis with diverse actions in cell recognition and differentiation. Endocr Rev. 2002;23:401–30.
38. Dell A, Morris R, Easton L, Panico M, Patankar M, Oehniger S, et al. Structural analysis of the oligosaccharides derived from glycodelin, a human glycoprotein with potent immunosuppressive and contraceptive activities. J Biol Chem. 1995;270:24116–26.
39. Dell A, Chalabi S, Easton L, Haslam M, Sutton-Smith M, Patankar S, et al. Murine and human zona pellucida 3 derived from mouse eggs express identical O-glycans. Proc Natl Acad Sci USA. 2003;100:15631–6.
40. Pang C, Tissot B, Drobnis Z, Sutovsky P, Morris R, et al. Expression of bisecting type and Lewisx/Lewisy terminated N-glycans on human sperm. J Biol Chem. 2007;282:36593–602.
41. Chiu C, Chung K, Koistinen R, Koistinen H, Seppala M, Ho C, et al. Glycodelin-A interacts with fucosyltransferase on human sperm plasma membrane to inhibit spermatozoa-zona pellucida binding. J Cell Sci. 2007;120:33–44.
42. Cross L, Morales P, Overstreet W, Hanson W. Induction of acrosome reactions by the human zona pellucida. Biol Reprod. 1988;38:235–44.
43. Lee A, Check H, Kopf A. Guanine nucleotide-binding regulatory protein in human sperm mediates acrosomal exocytosis induced by the human zona pellucida. Mol Reprod. 1992;31:78–86.
44. Franken DR, Morales J, Habenicht F. Inhibition of G protein in human sperm and its influence on acrosome reaction and zona pellucida binding. Fertil Steril. 1996;66:1009–11.
45. Schuffner A, Bastiaan S, Duran E, Lin Y, Morshedi M, et al. Zona pellucida-induced acrosome reaction in human sperm: dependency on activation of pertussis toxin-sensitive G(i) protein and extracellular calcium, and priming effect of progesterone and follicular fluid. Mol Hum Reprod. 2002;8:722–7.
46. Lefièvre L, Conner SJ, Salpekar A, Olufowobi O, Ashton P, Pavlovic B, et al. Four zona pellucida glycoproteins are expressed in the human. Hum Reprod. 2004;19:1580–6.
47. Conner J, Lefievre L, Hughes C, Barratt L. Cracking the egg: increased complexity in the zona pellucida. Hum Reprod. 2005;20:1148–52.
48. Bedford M. Ultrastructural changes in the sperm head during fertilization in the rabbit. Am J Anat. 1968;123:329–58.
49. Stein KK, Primafoff P, Myles D. Sperm-egge fusion: events at the plasma membrane. J Cell Sci. 2004;117:6269–74.
50. Snell J, White M. The molecules of mammalian fertilization. Cell. 1996;85:629–37.
51. Cowan E, Koppel E, Vargas A, Hunnicutt R. Guinea pig fertilin exhibits restricted lateral mobility in epididymal sperm and becomes freely diffusing during capacitation. Dev Biol. 2001;15:502–9.
52. Primakoff P, Myles DG. The ADAM gene family: surface proteins with adhesion and protease activity. Trends Genet. 2000;16:83–7.
53. Fusi F, Montesano M, Bernocchil N, Panzeri C, Ferrara F, Villa A, Bronson R. P-selectin is expressed on the oolemma of human and hamster oocytes following sperm adhesion and is also detected on the equatorial region of acrosome-reacted human spermatozoa. Mol Hum Reprod. 1996;2:341–7.
54. Cohen J, Ros D, Busso D, Maldera J, Goldweic N, Cuasnicu S. Molecular mechanisms involved in gamete interaction. Anim Reprod. 2006;3:127–9.
55. Toshimori K, Saxena DK, Tanii I, Yoshinaga K. An MN9 antigenic molecule, equatorin, is required for successful sperm-oocyte fusion in mice. Biol Reprod. 1998;59:22–9.
56. Miyado K, Yamada G, Yamada S, Hasuwa H, Nakamura Y, Ryu F, Mekada E, et al. Requirement of CD9 on egg plasma membrane for fertilization. Science. 2000;287:321–4.
57. Kaji K, Oda S, Shikano T, Ohnuki T, Uematsu Y, Sakagami J, et al. The gamete fusion process is

defective in eggs of CD9-deficient mice. Nature Genet. 2000;24:279–82.
58. Inoue N, Ikawa M, Isotanil A, Okabe M. The immunoglobulin superfamily protein Izumo is required for sperm to fuse with eggs. Nature. 2005;434:234–8.
59. Inoue N, Ikawa M, Okabe M. Putative sperm fusion protein Izumo and the role of N-glycosylation. Biochem Biophys Res Commun. 2008;377(3):910–4.
60. Vjugina U, Evans JP. New insights into the molecular basis of mammalian sperm-egg membrane interactions. Front Biosci. 2008;13:462–76.
61. Dale B, DeFelice LJ, Ehrenstein G. Injection of a soluble sperm extract into sea urchin eggs triggers the cortical reaction. Experientia. 1985;41:1068–70.
62. Fissore A, Reis M, Palermo D. Isolation of the Ca^{2+} releasing component(s) of mammalian sperm extracts: the search continues. Mol Hum Reprod. 1999;5:189–92.
63. Kline D, Simoncini L, Mandel G, Maue RA, Kado RT, Jaffe LA. Fertilization events induced by neurotransmitters after injection of mRNA in Xenopus eggs. Science. 1988;241:464–7.
64. Jaffe F. Sources of calcium in egg activation: a review and hypothesis. Dev Biol. 1983;99:265–76.
65. Parrington J, Swann K, Shevchenko VI, Sesay AK, Lai FA. Calcium oscillations in mammalian eggs triggered by a soluble sperm protein. Nature. 1996;379:364–8.
66. Tesarik J. Sperm-induced calcium oscillations. Oscillin—reopening the hunting season. Mol Hum Reprod. 1998;4:1007–12.
67. Saunders M, Larman G, Parrington J, Cox J, Royse J, Blayney M, et al. PLC zeta: a sperm-specific trigger of Ca(2+) oscillations in eggs and embryo development. Development. 2002;129:3533–44.
68. Kouchi Z, Fukami K, Shikano T, Oda S, Nakamura Y, et al. Recombinant phospholipase Czeta has high Ca^{2+} sensitivity and induces Ca^{2+} oscillations in mouse eggs. J Biol Chem. 2004;279:10408–12.
69. Swann K, Larman G, Saunders M, Lai A. The cytosolic sperm factor that triggers Ca^{2+} oscillations and egg activation in mammals is a novel phospholipase C: PLCzeta. Reproduction. 2004;127:431–9.
70. Saunders CM, Swann K, Lai FA. PLCzeta, a sperm-specific PLC and its potential role in fertilization. Biochem Soc Symp. 2007;74:23–36.
71. Dupont G. Theoretical insights into the mechanism of spiral Ca^{2+} wave initiation in Xenopus oocytes. Am J Physiol. 1998;275:C317–22.
72. Eliyahu E, Shalgi R. A role for protein kinase C during rat egg activation. Biol Reprod. 2002;67:189–95.
73. Talmor-Cohen A, Tomashov-Matar R, Eliyahu E, Shapiro R, Shalgi R. Are Src family kinases involved in cell cycle resumption in rat eggs? Reproduction. 2004;127:455–63.
74. Sette C, Bevilacqua A, Bianchini A, Mangia F, Geremia R, Rossi P. Parthenogenetic activation of mouse eggs by microinjection of a truncated c-kit tyrosine kinase present in spermatozoa. Development. 1997;124:2267–74.
75. Sette C, Paronetto MP, Barchi M, Bevilacqua A, Geremia R, Rossi P. Tr-kit-induced resumption of the cell cycle in mouse eggs requires activation of a Src-like kinase. EMBO J. 2002;21:5386–95.
76. Wu A, Sutovsky P, Manandhar G, Xu W, Katayama M, Day BN, et al. PAWP a sperm-specific WW domain-binding protein, promotes meiotic resumption and pronuclear development during fertilization. J Biol Chem. 2007;282:12164–75.
77. Hewitson L, Simerly CR, Schatten G. Fate of sperm components during assisted reproduction: implications for infertility. Hum Fertil (Camb). 2002;5:110–6.
78. Schatten G. The centrosome and its mode of inheritance: the reduction of the centrosome during gametogenesis and its restoration during fertilization. Dev Biol. 1994;165:299–335.
79. Allan V. Role of motor proteins in organizing the endoplasmic reticulum and Golgi apparatus. Semi Cell Dev Biol. 1996;7:335–42.
80. Payne C, Rawe V, Ramalho-Santos J, Simerly C, Schatten G. Preferentially localized dynein and perinuclear dynactin associate with nuclear pore complex proteins to mediate genomic union during mammalian fertilization. J Cell Sci. 2003;116:4727–38.
81. Helfand T, Mikami A, Vallee B, Goldman D. A requirement for cytoplasmic dynein and dynactin in intermediate filament network assembly and organization. J Cell Biol. 2002;157:795–806.
82. Sheeman B, Carvalho P, Sagot I, Geiser J, Kho D, et al. Determinants of S. cerevisiae dynein localization and activation: implications for the mechanism of spindle positioning. Curr Biol. 2003;13:364–72.
83. Ostermeier C, Miller D, Huntriss D, Diamond P, Krawetz A. Reproductive biology: delivering spermatozoan RNA to the oocyte. Nature. 2004;429:154.
84. Ostermeier C, Goodrich J, Moldenhauer S, Diamond P, Krawetz A. A suite of novel human spermatozoal RNAs. J Androl. 2005;26:70–4.
85. Miller D. RNA in the ejaculate spermatozoon: a window into molecular events in spermatogenesis and a record of the unusual requirements of haploid gene expression and post-meiotic equilibration. Mol Hum Reprod. 1997;3:669–76.
86. Dadoune JP, Pawlak A, Alfonso MF, Siffro JP. Identification of transcripts by macroarrays, RT—PCR and in situ hybridization in human ejaculate spermatozoa. Mol Hum Reprod. 2005;11:133–40.
87. Avendaño C, Franchi A, Oehninger S. Pregnancy-specific {beta}-1-glycoprotein 1 and human leukocyte antigen-E mRNA in human sperm: differential expression in fertile and infertile men and evidence of a possible functional role during early development. Hum Reprod. 2009;24:270–7.
88. Hall JE. Female physiology before pregnancy and female hormones. In: Guyton and Hall Textbook of Medical Physiology. 12th ed. Philadelphia: W.B. Saunders; 2011.
89. Andrews CJ. Migrating Grafenberg contraception ring. J Am Med Assoc. 1936;107:279.

90. Beitins IZ, McArthur JW, Turnbull BA, Skrinar GS, Bullen BA. Exercise induces two types of human luteal dysfunction: confirmation by urinary free progesterone. J Clin Endocrinol Metab. 1991;72:1350–8.
91. Kossman DA, Williams NI, Domchek SM, Kurzer MS, Stopfer JE, Schmitz KH. Exercise lowers estrogen and progesterone levels in premenopausal women at high risk of breast cancer. J App Physiol. 2011;111:1687–93.
92. DeSouza MJ. Menstrual disturbances in athletes: a focus on luteal phase defects. Med Sci Sport Exerc. 2003;35:1553–63.
93. Bullen BA, Skrinar HS, Beitins IZ, von Mering G, Turnbull BA, McArthur JW. Induction of menstrual disorders by strenuous exercise in untrained women. N Engl J Med. 1985;312:1349–53.
94. Williams NI, Caston-Bolderrama AL, Helmreich DL, Parfitt DB, Nosbisch C, Cameron JL. Longitudinal changes in reproductive hormones and menstrual cyclicity in cynomolgus monkeys during strenuous exercise training: abrupt transition to exercise-induced amenorrhea. Endocrinology. 2001;2:2381–9.
95. Williams NI, Helmreich DL, Parfitt DB, Caston-Balderrama A, Cameron JL. Evidence for a causal rol of low energy availability in the induction of menstrual cycle disturbances during strenuous exercise training. J Clin Endocrinol Metab. 2001;86:5184–93.
96. Loucks AB, Thuma JR. Luteinizing hormone pulsatility is disrupted at a threshold of energy availability in regularly menstruating women. J Clin Endocrinol Metab. 2003;88:297–311.
97. Williams NI. Lessons from experimental disruptions of the menstrual cycle in humans and monkeys. Med Sci Sports Exerc. 2003;35:1564–72.
98. Loucks AB, Thuma JR. Luteinizing hormone pulsatility is disrupted at a threshold of energy availability in regularly menstruating women. J Clin Endocrinol Metab. 2003;88:297–311.
99. Zalányi S. Progesterone and ovulation. Eur J Obstet Gynecol Reprod Biol. 2001;98:152–9.
100. Usandizaga JA, De La, Fuente P. *Obstetricia y Ginecología*. 4th ed. Madrid: Marban; 2011.
101. Cunningham FG, Leveno KJ, Bloom SL, Hauth JC, Rouse DJ, Spong CY. Williams obstetrics. 23rd ed. New York: The McGraw-Hill Companies, Inc.; 2010.
102. Friedman EA. Primigravid labor; a graphicostatistical analysis. Obstet Gynecol. 1955;6:567–89.
103. Matorras R, Remohi J, Serra V. Casos Clínicos de Ginecología y Obstetricia. Editorial *Médica Panamericana*, Madrid; 2011.
104. Bonica JJ. Principles and practice of obstetric analgesia and anesthesia. Philadelphia: FA Davis; 1967. p. 24.

Conceptual and Terminological Foundations for the Sciences of Physical Exercise: New Perspectives

4

Marzo Edir Da Silva-Grigoletto and Juan Ramón Heredia Elvar

Introduction

The aim of this chapter is to introduce the reader to some of the general aspects of the terminology and basic concepts related to the practice of physical exercise and sports training. A working understanding of these concepts enables the practice of physical exercise and its relationship to fertility in men and women to be placed in the correct context.

Such knowledge is fundamental for an in-depth analysis of the adaptive responses that take place as a consequence of training and their relationship with performance, but it also enables the relationships to be established between physical exercise and improvement in health, both in a sportsperson and a physically active individual. It is a well-established fact that an active lifestyle has important benefits for people's quality of life [1], and that sedentary habits are associated with a deterioration of health in general [2]. Intense sporting activity, however, as opposed to light exercise undertaken on a regular basis for recreational purposes, entails by its very nature a certain level of risk that needs to be eliminated, or at least reduced, if it is to become a healthy and non-harmful occupation for the sportsperson.

In this chapter, certain aspects of these points will be addressed that allow a new perspective on all these concepts, from a point of view that is more in line with the actual needs of health-related interventions in the prescription of physical activity. Finally, some proposals will be put forward, enabling improved oversight of the exercise "dose" as a fundamental factor for understanding the relationship between physical exercise, health, and fertility.

What Are Physical Activity, Physical Exercise, and Sport?

It appears to be common in popular culture to use the word "sport" as a way of referring to any "type" of physical exercise; even in other areas of knowledge, the term is applied regardless of context and without any truly objective benchmark, which makes it essential to define this term at the outset and specify the limits of its use even more strictly in relation to others such as "physical activity" and "physical exercise."

Regrettably, many studies suffer from a degree of confusion or lack of definition of some of the parameters that determine the concept of physical exercise, as well as its application. To this end, the following are offered as operation definitions to clarify potential misunderstandings.

M. E. Da Silva-Grigoletto (✉)
Department of Physical Education, Universidade Federal de Sergipe, Rua Napoleao Dorea, 165 (casa 03), Aracaju, SE 49037-460, Brazil
e-mail: pit_researcher@yahoo.es

J. R. Heredia Elvar
Department of Fitness and Health, International Institute for Exercise Science and Health, Alfàs del Pi, Spain

© Springer Science+Business Media New York 2016

D. Vaamonde et al. (eds.), *Exercise and Human Reproduction,* DOI 10.1007/978-1-4939-3402-7_4

Sport may be understood as "physical activity, undertaken as a game or competition, the practice of which involves training and submission to rules," whether performed as a professional occupation or as an activity oriented towards recreation, pastime, pleasure, or diversion for those who engage in it.

Sport

Sport may be defined as an activity that is played (all sports start off as games, with a playful character); with specific motor requirements (they entail physical and motor demands limited to the selfsame determinants of the activity); is competitive (there is a need to exceed or overcome a score or one or more adversaries); and has codified and standardized rules and a high degree of institutionalization (they are governed by official institutions) [3].

Physical Activity and Physical Exercise

Physical activity is regarded as any bodily movement generated by skeletal muscles that requires the expenditure of energy [4]. Taking this definition as one's starting point, it is important to differentiate clearly between "physical activity" and "physical exercise," since the latter entails a physical activity with a goal (maintaining, improving, or recovering physical condition and health) and pays strict attention to questions of programming, periodicity, and prescription to this end.

The term "physical exercise" (from the Latin, *exercitĭum*) is defined as: "a set of bodily movements that are carried out to maintain or improve physical fitness." A bodily "movement" may therefore only be considered as exercise when the act of choosing it and its execution variables (the "dose"), integrated into the context of a training program, fulfill appropriate and attested criteria involving sufficient stimulation to be able to maintain, improve or recover physical fitness and health [4].

Classical Control Parameters for Training Workloads

From the classical or traditional point of view, the training "workload" has been defined in terms of four fundamental variables: frequency, volume, intensity, and recovery. Although it may be necessary to modify some of these parameters, what follows is an attempt to give a brief description of the parameters from the classical perspective [5–12]. The appropriate management of these factors will cause an adaptive response in the sportsperson's organism, which should have direct repercussions on sporting performance [13–15].

The variables of frequency, volume, and recovery are relatively easy to ascertain and quantify (especially when dealing with endurance events), whereas the intensity variable turns out to be a more complicated parameter, despite being a key determinant in the adaptations that come from training [16]. Thus, it is necessary not only to give a definition of these factors but also relate them to the type of sport being undertaken (endurance or resistance), given that this governs the very definition and the means of ascertaining the factors.

Volume

This is a training variable that proves to be relatively easy to define and quantify from a classical perspective, since it is related to mainly quantitative factors [17–21].

- In endurance training, it is defined as the distance covered or the number of hours of training during a period or cycle of the planned work program (session, microcycle, mesocycle, macrocycle, or season);
- In resistance training, it is defined on the basis of the number of tons, kilos, sets, or repetitions completed during a period of time or cycles of the training program.

Frequency

Frequency of training is a variable that refers to the number of times a sportsperson trains within a given period of time [17]. There is a close connection between the variables of frequency and volume, in that the latter can rise and fall owing to variations in the former.

Intensity

Owing to the fact that intensity, in contrast with volume, is a variable related to qualitative aspects, it has certain characteristics that make its definition and determination more difficult [17, 21].

- In endurance training, it is defined as speed or a percentage (%) of the maximum value of one of the following parameters: maximum heart rate, heart rate reserve, maximum oxygen uptake, oxygen uptake reserve, ventilator thresholds, as well as on the basis of measures of blood lactate concentration and maximum heart reserve;
- In resistance training, it is common to refer to values relative to a force applied against a resistance that is impossible to move (maximum isometric force) or a resistance that is possible to move only once (maximum repetition) obtained through a specific test or by applying indirect estimation formulas.
- Another possibility for establishing intensity involves using various perceive exertion scales of subjective perception of effort that have been validated for both endurance (Borg Scale) and resistance Omni-Resistance Scale (OMNI-RES) events [20].

Recovery
This refers to the time that elapses between stimuli, with the character of the recovery also needing to be taken into account, in other words the activity that is carried out in this period (active vs. passive). It is directly related to the capacity to undertake or repeat activations of a certain intensity [17, 21]. Similarly, the type of recovery (active or passive) that is used needs to be considered. Recovery is a variable that is used in a similar way, with regard to the physiological objective, for both endurance and resistance events.

Why Is It Necessary to Vary the Stimuli to Acquire Adaptations?

The aforementioned training parameters and factors need to be used appropriately with the aim of providing constant and sufficient levels of stimuli to ensure the desired changes. It is advisable that they are varied in form, intensity, and volume in order to avoid standstills in the response being sought. To this end, there exists a set of operational strategies that allow not only the stimulus to be controlled and graduated, but also a succession of stimuli to be organized, enabling suitable synergies between them. These conceptual approaches are relevant to understanding the relationship between physical exercise or sport and their impact on the psychobiological system and especially how these activities affect the reproductive system.

In this respect, it is necessary to be acquainted with some of these methodological strategies, which will be fundamentally defined on the basis of organizational and functional parameters [22–26].

Planning
"Planning" processes refer to the first phase of drawing up a training program. This involves the establishing of the general operative plan in relation to the individual subject, his or her level of physical fitness and health, the objectives and considering the various organizational structures.

As far as training for sports performance is concerned, the planning structures can span multiyear and/or yearly cycles (seasons); in the domain of training for health however, such structures can only realistically and in practice extend to monthly or multi-monthly cycles, annual cycles being too difficult to arrange. The aforementioned yearly period is usually divided into smaller structures spanning various months, known as "macrocycles." These macrocycles in turn contain various intermediate structures known as mesocycles, which have a duration of various weeks. Similarly, the mesocycles are operationally subdivided into more elemental structures known as microcycle, the duration of which normally corresponds to a number of days close to a week.

Within the context of sporting performance, it is also common to find another operational process known as "periodization" and which is related more to the sequencing and variation of the training load.

Periodization
This is defined as the aspect devoted to sequencing the activities that make up the training cycle, in particular periods of time, with well-estab-

lished objectives and contents. Similarly, the expression "periodize" refers to the systematic and planned variation of specific components or variables in the training activity.

Reflections regarding a new proposal for the definition and control of the variables in the training dose.

As indicated above, in order to be able to intervene appropriately with a training program, and achieve the psychobiological adaptations sought, it is necessary to differentiate between training programs oriented towards high-performance athletes and those applied to a health-seeking population (on the understanding that in the latter case the sole objective is to maintain suitable levels of physical fitness, without being influenced by the need to obtain a maximum level of performance in a sporting specialty).

Correctly understanding the possible limitations of this reality marks the step in being able to put forward a more nuanced reflection on the subject under study. The nonsporting individual does not possess the same temporal availability, aims, motivation, or potential capacity for response-adaptation, or seek to achieve high levels of fitness. All these factors significantly limit the capacity to operate in relation to many of the organizational structures mentioned above.

Thus, it is difficult (not to say impossible) to be able to operate with long-term structures (1 year or longer) in populations that have as their aim the maintenance or improvement of their health. Neither their availability, nor their capacity or motivation is comparable. As a consequence, the dose–response relationship in training workloads exhibits significant differences that should always to be taken into account in designing training programs and the possible effects that these will have on the sportsperson's organism.

From this perspective, the traditional definition of these variables is found to provide somewhat limited information, which is inadequate for operating effectively or even properly comparing different interventions to establish the most appropriate in the context of health.

So with regard to the aforementioned variables, we propose the following definition:

Frequency

Although sportspeople find this parameter easy to manipulate (owing to their availability), it is something that is often less flexible in health-based programs, because the individuals involved do not enjoy complete availability and it depends upon the free time that they have at their disposal in their daily lives. Despite this, its definition remains broadly similar to the classical conception of the number of training units or sessions during a fixed period of time (normally a microcycle).

Volume

The authors find certain shortcomings and a lack of value in the measures used to define this variable. Considering only the number of kilos, tons, sets, repetitions, or kilometers does not sufficiently capture a variable that is so important for periodization.

It is therefore suggested that the volume variable be defined more concretely and operatively, differentiating according to the type of training:

- In the case of endurance training: the duration of this type of training, the total time of each stimulus, and the number of stimuli should be considered.

Total duration/number of blocks or sets × stimulus duration

- In the case of resistance training: the duration of this type of training, the number of exercises, and the number of sets should be considered.

Total duration/number of exercises × number of set

Intensity

In the case of this variable, it is necessary to delve deeper into the method proposed for resistance training, given that it has been developed by estimating the hypothetical value of 1 repetition maximum (RM), and it is a parameter that is too variable to be given such a specific value. Similarly, with regard to endurance training, the ability to complement a suitable check by means of other components that supplement measurements of heart rate or maximal oxygen uptake is indispensable. It is currently highly advisable to define and monitor such a key variable in training in a broader way.

- For endurance training, intensity may be defined in terms of the classic values of maximum heart rate, heart rate reserve, maximal oxygen uptake, oxygen uptake reserve, breathing thresholds, as well as by using values for the concentration of blood lactate and maximum heart reserve, complemented by the use of perceived exertion scales. From a practical point of view, however, monitoring on the basis of more accessible parameters is proposed, such as percentages of heart rate (HR; maximum or reserve) and the use of perceived exertions scales (PES).

$\%\ HR_{max}$ or $VO_{2max}\ldots + PES$

- The resistance training variable could be defined on the basis of estimating the number of repetitions carried out against a resistance with respect to a speed or cadence of execution and linking it to a perceived exertion scale of the OMNI-RES type.

Number of repetitions × speed of execution + OMNI-RES

Density
This would be defined as the relationship between the duration of the exertion and the length (duration) of the break period for recovery or rest.

Although it is a key factor in determining training workloads, this is a parameter that is frequently overlooked or undervalued in studies. The alteration of this relationship, lengthening or shortening the duration of the recovery period compared to the duration of the exertion will affect the intense responses (metabolic, hormonal, and cardiovascular) and the adaptations caused by the training stimuli. Therefore, such a relationship (stimulus/break) will be dependent on the physiological aim and the exercise training level of the subject concerned.

Conclusion

In conclusion, these reflections and proposals for the definition and determination of variables/factors is only a simplified version of the suggestions developed by our research group to improve the way in which the training dose is established (quantified) in physical exercise programs used for the improvement of health and quality of life. For a more detailed proposal, in which the means of establishing the variables are set out in greater depth, we invite readers to consult the document entitled "Reflection and new proposals for defining and controlling the dose in physical exercise and health programs" [2].

References

1. Diehl JJ, Choi H. Exercise: the data on its role in health, mental health, disease prevention, and productivity. Prim Care: Clin Off Pract. 2008;35(4):803–16.
2. Heredia-Elvar, JR, Peña García-Oreo, G, Isidro, F, Mata, F, Da Silva Grigoletto, ME. Reflection and new proposals for defining and controlling the dose in physical exercise and health programs. Rev Andal Med Dep. In Press.
3. Hernández Moreno J. Fundamentos del deporte. Análisis de las estructuras del juego deportivo. Barcelona: INDE; 1994.
4. World Health Organization (WHO). Global strategy on diet, physical activity and health: Physical activity. 2014. http://www.who.int/dietphysicalactivity/pa/en/. Consulted 24/02/2013. Accessed 15 Dec 2014.
5. DeLorme TL, Watkins AL. Techniques of progressive resistance exercise. Arch Phys Med. 1948;29:263–73.
6. Verjonshanki, IV. Entrenamiento Deportivo: Planificación y Programación. Barcelona: Ediciones Martínez Roca.1990.
7. Grosser M, Starischa S. Principios del entrenamiento deportivo. Barcelona: Martínez y Roca; 1988.
8. Bompa T. Theory and methodology of training. Dubuque: Kendal/Hunt; 1994.
9. Platonov VN. El entrenamiento deportivo, teoría y metodología. 4th ed. Barcelona: Paidotribo; 1995.
10. Kraemer WJ. Exercise prescription in weight training: manipulating program variables. Natl Strength Cond Assoc J. 1983;5:58–61.
11. Viru A. About training loads. Mod Athl Coach. 1993;31(4):32–6.

12. Zatsiorsky VM. Science and practice of strength training. Champaign: Human Kinetics; 1995.
13. Viru A. Mecanismos de adaptación biológica y entrenamiento. Rev Entrenamiento Deportivo. 1996;9(2):6–11.
14. Kraemer WJ. Exercise prescription in weight training: manipulating program variables. Natl Strength Cond Assoc J. 1983;5:58–61.
15. Zintl F. Entrenamiento de la Resistencia. Fundamentos, métodos y dirección del Entrenamiento. Barcelona: Ediciones Martinez Roca; 1991.
16. Kraemer WJ, Deschenes MR, Fleck SJ. Physiological adaptations to resistance exercise. Implications for athletic conditioning. Sports Med. 1988;6:246–56.
17. Baechle TR, Earle RW, Wathen D. Resistance training. In: Baechle TR, Earle RW, editors. Essentials of strength training and conditioning. 2nd ed. Champaign: Human Kinetics; 2000. p. 395–425.
18. Feigenbaum MS, Pollock ML. Prescription of resistance training for health and disease. Med Sci Sports Exerc. 1999;31(38–45):11.
19. Tan B. Manipulating resistance training program variables to optimize maximum strength in men: a review. J Strength Cond Res. 1999;13:289–304.
20. Knuttgen HG, y Kraemer WJ. Terminology and measurement in exercise performance. J Appl Sports Sci Res. 1987;1:1–10.
21. United States Department of Health and Human Services. Physical activity guidelines for Americans. Be active, healthy, and happy! Washington, DC: U.S. Dept. of Health and Human Services; 2008.
22. Bompa TO. Periodization of strength training: the new wave in strength training. Toronto: Veritas Publis. Inc; 1993.
23. Bompa TO. Variations of periodization of strength. Strength Cond. 1996;18(3):58–61.
24. Stone MH, O'bryant H, Garhammer J, Mcmillan J, Rozenek R. A theoretical model of strength training. NSCA J. 1982;4:36–9.
25. Rhea MR, Ball SD, Phillips WT, Burkett A. A comparison of linear and daily undulating periodized programs with equated volume and intensity for strength. J Strength Cond Res. 2002;16(2):250–5.
26. Rhea MR, Alvar BA, Burkett LN, Ball SD. A meta-analysis to determine the dose response for strength development. Med Sci Sport Exerc. 2003;35:456–64.

Sports Physiology and Endocrinology (Endurance vs. Resistance Exercise)

5

Anthony C. Hackney and Mehis Viru

Introduction

In the past few years, there has been a growing realization that increased amounts of physical activity and exercise training in an individual's life offers health benefits from both a preventative and intervention perspective. To those unfamiliar with the scientific discipline of Exercise Physiology, the terms "physical activity" and "exercise training" may seem mutually inclusive; however, that is not entirely the case. Physical activity refers to all forms of muscular activity encountered in daily life, which could be as simple as walking to the bus stop, working in a garden, cleaning in one's home, or going for a stroll with your dog in the park. Exercise training, however, refers to specific time set aside to perform muscular activity with the intent of improving one's physical performance or fitness by conducting such activity. Exercise training therefore can be associated with individuals wishing to improve just overall general health and well-being or for those desiring to enhance sporting performance, that is, individuals who are athletes.

A. C. Hackney (✉)
Department of Exercise & Sport Science, Department of Nutrition, University of North Carolina, 203 Fetzer Hall, South Rd., Chapel Hill, NC 27599, USA
e-mail: ach@email.unc.edu

M. Viru
Faculty of Exercise and Sport Sciences, University of Tartu, Tartu, Estonia

Individuals involved with exercise for the intent of improving health and well-being may typically carry out a training "exercise prescription" comprising 3–5 days a week of activity, for 30–60 min in duration at a moderate to moderately vigorous intensity [1]. This 1.5–5 h commitment per week is challenging for many average people to achieve. In the case of elite athletes, this volume of activity might represent what they typically do in a single day of their exercise training regimen. Such large dosages of exercise in athletes, when administered chronically, bring about large and substantial physiological adjustment and adaptation, which many experts feel is necessary to enhance sporting performance to the highest levels [2, 3].

Achieving the highest levels of sport performance is dependent on adjustments and adaptations in a multitude of physiological systems including: the cardiovascular, respiratory, metabolic, muscular, and endocrine systems. The latter, the endocrine system, is critical and highly influential in numerous capacities to induce and regulate the responses being pursued through exercise training. To this end, this chapter will review the responses and adjustments/adaptation of the endocrine system with respect to exercise training in athletes involved in endurance training versus those involved in resistance training sporting activities. Table 5.1 presents several examples of sporting activities that fit into each of these categories.

To aid in the clear and concise discussion of this topic, it is important to present some opera-

© Springer Science+Business Media New York 2016
D. Vaamonde et al. (eds.), *Exercise and Human Reproduction*, DOI 10.1007/978-1-4939-3402-7_5

Table 5.1 Examples of sporting activities that can be categorized as endurance versus resistance based upon the emphasis placed in the exercise training for an athlete

Sporting activity	
Endurance	Resistance
5000–10,000 m run	Shot put
Half marathon—marathon	Discus throw
20–50 km race walk	Javelin throw
Olympic distance triathlon	Hammer throw
Ironman triathlon	Olympic style weightlifting
Cycling—road racing	Power lifting
Cycling—individual time trial	Wrestling

tional definitions of terms and concepts for the reader. *Sport physiology* is the application of the discipline of exercise physiology to the special demands of sport. Specifically, it involves applying the concepts derived from exercise physiology to optimize the training of athletes and enhance their physical performance (i.e., competition). *Endocrinology* is that branch of physiological–medical sciences that deals with the endocrine-related activities of glands and tissues that release hormones. In turn, a *hormone* is a chemical substance, formed in one gland/tissue of the body and carried in the blood to another gland/tissue where it exerts functional effects (i.e., endocrine function). Additionally, this definition of hormones has been recently broadened to include chemical substances formed by cells of the tissue, which in turn act on neighboring cells (i.e., paracrine function) or the same cells that produce them (i.e., autocrine function). In assessing and quantifying exercise training, it is critical to understand the concept of exercise dosage. *Exercise dosage* consists of "how much" exercise an individual is being exposed to in their training regime. The components which are manipulated to modulate the dosage are the duration (volume) of an exercise session, the frequency of exercise sessions per day–week, and the intensity of effort within a respective exercise session. The first two components of dosage are self-explanatory, but intensity is somewhat more complex. Classically, the perception of how difficult intense exercise is has been linked to cardiovascular responses, usually expressed as a percentage of maximal heart rate (HR_{max}) or maximal oxygen uptake (VO_{2max}, which represents the amount of oxygen being utilized by body tissues which is proportional to overall energy expenditure; VO_2 = (heart rate × stroke volume) × arteriovenous oxygen content differential; [4, 5]). For endurance-based sport activities (e.g., 10,000 m distance run), there is a high reliance on the cardiovascular system and aerobic energy metabolism to determine performance capacity. This means for such activities, the expressing of intensity relative to VO_{2max} or HR_{max} is appropriate, although VO_{2max} is recognized as the "gold standard." On the other hand, resistance-based sport activities are highly explosive in muscular force–power output (e.g., shot put, hammer throw) and performance is far less dependent upon cardiovascular functioning and much more so on anaerobic energy production pathways. For such activities, the expression of intensity based upon VO_{2max} or HR_{max} are far less valid (although, in some situations the intensity of some such activities is still expressed relative to VO_{2max}; [5]). In the latter sporting activities, since resistance exercise training is a predominant component, the expression of exercise intensity is based upon percentage of maximal performance relative to a resistance task (i.e., the lifting of a specific amount of weight). The reference criterion here is the 1 repetition maximum (1 RM). This represents the maximal weight–force that can be generated for that task and signifies an intensity capacity of 100 %. Thus, submaximal intensity efforts are a percentage of the maximal weight–force generated (e.g., task, bench press → 1 RM = 120 kg; therefore, 60 % effort = 72 kg; [6]).

Table 5.2 presents some examples, explanation and terminology to aid in understanding the intensity concept and how this aspect of dosage is quantified in the sport physiology research literature [1, 7, 8]. On reviewing the table, it is obvious that team sport activities such as football (soccer) or field hockey are not represented. These sports activities are multidimensional in the demands that are placed on the physiology of the athlete and the intensity of their efforts (i.e., highly variable)—influenced by the position of play of the athlete, the competitiveness of the

Table 5.2 Examples of endurance and resistance exercise actives classified by different levels of intensity

Category term	Effort perception	Relative intensity	Energy pathway predominating	Representative duration (minute)	Other terminology	Sporting examples
Endurance						
Light exercise	Easy	<35% VO_{2max}	Aerobic	>30	Short term, submaximal	Warm-up activities
Moderate exercise	Modest difficulty	<70>35% VO_{2max}	Aerobic	30–180	Submaximal, prolonged	Cycle-run training
Heavy exercise	Difficult	<100>70% VO_{2max}	Aerobic–anaerobic	≤120	Submaximal, prolonged, high intensity	10,000 m, marathon run, triathlons
Maximal exercise	Strenuous	100% VO_{2max}	Aerobic–anaerobic	<15	Maximal or max, high intensity	1500–5000 m runs
Supramaximal exercise	Extremely strenuous	>100% VO_{2max}	Anaerobic	<1	All out, power	100–400 m sprints
Resistance						
Submaximal exercise	Modest—difficult	<70>35% 1 RM	Aerobic–anaerobic	≥1	Submaximal	Circuit resistance training
Maximal exercise	Extremely strenuous	~100% 1 RM	Anaerobic	<0.1	All out, power	Shot put, javelin, Olympic lifts
Supramaximal exercise	Extremely strenuous	>100% 1 RM	Anaerobic	≤0.1	Negatives	Eccentric resistance training

game, and action-events in the game. Thus, quantifying intensity in such sports gaming activities is extremely difficult. This difficulty makes it a highly complex area to study in sports physiology, and far more research is needed in the area of team sports.

Endocrine Responses

Acute Exercise

The acute responses of the major physiological systems to a single bout of exercise (training) or a sporting event (competition) can be large and robust and are usually proportional to the intensity of the exercise (most certainly for endurance events), although it is important to recognize that the relationship of this proportional response(s) is not always linear in nature [7]. Table 5.3 presents the major physiological systems and some of the key parameters reflective of the respective systems and how these parameters change in response to an exercise session/sports event based upon the emphasis of the activity being either endurance or resistance based in nature.

As noted earlier, the primary focus in this chapter is the endocrine system responses to exercise. Table 5.3 illustrates the general changes for a variety of hormones in response to endurance–resistance exercise. It is important to recognize, however, that many of these hormonal responses are and not independent of one another but highly interrelated. To illustrate this point, Dr. Henrik Galbo devised an explanatory model of the hormonal responses to exercise consisting of three interactive phases [9, 10]. The first phase of this model deals with the hormonal response immediately at the onset of exercise, with these responses taking just seconds to occur. These responses revolve around the increased sympathetic nervous system (SNS) activation that occurs with the onset of body motion. This increased SNS activity can also be a result of anticipation to the stress of the ensuing exercise, which is most certainly the case in sport competition scenarios. This increased SNS activity results in catecholamine (norepinephrine) release at target tis-

Table 5.3 Physiological responses to an acute exercise session based upon whether the activity is predominating involved with endurance or resistance forms of exercise activity. It is important to note that the changes in measure/parameter denoted here are relative to before versus immediately after the activity. It is well documented that as an athlete moves into the recovery period from exercise measure/parameter changes can be different from those observed at the completion of exercise [8, 9, 77]

Physiological systems	Measure/parameter	Exercise-sport activity predominating training component	
		Endurance	Resistance
Cardiovascular	Heart rate	↑	↑
	Stroke volume	↑	↑↓
	Cardiac output	↑	↑↓
	Arteriovenous O_2 difference	↑	↑↓
Respiratory	Tidal volume	↑↑	↑
	Breathing frequency	↑↑	↑
	Minute ventilation	↑↑	↑
Metabolic	ATP → ADP + Pi + energy	↑	↑↑
	CP → creatine + phosphate + energy	↑	↑↑
	Anaerobic glycolysis	↑	↑↑
	Aerobic glycolysis	↑↑	↑↓
	Tricarboxylic acid cycle	↑↑	↑↓, nc
	β-oxidation cycle	↑↑	↑↓, nc
Muscle	Force	↑	↑↑
	Power	↑	↑↑
	Endurance	↑↑	↑
Endocrine	Adrenocorticotrophic hormone (ACTH)	↑	↑
	Aldosterone	↑	↑
	Angiotensin	↑	↑
	Antidiuretic hormone (ADH)	↑	↑↓
	Cortisol	↑	↑
	Dehydroepiandrosterone (DHEA)	↑	↑
	β-Endorphin	↑	↑
	Epinephrine (adrenaline)	↑↑	↑↑
	Estrogens	↑	↑
	Follicle-stimulating hormone (FSH)	↑↓, nc	↑↓, nc
	Glucagon	↑	↑
	Growth hormone (GH)	↑	↑
	Insulin	↓	↑↓, nc
	Insulin-like growth factor-1 (IGF-1)	↑, nc	↑, nc
	Leptin	↑↓, nc	↑↓, nc
	Luteinizing hormone (LH)	↑↓, nc	↑↓, nc
	Norepinephrine (noradrenaline)	↑↑	↑↑
	Progesterone	↑	↑
	Prolactin (PRL)	↑	↑
	Testosterone	↑	↑
	Thyroxine (T4)	↑	↑
	Triiodothyronine (T3)	↑	↑
	Vitamin D	↑	?

ATP adenosine triphosphate, *ADP* adenosine diphosphate, *CP* creatine phosphate, *Pi* phosphate, ↑ increase, ↑↑ large increase, ↓ decrease, ↑↓ possible increase or decrease, *nc* no change, *?* unresolved

sues directly as well as elevations in circulating catecholamine from so-called sympathetic spill-over effects [9–11]. This effect is further amplified by the sympathetic connection to the adrenal medullary gland, which in turn adds to the circulating catecholamine (epinephrine) response [10, 12]. Concurrent with these sympathetic–adrenal actions, pancreatic insulin secretion begins to be inhibited while glucagon secretion becomes stimulated [10]. This entire process involves a feed-forward mechanism of the central nervous system to drive these initial responses, although the events are also modified by peripheral afferent neural input from sensory receptors in particular those of skeletal muscle [12, 13].

The intermediate or secondary phase takes slightly longer to develop but is still typically very fast, beginning usually in much less than a minute from the onset of exercise. In this stage, the hypothalamus begins the process of releasing its hormones such as thyrotropin-releasing factor, corticotropin-releasing factor (CRF), and growth hormone-releasing factor (GHRF) in an attempt to provoke changes at the anterior pituitary gland to stimulate the release of select hormones. As the pituitary begins to respond to the hypothalamic stimulus, its "trophic hormones" begin to be added to the circulation, and these hormones begin to act upon their specific peripheral target glands to stimulate additional hormonal release. One of the most rapidly acting in this cascade of events is the hypothalamic–pituitary–adrenocortical interaction where CRF brings about adrenocorticotrophic hormone (ACTH) release and that in turn brings about cortisol release [8, 13, 14].

If the duration of an exercise session continues, there is a transition beyond the intermediate phase into a third phase of response which is a more prolonged state. In this third phase, the responses of the sympathetic–adrenal axis are being augmented by other hormones from the anterior and posterior pituitary (e.g., ADH, GH, PRL; see Table 5.3 for hormonal abbreviations) and the peripheral endocrine glands subordinated to pituitary regulation (testosterone, T4, T3, IGF-1; [7, 8]). Additionally, during this phase, the skeletal muscle begins to release select cytokines (e.g., interleukin-6, IL-6), hormonal-like agents, into the circulation, which affect other hormones to be released (IL-6 $\Rightarrow$ cortisol; [15]).

Phase one and two of the model propose that neural factors are the primary stimuli regulating the hormonal responses to exercise; however, in the third phase of response, there is an ever-increasing influence of the humoral and hormonal factors that regulate the overall responses due to the changes in the "internal milieu" [10]. This shifting of primary regulatory factors allows an increasing reliance upon feedback rather than feed-forward control mechanism to determine the magnitude of the hormonal response. The influence of humoral and hormonal stimuli in modulating the hormonal levels are magnified as the exercise duration is extended, and energy substrate availability issues cause shifts in energy fuel usage (i.e., $\downarrow$ carbohydrate $\Rightarrow\uparrow$ lipid) or hydration issues (i.e., hemoconcentration and/or dehydration), which begin compromising the thermoregulatory ability and lead to greater heat storage within the body affecting hormonal responses (e.g., $\uparrow$ heat storage $\Rightarrow\uparrow$ norepinephrine, epinephrine; [4, 12, 13]). A need for conciseness does not allow for a more extensive discussion of all of the intricate details of hormonal responses to exercise, but the model of Galbo does illustrate that endocrine actions are highly interactive and complex [9, 10].

Chronic Exercise

The general responses of the body's various physiological systems to an exercise bout/session after performing a progressive exercise training regime (chronic exposure) are similar to those as before such training. In other words, an acute bout of exercise after chronic training is still a stimulus to the physiology of the body. However, at all exercise intensities, less than the maximal level, such responses are typically attenuated to some extent. The greater the training adaption incurred due to the training regime, the greater is the attenuation of the response. The exception to this occurrence is maximal or supramaximal exercise. In such situations, the training adaptations result in a great level of workload performed at maximal/supramaximal efforts, for example, the athlete can run further or run faster over a fixed distance or lift a greater maximal amount weight, etc. The greater absolute maximal workload achievement in turn produces a greater physiological stimulus and thus comparable (or greater) maximal responses in the measures/parameters of the physiological systems, in other words, typically not an attenuation of responses. A noted allowance to this generalization is HR_{max}, as it is common for this parameter to be slightly lower or unchanged after a well-executed training regime even when there is substantial and further cardiovascular adaptation [4, 5, 13].

Relative to the endocrine system, typically after an adaptation and physical improvement to a training program, an exercise session (endurance or resistance based) still provokes a hormonal response. But, just as noted above, the responses tend to be attenuated. These attenuated responses come about by a greater sensitivity of target tissue to the hormonal stimulus and because the level of neural, humoral, and hormonal stimuli disturbances in the blood that influence the various endocrine glands become far less [13]. Also, relative to the former point (i.e., sensitivity), in response to an exercise training regime, many target tissues increase the expression of functional hormone receptors, receptor affinity for hormones become increased, and post-receptor amplification mechanisms in the cells of target tissues are typically increased. Essentially all these changes result in a target tissue needing less amount of a hormone to bring about a physiological outcome/change.

Maladaptation in the Exercise Training Process

Many athletes have met stagnation or decline of their performance in their career though they are training hard and pushing as much as possible. Athletes, especially elite athletes, wish to enhance their performance by constantly increasing their training loads. It has been estimated that the exercise training loads of athletes have increased on average by 20–25% over the past decade [16–18]. The result of such training approaches is that sooner or later an athlete reaches the limit of his/her individual abilities. When this occurs, there are two possibilities, first an athlete's training plan prescribes adequate amount of rest and the athlete develops due to supercompensation. Secondly, the athlete keeps on training with high loads and loses an optimal balance between training stressors (plus non-sport stressors affecting them) and recovery. The second way pushes the athlete in the direction of developing a state of overreaching and/or the overtraining syndrome (OTS).

Because there is a lack of common and consistent terminology in this research field, the following definitions are presented to aid the reader, as they are somewhat widely used definitions [19]:

> *Overreaching*—an accumulation of training and/or non-training stress resulting in short-term decrement in performance capacity with or without related physiological and psychological signs and symptoms of maladaptation in which restoration of performance capacity may take several days to several weeks.
>
> *Overtraining*—an accumulation of training and/or non-training stress resulting in long-term decrement in performance capacity with or without related physiological and psychological signs and symptoms of maladaptation in which restoration of performance capacity may take several weeks or months.

These definitions emphasize that the difference between overreaching and overtraining is the amount of time needed for performance restoration and not the type or duration of training stress or degree of impairment. This opinion was recently updated by leading sports science organization American College of Sports Medicine (ACSM) and European Congress of Sport Science (ECSS) Joint Consensus Statement [20].

According to the consensus statement, *overtraining* is used as a process of intensified training with possible outcomes of short-term overreaching (functional OR (FOR)), extreme overreaching (nonfunctional OR (NFOR)), or OTS. Overreaching is often used by athletes during a typical training cycle to enhance performance. Intensified training can result in a decline in performance; however, when appropriate periods

Table 5.4 Development of functional overreaching (FOR), nonfunctional overreaching (NFOR), and overtraining syndrome (OTS)

Process	Training	Intensified training →		
Outcome	Acute fatigue	Functional overreaching (FOR) (short-term)	Non – functional overreaching (NFOR)	Overtraining syndrome
Recovery	Days	Days – weeks	Weeks - months	Months - ...?
Performance	Increase	Temporary performance decrement	Stagnation Decrease	Decrease

? Unknown

of recovery are provided, a supercompensation effect may occur with the athlete exhibiting an enhanced performance compared with baseline levels.

This form of short-term OR can also be called FOR. When this intensified training continues, the athletes can evolve into a state of extreme OR or NFOR, which will lead to a stagnation or decrease in performance that will not resume for several weeks or months. At this stage, the first signs and symptoms of prolonged training distress such as performance decrements, psychological disturbance (decreased vigor, increased fatigue), and hormonal disturbances will occur, and the athletes will need weeks or months to recover. Several confounding factors such as inadequate nutrition, illness, and sleep disorders may be present. All of these factors combine to add to the total stress placed upon the athlete and in doing so can impact the effect of training process (Table 5.4 illustrates and summarizes these points).

The distinction between NFOR and OTS is very difficult and will depend on the clinical outcome and exclusion diagnosis. The athlete will often show the same clinical, hormonal, and other signs and symptoms. Therefore, the diagnosis of OTS can often only be made retrospectively when the time course can be overseen. The physiological cause to OTS is known—the exercise training load placed upon an athlete is too great, the stress level exceeds their ability to adapt [9, 18, 20]. Still it is difficult to determine on an individual basis how much is too much stress.

Some researchers have proposed there may be two discrete neuroendocrine varieties [21, 22], that is, OTS consists of a hyper-arousal and/or a hypo-arousal form. This conclusion is based upon the finding that in certain physiological parameters, diverging symptomology exists. The hyper-arousal form is also referred to as the "sympathetic" or "Basedow's" OTS. It is commonly observed in "power" athletes (e.g., sprinters, jumpers, weight lifters) and occurs less frequently than the hypo-arousal disorder. The hypo-arousal form is more common and is also referred to as "parasympathetic" or "Addison's" OTS. This form of the disorder is frequently observed in endurance-trained athlete (e.g., long-distance runners, rowers, cross-country skiers, cyclists, swimmers). Each form of the disorder has some similar characteristics and symptoms (i.e., in particular declining physical performance), but there also are obvious psychophysiological differences (see Table 5.5; [22]).

OTS reflects the attempt of the human body to cope with physiological and other stressors. Several studies have revealed that OTS represents the sum of multiple life stressors, such as physical training, sleep loss, exposure to environmental stresses (e.g., exposure to heat, high humidity, cold, and high altitude), occupational pressures, change of residence, and interpersonal difficulties. Thus, OTS can be understood partly within the context of the General Adaptation Syndrome of Selye [23]. Concomitant to this "stress disturbance," the endocrine system is called upon to counteract the stress situation. The primary hormone products (adrenaline, noradrenaline, and cortisol) all serve to redistribute metabolic fuels, maintain blood glucose, and enhance the responsiveness of the cardiovascular system [20].

The endocrine system is one of the major systems involved in the responses to acute stress and the adaptation to chronic stress. A great diversity of mechanisms is involved in such adaptation, acting at potentially all levels in the cascade of physiological events, leading to the biological events regulated by hormones. A keyword in the recognition of OTS might be prolonged malad-

Table 5.5 Pathophysiologic findings in hyper-arousal versus hypo-arousal forms of the overtraining syndrome (OTS)

Parasympathetic, hypo-arousal	Sympathetic, hyper-arousal
Decrease in physical performance	Decrease in physical performance
Easily fatigued	Easily fatigued
Depression	Hyperexcitability
Normal sleep	Disturbed sleep
Normal constant weight	Weight loss
Low resting HR	Increased resting HR and blood pressure
Hypoglycemia during exercise	Slow recovery of HR and BP after exercise
Loss of competitive desire	Loss of competitive desire
Gonadal–reproductive function normal (?)	Amenorrhea in women
	Hypogonadism in men
Increased incidence of infections	Increased incidence of infections
Decreased maximal lactate response to exercise	Decreased maximal lactate response to exercise

HR heart rate, BP blood pressure, ? inconclusive findings

aptation of the athletic performance and several biological, neurochemical, and hormonal regulation mechanisms. Most of the literature agrees that FOR, NFOR, and OTS must be viewed on a continuum with a disturbance, an adaptation, and finally a maladaptation of the hypothalamic–pituitary–adrenal (HPA) axis, resulting in an altered hormonal response to intense training and competition.

The hypothalamus is under the control of several higher brain centers, and several neurotransmitters are known to play a major role in various neuroendocrine and behavioral functions, for example, activation of the HPA axis, feeding, and locomotion. Therefore, the typical HPA-axis-related hormones—cortisol, testosterone, ACTH, prolactin (PRL), and human growth hormone (hGH)—are usually followed in overtraining studies [24]. Besides basal hormone levels, hormonal responses to one or two bouts of test exercise are followed to better distinguish between FOR, NFOR, and OTS.

The clinical patho-phenomena related to either adrenal cortex or thyroid gland disorders in clinical meaning have been never evidenced in overtrained athletes. Nonetheless, the dysfunction of endocrine system is usual [25]. According to Lehmann and coworkers [26–29], the first step to NFOR, inducing OTS, is depressed adrenal responsiveness to corticotropin (i.e., another term used to refer to ACTH), obviously caused by downregulation of corticotropin receptors on adrenocortical cells. They interpreted this change as a protective mechanism against chronic overload [28, 29]. The positive feedback influence or other mechanisms increase the secretion of corticotropin. Increased corticotropin level has been found at the influence of overload exercise. However, the increased corticotropin release fails to overcome the depressed adrenal responsiveness and cortisol secretion decreases, particularly during an exercise. In an advanced stage of overtraining, the pituitary corticotropin and GH responses reduce [30].

The possibility of disbalance in endocrine control has been supported by the fact that after the intensive training stage, the release of corticotropin caused by exogenous administration of corticotropin-releasing hormone (CRH) was 60 % higher but the increase in blood cortisol level 30 % lower than before the strenuous training stage [22]. Several studies have indicated that high-workload training period for several weeks increased serum cortisol basal level. Some scientists consider this change as a response to hard training, the others as an indication of overtraining [31, 32]. In these studies, the training situation appears to resemble more overreaching than overtraining. On the other hand, overtraining has been associated with decreased cortisol basal level [22, 33] and/or reduced or inversed cortisol responses in exercise tests [34–36].

A typical overtraining effect is low testosterone levels in the blood [31, 35, 37]. Some scientists have focused on the associated increase in cortisol levels to overtraining. Therefore, the resultant testosterone/cortisol ratio is also low in this situation. Adlercreutz and coauthors [38] recommended using the ratio between free testosterone and cortisol as an indication of the overtraining if the ratio decreases more than 30 % or if the ratio is $<0.35 \times 10^{-3}$. However, even if the ratio decreases more than 30% or it is $<0.35 \times 10^{-3}$, there may be no indications of overtraining [16, 35, 39]. The physiological meaning of the altered ratio is different if it is by decrease in testosterone or a lack of cortisol increase, by less pronounced increase of testosterone than increase of cortisol, or by more pronounced decrease of cortisol than of testosterone. Instead of the expected testosterone decrease and cortisol increase, Urhausen et al. [40] found decreased testosterone/cortisol ratio due to reduction in testosterone concentration while cortisol level remained unchanged.

Thus, in NFOR and OTS, the cortisol increase appears as an exception. Therefore, the usage of ratio testosterone/cortisol for overtraining diagnostics appears meaningless. Mostly, the decrease in testosterone level in conjunction with the increase in the cortisol level takes place during intensive training stages. These changes indicate overreaching but not overtraining. The conclusion of Urhausen and coauthors [35] is that the behavior of testosterone and cortisol is rather a physiological indicator of the current training load, but it does not necessarily indicate OTS status. Furthermore, Lane and associates [41] have noted the ratio is highly sensitive to diet. They demonstrated that as little as 3 days of low dietary carbohydrate intake during intensive FOR training substantially lowered the ratio than similar intensive FOR training with moderate–high carbohydrate intake (~60 % daily caloric intake).

Hug et al. [42] followed hormonal changes in male elite cyclists during intensive training period at high altitude. The levels of free testosterone, testosterone and testosterone/serum sex hormone-binding globulin (SHBG) ratio were reduced—in contrast to the normoxia training group. ACTH responsiveness seemed to be reduced in the subjects as cortisol responses decreased. In trained runners, 10 days of twice-daily interval training sessions resulted in a significant fall in performance and several mood changes that persisted at least for 5 days. Cortisol level began to decrease for the end of the 10-day exercise period, and the low level persisted during 5 days into recovery. Testosterone, luteinizing hormone (LH), and follicle-stimulating hormone (FSH) levels did not change significantly [43].

Recently, Taskanen et al. [44] showed that SHBG and cortisol concentrations were associated with overreaching during 8-week strenuous military training. Basal SHBG increased, and insulin-like growth factor-1 (IGF-1) and cortisol decreased. Furthermore, submaximal exercise-induced increases in cortisol, maximum heart rate, and postexercise increase in blood lactate were blunted. Suppressed adrenocortical activity reflects a general disbalance induced by overtraining either on the level of hypothalamic neurosecretion or in function of anterior pituitary. In overtrained distance runners, the responses of cortisol, corticotropin, growth hormone (GH), and PRL to insulin-hypoglycemia were reduced [30]. Overtrained weight lifters exhibited a moderate increase in testosterone response and pronounced decrease in cortisol response to test exercise in conjunction with 1-RM strength decrements [45]. Keizer and collaborators [46] found that exhaustive running training reduces the ß-endorphin response to an incremental treadmill running and also blunted ß-endorphin response to human CRH. Other changes, typical to overtraining, are decreased ß-adrenoreceptor density and, thereby, diminished sensitivity to catecholamines and decreased intrinsic sympathetic activity [28, 29]. These changes are also considered as a part of mentioned protective mechanism against chronic overload [29]. Altered autonomic balance is expressed by low nocturnal catecholamine excretion [26]. In male middle- and long-distance runners, an exhaustive training stage increased norepinephrine levels at rest and during submaximal but not during maximal exercise; epinephrine and dopamine levels did not change [26]. Uusitalo et al. [47] found decreased epinephrine level in blood at maximal and decreased norepinephrine level at submaximal exercises in overtrained female athletes. However, the resting catecholamine level and exercise-induced responses were found increased in overtrained athletes in several other studies [28]. Increased norepinephrine level was confirmed in overtrained swimmers, whereas high norepinephrine level remained when usual training was substituted by tapering [48]. The decreased sensitivity to catecholamines and altered responsiveness of various links in pituitary–adrenocortical system has been demonstrated in several studies. Increased catecholamine level may point on the hyperadrenergic type of overtraining. The exaggerated drop in insulin during an exercise has also been linked with this type of overtraining [34]. Keizer and associates [46] studied LH secretion in female amenorrheic athletes before and after a test exercise. When training volume or intensity was promptly increased during an ovarian-menstrual cycle, LH pulse frequency was not altered, but the amplitude of secretory bursts was decreased. These results support the suggestion that menstrual disorders in endurance female athletes are caused by overload training. Possibilities to follow changes in ghrelin, leptin, adiponectin, and IL-6 levels as biomarkers for training monitoring were tested. The authors concluded that although some of these parameters may provide information about energetic regulatory mechanisms and may change after intensive training or in OR, there are no studies supporting the possible suitability of these variables as markers of training stress or for the prevention or diagnosis of OR and OTS [49].

According to the review by Purvis et al. [50], the hormonal biomarker for detection of OR and OTS might be the decrease in maximal cortisol responses in OR. They pointed out that the findings in total and free testosterone levels during OR were contradictory; the testosterone/cortisol ratio was unchanged in OR; reports of resting ACTH levels were highly variable (increase, decrease, and no change). Purvis et al. [50] concluded that there is a great need for further research in this field.

Viru and Viru [13] concluded that the main hormonal indicators of the overtraining status are the suppressed productions of cortisol, testosterone, and GH and of nocturnal excretion of catecholamines as well as decreased tissue sensitivity to hormones. They suggested that the hormonal indicators of overtraining have power only in conjunction with the decrease in performance level and mood changes. When hormonal indicators appear without performance and mood alterations, they inform about the high risk of the appearance of overtraining. Detection of this situation gives a great value to hormonal monitoring because it timely informs coaches about the necessity to decrease the training workload and increase the time for recovery. This situation requires special attention if it appears in association with stagnation in training progress.

Meeusen et al. [20] explained that conflicting results in resting hormone concentrations were, at least partly, because of a lack of standardization in both the way overtraining was measured and in the hormone measurement protocols used among studies. Therefore, Meeusen and associates concluded that resting hormone concentrations are not sensitive enough to diagnose unexplained underperformance in athletes [20]. However, that view is not shared by all researchers who study overtraining [21, 51].

Many factors affect blood hormone concentrations and that may complicate the interpretation of hormonal data. These factors are linked to sampling conditions and storage of samples; techniques used to measure hormone levels; intra- and interassay coefficient of variability; food intake of an athlete; pulsatility of the secretion of some hormones, which modulates the tissue sensitivity to these hormones; the phase of the menstrual cycle in female athletes; diurnal and seasonal variations of the hormones; type of test protocol (aerobic and resistance protocols typically elicit different endocrine responses) [20].

In addition to the need to study different hormonal axes in parallel, it is also important to consider the dynamics of hormonal responses. The hormonal responses during exercise influence the hormonal responses during exercise recovery, and it is therefore important to study both phases of exercise. For this reason, a multiple exercise test that not only gives the opportunity to measure the recovery capacity of the athlete but also can assess the ability to normally perform the second bout of exercise could be useful to detect signs of OTS and distinguish them from normal training responses or FOR. According to Meeusen et al. [52], a hallmark feature of OTS is the inability to sustain intense exercise and recover for the next training or competition session. Therefore they used a test protocol utilizing two bouts of maximal work to establish the difference in hormonal responses between the training statuses of trained and OR athletes. Performance decreased by 6% between the first and the second exercise test in the OR group. The hormonal responses (cortisol, ACTH, PRL, GH) to the second exercise test were different between the trained and OR athletes (the increase in the T group was higher than in the OR). In 2010, in a similar study by Meeusen and associates [24], the subjects were underperforming athletes who were diagnosed with the suspicion of NFOR or OTS. Resting concentrations of cortisol, ACTH, and PRL concentrations were higher. However, sensitivity of these measures was low. The ACTH and PRL reactions to the second exercise bout were much higher in NFOR athletes compared with OTS and showed the highest sensitivity for making the distinction. Meeusen et al.'s conclusion was that this protocol could be a useful tool for diagnosing NFOR and OTS; however, it is advisable that more data should be collected before this test can be used as the gold standard [24, 52].

Drug Abuse

Since ancient times, some unethical athletes have attempted to gain an unfair competitive advantage through the use of doping substances. The use of enhancement substances for sporting events dates back to the ancient Greeks. A list of doping substances and methods banned in sports is published yearly by the World Anti-Doping Agency (WADA) [53]. A substance or method might be included in the list if it fulfills at least two of the following criteria: enhances sports performance, represents a risk to the athlete's health, or violates the spirit of sports. Among the substances included are steroidal and peptide hormones and their modulators, stimulants, glucocorticosteroids, β_2-agonists, diuretics and masking agents, narcotics, and cannabinoids. From all these, hormones constitute the highest number of adverse analytical findings reported by anti-doping laboratories. Although to date most are due to anabolic steroids, the development of molecular biology techniques has made recombinant peptide hormones also available for misuse. Peptide hormones, such as hGH or GH, IGF-1, insulin, and erythropoietin (EPO), are presumed to be widely abused for performance enhancement [54].

The prohibited substances have different origins—endogenous or exogenous in nature. The endogenous substances are naturally produced by the body (e.g., testosterone, dehydroepiandrosterone (DHEA), GH, insulin, IGF-1, and EPO). The members of other group are exogenous substances that are not ordinarily produced by the body (e.g., synthetic anabolic androgenic steroids (AAS), stimulants, diuretics and narcotics).

AAS

AAS are related to the male hormone testosterone. These compounds enhance athletic performance by promoting increase of muscle mass and strength and enhance recovery during training process. Anabolic steroids are believed to exert their effects by binding to androgen receptors at the cellular level, which translocate to binding sites on chromatin, promoting gene transcription, stimulating production of mRNA, and ultimately increasing protein synthesis [55]. AAS are misused by competitive but also by recreational athletes.

The therapeutic use of AAS is limited and may vary between steroids. The most important indications are endocrine dysfunction of the testes and of the hypothalamus–pituitary–gonadal axis (i.e., male hypogonadism and growth retardation). AAS are used to treat disturbances of nitrogen balance and muscular development and several other non-endocrine diseases, including several forms of anemia, hereditary angioneuroticedema, breast carcinoma, male infertility, and osteoporosis. Additionally, AAS stimulation of protein nitrogen balance is used in treating polytrauma patients, after abdominal surgery and burn injury, in chronic obstructive pulmonary disease and in HIV patients [56].

Effects of AAS

AAS exert essential effect on the sex hormones and reproductive system. AAS disturb the endogenous production of testosterone, LH, and FSH as they suppress the hypothalamic–pituitary–gonadal axis. According to Bhasin et al. [57], a close dose–response relationship exists between the administered dose of testosterone and serum level of testosterone. Administration of high weekly doses of intramuscular testosterone (>300 mg) increase serum levels of free and total testosterone, whereas 50 mg per week resulted in lower serum levels. Serum concentrations of androstenedione, estradiol, and dihydrotestosterone follow the same pattern of response [58, 59] that can be explained by peripheral conversion of AAS [60].

Altered glucose tolerance with increased insulin resistance, increased GH levels, as well as decreases in thyroid hormones and ACTH and no change in cortisol levels have also been reported with anabolic steroid use in male athletes [61–63]. Another study showed decrease in serum pregnenolone, progesterone, SHBG levels, and no change in cortisol-binding globulin (CBG) levels in power athletes during 26 weeks of steroid self-administration [59].

In women using anabolic steroids for a prolonged period of time, masculinization may be manifested as hirsutism, deepening of the voice, and menstrual irregularities that are caused by steroid use, but which may be irreversible once the drugs are discontinued [55].

AAS Administration Effects on Endocrine System

- Testosterone ↓ (low dose)
- Testosterone ↑ (high dose)
- Androstenedione ↑
- Dihydrotestosterone ↑
- DHEA ↓
- SHBG ↓
- Pregnenolone ↓
- Progesterone ↓
- Estradiol and estrone ↑
- LH ↓
- FSH ↓
- Thyroid hormones (TSH, T3, T4) ↓
- EPO ↑
- GH ↑
- ACTH ↓
- Cortisol—no change
- CBG—no change

Glucocorticosteroids

Athletes have misused glucocorticosteroids for many decades to enhance performance by stimulation of gluconeogenesis and mobilization of amino acids and fatty acids. Except for the believed performance enhancement, athletes may also take glucocorticosteroids to alleviate pain and reduce tiredness, ignoring the possible adverse effects, such as diabetes mellitus, myopathy, and growth retardation [64].

Glucocorticosteroids Administration Effects on Endocrine System

- CRH ↓
- ACTH ↓
- Testosterone ↓

Peptide Hormones

Several endogenous peptide hormones with potential performance-enhancing properties are listed in WADA's List of Prohibited Substances [53]. The following substances are the most well known and most widely spread: EPO, GH, IGF-1s and mechano-growth factors (MGF), gonadotropins (e.g., LH, human chorionic gonadotropin (hCG)), insulins, and corticotrophins [65].

Erythropoietin

EPO was granted license in 1988 as a therapeutic agent for correcting anemia of chronic kidney disease or other similar type conditions. The hormone is a member of the type I cytokine family, and it stimulates erythroid progenitors within the bone marrow to mature into erythrocytes. The main site of production of EPO is the kidney and to a lesser extent liver. Some studies also suggest the important role of proximal tubular cells in this process [66]. Some athletes and their coaches abuse recombinant EPO (rhEPO) because it increases the oxygen (O_2) supply to the muscles and boosts performance in endurance sports. The most important recombinant EPO and analogues misused in sport are rhEPO, darbepoetin alpha, and continuous erythropoietin receptor activator (CERA).

Clinical applications of rhEPO are chronic kidney disease, rheumatoid arthritis, HIV, hepatitis C, and cancer/chemotherapy-related anemia [66]. The presence of EPO and its receptors in several central nervous system regions indicates additional functions beside its hematopoietic role. A study by Markianos et al. [67] showed that EPO administration caused a significant reduction in PRL levels, suggesting that EPO may promote dopamine release in humans. Acute EPO administration to cancer patients showed no significant changes in serum levels of FSH, LH and TSH, but both GH and IGF-1 levels become significantly decreased [68]. This study shows that EPO may inhibit GH secretion from the pituitary gland and IGF-1 production. Since GH would stimulate EPO release, the results of this study may suggest the existence of feedback mechanism operating between GH secretion and EPO production, with inhibitory effect of EPO on GH secretion, and stimulatory action of GH on EPO production [68].

EPO Administration Effects on Endocrine System

- PRL ↓
- GH ↓
- IGF-1 ↓
- FSH—no change
- LH—no change
- TSH—no change

GH and IGF-1

hGH is a protein synthesized, stored, and released endogenously mostly from the somatotropes of the anterior pituitary gland. GH is the most abundant pituitary hormone and is secreted in a pulsatile manner under the control of the hypothalamic hormones, GH-releasing hormone, somatostatin, and ghrelin. GH plays an important role in body composition, well-being, physical performance, and cardiovascular health. GH exerts its multiple metabolic and anabolic actions through binding to specific GH receptors that are found on every cell of the body [65, 69].

GH Administration Effects on Endocrine System

- GH ↑
- IGF-1 ↑
- IGFBP-3 ↑
- Insulin ↑
- free T4 ↓

IGF-1 is a small single-chain polypeptide that has shown anabolic effects on cytoskeletal muscles. The actions of GH that interest athletes are anabolic and lipolytic, leading to an increase in lean body mass and reduction in fat mass. GH exerts most of its anabolic actions through the generation of circulating IGF-1. However, the prevalence of IGF-1 abuse is probably much lower than for GH because of its poor commercial availability. Circulating IGF-1 reduces GH secretion through classical negative endocrine feedback [69].

IGF-1 Administration Effects on Endocrine System

- IGF-1 ↑
- GH ↓
- Insulin ↓
- Glucagon ↓

Insulin

Insulin is produced by β cells in pancreatic islets through a complex proteolytic process involving the enzymatic cleavage of proinsulin into insulin and C-peptide. Insulin is mainly used to treat insulin-deficient patients suffering from type 1 diabetes mellitus. Due to its influence on many metabolic processes, insulin is a potential performance-enhancing agent. Insulin increases the rate of glucose uptake into adipose and muscle tissues and stimulates glycogenesis, thus increasing the intramuscular energy reserves. Insulin works in synergy with steroids. Steroids increase muscular mass and strength, whereas insulin inhibits catabolism in muscle and liver by increasing the synthesis of glycogen and proteins and promoting the entry of glycogen and amino acids into muscle cells. The combination of short-acting insulin and high carbohydrate diets has an anabolic effect on muscle mass through the inhibition of protein breakdown. The use of insulin could also improve post-competition recovery [54].

Insulin Administration Effects on Endocrine System

- Glucagon ↓
- LH ↑
- IGF-1 ↑

Leptin

Leptin, discovered through positional cloning process approximately 15 years ago, is an adipocyte-secreted hormone with pleiotropic effects in the physiology and pathophysiology of energy homeostasis, endocrinology, and metabolism. Leptin is produced predominantly in the adipose tissue but is also expressed in a variety of other tissues, including placenta, ovaries, mammary epithelium, bone marrow, and lymphoid tissues. The release of leptin into the circulation is pulsatile, and leptin concentrations follow a circadian rhythm and are affected by sleep patterns. Studies have shown that leptin contributes to the regulation of energy homeostasis, neuroendocrine function, metabolism, immune function, and bone metabolism [70, 71].

Leptin Administration Effects on Endocrine System

- LH ↑
- FSH ↑
- Gonadotropins ↑
- Estradiol ↑
- Testosterone ↑
- Cortisol ↓
- T3 and T4 ↑
- IGF-1 and IGFBP3 ↑

Gonadotropins

hCG is a glycoprotein produced at high concentrations by the placenta trophoblasts, during pregnancy. The hormones hCG and LH exert the same activity, through the LH receptor, which is the stimulation of testosterone production in the male testicles and progesterone and estradiol production in the female ovaries, respectively. Parenteral administration of hCG or LH stimulates the production of testosterone in males, and these gonadotropins can therefore be used by athletes to enhance muscle strength, although they are more expensive and less efficient than testosterone and anabolic steroids [65]. Therefore, their main use is probably to stimulate gonadal testosterone production during and after self-administration of testosterone or anabolic steroids. In women, hCG has not been shown to provide a clear beneficial effect on athletic performance; furthermore, detection of hCG is considered an intrusion on the privacy of a pregnant athlete. Thus, the use of gonadotropins is therefore prohibited only in males but not in females [64].

hCG and LH Administration Effects on Endocrine System

- Testosterone ↑
- Progesterone ↑
- Estradiol ↑

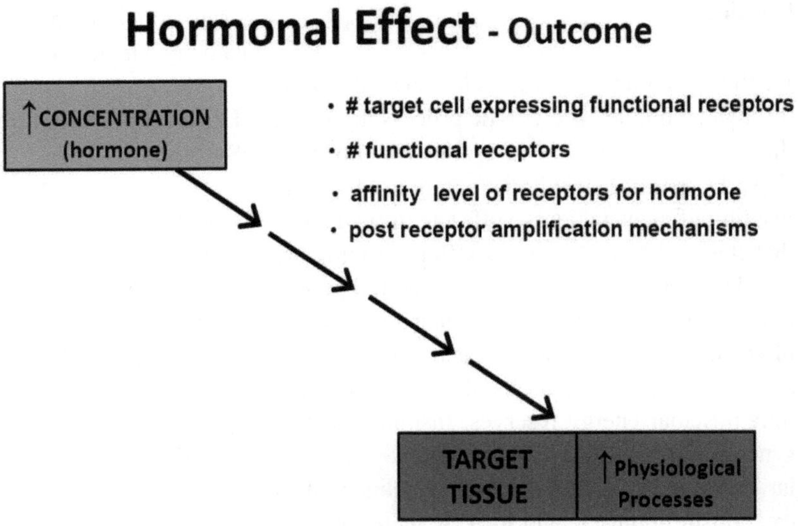

Fig. 5.1 The sequence of events and conditions necessary for a change (increase ⇒↑) in the circulating hormonal concentration to induce an effect on a target tissue to result in physiological process changes [77]

Future—Conclusions

The area of exercise-sports endocrinology is one in which there has been a constantly changing body of knowledge. Technological advancement and increasing rigorous experimental approaches have allowed for new discoveries in the existence of new hormones, hormonal interactions, and the hormonal-like effects of many substances released from both glandular and non-glandular tissues. For these reasons, the last 20 years have been an extremely exciting time in this field of endeavor. That being said, there is still a tremendous amount of uncertainty and questions in need of addressing. In particular, the scientists who work in exercise-sport aspect of endocrinology need to focus on not just "what" happens with exercise but "why" it happens, and what are the "consequences" of it happening. Research studies have well defined what the acute and chronic effects of exercise are to either increase or decrease the presence of many known hormones, but the specific regulatory events to induce such actions and outcomes from the hormonal change induced are not completely resolved and are an issue of continued debate [72–76]. This later point is illustrated by the prevalent misconception within some exercise researchers that an increase in the circulating levels of a hormone(s) always leads to a resultant change in a physiological process, for example, elevated concentrations of testosterone result in increased protein synthesis rates in skeletal muscle tissue [77]. Such a consequence is certainly a possibility, however, Fig. 5.1 illustrates that a number of conditions need to be met relative to receptor functionality and post-receptor mechanism (e.g., amino acid availability, endoplasmic reticular functionality, etc.) before such an event could occur. The new generation of scientists working in exercise-sport endocrinology must develop studies to address such points of "why," "how," and the "consequences of" if we are to gain a true understanding of how the integral and interacting aspect of acute and chronic exercise completely affects the endocrine system and those process under its control. This approach to future research presents challenges, but exciting opportunities, for scientists.

References

1. Garber CE et al. American College of Sports Medicine (ACSM) position stand. Quantity and quality of exercise for developing and maintaining cardiorespiratory, musculoskeletal, and neuromotor fitness in apparently healthy adults: guidance for prescribing exercise. Med Sci Sports Exerc. 2011;43(7):334–1359.
2. Joyner MJ. Physiologic limiting factors and distance running: influence of gender and age on record performances. Exerc Sport Sci Rev. 1993;21:103–33.

3. Joyner MJ, Coyle EF. Endurance exercise performance: the physiology of champions. J Physiol. 2008;586(1):35–44.
4. Rowell LB. Cardiovascular adjustments to thermal stress. Handbook of physiology, the cardiovascular system, peripheral circulation and organ blood flow (Suppl 8). New York: Wiley-Blackwell; 1983.
5. Saltin B, Astrand PO. Maximal oxygen uptake in athletes. J Appl Physiol. 1967;23:353–8.
6. Kraemer WJ, Fleck SJ, Evans WJ. Strength and power training: physiological mechanisms of adaptation. Exerc Sport Sci Rev. 1996;24:363–97.
7. Hackney AC. Exercise as a stressor to the neuroendocrine system. Medicina (Kaunas). 2006;42(10):788–97.
8. Hackney AC. Stress and the neuroendocrine system: the role of exercise as a stressor and modifier of stress. Expert Rev Endocrinol Metab. 2006;1(6):783–92.
9. Galbo H. Hormonal and metabolic adaptation to exercise. Stuttgart: Thieme Verlag; 1983.
10. Galbo H. The hormonal response to exercise. Diabetes Metab Rev. 1986;1(4):385–408.
11. Kjaer M, Secher NH, Galbo H. Physical stress and catecholamine release. Baillieres Clin Endocrinol Metab. 1987;1(2):279–98.
12. Viru A. Plasma hormones and physical exercise. Int J Sports Med. 1992;13(3):201–9.
13. Viru A, Viru M. Biochemical monitoring of sport training. Champaign: Human Kinetics; 2001.
14. Davies CT, Few JD. Effects of exercise on adrenocortical function. J Appl Physiol. 1973;35(6):887–91.
15. Steenberg A, Fischer CP, Keller C, Møller K, Pedersen BK. IL-6 enhances plasma IL-1ra, IL-10, and cortisol in humans. Am J Physiol (Endocrinol Metab). 2003;285(2):433–7.
16. Kuipers H, Keizer HA. Overtraining in elite athletes: review and directions for the future. Sports Med. 1988;6:79–92.
17. Kraemer WJ. Endocrine response to resistance exercise. Med Sci Sports Exerc. 1988;20:152–7.
18. Hackney AC, Koltun KJ. The immune system and overtraining in athletes: clinical implications. Acta Clin Croat. 2012;51(4):633–41.
19. Kreider R, Fry AC, O'Toole M. Overtraining in sport: terms, definitions, and prevalence. In: Kreider R, Fry AC, O'Toole M, editors. Overtraining in sport. Champaign: Human Kinetics; 1998.
20. Meeusen R, Duclos M, Foster C, Fry A, Gleeson M, Nieman D, Raglin J, Rietjens G, Steinacker J, Urhausen A. Prevention, diagnosis, and treatment of the overtraining syndrome: joint consensus statement of the European College of Sport Science and the American College of Sports Medicine. Med Sci Sports Exerc. 2013;45(1):186–205.
21. Hackney AC, Battaglini C. The overtraining syndrome: neuroendocrine imbalances in athletes. Braz J Biomotricity. 2007;1(2):34–44.
22. Lehmann M, Foster C, Keul J. Overtraining in endurance athletes: a brief review. Med Sci Sports Exerc. 1993;25:854–62.
23. Selye H. Stressand the general adaptation syndrome. Br Med J. 1950;1(4667):1383–92.
24. Meeusen R, Nederhof E, Buyse L, Roelands B, de Schutter G, Piacentini MF. Diagnosing overtraining in athletes using the two-bout exercise protocol. Br J Sports Med. 2010;44(9):642–8.
25. Foster C, Lehmann M. Overtraining syndrome. In: Guten GN, editor. Running injuries. Philadelphia: Saunders; 1997.
26. Lehmann M, Schnee W, Scheu R, Stockhausen W, Bachl N. Decreased nocturnal catecholamine excretion: parameter for an overtraining syndrome in athletes? Int J Sports Med. 1992;13:236–42.
27. Lehmann M, Baumgarte P, Wiesenack C, Seidel A, Baumann H, Fisher S, Spöri U, Gendrish G, Kaminski R, Keul J. Training-overtraining: influence of a defined increase in training volume vs. training intensity on performance catecholamines and some metabolic parameters in experienced middle- and long-distance runners. Eur J Appl Physiol. 1992;64:169–77.
28. Lehmann M, Foster C, Netzer N, Lormes W, Steinacker JM, Liu Y, Opitz-Gress A, Gastmann U. Physiological responses to short- and long-term overtraining in endurance athletes. In: Krieder RB, Fry AC, O'Toole ML, editors. Overtraining in sports. Champaign: Human Kinetics; 1998.
29. Lehmann M, Gastmann U, Baur S, Liu Y, Lormes W, Opiz-Gress A, Reißnecker S, Simisch C, Steinacker JM. Selected parameters and mechanisms of peripheral and central fatigue and regeneration in overtrained athletes. In: Lehmann M, Foster C, Gastmann U, Keizer H, Steinacker JM, editors. Overload, performance and regeneration in sport. New York: Springer; 1999.
30. Barron GL, Noakes TD, Levy W, Smith C, Millar RP. Hypothalamic dysfunction in overtrained athletes. J Clin Endorcrinol Metab. 1985;60:803–6.
31. Roberts AC, McClure RD, Weiker RI, Brooks GA. Overtraining affects male reproductive status. Fertil Steril. 1993;60:686–92.
32. Stray-Gundersen J, Videman T, Snell PG. Changes in selected objective parameters during overtraining. Med Sci Sports Exerc. 1986;18(Suppl): 54–5.
33. Snyder AC, Kuipers H, Cheng B, Servais R, Fransen E. Overtraining followed intensified training with normal muscle glycogen. Med Sci Sports Exerc. 1995;27:1063–70.
34. Urhausen A, Kindermann W. Monitoring of training by determination of hormone concentration in the blood. In: Liesen H, Weiß MM, Baum M, editors. Regulations und Repairmechanismen. Köln: Deutche Ärzte-Verlag; 1994. pp. 551–4.
35. Urhausen A, Gabriel H, Kindermann W. Blood hormones as markers training stress and overtraining. Sport Med. 1995;20:351–76.
36. Urhausen A, Gabriel HHW, Kindermann W. Impaired pituitary hormonal responses to exhaustive exercise in overtrained athletes. Med Sci Sports Exerc. 1998;30:407–14.

37. Kraemer WJ, Nindl BC. Factors involved with overtraining for strength and power. In: Kreider RB, Fry AC, O'Toole ML, editors. Overtraining in sport. Champaign: Human Kinetics; 1998. pp. 69–86.
38. Adlercreutz H, Härkönen M, Kuoppasalmi K, Näveri H, Huthaniani I, Tikkanen H, Remems K, Dessypris A, Karvonen J. Effect of training on plasma anabolic and catabolic steroid hormones and their response during physical exercise. Int J Sports Med. 1986;7(Suppl 1):27–8.
39. Vervoorn C, Vermlust LJM, Boelens-Quist AM, Koppeschaar HPF, Erich WBM, Thijssen JHH, Vries WR. Seasonal changes in performance and free testosterone: cortisol ratio of elite female rowers. Eur J Appl Physiol. 1992;64:14–21.
40. Urhausen A, Kullmer T, Kindermann W. A 7-week follow-up study of the behaviour of testosterone and cortisol during the competition period in rowers. Eur J Appl Physiol Occup Physiol. 1987;56(5):528–33.
41. Lane AR, Duke JW, Hackney AC. Influence of dietary carbohydrate intake on the free testosterone: cortisol ratio responses to short-term intensive exercise training. Eur J Appl Physiol. 2010;108(6):1125–31.
42. Hug M, Mullis PE, Vogt M, Ventura N, Hoppler H. Training modalities: over-reaching and overtraining in athletes, including a study of the role of hormones. Best Pract Res Clin Endocrinol Metab. 2003;17(2):191–209.
43. Fry RW, Morton AR, Garcia-Webb P, Crawford GP, Keast D. Biological responses to overload training in endurance sports. Eur J Appl Physiol. 1992;64:335–44.
44. Tanskanen MM, Uusitalo AL, Kinnunen H, Häkkinen K, Kyröläinen H, Atalay M. Association of military training with oxidative stress and overreaching. Med Sci Sports Exerc. 2011;43(8):1552–1560.
45. Fry AC, Kraemer WJ, Ransay CT. Pituitary-adrenal-gonadal responses to high-intensity resistance exercise overtraining. J Appl Physiol. 1998;85:2352–9.
46. Keizer HA, Platen P, Kuoppeschaar H, de Vries WR, Vervoon C, Geurten P, von Kraneburg G. Blunted ß-endorphin response to corticotropin releasing hormone and exercise after exhaustive training. Int J Sports Med. 1991;12:97.
47. Uusitalo ALT, Huttunen P, Hanin Y, Uusitalo AJ, Rusko HK. Hormonal responses to endurance training and overtraining in female athletes. Clin J Sports Med. 1998;8:178–86.
48. Hooper S, MacKinnon LT, Gordon RD, Bachmann AW. Hormonal responses of elite swimmers to overtraining. Med Sci Sports Exerc. 1993;25:741–7.
49. Jürimäe J, Maestu J, Jürimäe T, Mangus B, von Duvillard S. Peripheral signals of energy homeostasis as possible markers of training stress in athletes: a review. Metabolism. 2011;60:335–50.
50. Purvis D, Gonsalves S, Deuster P. Physiological and psychological fatigue in extreme conditions: overtraining and elite athletes. Phys Med Rehabil. 2010;2:442–50.
51. Hackney AC. Hormonal changes at rest in overtrained endurance athletes. Biol Sport. 1991;8(2):49–56.
52. Meeusen R, Piacentini MF, Busschaert B, Buyse L, De Schutter G, Stray-Gundersen J. Hormonal responses in athletes: the use of a two bout exercise protocol to detect subtle differences in (over)training status. Eur J Appl Physiol. 2004;91(2–3):140–146.
53. World Anti-Doping Agency. The 2013 prohibited list: international standard. The world anti-doping code. September 10 2012. 2014. http://www.wada-ama.org/Documents/WorldAnti-DopingProgram/WADP-Prohibited-list/2013/WADA-Prohibited-List-2013-EN.pdf. Accessed 30 July 2014.
54. Barroso O, Mazzoni I, Rabin O. Hormone abuse in sports: the antidoping perspective. Asian J Androl. 2008;10(3):391–402.
55. Bahrke MS, Yesalis CE. Abuse of anabolic-androgenic steroids and related substances in sport and exercise. Curr Opin Pharmacol. 2004;4:614–20.
56. Hartgens F, Kuipers H. Effects of androgenic-anabolic steroids in athletes. Sports Med. 2004;34(8):513–554.
57. Bhasin S, Woodhouse L, Casaburi R, Singh AB, Bhasin D, Berman N, Chen X, Yarasheski KE, Magliano L, Dzekov C, Dzekov J, Bross R, Phillips J, Sinha-Hikim I, Shen R, Storer TW. Testosterone dose-response relationships in healthy young men. Am J Physiol (Endocrinol Metab). 2001;281:E1172–81.
58. Alen M, Rahkila P, Reinila M, Vihko. Androgenic-anabolic steroid effects on serum thyroid, pituitary and steroid hormones in athletes. Am J Sports Med. 1987;15:357–61.
59. Ruokonen A, Alen M, Bolton N, Vihko R. Response of serum testosterone and its precursor steroids, SHBG and CBG to anabolic steroid and testosterone self-administration in man. J Steroid Biochem. 1985;23:33–8.
60. Matsumine H, Hirato K, Ynaihara T, Tamada T, Yoshida M. Aromatization by skeletal muscle. J Clin Endocrinol Metab. 1986;63:717–20.
61. Alen M, Reinilä M, Vihko R. Response of serum hormones to androgen administration in power athletes. Med Sci Sports Exerc. 1985;17(3):354.
62. Cohen JC, Hickman R. Insulin resistance and diminished glucose tolerance in powerlifters ingesting anabolic steroids. J Clin Endocrinol Metab. 1987;64:960–3.
63. Shahidi NT. A review of the chemistry, biological action, and clinical applications of anabolic-androgenic steroids. Clin Ther. 2001;23:1355–90.
64. Nikolopoulos DD, Spiliopoulou C, Theocharis SE. Doping and musculoskeletal system: short-term and long-lasting effects of doping agents. Fund Clin Pharmacol. 2001;25(5):535–63.
65. Hackney AC, Dobridge J. Exercise and male hypogonadism: testosterone, the hypothalamic-pituitary-testicular axis and physical exercise. In: Winter S,

editor. Male hypogonadal disorders: contemporary endocrinology series. New York: Humana Publishing; 2003.

66. John MJ, Jaison V, Jain K, Kakkar N, Jacob JJ. Erythropoietin use and abuse. Indian J Endocrinol Metab. 2012;16(2):220–7.
67. Markianos M, Kosmidis ML, Sfagos C. Reductions in plasma prolactin during acute erythropoietin administration. Neuro Endocrinol Lett. 2006;3:355–8.
68. Lissoni P, Perego M, Veronese E, Fumagalli G, Brivio F, Colciago M, Messina G, Rovelli F, Brivio R, Gardani G. Endocrine effects of erythropoietin in cancer patients. Hematology. 2004; 9(5–6): 363–7.
69. Holt RI, Sönksen PH. Growth hormone, IGF-I and insulin and their abuse in sport. Br J Pharmacol. 2008;154(3):542–56.
70. Mantzoros CS, Magkos F, Brinkoetter M, Sienkiewicz E, Dardeno TA, Kim SY, Hamnvik OP, Koniaris A. Leptin in human physiology and pathophysiology. Am J Physiol (Endocrinol Metab). 2011; 301(4): E567–84.
71. Lacquemant C, Vasseur F, Leprete F, Froguel P. Adipocytokines, obesity and development of type 2 diabetes. Med Sci (Paris). 2003;19(8–9):809–17.
72. Widmaier EP. Metabolic feedback in mammalian endocrine systems. Horm Metab Res. 1992;24 (4):147–53.
73. Viru A. The mechanism of training effects: a hypothesis. Int J Sports Med. 1985;5(5):219–27.
74. West DW, Phillips SM. Anabolic processes in human skeletal muscle: restoring the identities of growth hormone and testosterone. Phys Sportsmed. 2010;38(3):97–104.
75. Vingren JL, Kraemer WJ, Ratamess NA, Anderson JM, Volek JS, Maresh CM. Testosterone physiology in resistance exercise and training: the up-stream regulatory elements. Sports Med. 2010;40(12):1037–53.
76. Fry AC, Kraemer WJ. Resistance exercise overtraining and overreaching: neuroendocrine responses. Sports Med. 1997;23(2):106–29.
77. Hackney AC, Viru A. Research methodology: issues with endocrinological measurements in exercise science and sport medicine. J Athl Train. 2008;43(6):631–9.

General Adaptations to Exercise: Acute Versus Chronic and Strength Versus Endurance Training

6

Michael I. Lambert

Introduction

A stressor is defined as anything that causes stress or elicits the stress response. A common feature of all stressors is that there is an acute phase, during which homeostatic adjustments occur; a more chronic phase, during which the stressor can be accommodated by the adaptations; and finally a phase of exhaustion, during which maladaptations occur [1]. According to this definition, exercise can be defined as a stressor, along with other examples such as food deprivation, exposure to hypo- or hyperthermia, or psychological and social challenges. The stress of exercise behaves in a biological way similar to other stressors. For example, at the start of exercise, there are acute physiological, metabolic, and neuromuscular changes that persist for the duration of the bout of exercise. These changes are in proportion to the increase in metabolic rate. During rest, oxygen consumption, which is a measure of metabolic rate, hovers around 3 ml oxygen/kg/min, and coinciding with exhaustive exercise, oxygen consumption may increase to around 50 ml oxygen/kg/min in a moderately active person and to around 70 ml oxygen/kg/min in a highly trained endurance athlete. Almost immediately after exercise ceases, oxygen consumption decreases returning to baseline levels a few hours later. These changes during exercise are transient. For example, the metabolic state a few hours after moderate exercise is indistinguishable from the metabolic state before the start of the exercise.

However, if the bout of exercise is repeated regularly, after a few weeks changes occur, which persist for longer than the transient acute changes. These more persistent changes, known as training-induced adaptations, are associated with an improvement in exercise performance. For example, a trained person has an increased capacity to resist fatigue, has stronger muscles, can generate more muscle power, or has more refined motor coordination or skill for a specific task. The exact nature of the adaptations depends on the type of exercise training. Consider, for example, a typical endurance training session where the active muscles are recruited several thousand times to contract at a relatively low intensity. Indeed the leg muscles of a jogger, at the end of a 10-km run, would have had to sustain over 6000 contractions. In contrast, a person undergoing resistance training in a gym may only contract a muscle 30 times at each training session; the difference being that each contraction is close to a maximal effort. It is therefore not surprising that the training-induced adaptations are different, considering the different types of training stimuli.

Following each training session, recovery has to occur before the next training session. The time course of recovery after exercise varies depending on the marker of recovery. For example,

M. I. Lambert (✉)
Division of Exercise Science and Sports Medicine
Department of Human Biology, University of Cape Town, 1 Boundary Rd, Newlands, Cape Town 7725, Western Cape, South Africa
e-mail: mike.lambert@uct.ac.za

© Springer Science+Business Media New York 2016

D. Vaamonde et al. (eds.), *Exercise and Human Reproduction*, DOI 10.1007/978-1-4939-3402-7_6

elevated heart rate, blood lactate concentrations, and breathing rate return to baseline levels within minutes after exercise, whereas metabolic rate may take hours. If the bout of exercise caused muscle damage, the changes may take weeks [2] or months [3] to revert to the pre-exercise values. Inadequate recovery between training sessions results in maladaptations with the accompanying symptoms of fatigue and impaired muscle function [4]. This is commonly known as overtraining and is something that has to be carefully managed, particularly with competitive athletes who are continually striving to improve performance by training hard with insufficient recovery between training sessions [5].

The principles of biology, particularly the principle of "dose and response" can be applied to exercise; the dose of exercise being the stimulus of a training session, and the response being the outcome from that training session. Coaches have learnt to apply this principle to training. Aligned to this principle is the concept of overload, which suggests that the biological stress has to be gradually increased for adaptations to occur. In practical terms, this translates to the weight lifted getting heavier, the distance run getting longer, or the intensity of the exercise increasing in a gradual, systematic way. This principle forms the basis of all training programs and assists athletes in reaching peak performances [6]. The next section will consider the biological signal in more detail.

Biological Stimulus

At rest, the physiological, metabolic, and endocrine systems in the body are in a state of equilibrium. This equilibrium is disturbed as soon as the muscles start contracting. This disturbance of homeostasis evokes several responses, all designed to meet the demands of the increased metabolic rate or the need to produce muscle power. Examples of these transient changes are [7]:

- Altered blood flow to the active muscles
- Increased heart rate
- Increased breathing rate
- Increased oxygen consumption
- Increased rate of sweating
- Increased body temperature
- Secretion of stress hormones such as adrenocorticotropic hormone (ACTH), cortisol, and catecholamines
- Increased glycolytic flux
- Altered recruitment of muscles

In short, these responses or homeostatic adjustments maintain the constancy of the body's internal milieu during exercise. The magnitude and type of responses to exercise are dependent on the interaction of several factors such as the type of muscle action, duration of activity, and whether the person has been exposed to the activity. The ambient conditions, such as temperature, altitude, and wind speed, also have an impact on the homeostatic response. Finally, there are significant intraindividual differences in responses to the same exercise stimulus [8]. This explains why some people seem to adapt at a much faster rate than others, after exposure to the same training stimulus. The reasons for this can be ascribed to pre-training phenotype and pre-training autonomic function. There is also evidence that the training response can be modulated by the timing and composition of the nutritional intake [8].

The exercise-associated signal that induces training-induced adaptations varies depending on the type of muscle contraction and the duration, frequency, and intensity of the bout of exercise. This mechanical signal is converted into primary and secondary messages for adaptation. These messages activate the pathways involved in protein synthesis or degradation, resulting in the adaptations that are associated with changes in performance. Also, the recovery period between exercise sessions can affect the signal. For example, the training-induced expression of messenger RNA (mRNA) of several oxidative enzymes are upregulated at 24 h after the bout of exercise [9].

A consequence of endurance training is that the muscle becomes more resistant to fatigue [10], whereas following resistance training, the muscles become stronger, more powerful, and in some cases bigger [11]. At the cellular level, the primary stimulus for exercise-induced adaptations is a combination of the load on the muscle, metabolic stress, and calcium flux [12]. The load of the muscle is dependent on the tension or strain and type of muscle action. For example, the muscle can shorten or lengthen under tension [13]. A muscle that lengthens under tension has unique activation patterns [14], which impact the mechanical signal. Increasing the load causes muscle hypertrophy through the activation of the pathways of protein synthesis and a suppression of the protein degradation pathways. This results in an increase in the amount of the myofibrillar contractile proteins (actin and myosin), with an increase in muscle cross-sectional area [11].

The metabolic stress stimulus varies depending on the intensity and type of exercise [15]. Metabolic stress is associated with a high rate of adenosine triphosphate (ATP) utilization and is influenced by the substrate availability in the muscle cell. The biochemical signals that activate adaptive cellular pathways include an increased ratio of adenosine monophosphate (AMP) to ATP (ATP), increased levels of reactive species of oxygen and nitrogen, depleted levels of muscle glycogen, and decreased oxygen tension [15].

The calcium flux refers to the rate at which calcium is released from the sarcoplasmic reticulum, binds to troponin C, and initiates muscle contraction [16]. During a single-muscle contraction, there is a transient increase in sarcoplasmic calcium concentration. However, as the rate of muscle contractions increases, the sarcoplasmic calcium concentrations are maintained at a higher level. The latter scenario is associated with a signal that results in mitochondrial biogenesis and an increase in the glucose transporter (GLUT 4) [17]. The increase in mitochondrial content and oxidative enzyme activity results in a reduced rate of glycogen utilization during exercise and an enhanced capacity to oxidize fat during submaximal exercise. This results in an increased capacity to resist to fatigue and is associated with enhanced endurance performance.

In summary, these three stimuli (load on the muscle, metabolic stress, and calcium flux) vary depending on the circumstances of the exercise. During endurance training, the load is low, the metabolic stress is high, and the calcium flux consists of short intermittent bursts for long periods. Under these conditions, there is an increase in mitochondrial mass and oxidative enzyme activity. During resistance training (i.e., few contractions in a training session, but these contractions are close to maximal power output), the load is high, the metabolic stress is moderate, and the calcium flux is high. This stimulus results in muscle fiber hypertrophy and neural changes. If the person exposed to resistance is untrained, almost all the changes in strength can be attributed to neural changes in the early phases of training. However, after 4–6 weeks of training, the first signs of hypertrophy become evident. This will be discussed in more detail in the section on resistance training.

Finally, there is evidence to suggest that a slightly elevated intramuscular temperature is an important part of the signal for inducing training adaptations. This was concluded after an experiment showed that training-induced adaptations were blunted if the muscles were cooled immediately after each training session [18].

Maladaptations

For competitors striving to improve performance, there is a fine line between doing insufficient training or too much training, with both resulting in underperformance. Insufficient training fails to induce appropriate adaptations necessary for peak performances. In contrast, too much training results in maladaptations or the failure to adapt, causing symptoms of fatigue and poor performance. This has been well researched and it is known that training-induced fatigue occurs on a continuum starting with "functional overreaching," which is overcome with a few days of rest [5]. Indeed some coaches will even induce this state intentionally to capitalize on the rebound and possible super compensatory effect as the athlete recovers. The next phase is "nonfunctional overreaching," which requires a longer rest period. This is regarded as a negative phase, which coaches try and avoid. If the training load persists, without adequate recovery, the athlete enters the overtraining phase [19]. A consistent symptom of overtraining is impaired performance. However, beyond this, the symptoms of overtraining are varied and may involve dysfunction in the neuromuscular, endocrine, metabolic, and immune systems. A common characteristic is the inability to accommodate the same training load that was possible before the development of the symptoms [20]. Symptoms of overtraining can be avoided if the athlete adopts a more systematic approach to training, ensuring the correct balance between training load and rest and recovery [21]. To facilitate this process, it is important to quantify both the training load and the fatigue arising from each session, so that the "dose/response" can be carefully manipulated [22]. This approach will increase the chances of the athlete peaking at the correct time coinciding with important competition. Researchers have attempted to identify a specific marker of overtraining—at present such a marker does not exist, possibly because of the varied and inconsistent responses [5].

Endurance Training

The main consequence of training-induced adaptations following endurance training is that resistance to fatigue increases. This means that after training more work can be done in the same time, compared to before training, or at the same submaximal intensity, the time to fatigue increases after training. Although the adaptations after endurance training are loosely referred to as aerobic adaptations, they have their origins in the skeletal muscle, in the cardiovascular system and in metabolism. Aerobic capacity is represented by the maximal oxygen uptake (VO_2max). As mentioned previously, the VO_2max of elite endurance athletes (males) is usually above 70 ml oxygen/kg/min, whereas it is about 10 % lower in elite females. Although VO_2max increases following endurance training, the changes are variable, possibly as a result of the athlete's genotype [15]. There are two schools of thought explaining the increase in VO_2max after training. The first view is that VO_2max increases as a result of the central adaptations that result in more oxygen being delivered to the muscles. According to this view, the changes in performance are a consequence of the increased oxygen delivery [23]. A second view is that the properties of the muscle change after training, enabling the person to achieve a higher workload in a VO_2max test. It follows that VO_2max increases as a consequence of the increased workload [24]. The latter interpretation seems to be the more popular and is supported by basic principles of exercise physiology [25].

If one considers a situation where an inactive person starts training systematically, there are a number of changes that take place. One of the first measureable changes is an increase in plasma volume [26]. This adaptation can also explain the increase in cardiac output and stroke volume and the decrease in heart rate, which occurs during submaximal exercise after training [27]. These changes are lost as soon as the regular training stops. Next, the capillaries in the active muscles proliferate. The capillary-to-fiber ratio increases by up to 20 % in a matter of weeks [28]. Another early adaptation evident after about 4 weeks of training is the increase in the mitochondrial mass with a concomitant increase in oxidative capacity [29].

At a fixed submaximal workload, the perception of effort decreases as the training status improves, or more work can be done at the same perception of effort. Indeed, this can be related to the reduced disturbance in homeostasis, which occurs at a fixed submaximal workload (before vs. after training). The athlete becomes more efficient and uses less oxygen at a fixed submaximal load [30]. This is supported by a slower breathing rate, lower heart rate, and lower blood lactate concentration. Also, more fat is used as fuel during submaximal exercise after training. This can be demonstrated quite easily in a laboratory if one measures the volume of carbon dioxide (CO_2) produced and the volume of oxygen (O_2) consumed. This ratio of CO_2/O_2, known as respiratory exchange ratio (RER), is close to 1.0 when glucose and glycogen are the main source of fuel, and the ratio decreases to 0.7 when free fatty acids are the predominant fuel during exercise [31]. An untrained person exercising at a submaximal intensity will have an RER of around 1.0, showing that they are using mainly glucose as fuel. This can be compared to an endurance-adapted athlete who will have an RER of between 0.8 and 0.9 during submaximal exercise, showing that both fatty acids and glucose are being oxidized for fuel. Under these conditions, the rate of glycogen utilization decreases during submaximal exercise. As a consequence, it takes longer for the glycogen stores to become depleted. This has important consequences for endurance performance because fatigue during such events is associated with glycogen depletion [32]. It therefore follows that if the depletion of glycogen can be delayed, the onset of fatigue will also occur at a later stage.

Strength Training

Many athletes striving to get stronger and more powerful practice strength training, also known as resistance training [6]. More recently, the health benefits of resistance training have been recognized, particularly to treat or manage conditions characterized by muscle weakness. Such conditions are sarcopenia (loss of muscle mass with ageing), neuromuscular skeletal disorders, and immobilization of a muscle following injury or following prolonged bed rest [33].

Muscle strength is defined as the ability of that muscle to produce force. This characteristic should be differentiated from muscle power, which is reflected in the ability to do work over time. In other words, muscle power is an interaction between the force of contraction and speed of contraction. Maximal power output usually coincides with between 40–70 % of the maximal weight lifted, depending on the type of muscle contraction. Normal daily activities require minimal strength, while performance in certain sports is dependent on high levels of strength. In particular, success in certain sports, such as weight lifting, is directly related to the strength of the muscle.

There are many forms of resistance training, for example:

- Free weights (e.g., dumbbells, barbells, and kettle bells)
- Machine weights (e.g., devices designed for particular muscle groups with adjustable seats using either weights on pulleys or hydraulics)
- Rubberized resistance bands
- Exercises using body weight

The overload, or specific resistance training stimulus, is applied by manipulating the number of repetitions, intensity (i.e., weight lifted), recovery period between repetitions and sets, and the frequency of training sessions [34]. The outcome of a resistance-training program can increase muscular endurance, hypertrophy, strength, or power. The final outcome depends on the manipulation of the variables associated with the overload stimulus. The choice of the application of the training load (free weight vs. machine weights) can also influence the type of adaptation.

The capacity of the skeletal muscle to generate a high level of force is a complex interplay between several factors. For example, the strength of a muscle depends on the muscle's fiber type, cross-sectional area, architecture, and neural drive [35]. In the initial phase of resistance training, strength can be increased without any change in muscle size, but it is always dependent on changes in the neural system. Sporting performance can benefit from increases in strength. The magnitude of the effect varies depending on the sport. For example, following a resistance training program in which the squat one-repetition maximum (1 RM) increased by 21 %, this increase in strength was accompanied by improvements in vertical jump performance (21 %) and sprinting speed (2.3 %) [36].

An untrained person starting a resistance training program will notice increases in strength almost immediately. There is no change in muscle size at this stage. Muscles only start showing signs of increasing size (hypertrophy) after about 4 weeks of consistent training, with the change in size being quiet significant after 8–12 weeks of resistance training [33]. For hypertrophy to occur, additional contractile proteins (actin and myosin) have to be manufactured and incorporated into the existing myofibrils. This increases the cross-sectional area of a muscle, which is directly proportional to the force the muscle can produce. Factors such as age, gender, and genotype affect the rate and size of muscle increases after training [37]. The exact time course for muscle fiber hypertrophy is not well documented but appears to require at least 6–7 weeks of regular resistance training at reasonably high intensity [38]. Increases in muscle protein synthesis occur following an isolated bout of resistance exercise [38]. The increase in muscle protein turnover can increase for up to 48 h after resistance training exercise [33, 39].

The size of muscles in the upper body of a previously untrained person increases at a faster rate after resistance training compared to the muscles in the lower body [33]. This can be explained because the muscles of the lower limbs have to bear weight continuously and are therefore recruited more frequently than the muscles of the upper body. Therefore, they can be considered more adapted than the muscles of the upper limbs in an untrained person.

Many shorter studies (6–10 weeks) report preferential hypertrophy of type 2 muscle fibers; however, the longer duration studies have also found hypertrophy of type 1 fibers [33]. In the early phase (2–3 months) following resistance training, there are subtle changes in fiber type, with an increase in type 2A fibers and a decrease in type 2X fibers [33].

While the expression of voluntary strength depends on the agonist muscles being maximally activated, there also has to be minimal activation of the antagonist muscles and appropriate support from synergistic and stabilizing muscles [40]. An untrained muscle cannot be activated fully [41]. A possible mechanism explaining this is that activation of the Golgi tendon organs inhibit the agonist muscle (via Ib inhibitory interneurons), while the antagonist muscles are facilitated by inhibition of the Ia inhibitory interneurons [41]. This inhibition seems to be overridden following strength training, through a process known as disinhibition. The increase in maximal voluntary contraction, particularly during the first 3–4 weeks after resistance training, is accompanied by increases in the surface electromyographic (EMG) activity of the agonist muscles, confirming a change in the neural drive to a muscle [33]. This indicates that more muscle fibers can be recruited compared to a maximal contraction before training. Once hypertrophy has occurred, fewer muscle fibers are recruited during a submaximal contraction—this is reflected in reduced EMG activity. Further evidence of neural adaptations after resistance training can be demonstrated by the "cross-over effect" where training one limb causes strength increases in the contralateral untrained limb [33].

Concurrent Strength and Endurance Training

For a long time, it has been known that the adaptations following a training program, which incorporates both endurance and strength training simultaneously, do not manifest to the same extent compared to when the training modalities are done on their own. In particular, expected gains in strength are reduced if additional endurance training occurs at the same time. The reduced gains in strength with concurrent training are partially due to a suppressed hypertrophic response in the muscle that may be related to an elevated catabolic state induced by endurance training [42]. It also appears that various molecular signaling responses induced in skeletal muscle by endurance exercise can inhibit pathways regulating protein synthesis and stimulate protein breakdown [43]. There is evidence, however, suggesting that aspects of vascularization and oxidative enzyme activity may be enhanced with concurrent training compared to either strength or endurance training alone. The practical application of this change has not been fully explored.

Cessation of Training

Detraining has been defined as the partial or complete loss of training-induced anatomical, physiological, and functional adaptations, as a consequence of training cessation [44]. The training-induced adaptations, which develop earliest (i.e., blood capillary proliferation, increased plasma volume), are usually the adaptations that revert first when training is reduced or stopped [45].

Athletes have to consider the loss of training adaptations when they prepare for competition. Their goal is twofold. First, they want to compete without residual training-induced fatigue. Second, they need to ensure they do not lose any training-induced adaptations before competing. This can be achieved by reducing the training volume (tapering) while maintaining a high training intensity during 2–3 weeks before the competition. The important features of the taper are the magnitudes of reduction in training volume, training intensity, duration, and interaction of the taper with the preceding phase of training [46]. The specifics of the taper vary according to how the training volume load is reduced and may be referred to as a linear taper, an exponential taper involving a fast or slow constant of decay (reduction) in training load, and a step taper. This approach reduces training-induced fatigue while maintaining the training-induced adaptations.

Practical Applications

Exercise-induced adaptations are varied depending on the primary stimulus of training. Muscle can be remodeled to be either fatigue resistant, stronger, bigger, and more powerful or better coordinated. These adaptations have application for sporting performance, rehabilitation after injury, and treatment of disease. The training adaptations persist provided that the training stimulus is applied consistently and systematically; however, they slowly regress to their pre-training state when the stimulus is removed.

References

1. Selye H. Stress without distress. London: Hodder and Stoughton Ltd; 1975.
2. Chambers C, Noakes TD, Lambert EV, Lambert MI. Time course of recovery of vertical jump height and heart rate versus running speed after a 90-km foot race. J Sport Sci. 1998;16(7):645–51.
3. Warhol M, Siegel A, Evans W, Silverman L. Skeletal muscle injury and repair in marathon runners after competition. Am J Pathol. 1985;118(2):331.
4. Kentta G, Hassmen P. Overtraining and recovery: a conceptual model. Sports Med. 1998;26(1):1–16.
5. Meeusen R, Duclos M, Foster C, Fry A, Gleeson M, Nieman D, et al. Prevention, diagnosis, and treatment of the overtraining syndrome: joint consensus statement of the European College of Sport Science and the American College of Sports Medicine. Med Sci Sports. 2013;45(1):186–205.
6. Rhea MR, Alderman BL. A meta-analysis of periodized versus nonperiodized strength and power training programs. Res Q Exerc Sport. 2004;75(4):413–22.
7. Brooks JA, Fahey TD. Exercise physiology: human bioenergetics and its applications. 4th ed. Mountain View: Mayfield; 2000.
8. Mann TN, Lamberts RP, Lambert MI. High responders and low responders: factors associated with individual variation in response to standardized training. Sports Med. 2014;44(8):1113–24.
9. Leick L, Plomgaard P, Grønløkke L, Al-Abaiji F, Wojtaszewski JFP, Pilegaard H. Endurance exercise induces mRNA expression of oxidative enzymes in human skeletal muscle late in recovery. Scand J Med Sci Sports. 2009;20(4):593–9.
10. Hood DA. Invited review: contractile activity-induced mitochondrial biogenesis in skeletal muscle. J Appl Physiol. 2001;90(3):1137–57.
11. Schoenfeld BJ. The mechanisms of muscle hypertrophy and their application to resistance training. J Strength Cond Res. 2010;24(10):2857–72.
12. Baar K. The signaling underlying FITness. Appl Physiol Nutr Metab. 2009;34(3):411–9.
13. Faulkner JA. Terminology for contractions of muscles during shortening, while isometric, and during lengthening. J Appl Physiol. 2003;95(2):455–9.
14. Enoka RM. Eccentric contractions require unique activation strategies by the nervous system. J Appl Physiol. 1996;81(6):2339–46.
15. Mann T, Lamberts RP, Lambert MI. Methods of prescribing relative exercise intensity: physiological and practical considerations. Sports Med. 2013;43(7):613–25.
16. Brooks SV. Current topics for teaching skeletal muscle physiology. Adv Physiol Educ. 2003;27(1–4):171–82.
17. Ojuka EO, Jones TE, Han D-H, Chen M, Holloszy JO. Raising Ca^{2+} in L6 myotubes mimics effects of exercise on mitochondrial biogenesis in muscle. FASEB J. 2003;17(6):675–81.
18. Yamane M, Teruya H, Nakano M, Ogai R, Ohnishi N, Kosaka M. Post-exercise leg and forearm flexor muscle cooling in humans attenuates endurance and resistance training effects on muscle performance and on circulatory adaptation. Eur J Appl Physiol. 2006;96(5):572–80.
19. Halson S, Jeukendrup A. Does overtraining exist?: an analysis of overreaching and overtraining research. Sports Med. 2004;34(14):967–81.
20. Grobler L, Collins M, Lambert M, Sinclair-Smith C, Derman W, St Clair Gibson A, et al. Skeletal muscle pathology in endurance athletes with acquired training intolerance. Br Med J. 2004;38(6):697.

21. Lambert M, Borresen J. A theoretical basis of monitoring fatigue: a practical approach for coaches. Int J Sport Sci Coach. 2006;1(4):371–88.
22. Borresen J, Lambert MI. The quantification of training load, the training response and the effect on performance. Sports Med. 2009;39(9):779–95.
23. Noakes T. Physiological models to understand exercise fatigue and the adaptations that predict or enhance athletic performance. Scand J Med Sci Sports. 2000;10(3):123–45.
24. Noakes TD. Implications of exercise testing for prediction of athletic performance: a contemporary perspective. Med Sci Sports. 1988;20(4):319–30.
25. Noakes TD. Testing for maximum oxygen consumption has produced a brainless model of human exercise performance. Br J Sports Med. 2008;42(7):551–5.
26. Green HJ, Jones LL, Painter DC. Effects of short-term training on cardiac function during prolonged exercise. Med Sci Sports. 1990;22(4):488–93.
27. Esfandiari S, Sasson Z, Goodman JM. Short-term high-intensity interval and continuous moderate-intensity training improve maximal aerobic power and diastolic filling during exercise. Eur J Appl Physiol. 2014;114(2):331–43.
28. Jensen L, Bangsbo J, Hellsten Y. Effect of high intensity training on capillarization and presence of angiogenic factors in human skeletal muscle. J Physiol (Lond). 2004;557(2):571–82.
29. Lambert MI, Noakes TD. Dissociation of changes in VO2 max, muscle QO2, and performance with training in rats. J Appl Physiol. 1989;66(4):1620–5.
30. Burgess TL, Lambert MI. The effects of training, muscle damage and fatigue on running economy. Int SportMed J. 2010;11(4):363–79.
31. Scott C. Misconceptions about aerobic and anaerobic energy expenditure. J Int Soc Sports Nutr. 2005;2:32–7.
32. Costill DL, Hargreaves M. Carbohydrate nutrition and fatigue. Sports Med. 1992;(2):86–92.
33. Folland JP, Williams AG. The adaptations to strength training: morphological and neurological contributions to increased strength. Sports Med. 2007;37(2):145–68.
34. Cannon J, Marino F. Early-phase neuromuscular adaptations to high-and low-volume resistance training in untrained young and older women. J Sport Sci. 2010;28(14):1505–14.
35. Bosquet L, Berryman N, Dupuy O, Mekary S, Arvisais D, Bherer L, et al. Effect of training cessation on muscular performance: a meta-analysis. Scand J Med Sci Sports. 2013;23(3):e140–9.
36. Young W. Transfer of strength and power training to sports performance. Int J Sports Physiol Perform. 2006;1(2):74.
37. Kraemer WJ, Häkkinen K, Newton RU, Nindl BC, Volek JS, McCormick M, et al. Effects of heavy-resistance training on hormonal response patterns in younger vs. older men. J Appl Physiol. 1999;87(3):982–92.
38. Phillips SM. Short-term training: when do repeated bouts of resistance exercise become training? Can J Appl Physiol. 2000;25(3):185–93. http://dxdoiorg/101139/h00-014. (NRC Research Press Ottawa, Canada)
39. Phillips SM, Tipton KD, Aarsland A, Wolf SE, Wolfe RR. Mixed muscle protein synthesis and breakdown after resistance exercise in humans. Am J Physiol Endocrinol Metab. 1997;273:E99–E107.
40. Sale DG, MacDougall JD, Upton AR, McComas AJ. Effect of strength training upon motoneuron excitability in man. Med Sci Sports. 1983;15(1):57–62.
41. Gabriel DA, Kamen G, Frost G. Neural adaptations to resistive exercise: mechanisms and recommendations for training practices. Sports Med. 2006;36(2):133–49.
42. Bell GJ, Syrotuik D, Martin TP, Burnham R, Quinney HA. Effect of concurrent strength and endurance training on skeletal muscle properties and hormone concentrations in humans. Eur J Appl Physiol. 2000;81(5):418–27.(Springer)
43. Fyfe JJ, Bishop DJ, Stepto NK. Interference between concurrent resistance and endurance exercise: molecular bases and the role of individual training variables. Sports Med. 2014;44(6):743–62.
44. Mujika II, Padilla S. Detraining: loss of training-induced physiological and performance adaptations. Part I. Sports Med. 2000;30(2):79–87. (Springer International Publishing)
45. Mujika I, Padilla S, Pyne D, Busso T. Physiological changes associated with the pre-event taper in athletes. Sports Med. 2004;34(13):891–927.
46. Pyne DB, Mujika I, Reilly T. Peaking for optimal performance: research limitations and future directions. J Sport Sci. 2009;27(3):195–202.

Impact of Physical Activity and Exercise on Male Reproductive Potential: Semen Alterations

7

Diana Vaamonde, Ashok Agarwal, Stefan S. du Plessis, Carolina Algar-Santacruz and Thinus Frans Kruger

Abbreviations

C	Cortisol
DHT	Dihydrotestosterone
FSH	Follicle-stimulating hormone
FT	Free testosterone
GnRH	Gonadotropin-releasing hormone
hCG	Human chorionic gonadotropin
HPG	Hypothalamic pituitary–gonadal axis
HPT	Hypothalamic pituitary–testicular axis
LH	Luteinizing hormone
SHBG	Sex hormone binding globulin
T	Testosterone
TRH	Thyrotropin-releasing hormone
TSH	Thyroid-stimulating hormone
TT	Total testosterone

D. Vaamonde (✉)
Department of Morphological Sciences, School of Medicine, University of Cordoba, International Network on Physical Exercise and Fertility (INPEF), Cordoba, Spain
e-mail: fivresearch@yahoo.com

A. Agarwal
American Center for Reproductive Medicine, Cleveland Clinic Foundation, Cleveland, OH, USA

S. S. du Plessis
Division of Medical Physiology, Department of Biomedical Sciences, Stellenbosch University, P.O. Box 19063, 7505 Tygerberg, Cape Town, South Africa
e-mail: ssdp@sun.ac.za

C. Algar-Santacruz
Scientific Sport Association, Nutrir, Nutrición Médica y Ejercicio, Córdoba, Spain

T. F. Kruger
Department of Obstetrics and Gynecology, Tygerberg Hospital, Stellenbosch University, Cape Town, Western Cape, South Africa

Introduction

Physical inactivity is a modifiable risk factor for cardiovascular disease and a widening variety of other chronic diseases, including diabetes mellitus, cancer, obesity, hypertension, bone and joint diseases, and depression [1–3]. Public health recommendations have evolved from emphasizing vigorous activity for cardiorespiratory fitness to including the option of moderate levels of activity for numerous health benefits [4].

Different international health organizations warn about the elevated degree of sedentarism in the general populations, especially in the most developed countries [5–7].

Therefore, it seems necessary to promote programs of physical activity that improve health and quality of life of citizens; however, not having adequate knowledge on how to perform these activities might, on occasion, lead to negative side effects (lesions, pathologies, etc.). Many subjects have different goals that, in some cases, may lead to addiction and/or extenuation which may lead to a wide variety of problems related to several systemic processes such as osteomuscular injuries and blood pressure. On the contrary, with an adequate knowledge, physical exercise may promote many benefits when performed on a regular and adequate basis.

Some inherent risks of physical activity and sports practice are linked to fertility in female and male athletes undergoing elevated and intense training volume. This is particularly relevant if we take into account that human fertility

© Springer Science+Business Media New York 2016

D. Vaamonde et al. (eds.), *Exercise and Human Reproduction*, DOI 10.1007/978-1-4939-3402-7_7

seems to have declined in subjects of fertile age in recent years. Over the past decade, a number of studies have been published on whether fertility has declined [8, 9]. It is known that the effects of lifestyle such as smoking, poor diet, alcohol abuse, obesity or psychological stress, and sedentary habits are important factors affecting male and female reproductive performance and fertility, and may have an impact on the fertility of their offspring [10]. Little is known about the beneficial and deleterious effects of physical exercise and sports on reproductive performance [11]. Indeed, exercise and physical activity could be good or bad depending on the several parameters inherent to exercise: type, intensity, volume, objective, organization, etc.

Many researchers have emphasized during the past decade the deleterious effect of exercise on reproductive functions, as in the case of elite female athletes, with problems in the reproductive system that may derive or turn into a wide range of pathologies such as delayed menarche, oligomenorrhea, amenorrhea, inadequate luteal phase, and, even, anovulatory cycles [12–15]. This association is obviously easier to assess in female athletes due to the unequivocal symptoms already mentioned, especially in runners [16, 17], cyclists [18], swimmers [19–21], gymnasts [22, 23], figure skaters [24], and ballet dancers [25].

In men, several investigators have demonstrated that prolonged exhaustive exercise may lead to adverse effects on physiological systems and, particularly, the reproductive system and fertility: altered reproductive hormone levels [26–36], atrophy of the testicular germinal epithelium and adverse effects on spermatogenesis [37–39], changes in semen parameters including abnormal sperm morphology [26, 27, 31, 34, 35, 40], and reduced sperm motility during multiple-stage bicycle race [40].

Some authors have postulated that there is a parallelism between the harmful effects produced on the female reproductive system and those produced on the male reproductive system, especially the chronic, or the so-called long-term effects [41], especially for exhaustive endurance exercise. It has been recently demonstrated that intensified exercise can cause oxidative stress and DNA damage in athletic male sperm [42–44].

In the early investigations, exercise volume was regarded as the variable most related to the negative effects on male reproduction, leading to the hypothesis of a volume threshold for reproductive disorders [26, 45]. However, it has been reported that exercise intensity is at least, if not more, equally deleterious for reproductive function [31, 46]. Inherent parameters linked to specific exercise modalities can also be responsible for negative effects on the reproductive system: friction from bike saddles [47] or from horseriding [48], the use of androgenic anabolic steroids [49, 50], abusive use of metals such as iron as an ergogenic help [51], etc.

Some others just seem to consider exercise as potentially harmful in the case of a previous existing pathology related to reproductive system [52, 53]. In Naessens's opinion, the interrelation in exercise–reproductive dysfunction may become such that athletes may even present a wide range of possibilities, from muscle recurrent lesions to loss of libido.

However, from a scientific standpoint, it is extremely complex to establish a clear and unequivocal affirmation of this interrelation due to the fact that male reproductive parameters are, "per se", the subject of ample variety [54, 55]. The reproductive system is, without any doubt, a complex system on which many factors act upon.

There is a notorious lack of consensus about the aforementioned relationship or interdependence, probably due to the fact that different parameters were used during the training sessions that athletes underwent.

Research in relation to the effect of physical fitness on reproduction is primarily focused on athletes rather than sedentary people who have a moderate level of fitness, independent of whether they are female or male. Rich-Edwards and colleagues [56] found that each hour of vigorous exercise per week was associated with a relative risk reduction of 5 % in ovulatory infertility; this association was not observed with moderate exercise. In contrast, when dealing with obese infertile women, just losing weight, improving physical fitness and psychological well-being resulted in significant improvement in ovulation and pregnancy rates [57]. More recently, in males, Vaamonde and colleagues have observed better semen parameters and hormone levels in physically active subjects when compared to sedentary males [58]. As a result, it seems possible that exercise does not only exert negative effects but may also exert beneficial ones on the reproductive potential.

Therefore, the aim of this chapter is to review the impact of physical exercise on reproductive performance and fertility. The authors have tried to summarize recent findings concerning the effect of physical activity and exercise on reproductive function and human semen in sedentary and sports practitioners.

Physical Activity and Exercise

In order to understand the relationship between physical exercise and fertility, it is necessary to have basic notions regarding physical activity and exercise as well as the different parameters and types of exercise so that the readers can more easily follow the information offered in the chapter. We must bear in mind that physical activity and physical exercise and sports training have different connotations, requirements, development, and objectives.

All these important concepts have been amply described in Chap. 4 (for more detailed information, refer to that chapter). Nevertheless, some basic notions are offered here for a more convenient understanding. Physical activity is any type of movement that requires us to contract our muscles. Exercise, although a physical activity, is a specific form of it. It is a purposeful and planned form and we perform it with the intention of acquiring health benefits and increasing our fitness level. Most of the papers to be discussed in this chapter will deal with sports training and, to a lesser extent, with physical exercise. The main two types of exercise that differ in several aspects are endurance exercise and strength exercise.

Endurance training involves many systemic processes and events as it induces many central (e.g., systolic volume, heart rate, and cardiac output) and peripheral (e.g., vascularization and mitochondrial density) physiological adaptations. Catabolic and oxidation events are crucial in these types of athletes so as to increase the capacity to use fat and glycogen to meet energetic demands (e.g., glycogenolysis, glycolysis, and lipolysis) as well as greater efficiency in oxygen transport and distribution. Typical examples of endurance sports are running events, cycling, and swimming. Combinations of these sports such as duathlon and triathlon are also endurance sports.

Strength training deals with using some sort of resistance with the objective of producing muscular contractions for increasing strength, and muscle size. It involves systemic processes that deal with bone and muscle metabolism and hormonal responses. Typical sports based on strength training are bodybuilding, weightlifting, and powerlifting.

Parameters Determining the Characteristics of Training Load

Load can be defined as a descriptive variable that characterizes the efforts imposed on an athlete during training and competition. It can be considered as physical, psychological, or cognitive. For the purpose of this chapter, we will deal with only physical load concepts because physical load is the one that imposes greater influence on the reproductive potential.

There are several parameters that are important to take into account with regard to sports training; although explained in detail in Chap. 4, they will be briefly commented subsequently. Training load is the quantitative amount of work developed during training. It mainly implies the degree of stimulation imposed on the body and that will lead to a series of changes and adaptations. Training load entails physical and mental activities performed by the sportsman in order to develop capacities and the addition of all training effects on organism.

- Training volume is a key element and it classically represents the amount of work performed (kilometers covered, kilograms lifted, number of repetitions, etc.).

- Training intensity, on the other hand, refers to the qualitative element of physical work. It is how "hard" the athlete will perceive the exercise. It is normally expressed as percentage of variables such as VO_{2max}, HR and 1RM).
- Training density expresses the relation between effort duration and recovery duration. This applies to intrasession (taking recovery times between repetitions) density or intersession density (recovery time between different training sessions). Training density will affect both acute and chronic responses induced by exercise.

Effect of Exercise on Male Reproductive Performance and Fertility

As mentioned before, exercise may affect male fertility. Its practice influences sexual hormones and the organs of the reproductive system through several pathways. The hypothalamic–pituitary–gonadal (HPG) axis, which is regulated by a negative feedback system, is central to male reproduction. The testes are the male gonads and are responsible for production of both steroid hormones (mainly testosterone) and sperm production. The hypothalamus releases in a pulsatile manner a hormone known as gonadotropin-releasing hormone (GnRH) which, in turn, stimulates luteinizing hormone (LH) and follicle-stimulating hormone (FSH) release from the pituitary—LH is responsible for testosterone (major regulatory hormone of the system) production by stimulating the interstitial cells of Leydig and FSH is pivotal in proper spermatogenesis. It is, therefore, easily understandable that altering this system somehow may affect fertility.

Hormonal Alterations

An intact hypothalamic–pituitary–testicular (HPT) axis is essential for qualitatively and quantitatively normal spermatogenesis to occur as the initiation and proper maintenance of process is highly dependent on androgens.

Endurance Training

Negative Effect

Acute and prolonged physical exercise may suppress endocrine functions at the hypothalamic and testicular levels. It has been reported that exercise induces suppression of both GnRH release and serum testosterone [59]. Therefore, this may alter the male reproductive system.

From the endurance point of view, training volume seems to be the most influencing parameter and it has certainly been the variable most used in the available literature. Many of the studies found could be categorized into *low-to-medium volume* or *high volume* of training; yet because of scarce data, in some of the studies, this categorization could be difficult. Thus, data in some of the studies are rather controversial as some report no alteration on the HPT axis or changes only appear in some of the hormones but not in others. If we deem, as previously mentioned, that testosterone is a major regulator of the HPT axis, we may categorize the studies into three categories: those that do not show changes in either testosterone (FT or TT) or any of the other HPT hormones [60–62], those that show no changes in testosterone (FT or TT) but show changes for any of the other HPT hormones [31, 63, 64], and those that show changes in testosterone (FT or TT) but there could be changes, or not, for any of the others [26, 27, 34, 65–70].

In the first scenario, it could be hypothesized that the training stimuli were not sufficient enough to alter the axis. In the case of the studies that do not detect changes in testosterone but detect changes for other hormones (FSH and LH), it can be noted that in McConnie's study LH values decrease but in Gutin's study both FSH and LH increase. It must be noted that in the McConnie study, a challenge test with human chorionic gonadotropin (hCG) resulted in an increase in testosterone whereas in the Gutin study there are two noteworthy characteristics: the low or moderate performance level of the subjects (VO_{2max} of 51 vs. 39 ml/kg/min) and the low volume used in the study (<40 km/week). Among works detecting changes in testosterone independent of changes, or not, in other hormones, the most habitual finding is changes in testosterone without changes in FSH or LH [26, 27, 34, 64, 69]. These findings may indicate alterations at the HPT axis at levels other than the hypothalamus or pituitary, compensatory mechanism such as less excretion, or even interrelations with other axis such as the hypothalamic–pituitary–adrenal or thyroid one. In fact, glucocorticoids directly alter steroidogenesis by having negative effects on LH receptor numbers in the interstitial cells of Leydig [71]. By means of several mechanisms (e.g., reduced excretion, adrenal-stimulated secretion, or even lactic acid buildup-stimulated secretion), testosterone could increase independent of LH [72].

At any rate, it seems evident that changes in testosterone take place when athletes undergo a high volume of training. In fact, some of the mentioned studies coined the "volume-threshold hypothesis" for observing alterations in testosterone levels and the HPT axis.

Although most of the available literature deals with runners, we cannot neglect other studies done with other endurance disciplines. In cyclists, results have also offered controversial and vague conclusions; while one study showed no differences in hormonal profiles of cyclists [40], other studies revealed that, in professional cyclist assessed in one of the main races of the season (Vuelta a España), competition period exerted a negative influence on testosterone, resulting in decreased values [73, 74]. Fernandez-Garcia and colleagues highlighted that those cyclists who came into competition with the greatest volume had testosterone levels lower than those of other cyclists. Other authors have suggested decreased TT as a result of training [29, 75]. Moreover, when comparing trained and untrained subjects who were subjected to 4 h of road bicycling at a performance level as high as possible, it was observed that FSH levels were higher in the trained subjects. Such findings may reveal a sign of compensated hypogonadism which could be the result of intensive chronic training or of Sertoli cell dysfunction [76].

In swimmers, there is also controversy regarding the effect of exercise on hormone levels. While one study has not reported any differences in hormonal levels (T and C) after increased training load during a period of 4 weeks [77], another study has reported changes in testosterone (both in bound and unbound forms) during exercise although these changes reverted back to initial values during recovery [62].

Many physiological adaptations, both positive (cardiovascular, cardiorespiratory, muscular system, and body composition) and negative (neuroendocrine system and reproductive health) are the result of ultraendurance exercise [29]. Mostly the effects of exercise on reproductive potential have been assessed on endurance-trained athletes. Nevertheless, recently, this effect has been assessed in male ultra-endurance-trained athletes. Hypogonadal states (low basal levels of testosterone) have been observed as a result of chronic ultraendurance training when athletes undergo running or cycling for 10–20 h/week [78]. Triathletes, whose normal training characteristics impose high volume in the three sports modalities composing this discipline, showed, significantly lower levels of estradiol and testosterone when compared to cyclists and recreationally active men [36]. Previous studies, however, have not observed such differences [40].

Rowing is another sports commonly used in assessing the effect of training on HPT. In most of the rowers, heavy training results in decreased free testosterone/cortisol ratio when compared to basal levels; nevertheless, values never drop below the threshold value of overstrain of 0.35×10^{-3} [79]. The same authors reported observing decreases greater than 30%. In a previous study, Urhausen et al. [80] observed that T, T/SHBG, and T/C decreased during a 7-week period; such decrease stopped with regenerative training of only 1 week. Two of the rowers had normalized values for T, T/SHBG, and T/C within several weeks of training discontinuation. Another study revealed that after a 2-week period of high-training volume, testosterone was significantly decreased 30 min after finishing a long-distance rowing test; the hormonal changes observed are indicative of decreased adaptivity [81]. Another work by Mäestu and colleagues [82] revealed also decreased adaptivity as evidenced by reduced basal FT and FT: C ratio as well as testosterone response to exercise challenge after a heavy training period of 3 weeks. Another study by Vinther and colleagues evidenced in elite male lightweight rowers values for serum TT, FT, and dihydrotestosterone (DHT) that, even though were within normal range, were in the lower part of the spectrum [83]. Therefore, as reported by some, testosterone and cortisol are altered as a result of changes in training volume, and the values of such hormones related to weekly training volume [84].

Skiing exercise has also proved that prolonged exercise imposes heavy physical stress which is evidenced by a significant drop in testosterone and LH and increase in cortisol, despite a relative stability in FSH. Therefore, the observed changes suggest that exercise alters both the adrenal and the HPT axes [85]. Also in skiers, a 75-km ski race resulted in decreased FSH, LH, and T as compared to values in a control day [76].

When taking intensity as the main differential parameter, it can be observed that this variable may also exert an influence on hormonal profiles. In this regard, Safarinejad and coworkers randomly allocated 286 subjects to either moderate-intensity exercise (60 % VO_{2max}) or high-intensity exercise (80 % VO_{2max}) groups. Both groups exercised for 60 weeks (running on a treadmill for 120 min, 5 sessions/week) followed by a low-intensity recovery period of 36 weeks. It was observed that after 12 weeks of training, serum TT and FT, as well as FSH and LH, began to decrease; conversely, sex hormone binding globulin (SHBG) began to increase with both protocols. Under a GnRH stimulation challenge, LH and FSH responses were blunted [34]. Although the response was similar in both groups, it was more marked in the high-intensity group, signifying that intensity has an effect on the hormonal response. In this study, hormonal levels returned to baseline after the recovery period.

In another study, maximal intensity exercise during a short period of time imposed on physically active subjects resulted in alterations in FSH, LH, prolactin (PRL), dehydroepiandrosterone (DHEA), and cortisol values; on the contrary, testosterone, progesterone, or estradiol did not vary significantly. Hormone values returned to those observed before training after 3 days during the recovery period (Fig. 7.1) [31]. Al-

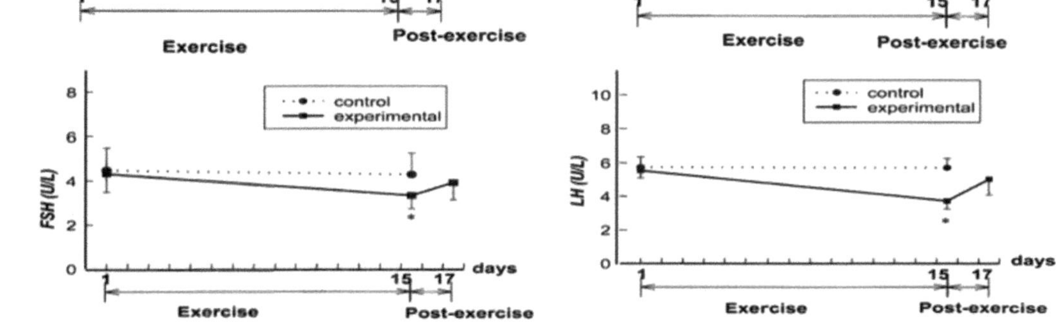

Fig. 7.1 Behavior of the most relevant hormones analyzed in relation to a 2-week intensive endurance exercise. (Reprinted from [31])

though both studies show the hormonal changes are transient, returning to normal values, it must be noted that changes may become nonreversible under certain conditions (e.g., not enough recovery periods, long-term training, and combination with high volume). These may be especially true for athletes starting heavy training at the pre- or peri-pubertal years, when it is even ethically controversial to control semen production and development. More recently, Mäestu et al. [82] proposed that decreased resting levels of free testosterone and lower maximal increases of the same hormone induced by exercise are the first sign for an athlete's decreased adaptability.

The effect of exercise volumes and intensities on male endocrine status is not well described in the literature; nevertheless, it would be important to know more precisely when the neuroendocrine system and, thus, male reproductive potential may be at risk.

The hormonal response to exercise is affected by both intensity and volume. The complexity in hormone feedback mechanisms and the disparity in results shown in the available literature demand that a consensus in study design and protocols be reached. The heterogeneity observed in different studies with regard, but not limited, to the type of athlete (sedentary vs. amateur vs. professional), the type of intervention (observational vs. modification of training or administration of exogenous hormones), etc., should be minimized.

In soccer, Grandi and Celani [86] have observed that both professional and nonprofessional players exhibit similar hormonal responses to training and to a gonadotropin-releasing hormone–thyrotropin-releasing hormone (GnRH–TRH) challenge test. Basal LH levels were higher in players during resting period than in sedentary men, but the response of LH to the challenge test was less in the players than in sedentary subjects. Although the training season did not seem to induce important hormone alterations, a strenuous soccer game induced an increase in prolactin basal levels. In basketball, it has been observed that TT increases during the season period while FT and T/C initially increase to later on start decreasing from mid-season until the end of the season [87].

Positive Effect

Most research have focused on the analysis of the acute response of the endocrine system to endurance loads, and longitudinal studies in which the long-term response to prolonged trainings is sought are sparser. Though most studies show an initial increase in levels of androgenic hormones as acute response to imposed training loads, if these are sustained in time and surpass the habitual training levels of the athletes, we could easily find with decreased basal levels of these hormones [88–91]. It is commonly accepted that the long-term effects of moderate training vary in relation to the characteristics of the used load, time of application, and the profile of the assessed athletes. Thus, it would be right to deal with the long-term effects as most likely we would find opposing results to those we find in short-term conditions [92, 93]. Frequently, we can find research concluding that middle-age subjects, or even older subjects, that perform physical activity present with testosterone basal levels that are higher than in sedentary subjects [94, 95]. However, it is necessary to understand that in order to find a response like this, it is necessary that the performed activity need not be either excessively prolonged nor it provokes great fatigue on the subject. It also has to be taken into account that the hormonal response of older subjects is not going to be as intense as in younger subjects; therefore, we may conclude that the latter have a more favorable anabolic response.

Moreover, securing a favorable hormonal response can be fulfilled with healthy life habits in which nutrition can be a key factor. In line with this, Tymchuk et al. analyzed the hormonal response to a light aerobic exercise along with a low-fat diet observing changes in the HPT axis that resulted mainly in increased SHBG [96]. Similar results have also been reported for men engaging in long-term exercise [97]. Also, in a 12-month randomized clinical study with aerobic exercise, intervention of moderate intensity in sedentary subjects resulted in increased serum DHT and SHBG [98]. In sedentary subjects submitted to low-volume exercise for 5 weeks, an increase in fT and decrease in SHBG was observed [99]. Also, when comparing sedentary subjects to physically active subjects, Vaamonde and colleagues have recently reported improved values for FSH, LH, T, and the T/C ratio. These findings further support that aerobic exercise can lead to an improved hormonal environment [58].

Resistance Training

Among the potential effects that can often be found in practitioners of resistance sports modalities (e.g., weightlifting, powerlifting, bodybuilding, and crossfit), we should distinguish those that depend on the activity itself and the intensity at which is practiced from others that are normally linked to nondesirable habits that these athletes normally follow (e.g., use of doping substances).

Use of Anabolic Androgenic Steroids

We need to bear in mind that this modality of exercise is specifically the one that we have to be careful about anabolic steroid use. Despite the fact the use of steroids significantly increases sports performance in resistance sports and provokes important increases in muscle mass of these athletes, we must not forget that the intensive and prolonged use of these substances is also linked to important androgenic effects that may derive in risks for the health of these athletes.

Although it is not the purpose of this chapter to discuss the use of anabolic steroids (for detailed information, refer to Chap. 10), due to the fact that their use is extensive among many athletes, we must note the dangerous side effects they pose for fertility and reproductive potential.

High doses of exogenous steroids alter the normal functioning of the HPT axis and inhibit the production of endogenous testosterone. The more prolonged the use of the synthetic steroid is, the more time endogenous testosterone secretion in suppressed and the longer the time for recovery to normal endogenous production may take. If the athlete wants to keep his performance level, he will enter a vicious cycle of steroid use with the risk for his own health and the possibility of being discovered and fined in an anti-doping control. When the functional situation is too adverse, it may be necessary to get the aid of a professional into trying to restore the organism's own capacities.

Hormonal Adaptive Response to Resistance Training

Hormonal responses constitute an essential part of the mechanisms that are activated in the processes of adaptation that take place with resistance training [100–102]. Resistance exercise elicits acute postexercise hormonal responses whereas prolonged, long-term training has an effect on basal or resting concentrations [103].

An adequate anabolic–catabolic balance allows for activation of protein synthesis and increase in muscle hypertrophy, which is one of the main objectives of resistance training. Hormones such as insulin, Insulin-like Growth Factor (IGF), growth hormone (GH), and testosterone are mainly anabolic, whereas cortisol, progesterone, and myostatin are catabolic or protein-synthesis-inhibiting hormones.

The circulating levels (and ratio) of such hormones, after a resistance training session, depend on the load (volume and intensity), the used muscle mass, and the impact that the session may impose on the organism [104]. Therefore, the exercise characteristics lead to an extremely complex functional response that results in specific adaptive processes in response to the type of load used. These adaptations are based on protein metabolism which conditions the metabolism of other substances in the organism. The protein metabolites generated during sports practice along with the developed neuroendocrine response are the causes that trigger differential protein synthesis in each training type.

Negative Effect

Some research have observed an increase in the resting levels of testosterone as an adjustment to strength training in the medium- to long-term (chronic) response, [105–108]. However, when resistance training becomes excessive and the athlete comes close to overtraining or deep fatigue levels, testosterone levels may remain close to or decrease from baseline levels [109–112].

The underlying mechanisms in this type of response are not well known; however, some authors hypothesize that it may be related to functional or anatomical alterations in areas of the central nervous system as a consequence of deficit of some amino acids [26]. Other studies link this to deficits or alterations in neurotransmitters related to nervous impulse (dopaminergic, noradrenergic, or serotoninergic), or the increase in the production of testosterone-inhibiting hormones (cortisol) [113]. The person's age may also influence the testosterone levels when trained subjects show advances in age and lowered training level [105, 112].

Positive Effect

Altering the levels of circulating anabolic hormones as well as the anabolic–catabolic ratio could be beneficial in males for several reasons. For an athlete, this can signify improving performance by increasing lean body mass and muscular strength and decreasing body fat [114]. Anabolic hormones and local autocrine/paracrine growth factors have a great effect on muscle adaptation to exercise. Since GH, IGF-I, and testosterone (T) promote muscle protein synthesis, they are directly involved in muscle adaptation. Although the effects are being described in terms of testosterone production, we have to be aware that the final result will depend on adequate interactions with the respective receptors.

Although there are some studies showing contradictory results, it is possible to assure that, generally, adequate resistance sessions provoke an increase in the testosterone levels (TT and fT) after one training session [101, 115–119].

The magnitude of changes in the levels of circulating testosterone after a resistance training session depends on different factors:

- Intensity of the load which is more elevated when reaching values greater than 70% of 1RM [102].
- Volume of work, since an elevated number of repetitions for exercise, work area, and session [120] increase endogenous testosterone production. Heavy resistance training can produce an increase in testosterone, which, in turn, can have a positive effect on male fertility. The acute response of testosterone is characterized by a brief increase followed by a decline to basal, or below basal, concentrations [121, 122].
- Incomplete recovery in micro and macro pauses (work:rest ratio between 0.5 and 3–5 min) [123].
- Trained muscle mass (big muscle groups).
- Athlete's age. A body that is still undergoing maturation shows an endocrine behavior different from that of an adult both in resting situation and when subjected to external loading that significantly alters his equilibrium status [124].
- Experience and performance level, in such way that the hormonal response is greater as years of training increase and the impact of the session elevated [111, 123, 124].
- The magnitude of the load used will determine the time that testosterone levels are elevated after training [110].

However, some authors hypothesize that blood testosterone levels are not real, but derived from diverse mechanisms that mask the real value, such as decreased hepatic clearance [125], theory not fully accepted [126], or an exercise-linked hemoconcentration [126].

Semen Alterations

Endurance Training

Negative Effect

Spermatozoa and Germ Cells

With regard to semen, studies also show controversial results regarding the effects of endurance exercise on sperm production. Nevertheless, there seems to be evidence of altered spermatogenesis and sperm output as a result of endurance training. Long-term exhaustive exercise seems to lower sperm quality and reproductive potential [35].

In runners, alterations in seminal quality have been reported by some authors, even up to 10% of the assessed athletes exhibiting severe oligospermia [65]; conversely, other authors postulate that differences between runners and control subjects are non-existing or merely subclinical [26, 45, 61]. An increase in non-sperm cells, such as round cells, has been reported by some authors

[26]; this fact would indicate possible infectious and/or inflammatory processes. Subjects with a higher training volume showed greatest differences in semen parameters [45]. Arce and colleagues [26] reported that athletes who exhibit differences in semen parameters are those with a minimum running volume of 100 km/week. Hall and coworkers reported no influence on sperm count, sperm morphology, and sperm motility after a gradually intensified training period of 6 weeks (186 % of normal training) followed by 2 weeks of detraining (50 % of normal training) [127].

Endurance-trained runners, but not resistance-trained athletes, showed altered values for sperm density, motility, morphology, and in vitro sperm penetration of standard cervical mucus [26]. Similar results have been found for high-intensity training athletes when compared to moderate-intensity ones [34]. It is worth mentioning that during recovery all parameters improved to pre-exercise levels [34].

When dealing with high-level athletes, it has to be considered that they have normally been training for many years; therefore, it becomes difficult to accurately estimate a threshold value for abnormal semen parameters. Nevertheless, a high cycling volume seems to be detrimental to sperm morphology [128]. Moreover, the same authors report that, in triathletes, a volume of 300 km/week in cycling correlates with serious fertility impairment from the sperm morphology point of view (Fig. 7.2).

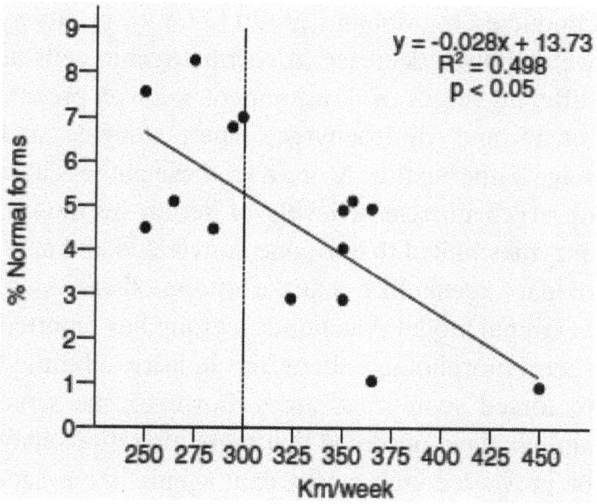

Fig. 7.2 Correlation between percentage of sperm with normal morphology and cycling weekly volume (expressed as km/week)

Competition period seems to be especially deleterious for semen parameters in cyclists; in fact, cyclists have shown during this period lower sperm motility (46.2 ± 19.5 %) than either recreational marathoners and sedentary subjects ($P<0.05$) or themselves at other season periods ($P<0.01$) [40]. Although this study does not reveal differences in sperm morphology, it is really striking to see that it reports morphology normalcy values above 95 %. Conversely, other authors have observed lower numbers of morphologically normal sperm in long-distance competitive cyclists (41.5 for controls vs. 19.5 for cyclists) whereas no changes were observed for semen volume, motility, viability, or concentration. Moreover, they found among the observed anomalies greater proportion of tapered forms [41]. Conversely, Vaamonde et al. showed that seminological values differed significantly even in recreational athletes when they exercised to the point of exhaustion (with morphology significantly decreasing from 17 % of normal forms to 12 %, total sperm count decreasing to half the original value, and percentage of immotile sperm significantly increasing with about 10 % of subjects developing necrozoospermia) [31]. The adverse effects of exercise especially become an aggravating factor in men whose sperm parameters are already compromised due to other pathologies such as varicocele [53].

Similar to what has been reported in endurance sports, ultraendurance athletes show significantly different values for sperm number/concentration, velocity, and morphology, as compared to physically active men or water polo players. Morphology was the parameter showing the greatest difference; this difference even reached clinical relevance for the triathletes (<5 % normal forms) for the reference values at the time of the study [35].

In animal models with rats, it has been observed that although rats maintain their reproductive capacity after swimming stress and the offspring shows normal morphology, the number of spermatids is reduced [129]. Several studies conducted by Manna's group [37–39], in rats as well, show a decrease in spermatogenic cells at different stages of development, such as preleptotene and midpachytene spermatocytes and stage 7 spermatids. Moreover, these authors also observed decreased levels of serum hormones, enzymes linked to hormone conversion and antioxidant agents like catalase among others. Also, in animal model, Vaamonde's group has reported sperm morphology alterations in mice submitted to forced swimming stress; however, the same authors have observed that these alterations may be prevented with antioxidant agents like n-acetyl cysteine and, more efficiently, with trans-resveratrol [130, 131].

Oxidative Stress and DNA Fragmentation

Information regarding the effect of exercise on oxidative stress and, especially, on semen oxidative stress and DNS fragmentation is very scarce. A study has recently evidenced that in comparison to recreationally active and nonactive men, resting seminal 8-isoprostane, Reactive Oxygen Species (ROS), Malondialdehyde (MDA), and sperm DNA fragmentation are higher in elite athletes and SOD, catalase, and TAC levels are lower [43]. As expected, sperm DNA fragmentation was shown to positively correlate to VO_{2max}, seminal 8-isoprostane, Reactive Oxygen Species (ROS), and Malondialdehyde (MDA) levels. These findings further support previous studies, suggesting that elite athletes are at greater risk of sperm dysfunction than recreational exercisers or, even, sedentary people [43]. In another work by the same group, a significant increase in seminal ROS and MDA levels and a significant decrease in seminal SOD, catalase, and total antioxidant capacity were demonstrated after 8 weeks of intensive cycling training in male road cyclists [42]. Although not in semen, it must be highlighted that there are some studies reporting a link between exercise and altered leucocyte number, especially in the case of overtrained subjects [132, 133].

Vaamonde's group has recently reported that, similar to what happens with sperm morphology, cycling volume positively correlates with sperm DNA fragmentation. As such, athletes undergoing greater annual mean weekly training volume showed the greatest percentage of sperm DNA damage [134]. From a practical point of view, Vaamonde and colleagues have analyzed a group of ultraendurance athletes, and found high correlation between training volume and sperm DNA fragmentation, percentage of morphological abnormalities, and TUNEL(+) cells (unpublished data).

Positive Effect

Spermatozoa and Germ Cells

There is still not much scientific evidence on whether exercise or physical activity may exert a beneficial effect on seminal parameters. In fact, scientific studies in this regard are scarce. In humans, Vaamonde and colleagues [58] have recently reported improved semen parameters in physically active men (PA) when compared to sedentary people (SE). Both total progressive motility (PA: 60.94 ± 5.03; SE: 56.07 ± 4.55) and morphology (PA: 15.54 ± 1.38, SE: 14.40 ± 1.15) showed statistically significant differences. Differences in seminological parameters were further supported by hormonal differences [58]. Similar results have been reported by Palmer et al. (2012) in an animal model (C57BL6 male mice) observing improved sperm motility (1.2-fold) and morphology (1.1-fold, $P < 0.05$) after a swimming training protocol of 8 weeks [135]. Also in mice, running training for 14 months (from 6 months old until they were 20 months old) induced positive effect on mice testicular health. Exercising mice exhibited uninterrupted seminiferous tubules as evidenced by complete number and type of cells at the different stages of the spermatogenic cycle and also a clear lumen with great sperm density. On the contrary, sedentary mice showed a disorganized germinal epithelium and no spermatocyte-stage cells. Sertoli cells were more abundant in the runners as compared to the sedentary subjects [136].

At any rate, even if it does not entail positive effects, it seems evident that exercise does not always induce alterations in the semen profile of endurance athletes. In line with this, Lucia et al. [40] report that average values of semen parameters are usually within normal limits in endurance-trained men. Other authors defend that when these alterations are present, they are subclinical in nature [26, 27, 61, 65]. Moreover, De Souza and co-workers [27] have reported the existence of a certain "training volume-threshold" (~100 km/week) for significant alterations to occur in male reproductive function. In their study, it was indeed shown that a high volume of endurance running (>104 km/week) was associated with subclinical alterations in both the profile of sex hormones (decreased levels of total and free testosterone) and the quality of semen (particularly decreased motility and increased number of immature cells).

Oxidative Stress and DNA Fragmentation

Exercise training seems to be able to exert modifying effects on oxidative stress, depending on the training load, training specificity, and the basal level of training. In fact, it has been reported that elite athletes have an augmented SOD capacity in comparison to recreationally active and sedentary control men [42]. The reason for this could be the greater aerobic capacity (VO_{2max}) of the subjects with greater performance in endurance, and this parameter correlates with elevated antioxidant enzyme activity in other tissues [137].

After comparing elite athletes and recreational active men, we have observed that the least active subjects have significantly higher levels of seminal antioxidant compounds (superoxide dismutase, catalase, and total antioxidant capacity) and lower levels of seminal ROS, malondialdehyde, and 8-isoprostane, and subsequently lower rate of sperm DNA fragmentation when compared with elite athletes ($P<0.001$) [43]. Significant negative correlation was observed between sperm DNA fragmentation with seminal SOD, catalase, and TAC levels ($P<0.001$). Significant positive correlation was observed between sperm DNA fragmentation with seminal 8-isoprostane, ROS, and MDA levels ($P<0.001$).

Also in animal models, it has been observed that, in mice, running training for 14 months (from 6 months old until they were 20 months old) reduces the levels of 8-isoprostane (marker of lipid peroxidation), nitrotyrosine, and protein carbonyl levels. Moreover, the levels of antioxidant-related enzymes such as SOD1 and GPX, among others, were increased in the runners. Therefore, lifelong running in this regard seemed to exert a positive effect [136]. Swimming exercise has also been proved beneficial to revert the pathophysiological effects of aging as changes in testosterone, and in biomarkers of inflammation and oxidative stress associated with age, were modulated by daily sessions of swimming for 15 min. The authors observed this effect in mice that started swimming early in life, at middle life, and later in life. Nevertheless, the effect was lesser when mice started exercising later in life [138]. This benefit related to age changes has also been reported by Joseph et al. in rat testes; 10-weeks of treadmill exercise induced beneficial adaptations increasing antioxidant capacity in mitochondria and decreasing DNA damage (phosphorylated histone H2AX) [139].

Even less training time (8 weeks of swimming exercise) is able to elicit a beneficial response in mice. Palmer and colleagues have observed a 1.5-fold reduction in sperm DNA damage, a 1.1-fold reduction in reactive oxygen species, and a 1.2-fold reduction in mitochondrial membrane potential [135].

As it has already been noted, exercise disrupts body homeostasis by increasing ROS and oxidative stress. As such, physically active people may suffer from ROS-induced damage that may lead to altered sperm parameters (motility, morphology, and DNA) and male subfertility. The effect is dependent on the mode, intensity, and duration of the exercise as well as the subject's antioxidant capacity. On the other hand, it has also been noted that training may have modifying effects on oxidative stress, depending on training load, training specificity, and the basal level of training. It seems that aerobic exercise training can result in a hormetic response, giving rise to an augmented SOD activity and reduced lipid peroxidation [140, 141]. According to the hormetic hypothesis, trained and athletic people have developed, as a result of intensive training, increased total antioxidant capacity, and in particular high levels of SOD, in several tissues [142, 143]. Despite having values of antioxidants in human semen in normal and infertile men [144, 145], knowledge on the behavior of antioxidant capacity in seminal plasma as a result of training is scarce and unclear.

Though not positive effects themselves, some studies point out that sports practice does not induce negative effects on semen parameters, especially if load is not too heavy, such as the threshold established by De Souza for volume (100 km/week) [27].

The positive or negative effect of aerobic work and the oxidative potential could very well be conditioned by the level of the athlete or his training experience [42, 143, 146, 147].

Resistance Training

Negative Effect

Spermatozoa and Germ Cells

Although to date, to the best of our knowledge, there are few/none studies reporting sperm quality as a result of resistance training under physiological (nonsteroid taking) conditions, there are some reports on the effect of concomitant use of androgenic anabolic steroids along with resistance training. In this case, first, we need to be aware that many anabolic-androgenic steroids (AAS) abusers do not disclose taking AAS; moreover, they normally concurrently take antiestrogens, aromatase inhibitors, and hCG to counteract the adverse effects of AAS, such as hypogonadotropic hypogonadism and gynecomastia, and perhaps avert the detection of their use [148]. By stimulating endogenous testosterone production and preventing testicular atrophy, hCG and clomifene were until recently concurrently abused by AAS users to avoid detection of exogenous testosterone [149].

Nevertheless, supraphysiologic levels of exogenous AAS actually exert negative feedback on the HPT axis and subsequently reduce FSH, LH, and intratesticular testosterone concentration. These hormonal changes can lead to azospermia, oligospermia, testicular atrophy, hypogonadotropic hypogonadism, and an increased percentage of morphologically abnormal sperm with amorphous spermatozoa and defects in the head and midpiece [150–152].

Usually, spermatogenesis recovers spontaneously within 4–6 months after cessation of AAS [153], although it has been reported to take up to 3 years or longer [154], maybe due to the wide variety of combinations and types of AAS. As a result of AAS abuse, there can be a transient impairment on semen quality with abnormal and hypokinetic spermatozoa [155].

It is difficult to study AAS use and its side effects because of the variable dosing as well as the prevalence of selection and information biases in research design.

In experiments performed in animal models (rats), apoptosis in the male germ line was characterized by TUNEL, caspase-3 assay, and transmission electron microscopy. The weights of the testes and accessory sex organs, as well as sperm parameters, significantly decreased in the experimental groups relative to the sham and control groups ($p <$ or $= 0.05$). Germ cell apoptosis and a significant decrease in the number of germ cell layers in nandrolone decanoate exercise-treated testes were observed ($p <$ or $= 0.05$). Exercise training seems to increase the extent of apoptotic changes caused by supraphysiological dose of nandrolone decanoate in rats, which, in turn, affects fertility [156].

Positive Effect

Spermatozoa and Germ Cells

The positive effect of resistance training on semen parameters has been scarcely addressed. In fact, there is no evidence that resistance training may improve semen profile; yet, Arce et al. [26] showed that sperm density, motility, morphology, and in vitro sperm penetration of standard cervical mucus were significantly altered in the endurance-trained runners, but not in the resistance-trained athletes. This seems to, at least, indicate that resistance training did not impose a detrimental effect on semen quality.

Morphofunctional Alterations of the Reproductive System

Endurance Training

Negative Effect

Testes Size and Accessory Ducts

It is difficult to examine the effect of exercise on testicular size and accessory glands and ducts in humans; however, one study on a soccer player reveals that the studied athlete exhibited testicular maldevelopment [52]. In this case, it is difficult to establish the clear cause–effect as the athlete had cryptorchidy. Nevertheless, all other symptoms worsened during periods of greater training load; therefore, it can be suspected that testicular features would also worsen during those time periods. Because of the special nature of these effects, the studies that have assessed the effect of exercise on morphofunctional characteristics of testes and accessory glands and ducts have been conducted in animal models. Manna et al. have observed the effect of different intensities of swimming exercise on testes and accessory glands and ducts, and found a decrease in testicular, epididymal, prostatic, and seminal vesicles somatic index [39].

Erectile Dysfunction, Microtrauma, and Varicocele

Erectile dysfunction (ED) or impotence has also been attributed to continuous strenuous exercise [157]. Tiredness and fatigue may reduce sexual desire and libido to the extent that it is impossible to get or sustain an erection. This phenomenon is highly associated with bicycling, as multiple studies repeatedly demonstrated the increased risk of ED in cyclists [52, 158–162] as they are more prone to suffer from microtrauma and compression due to the friction that the bike saddle imposes on the genital area. It becomes more apparent that it is not a simple fact of exercise leading to infertility, but rather that inherent parameters of exercise such as the type, volume, and intensity must also be taken into consideration and carefully analyzed.

As in the case of the studies assessing hormones, training volume was variable in the studies assessing seminal quality. Despite this inconvenience, it seems evident that subjects with a higher training volume showed greater differences. We have to bear in mind though that the reversible deleterious effects may not be reversible if athletes have been training for longer periods of time (years) or had started training around puberty.

Positive Effect

Testes Size and Accessory Ducts

Testicular atrophy is a well-known feature of the aging process; this testicular atrophy is characterized by many histological features; however, these changes seem to be dampened by exercise in animal models. As a result of a 14-month running training (from 6 months old to 20 months old), mice in the running group exhibited lower weight of both seminal vesicles and testes when compared to sedentary mice. Histological features observed in the testes of sedentary mice included areas of focal and diffused sclerosis; such findings clearly evidence tissue inflammation and degeneration [136]. Rats submitted to treadmill exercise for 10 weeks exhibited attenuated testicular atrophy, which is typical of older sedentary animals as a result of changes in mitochondria and oxidative stress profile [139].

Erectile dysfunction, Microtrauma, and Varicocele

Derby and colleagues have observed that ED may be improved by modifying unhealthy lifestyles [163]. Becoming physically active (at least 200 kcal/day) significantly improved ED condition in subjects that had been previously sedentary. So, by becoming physically active, subjects had less chance to suffer from ED than those that stayed sedentary and the chance was similar to that in subjects that were already physically active at the beginning of the study. Further studies have also observed and supported the notion that physically active subjects have less chances of suffering from ED [164, 165]. It is worth mentioning that the subjects in this study were middle-aged physically active subjects and not athletes.

Resistance Training

Negative Effect

Testes Size and Accessory Ducts

The deleterious effects of AAS, such as nandrolone decanoate, have already been mentioned. They can affect testicular ultrastructure as evidenced by transmission electron microscopy. It has been observed that these alterations include decreased number and size of Leydig cells, altered germinal epithelium (basal membrane with increased thickness and irregular wavy multilaminar appearance), and cytologic alterations (vacuoles, lipid droplets, altered mitochondria, etc.). Apoptotic features in germ were extensively observed. Though the study assessed swimming exercise, due to the fact that AAS use and abuse is common in resistance exercise, the observations have been included here. All alterations were more evident in the group of rats that were submitted to swimming exercise besides being treated with nandrolone decanoate; therefore, exercise seems to aggravate the extent of the damage induced by the steroids [166].

Mixed Modalities

There are some sports (soccer, basketball, rugby, handball, etc.) that cannot be considered as purely endurance or resistance sports, but they are to be considered as mixed modalities. From an effectiveness standpoint, these sports are based on technical actions with great dependence on strength and, therefore, anaerobic metabolism; yet, from a competition standpoint, the sports acts have an energetic dependence on fat and carbohydrates via aerobic metabolism.

Athletes engaging in mixed modalities have also been shown to have altered values for both hormones and semen parameters. Especially, exercise seems to be an aggravating factor in the case of previous existing pathologies [52, 53]. Di Luigi's group reported that exercise aggravated the varicocele condition of athletes. Naessen's group reported that a soccer player's previous existing HPG axis alteration was aggravated by physical exercise, especially as a result of increased training load, typical of competition periods. Moreover, this subject showed recurrent muscle problems and decreased libido [52]. In another study, it was observed that sperm motility was in soccer players as compared to sedentary subjects [86]. Increased C and decreased T values have been observed in rugby players during competition; conversely, these changes would revert during the post-competition period with T values increasing above basal values and C values decreasing until the fifth day post-competition [167]. It must be noted that in mixed modalities, however, it is difficult to establish clear causal and correlational relationships between volume and intensity, and even with regard to metabolic route employed as the imposed demands normally vary with regard to the type of training undertaken.

Volume-Threshold Hypothesis: True or Not?

Some of the studies have postulated the existence of a minimum volume, the so-called volume threshold, for reproductive alterations (either hormonal or seminological) to appear. The first authors in describing this were the group of De Souza [26, 27].

Afterward, although not stating a definite number of kilometers or hours of training, other authors have observed how athletes tend to show a decrease in seminal and/or hormonal parameters during competition or post-competition periods. It seems rather plausible that a threshold exists; in line with this, recent findings support this theory by showing, in triathletes, that those with the highest volume of cycling show the worst semen parameters. Interestingly enough, when assessing triathletes, Vaamonde and colleagues could observe that the athlete showing the greatest performance level of those they could analyze followed a low-volume, high-intensity training; in such a case, the semen parameters were as bad, or even worse, as those of other athletes with high training volume; moreover, this athlete exhibited low morphology, high DNA fragmentation, and TAC values in the lower end of the spectrum [44].

Even though it certainly seems a threshold exists, the wrong models have been adopted so far to prove this theory as the way it should be done would be by allocating different groups to different training volumes. However, it seems clear that intensity, as well as volume, may affect the hormonal and seminological response. Moreover, the other parameters and characteristics inherent to training (frequency, clothing, environmental temperature, possible damage to pelvic area and tendinitis, infections and/or inflammations, etc.) may also play a role. In line with this, and as in any other physiological process, the subject's own characteristics and how his adaptive systems are prepared for the challenge will determine the final response. Those practitioners systematically undergoing high training loads presented with altered values for semen parameters. Due to the fact that exercise may produce, or aggravate previously existing, reproductive profile pathologies, such as hormonal and seminological alterations, it would be appropriate to further assess this relationship.

Conclusions

In spite of the many benefits promoted by physical exercise, we must be aware that, especially when excessively practiced, it may actually exert negative effects on the endocrine and reproductive systems and, thus, may compromise fertility [15, 168, 169]. The positive or negative impact and oxidative potential of exercise, especially that of aerobic nature, could well be conditioned by the level of the athlete and his training experience [42, 143, 146, 147]. Both intensity and volume seem to exert an effect on the hormonal and seminal response. Yet other parameters and characteristics related to training cannot be ruled out. The final outcome will depend on how the subjects' adaptive systems are able to respond to the exercise challenge. Results from different studies and researchers are not in full agreement as to what is the effect of exercise on these systems. Nevertheless, evidence suggests a relationship between high-load exercise and a negative impact on male fertility. The severity of the effect seems dependent on the duration, intensity, and type of modalities. Moreover, as it happens with any condition, the athletes' own features such as fitness level and adaptive capacity will also have an important modulating effect. Whatever the underlying mechanism may be, exercise may lead to altered semen parameters and fertility potential, especially in the case of previously existing pathologies that are aggravated by exercise. Yet, most of the studies have revealed either subclinical alterations or restoration to normal, or almost normal, values upon cessation of exercise. With regard to future studies, it is clear that well-designed studies with standardization regarding testing and exercise conditions and characteristics are a must. Also, potential confounding factors should be carefully addressed.

In order to clearly establish the interrelation between exercise and fertility, careful attention ought to be paid to the main exercise parameters that were briefly defined earlier in this chapter and are given in more detail in Chap. 4. These important parameters are intensity and volume and they should be carefully addressed not only in studies but also when trying to preserve the athlete's fertility potential. Awareness must be raised so that the diverse professionals dealing with athletes will know that exercise (though dependent on volume, intensity, and modality) is really a potential cause for urological and andrological disorders that could compromise male fertility [162]. Therefore, as suggested previously, we deem necessary to have high-load training included as a component of male factor infertility [26]. Also, future studies should assess the addition of antioxidant supplements to the exercise routine of athletes [26], and even in the case of recreational regular exercisers. Unless these measures are taken, the relationship between exercise and fertility will remain a strange paradox. It seems somewhat clearer that being physically active elicits beneficial effects that seem to outweigh possible deleterious effects. However, further information as to the effects of moderate- and low-level exercise on reproductive performance is needed. Evidence points out that, as well as it happens with general health benefits, moderate levels of exercise along with a well-balanced diet could also have a beneficial effect on fertility. Therefore, such lifestyle practices could help couples in achieving pregnancy and should be recommended.

Nevertheless, we must be cautious and acknowledge that exercise may be a cause, solely or coadjuvant, for fertility problems, and if we see a patient with idiopathic male infertility, it could be wise to advise him to decrease the exercise load as a preventive measure (Fig. 7.3) [170].

The clinician handling an athlete with infertility must first see him in the same way as any other infertility patient. Taking a detailed history and performing a thorough physical examination, as well as taking the female infertility factors into consideration, is always the mainstay of the approach. An important principle is to looking at the fertility picture holistically and planning with the male and female infertility factors in mind.

Extra information on the use of supplements, smoking, alcohol, the specific diet, and the use of androgens is of course of utmost importance in these men. The type of sport and excessive exercise can also play a role in the fertility profile and must be noted. After the physical examination, a semen analysis will be of great help. A hormonal evaluation (e.g., testosterone, FSH, thyroid-stimulating hormone (TSH), and prolactin) can be of value in some patients but should be done as a routine at the first consultation, especially in athletes. If the semen analysis is abnormal, a recognized andrology laboratory should perform a repeat evaluation after 8 weeks. This simple holistic approach will assist the fertility specialist to work out a plan for both partners. It is often necessary to give advice on supplements, drugs, and diet to these men that can assist greatly in achieving a pregnancy.

If infertility is the complaint and extreme sport is the only factor and the semen parameters are in

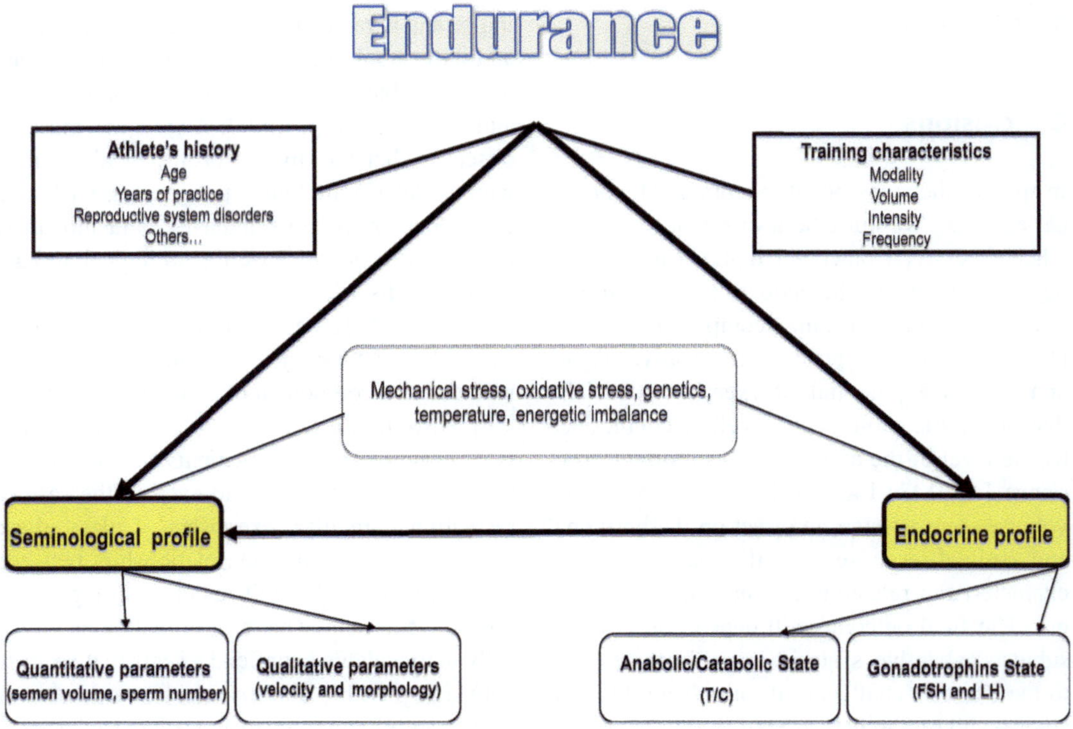

Fig. 7.3 Factors related to the relationship between endurance exercise and fertility. (Modified from Vaamonde et al. 2015. In Press)

the subfertile ranges, a decrease in activity can be of value for a specific couple. However, more studies like the ones conducted by the group of Vaamonde are needed to assist in understanding the impact of different sports on semen quality and fertility. In an attempt to help standardize future studies and aid clinicians assess the possible effect of exercise on fertility, a questionnaire has been developed by Vaamonde and colleagues [170].

References

1. Lee IM, Skerrett PJ. Physical activity and all-cause mortality: what is the dose-response relation? Med Sci Sports Exerc. 2001;33(6 Suppl):S459–71.
2. Warburton DE, Nicol CW, Bredin SS. Health benefits of physical activity: the evidence. CMAJ. 2006;174(6):801–9.
3. Blair SN, Morris JN. Healthy hearts and the universal benefits of being physically active physical activity and health. Ann Epidemiol. 2009;19:253–6.
4. Haskell WL, Lee IM, Pate RR, Powell KE, Blair SN, Franklin BA, Macera CA, Heath GW, Thompson PD, Bauman A. Physical activity and public health: updated recommendation for adults from the American College of Sports Medicine and the American Heart Association. Med Sci Sports Exerc. 2007;39(8):1423–34.
5. United States. Public Health Service. Office of the Surgeon General, National Center for Chronic Disease Prevention, Health Promotion (US), President's Council on Physical Fitness, & Sports (US). Jones & Bartlett Learning. Physical activity and health: a report of the surgeon general. 1996.
6. World Health Organization (WHO). Physical inactivity: a global public health problem. Geneva: World Health Organization; 2008
7. Go AS, Mozaffarian D, Roger VL, Benjamin EJ, Berry JD, Borden WB, Bravata DM, Dai S, Ford ES, Fox CS, Franco S, Fullerton HJ, Gillespie C, Hailpern SM, Heit JA, Howard VJ, Huffman MD, Kissela BM, Kittner SJ, Lackland DT, Lichtman JH, Lisabeth LD, Magid D, Marcus GM, Marelli A, Matchar DB, McGuire DK, Mohler ER, Moy CS, Mussolino ME, Nichol G, Paynter NP, Schreiner PJ, Sorlie PD, Stein J, Turan TN, Virani SS, Wong ND, Woo D, Turner MB; American Heart Association Statistics Committee and Stroke Statistics Subcommittee. Heart disease and stroke statistics update: a report from the American Heart Association. Circulation. 2013;127:e6–e245.
8. Olsen J, Zhu JL, Ramlau-Hansen CH. Has fertility declined in recent decades? Acta Obstet Gynecol Scand. 2011;90(2):129–35.
9. Yoldemir T, Oral E. Has fertility declined in recent decades? Curr Opin Obstet Gynecol. 2012;24(3):119–26.
10. Homan GF, Davies M, Norman R. The impact of lifestyle factors on reproductive performance in the general population and those undergoing infertility treatment: a review. Hum Reprod Update. 2007;13(3):209–23.
11. Du Plessis S, Kashou A, Vaamonde D, Agarwal A. Is there a link between exercise and male factor infertility? Open Reprod Sci J. 2011;3:105–13.
12. De Souza MJ, Maguire MS, Maresh CM, Kraemer WJ, Rubin KR, Loucks AB. Adrenal activation and the prolactin response to exercise in eumenorrheic and amenorrheic runners. J Appl Physiol (1985). 1991;70(6):2378–87.
13. Warren MP, Perlroth NE. The effects of intense exercise on the female reproductive system. J Endocrinol. 2001;170(1):3–11.
14. Redman LM, Loucks AB. Menstrual disorders in athletes. Sports Med. 2005;35(9):747–55.
15. Olive DL. Exercise and fertility: an update. Curr Opin Obstet Gynecol. 2010;22(4):259–63.
16. Dusek T. Influence of high intensity training on menstrual cycle disorders in athletes. Croat Med J. 2001;42(1):79–82.
17. Thompson SH. Characteristics of the female athlete triad in collegiate cross-country runners. J Am Coll Health. 2007;56(2):129–36.
18. Haakonssen EC, Martin DT, Jenkins DG, Burke LM. Race weight: perceptions from elite female road cyclists. Int J Sports Physiol Perform. 2014. (Epub ahead of print). 2015;10(3):311–7.
19. Constantini NW, Warren MP. Menstrual dysfunction in swimmers: a distinct entity. J Clin Endocrinol Metab. 1995;80(9):2740–4.
20. Schtscherbyna A, Soares EA, de Oliveira FP, Ribeiro BG. Female athlete triad in elite swimmers of the city of Rio de Janeiro, Brazil. Nutrition. 2009;25(6):634–9.
21. Vanheest JL, Rodgers CD, Mahoney CE, De Souza MJ. Ovarian suppression impairs sport performance in junior elite female swimmers. Med Sci Sports Exerc. 2014;46(1):156–66.
22. Klentrou P, Plyley M. Onset of puberty, menstrual frequency, and body fat in elite rhythmic gymnasts compared with normal controls. Br J Sports Med. 2003. 37(6):490–4.
23. Maïmoun L, Coste O, Georgopoulos NA, Roupas ND, Mahadea KK, Tsouka A, Mura T, Philibert P, Gaspari L, Mariano-Goulart D, Leglise M, Sultan C. Despite a high prevalence of menstrual disorders, bone health is improved at a weight-bearing bone site in world-class female rhythmic gymnasts. J Clin Endocrinol Metab. 2013;98(12):4961–9.
24. Vadocz EA, Siegel SR, Malina RM. Age at menarche in competitive figure skaters: variation by competency and discipline. J Sports Sci. 2002;20(2):93–100.
25. Hincapié CA, Cassidy JD. Disordered eating, menstrual disturbances, and low bone mineral density in

dancers: a systematic review. Arch Phys Med Rehabil. 2010;91(11):1777–89.
26. Arce JC, De Souza MJ, Pescatello LS, Luciano AA. Subclinical alterations in hormone and semen profile in athletes. Fertil Steril. 1993;59(2):398–404.
27. De Souza MJ, Arce JC, Pescatello LS, Scherzer HS, Luciano AA. Gonadal hormones and semen quality in male runners. A volume threshold effect of endurance training. Int J Sports Med. 1994;15(7):383–91.
28. Viru AM, Hackney AC, Valja E, Karelson K, Janson T, Viru M. Influence of prolonged continuous exercise on hormone responses to subsequent exercise in humans. Eur J Appl Physiol. 2001;85:578–85.
29. Maimoun L, Lumbroso S, Manetta J, Paris F, Leroux JL, Sultan C. Testosterone is significantly reduced in endurance athletes without impact on bone mineral density. Horm Res Paediatr. 2003;59(6):285–92.
30. Hackney AC. Exercise as a stressor to the human neuroendocrine system. Medicina (Kaunas). 2006;42:788–97.
31. Vaamonde D, Da Silva ME, Poblador MS, Lancho JL. Reproductive profile of physically active men after exhaustive endurance exercise. Int J Sports Med. 2006;27:680–9.
32. Hackney AC. Effects of endurance exercise on the reproductive system of men: the "exercise-hypogonadal male condition". J Endocrinol Invest. 2008;31:932–38.
33. Hill EE, Zack E, Battaglini C, Viru M, Viru A, Hackney AC. Exercise and circulating cortisol levels: the intensity threshold effect. J Endocrinol Invest. 2008;31:587–91.
34. Safarinejad MR, Azma K, Kolahi AA. The effects of intensive, long-term treadmill running on reproductive hormones, hypothalamus-pituitary-testis axis, and semen quality: a randomized controlled study. J Endocrinol. 2009;200(3):259–71.
35. Vaamonde D, Da Silva-Grigoletto ME, García-Manso JM, Vaamonde-Lemos R, Swanson RJ, Oehninger SC. Response of semen parameters to three training modalities. Fertil Steril. 2009;92:1941–6.
36. Fitzgerald LZ, Robbins WA, Kesner JS, Xun L. Reproductive hormones and interleukin-6 in serious leisure male athletes. Eur J Appl Physiol. 2012;112(11):3765–73.
37. Manna I, Jana K, Samanta PK. Effect of intensive exercise-induced testicular gametogenic and steroidogenic disorders in mature male Wistar strain rats: a correlative approach to oxidative stress. Acta Physiol Scand. 2003;178(1):33–40.
38. Manna I, Jana K, Samanta PK. Intensive swimming exercise-induced oxidative stress and reproductive dysfunction in male Wistar rats: protective role of alpha-tocopherol succinate. Can J Appl Physiol. 2004;29(2):172–85.
39. Manna I, Jana K, Samanta PK. Effect of different intensities of swimming exercise on testicular oxidative stress and reproductive dysfunction in mature male albino Wistar rats. Indian J Exp Biol. 2004;42:816–22.
40. Lucía A, Chicharro JL, Pérez M, Serratosa L, Bandrés F, Legido JC. Reproductive function in male endurance athletes: sperm analysis and hormonal profile. J Appl Physiol (1985). 1996;81(6):2627–36.
41. Gebreegziabher Y, Marcos E, McKinon W, Rogers G. Sperm characteristics of endurance trained cyclists. Int J Sports Med. 2004;25(4):247–51.
42. Tartibian B, Maleki BH. Correlation between seminal oxidative stress biomarkers and antioxidants with sperm DNA damage in elite athletes and recreationally active men. Clin J Sport Med. 2012;22(2):132–9.
43. Tartibian B, Maleki BH. The effects of honey supplementation on seminal plasma cytokines, oxidative stress biomarkers, and antioxidants during 8 weeks of intensive cycling training. J Androl. 2012;33(3):449–61.
44. Vaamonde D, Da Silva-Grigoletto ME, Fernandez JM, Algar-Santacruz C, García-Manso JM. Findings on sperm alterations and DNA fragmentation, nutritional, hormonal and antioxidant status in an elite triathlete. Case report. Rev Andal Med Deporte. 2014;7(4):143–8.
45. De Souza MJ, Miller BE. The effect of endurance training on reproductive function in male runners. A "volume threshold" hypothesis. Sports Med. 1997;23:357–73.
46. Jensen CE, Wiswedel K, McLoughlin J, van der Spuy Z. Prospective study of hormonal and semen profiles in marathon runners. Fertil Steril. 1995;64:1189–96.
47. Brock G. Erectile function of bike patrol officers. J Androl. 2002;23:758–9.
48. McAleer IM, Kaplan GW, LoSasso BE. Renal and testis injuries in team sports. J Urol. 2002;168:1805–7.
49. Karila T, Hovatta O, Seppala T. Concomitant abuse of anabolic androgenic steroids and human chorionic gonadotrophin impairs spermatogenesis in power athletes. Int J Sports Med. 2004;25:257–26.
50. Shokri S, Hemadi M, Bayat G, Bahmanzadeh M, Jafari-Anarkooli I, Mashkani B. Combination of running exercise and high dose of anabolic androgenic steroid, nandrolone decanoate, increases protamine deficiency and DNA damage in rat spermatozoa. Andrologia. 2014;46(2):184–90.
51. Aydemir B, Kiziler AR, Onaran I, Alici B, Ozkara H, Akyolcu MC. Impact of Cu and Fe concentrations on oxidative damage in male infertility. Biol Trace Elem Res. 2006;112(3):193–203.
52. Naessens G, De Slypere JP, Dijs H, Driessens M. Hypogonadism as a cause of recurrent muscle injury in a high level soccer player. A case report. Int J Sports Med. 1995;16(6):413–7.
53. Di Luigi L, Gentile V, Pigozzi F, Parisi A, Giannetti D, Romanelli F. Physical activity as a possible aggravating factor for athletes with varicocele: impact on the semen profile. Hum Reprod. 2001;16(6):1180–4.
54. Word Health Organization editor. WHO laboratory manual for examination of human semen and sperm-cervical mucus interaction. 4th ed. In: World Health Organization. Cambridge: Cambridge University Press; 1999.

55. NAFA-ESHRE. Manual on basic semen analysis. NAFA and ESHRE-SIGA. 2002.
56. Rich-Edwards JW, Spiegelman D, Garland M, Hertzmark E, Hunter DJ, Colditz GA, Willett WC, Wand H, Manson JE. Physical activity, body mass index, and ovulatory disorder infertility. Epidemiology. 2002;13(2):184–90.
57. Clark AM, Ledger W, Galletly C, Tomlinson L, Blaney F, Wang X, Norman RJ. Weight loss results in significant improvement in pregnancy and ovulation rates in anovulatory obese women. Hum Reprod. 1995;10:2705–12.
58. Vaamonde D, Silva-Grigoletto ME D, García-Manso JM, Barrera N, Vaamonde-Lemos R. Physically active men show better semen parameters and hormone values than sedentary men. Eur J Appl Physiol. 2012;112(9):3267–73.
59. Kujala UM, Alen M, Huhtaniemi IT. Gonadotrophin-releasing hormone and human chorionic gonadotrophin tests reveal that both hypothalamic and testicular endocrine functions are suppressed during acute prolonged physical exercise. Clin Endocrinol. 1990;33:219–25.
60. Mathur DN, Toriola AL, Dada OA. Serum cortisol and testosterone levels in conditioned male distance runners and nonathletes after maximal exercise. J Sports Med Phys Fitness. 1986;26(3):245–50.
61. Bagatell CJ, Bremner WJ. Sperm counts and reproductive hormones in male marathoners and lean controls. Fertil Steril. 1990;53(4):688–92.
62. Flynn MG, Pizza FX, Boone JB Jr, Andres FF, Michaud TA, Rodriguez-Zayas JR. Indices of training stress during competitive running and swimming seasons. Int J Sports Med. 1994;15(1):21–6.
63. Gutin B, Alejandro D, Duni T, Segal K, Phillips GB. Levels of serum sex hormones and risk factors for coronary heart disease in exercise-trained men. Am J Med. 1985;79(1):79–84.
64. MacConnie SE, Barkan A, Lampman RM, Schork MA, Beitins IZ. Decreased hypothalamic gonadotropin-releasing hormone secretion in male marathon runners. N Engl J Med. 1986;315(7):411–7.
65. Ayers JW, Komesu Y, Romani T, Ansbacher R. Anthropomorphic, hormonal, and psychologic correlates of semen quality in endurance-trained male athletes. Fertil Steril. 1985;43(6):917–21.
66. Hackney AC1, Sinning WE, Bruot BC. Reproductive hormonal profiles of endurance-trained and untrained males. Med Sci Sports Exerc. 1988;20(1):60–5.
67. McColl EM, Wheeler GD, Gomes P, Bhambhani Y, Cumming DC. The effects of acute exercise on pulsatile LH release in high-mileage male runners. Clin Endocrinol. 1989;31(5):617–21.
68. Hackney AC, Sinning WE, Bruot BC. Hypothalamic-pituitary-testicular axis function in endurance-trained males. Int J Sports Med. 1990;11(4):298–303.
69. Wheeler GD, Singh M, Pierce WD, Epling WF, Cumming DC. Endurance training decreases serum testosterone levels in men without change in luteinizing hormone pulsatile release. J Clin Endocrinol Metab. 1991;72(2):422–5.
70. Roberts AC, McClure RD, Weiner RI, Brooks GA. Overtraining affects male reproductive status. Fertil Steril. 1993;60(4):686–92.
71. Bambino TH, Hsueh AJ. Direct inhibitory effect of glucocorticoids upon testicular luteinizing hormone receptor and steroidogenesis in vivo and in vitro. Endocrinology. 1981;108(6):2142–8.
72. Raastad T, Bjøro T, Hallén J. Hormonal responses to high- and moderate-intensity strength exercise. Eur J Appl Physiol. 2000;82(1–2):121–8.
73. Lucía A, Díaz B, Hoyos J, Fernández C, Villa G, Bandrés F, Chicharro JL. Hormone levels of world class cyclists during the Tour of Spain stage race. Br J Sports Med. 2001;35(6):424–30.
74. Fernández-Garcia B, Lucía A, Hoyos J, Chicharro JL, Rodriguez-Alonso M, Bandrés F, Terrados N. The response of sexual and stress hormones of male pro-cyclists during continuous intense competition. Int J Sports Med. 2002;23(8):555–60.
75. Hoogeveen AR, Zonderland ML. Relationships between testosterone, cortisol and performance in professional cyclists. Int J Sports Med. 1996;17(6):423–8.
76. Vasankari TJ, Kujala UM, Heinonen OJ, Huhtaniemi IT. Effects of endurance training on hormonal responses to prolonged physical exercise in males. Acta Endocrinol (Copenh). 1993;129(2):109–13.
77. Mackinnon LT, Hooper SL, Jones S, Gordon RD, Bachmann AW. Hormonal, immunological, and hematological responses to intensified training in elite swimmers. Med Sci Sports Exerc. 1997;29(12):1637–45.
78. Hackney AC, Moore AW, Brownlee KK. Testosterone and endurance exercise: development of the exercise-hypogonadal male condition. Acta Physiol Hung. 2005;92(2):121–37.
79. Vervoorn C, Quist AM, Vermulst LJM, Erich WBM, De Vries WR, Thijssen JHH. The behaviour of the plasma free testosterone/cortisol ratio during a season of elite rowing training. Int J Sports Med. 1991;12(03):257–63.
80. Urhausen A, Kullmer T, Kindermann W. A 7-week follow-up study of the behaviour of testosterone and cortisol during the competition period in rowers. Eur J Appl Physiol Occup Physiol. 1987;56(5):528–33.
81. Rämson R, Jürimäe J, Jürimäe T, Mäestu J. Behavior of testosterone and cortisol during an intensity-controlled high-volume training period measured by a training task-specific test in men rowers. J Strength Cond Res. 2009;23(2):645–51.
82. Mäestu J, Jürimäe J, Jürimäe T. Hormonal response to maximal rowing before and after heavy increase in training volume in highly trained male rowers. J Sports Med Phys Fitness. 2005;45(1):121–6.
83. Vinther A, Kanstrup IL, Christiansen E, Ekdahl C, Aagaard P. Testosterone and BMD in elite male lightweight rowers. Int J Sports Med. 2008;29(10):803–7.
84. Purge P, Jürimäe J, Jürimäe T. Hormonal and psychological adaptation in elite male rowers during prolonged training. J Sports Sci. 2006;24(10):1075–82.

85. Väänänen I, Vasankari T, Mäntysaari M, Vihko V. Hormonal responses to 100 km cross-country skiing during 2 days. J Sports Med Phys Fitness. 2004;44(3):309–14.
86. Grandi M, Celani MF. Effects of football on the pituitary-testicular axis (PTA): differences between professional and non-professional soccer players. Exp. Clin Endocrinol. 1990;96(3):253–9.
87. Martínez AC, Seco Calvo J, Tur Marí JA, Abecia Inchaurregui LC, Orella EE, Biescas AP. Testosterone and cortisol changes in professional basketball players through a season competition. J Strength Cond Res. 2010;24(4):1102–8.
88. Bonifazi M, Bela E, Carli G, Lodi L, Martelli G, Zhu B, Lupo C. Influence of training on the response of androgen plasma concentrations to exercise in swimmers. Eur J Appl Physiol Occup Physiol. 1995;70(2):109–14.
89. Hackney AC, Premo MC, McMurray RG. Influence of aerobic versus anaerobic exercise on the relationship between reproductive hormones in men. J Sports Sci. 1995;13(4):305–11.
90. Kraemer WJ, Hakkinen K, Newton RU, McCormick M, Nindl BC, Volek JS, Gotshalk LA, Fleck SJ, Campbell WW, Gordon SE, Farrell PA, Evans WJ. Acute hormonal responses to heavy resistance exercise in younger and older men. Eur J Appl Physiol Occup Physiol. 1998;77(3):206–11.
91. Willoughby DS, Taylor L. Effects of sequential bouts of resistance exercise on androgen receptor expression. Med Sci Sports Exerc. 2004;36(9):1499–506.
92. Herbst KL, Bhasin S. Testosterone action on skeletal muscle. Curr Opin Clin Nutr Metab Care. 2004;7(3):271–7.
93. Kraemer WJ, Ratamess NA. Hormonal responses and adaptations to resistance exercise and training. Sports Med. 2005;35(4):339–61.
94. Muller M, den Tonkelaar I, Thijssen JH, Grobbee DE, van der Schouw YT. Endogenous sex hormones in men aged 40–80 years. Eur J Endocrinol. 2003;149(6):583–9.
95. Ari Z, Kutlu N, Uyanik BS, Taneli F, Buyukyazi G, Tavli T. Serum testosterone, growth hormone, and insulin-like growth factor-1 levels, mental reaction time, and maximal aerobic exercise in sedentary and long-term physically trained elderly males. Int J Neurosci. 2004;114(5):623–37.
96. Tymchuk CN, Tessler SB, Aronson WJ, Barnard RJ. Effects of diet and exercise on insulin, sex hormone-binding globulin, and prostate-specific antigen. Nutr Cancer. 1998;31(2):127–31.
97. Cooper CS, Taaffe DR, Guido D, Packer E, Holloway L, Marcus R. Relationship of chronic endurance exercise to the somatotropic and sex hormone status of older men. Eur J Endocrinol. 1998;138(5):517–23.
98. Hawkins VN, Foster-Schubert K, Chubak J, Sorensen B, Ulrich CM, Stancyzk FZ, Plymate S, Stanford J, White E, Potter JD, McTiernan A. Effect of exercise on serum sex hormones in men: a 12-month randomized clinical trial. Med Sci Sports Exerc. 2008;40(2):223–33.
99. Grandys M, Majerczak J, Duda K, Zapart-Bukowska J, Kulpa J, Zoladz JA. Endurance training of moderate intensity increases testosterone concentration in young, healthy men. Int J Sports Med. 2009;30(7):489–95.
100. Craig BW, Brown R, Everhart J. Effects of progressive resistance training on growth hormone and testosterone levels in young and elderly subjects. Mech Ageing Dev. 1989;49(2):159–69.
101. Jensen J, Oftebro H, Breigan B, Johnsson A, Ohlin K, Meen HD, Strømme SB, Dahl HA. Comparison of changes in testosterone concentrations after strength and endurance exercise in well-trained men. Eur J Appl Physiol. 1991;63:467–71.
102. Häkkinen K, Pakarinen A. Acute hormonal responses to two different fatiguing heavy-resistance protocols in male athletes. J Appl Physiol (1985). 1993;74(2):882–7.
103. Deschenes MR1, Kraemer WJ. Performance and physiologic adaptations to resistance training. Am J Phys Med Rehabil. 2002;81(11 Suppl):S3–S16.
104. Häkkinen K, Pakarinen A. Serum hormones in male strength athletes during intensive short term strength training. Eur J Appl Physiol Occup Physiol. 1991;63(3–4):194–9.
105. Nicklas BJ, Ryan AJ, Treuth MM, Harman SM, Blackman MR, Hurley BF, Rogers MA Testosterone, growth hormone and IGF-I responses to acute and chronic resistive exercise in men aged 55–70 years. Int J Sports Med. 1995;16(7):445–50.
106. Raastad T, Glomsheller T, Bjøro T, Hallén J. Recovery of skeletal muscle contractility and hormonal responses to strength exercise after two weeks of high-volume strength training. Scand J Med Sci Sports. 2003;13(3):159–68.
107. Tsolakis CK, Vagenas GK, Dessypris AG. Strength adaptations and hormonal responses to resistance training and detraining in preadolescent males. J Strength Cond Res. 2004;18(3):625–9.
108. Izquierdo M, Ibañez J, González-Badillo JJ, Häkkinen K, Ratamess NA, Kraemer WJ, French DN, Eslava J, Altadill A, Asiain X, Gorostiaga EM. Differential effects of strength training leading to failure versus not to failure on hormonal responses, strength, and muscle power gains. J Appl Physiol (1985). 2006;100(5):1647–56.
109. Häkkinen K, Pakarinen A, Kallinen M. Neuromuscular adaptations and serum hormones in women during short-term intensive strength training. EurJ Appl Physiol. 1992;64:106–11.
110. Izquierdo M, Häkkinen K, Ibañez J, Garrues M, Antón A, Zúñiga A, Larrión JL, Gorostiaga EM. Effects of strength training on muscle power and serum hormones in middle-aged and older men. J Appl Physiol. 2001;90(4):1497–507.
111. Ahtiainen JP, Pakarinen A, Alen M, Kraemer WJ, Häkkinen K. Muscle hypertrophy, hormonal adaptations and strength development during strength training in strength-trained and untrained men. Eur J Appl Physiol. 2003;89(6):555–63.

112. Cadore EL1, Lhullier FL, Brentano MA, da Silva EM, Ambrosini MB, Spinelli R, Silva RF, Kruel LF. Hormonal responses to resistance exercise in long-term trained and untrained middle-aged men. J Strength Cond Res. 2008;22(5):1617–24.
113. Kuoppasalmi K, Adlercreutz H. "Interaction between catabolic and anabolic steroid hormones in muscular exercise." Exercise endocrinology. Berlin: Walter de Gruyter; 1985. p. 65–98.
114. Myhal M, Lamb DR. Hormones as performance enhancing drugs. In: Warren MP, Constantini NW, editors. Sport endocrinology. Totowa: Humana; 2000. p. 433–76.
115. Häkkinen K, Pakarinen A, Newton RU, Kraemer WJ. Acute hormone responses to heavy resistance lower and upper extremity exercise in young versus old men. Eur J Appl Physiol Occup Physiol. 1998;77(4):312–9.
116. Kraemer WJ, Volek JS, Bush JA, Putukian M, Sebastianelli WJ. Hormonal responses to consecutive days of heavy-resistance exercise with or without nutritional supplementation. J Appl Physiol. 1998;85:1544–55.
117. Pullinen T, Mero A, Huttunen P, Pakarinen A, Komi PV. Resistance exercise-induced hormonal responses in men, women, and pubescent boys. Med Sci Sports Exerc. 2002;34:806–13.
118. Tremblay MS, Copeland JL, Van Helder W. Effect of training status and exercise mode on endogenous steroid hormones in men. J Appl Physiol. 1985, 2004;96(2):531–9.
119. Kon M, Ikeda T, Homma T, Suzuki Y. Effects of low-intensity resistance exercise under acute systemic hypoxia on hormonal responses. J Strength Cond Res. 2012;26(3):611–7.
120. Ostrowski KJ, Wilson GJ, Weatherby R, Murphy PW, Lyttle AD. The effect of weight training volume on hormonal output and muscular size and function. J Strength Cond Res. 1997;11(3):148–54.
121. Bloomer RJ, Sforzo GA, Keller BA. Effects of meal form and composition on plasma testosterone, cortisol, and insulin following resistance exercise. Int J Sport Nutr Exerc Metab. 2000;10:415–24.
122. Kraemer WJ, Spiering BA, Volek JS, Ratamess NA, Sharman MJ, Rubin MR, French DN, Silvestre R, Hatfield DL, Van Heest JL, Vingren JL, Judelson DA, Deschenes MR, Maresh CM. Androgenic responses to resistance exercise: effects of feeding and L-carnitine. Med Sci Sports Exerc. 2006;38(7):1288–96.
123. Kraemer WJ, Marchitelli L, Gordon SE, Harman E, Dziados JE, Mello R, Frykman P, McCurry D, Fleck SJ. Hormonal and growth factor responses to heavy resistance exercise protocols. J Appl Physiol. 1990;69:1442–50.
124. Cadore EL, Lhullier FL, Alberton CL, Almeida AP, Sapata KB, Korzenowski AL, Kruel LF. Salivary hormonal responses to different water-based exercise protocols in young and elderly men. J Strength Cond Res. 2009;23(9):2695–701.
125. Cadoux-Hudson TA, Few JD, Imms FJ. The effect of exercise on the production and clearance of testosterone in well trained young men. Eur J Appl Physiol Occup Physiol. 1985;54(3):321–5.
126. Kuoppasalmi K. Plasma testosterone and sex-hormone-binding globulin capacity in physical exercise. Scand J Clin Lab Invest. 1980;40(5):411–8.
127. Hall HL, Flynn MG, Carroll KK, Brolinson PG, Shapiro S, Bushman BA. Effects of intensified training and detraining on testicular function. Clin J Sport Med. 1999;9:203–8.
128. Vaamonde D, Da Silva-Grigoletto ME, García-Manso JM, Cunha-Filho JS, Vaamonde-Lemos R. Sperm morphology normalcy is inversely correlated to cycling kilometers in elite triathletes. Revista Andaluza de Medicina del Deporte. 2009;02:43–6.
129. Mingoti GZ, Pereira RN, Monteiro CM. Fertility of male adult rats submitted to forced swimming stress. Braz J Med Biol Res. 2003;36:677–81.
130. Vaamonde D, Diaz A, Rodriguez I. Preliminary results of trans-resveratrol as an effective protector against exercise-induced morphology abnormalities on mice sperm. Fertil Steril. 2011;96(3 Suppl):S166–7.
131. Rodriguez I, Diaz A, Vaamonde D. Assessment of the effect of prolonged forced swimming on CD1 mice sperm morphology with and without antioxidant supplementation. Andrologia. 2015. (In Press).
132. Ferry A, Picard F, Duvallet A, Weill B, Rieu M. Changes in blood leucocyte populations induced by acute maximal and chronic submaximal exercise. Eur J Appl Physiol Occup Physiol. 1990;59(6):435–42.
133. Lehmann M, Dickhuth HH, Gendrisch G, Lazar W, Thum M, Kaminski R, Aramendi JF, Peterke E, Wieland W, Keul J. Training-overtraining. A prospective, experimental study with experienced middle- and long- distance runners. Int J Sports Med. 1991;12(5):444–52.
134. Vaamonde D, Da Silva-Grigoletto ME, Abbasi A, Barrera-Hurtado N, García-Manso JM. Sperm DNA fragmentation as a result of ultra-endurance exercise training. J Sci Med Sport. 2015. (In Press).
135. Palmer NO, Bakos HW, Owens JA, Setchell BP, Lane M. Diet and exercise in an obese mouse fed a high-fat diet improve metabolic health and reverse perturbed sperm function. Am J Physiol Endocrinol Metab. 2012;302(7):E768–80.
136. Chigurupati S, Son TG, Hyun DH, Lathia JD, Mughal MR, Savell J, Li SC, Nagaraju GP, Chan SL, Arumugam TV, Mattson MP. Lifelong running reduces oxidative stress and degenerative changes in the testes of mice. J Endocrinol. 2008;199(2):333–41.
137. Jenkins RR, Friedland R, Hownld H. The relationship of oxygen uptake to Superoxide dismutase and catalase activity in human muscle. Int J Sports Med. 1984;95:11–4.
138. Zhao X, Bian Y, Sun Y, Li L, Wang L, Zhao C, Shen Y, Song Q, Qu Y, Niu S, Wu W, Gao F. Effects of

moderate exercise over different phases on age-related physiological dysfunction in testes of SAMP8 mice. Exp Gerontol. 2013;48(9):869–80.
139. Joseph AM, Nguyen LM, Welter AE, Dominguez JM 2nd, Behnke BJ, Adhihetty PJ. Mitochondrial adaptations evoked with exercise are associated with a reduction in age-induced testicular atrophy in Fischer-344 rats. Biogerontology. 2014;15(5):517–34.
140. Ortenblad N, Madsen K, Djurhuus MS. Antioxidant status and lipid peroxidation after short-term maximal exercise in trained and untrained humans. Am J Physiol. 1997;272(4 Pt 2):R1258–63.
141. Niess AM, Simon P. Response and adaptation of skeletal muscle to exercise–the role of reactive oxygen species. Front Biosci. 2007;12:4826–38.
142. Banfi G, Malavazos A, Iorio E, Dolci A, Doneda L, Verna R, Corsi MM. Plasma oxidative stress biomarkers, nitric oxide and heat shock protein 70 in trained elite soccer players. Eur J Appl Physiol. 2006;96(5):483–6.
143. Dekany M, Nemeskeri V, Györe I, Harbula I, Malomski J, Pucsok J. Antioxidant status of interval-trained athletes in various sports. Int J Sports Med. 2006;27(2):112–6.
144. Kobayashi T, Miyazaki T, Natori M, Nozawa S. Protective role of superoxide dismutase in human sperm motility: superoxide dismutase activity and lipid peroxide in human seminal plasma and spermatozoa. Hum Reprod. 1991;6(7):987–91.
145. Zini A, de Lamirande E, Gagnon C. Reactive oxygen species in semen of infertile patients: levels of superoxide dismutase and catalase-like activities in seminal plasma and spermatozoa. Int J Androl. 1993;16:183–8.
146. Powers SK, Ji LL, Leeuwenburgh C. Exercise training-induced alterations in skeletal muscle antioxidant capacity: a brief review. Med Sci Sports Exerc. 1999;31(7):987–97.
147. Fatouros IG, Jamurtas AZ, Villiotou V, Pouliopoulou S, Fotinakis P, Taxildaris K, Deliconstantinos G. Oxidative stress responses in older men during endurance training and detraining. Med Sci Sports Exerc. 2004;36(12):2065–72.
148. Kanayama G, Brower KJ, Wood RI, Hudson JI, Pope HG Jr. Anabolic-androgenic steroid dependence: an emerging disorder. Addiction. 2009;104:1966–78.
149. Hoffman JR, Kraemer WJ, Bhasin S, Storer T, Ratamess NA, Haff GG, Willoughby DS, Rogol AD. Position stand on androgen and human growth hormone use. J Strength Cond Res. 2009;23(5 suppl):S1–59.
150. Schurmeyer T, Knuth UA, Belkien L, Nieschlag E. Reversible azoospermia induced by the anabolic steroid 19-nortestosterone. Lancet. 1984;1:417–20.
151. Torres-Calleja J, Gonzalez-Unzaga M, DeCelis-Carrillo R, Calzada- Sanchez L, Pedron N. Effect of androgenic anabolic steroids on sperm quality and serum hormone levels in adult male bodybuilders. Life Sci. 2001;68:1769–74.
152. Bonetti A, Tirelli F, Catapano A, Dazzi D, Dei Cas A, Solito F, Ceda G, Reverberi C, Monica C, Pipitone S, Elia G, Spattini M, Magnati G. Side effects of anabolic androgenic steroids abuse. Int J Sports Med. 2008;29:679–87.
153. Knuth UA, Maniera H, Nieschlag E. Anabolic steroids and semen parameters in bodybuilders. Fertil Steril. 1989;52(6):1041–47.
154. Schurmeyer-Menon DK. Successful treatment of anabolic steroid-induced azoospermia with human chorionic gonadotropin and human menopausal gonadotropin. Fertil Steril. 2003;79(Suppl 3):1659–61.
155. Karila T, Hovatta O, Seppala T. Concomitant abuse of anabolic androgenic steroids and human chorionic gonadotrophin impairs spermatogenesis in power athletes. Int J Sports Med. 2004;25:257–63.
156. Shokri S, Aitken RJ, Abdolvahhabi M, Abolhasani F, Ghasemi FM, Kashani I, Ejtemaeimehr S, Ahmadian S, Minaei B, Naraghi MA, Barbarestani M. Exercise and supraphysiological dose of nandrolone decanoate increase apoptosis in spermatogenic cells. Basic Clin Pharmacol Toxicol. 2010;106(4):324–30.
157. Burge MR, Lanzi RA, Skarda ST, Eaton RP. Idiopathic hypogonadotropic hypogonadism in a male runner is reversed by clomiphene citrate. Fertil Steril. 1997;67(4):783–5.
158. Marceau L, Kleinman K, Goldstein I, McKinlay J. Does bicycling contribute to the risk of erectile dysfunction? Results from the Massachusetts Male Aging Study (MMAS). Int J Impot Res. 2001;13(5):298–302.
159. Sommer F, Schwarzer U, Klotz T, Caspers HP, Haupt G, ngelmann U. Erectile dysfunction in cyclists. Is there any difference in penile blood flow during cycling in an upright versus a reclining position? Eur Urol. 2001;39(6):720–3.
160. Southorn T. Great balls of fire and the vicious cycle: a study of the effects of cycling on male fertility. J Fam Plann Reprod Health Care. 2002;28(4):211–3.
161. Dettori JR, Koepsell TD, Cummings P, Corman JM. Erectile dysfunction after a long-distance cycling event: associations with bicycle characteristics. J Urol. 2004;172(2):637–41.
162. Leibovitch I, Mor Y. The vicious cycling: bicycling related urogenital disorders. Eur Urol. 2005;47(3):277–86.
163. Derby CA, Mohr BA, Goldstein I, Feldman HA, Johannes CB, McKinlay JB. Modifiable risk factors and erectile dysfunction: can lifestyle changes modify risk? Urology. 2000;56(2):302–6.
164. Bacon CG, Mittleman MA, Kawachi I, Giovanucci E, Glasser DB, Rimm EB. Sexual function in men older than 50 years of age: results from the health professionals follow-up study. Ann Intern Med. 2003;139:161–8.
165. Nicolosi A, Glasser DB, Moreira ED, Villa M. Prevalence of erectile dysfunction and associated factors among men without concomitant diseases: a population study. Int J Impot Res. 2003;15:253–7.

166. Naraghi MA, Abolhasani F, Kashani I, Anarkooli IJ, Hemadi M, Azami A, Barbarestani M, Aitken RJ, Shokri S. The effects of swimming exercise and supraphysiological doses of nandrolone decanoate on the testis in adult male rats: a transmission electron microscope study. Folia Morphol (Warsz). 2010;69(3):138–46.
167. Elloumi M, Maso F, Michaux O, Robert A, Lac G. Behaviour of saliva cortisol [C], testosterone [T] and the T/C ratio during a rugby match and during the post-competition recovery days. Eur J Appl Physiol. 2003;90(1–2):23–8.
168. Mastaloudis A, Yu TW, O'Donnell RP, Frei B, Dashwood RH, Traber MG. Endurance exercise results in DNA damage as detected by the comet assay. Free Radic Biol Med. 2004;36:966–75.
169. Scharhag J, Herrmann M, Urhausen A, Haschke M, Herrmann W, Kindermann W. Independent elevations of N-terminal pro-brain natriuretic peptide and cardiac troponins in endurance athletes after prolonged strenuous exercise. Am Heart J. 2005;150:1128–34.
170. Vaamonde D, Hackney AC, Garcia-Manso JM. Impact of physical activity and exercise on male reproductive potential. Rev Andal Med Deporte. 2015. (In press).

Hormonal Changes Associated with Physical Activity and Exercise Training

8

Anthony C. Hackney, William J. Kraemer and David R. Hooper

Introduction

The nature of the human body is such that its survival is dependent on having effective and efficient internal communication systems. The two major such systems are the nervous system and the endocrine system. The former responds rapidly by using specific neural pathways to receive and send information throughout the body. The endocrine system, a series of glandular and non-glandular tissues which secrete hormones, typically processes at a much slower rate than the nervous system to bring about change in physiological systems (though, there are aspects of the endocrine system that are remarkably rapid in responsiveness). The endocrine tissues of the body use the circulatory system (i.e., the blood) as a principal means of carrying/delivering hormones to the target tissues to induce an "endocrine" effect on those tissues, although many hormones have "paracrine" and "autocrine" actions too. Through the interaction of these two communication systems, the body maintains a homeostatic balance and the ability to respond to any stress that disrupts homeostasis. This chapter provides an overview of how one of these systems, the endocrine, responds to the homeostatic challenge and stress of physical activity—exercise—by altering hormonal release. A special emphasis in this discussion is given on reproductive hormones of the endocrine system.

Different types of physical activities can be classified as exercise and each of these activities has varying and unique degrees of muscular movement patterns, force development, and contractile characteristics associated with them. These unique and varying aspects of movement patterns influence the hormonal response to exercise. Space limitations do not allow for a full-fledged discussion of the intricacies of these responses for the complete gambit of movement patterns that exist within different physical activities and exercise. Therefore, we have chosen to delimit and organize this discussion on hormones by using a simple dichotomous approach in which responses will be characterized by those associated with (i) resistance–power activities-exercise and (ii) endurance/aerobic activities-exercise.

Resistance Exercise and Training

A dearth of information exists regarding the role of resistance exercise in male or female reproductive functions, including fertility, menstrual

A. C. Hackney (✉)
Department of Exercise & Sport Science, Department of Nutrition, University of North Carolina, 203 Fetzer Hall, South Rd., Chapel Hill, NC 27599, USA
e-mail: ach@email.unc.edu

W. J. Kraemer
Department of Kinesiology, Physiology, Neurobiology, Medicine, University of Connecticut, Storrs, CT, USA

D. R. Hooper
Department of Kinesiology, University of Connecticut, Storrs, CT, USA

© Springer Science+Business Media New York 2016

D. Vaamonde et al. (eds.), *Exercise and Human Reproduction*, DOI 10.1007/978-1-4939-3402-7_8

cycle changes, menopause, gonadopause, etc. Thus, most of the influences of resistance exercise and reproductive system changes may well be related to the tangential effects on fitness, adaptive capabilities of tissues, and recovery aspects of function. Cell signaling systems, including hormonal signals and interactions, are both complex and redundant and are just starting to be unraveled but are further complicated by epigenomics interactions as well. The hypothalamic–pituitary–gonadal axis (HPG axis) plays many different roles in the homeostatic regulation and physiological signaling related to target tissues (e.g., skeletal muscle and connective tissue) beyond the obvious reproductive functions. Due to the systematic integration of this axis, it has typically been viewed as an integrated system. Gonadotropin-releasing hormone (GnRH) is produced and released by the hypothalamus and the anterior pituitary gland synthesizes and secretes luteinizing hormone (LH) and follicle-stimulating hormone (FSH) that together allow the gonads to produce estrogen and testosterone. LH has been documented as the primary "pulse generator" of the endocrine system. Closely related to this system are the hormones stimulated by hypothalamic releasing hormones causing release of hormones from the anterior pituitary and adrenal glands resulting in an integrated stress–response system outside of the obvious reproductive functions played by the HPG axis. With exercise, and more specifically resistance exercise, this set of integrated systems plays vital roles in the signaling of target tissues, allowing acute homeostatic regulation and chronic adaptations to occur. In this section, we overview some of the basic issues in resistance training and also some of the major hormones involved with hormonal cell signaling. In essence, the hormonal signals are but part of a more extensive signaling network. Thus, circulatory concentrations and their changes are but part of a complex cybernetic pathway for stimulating acute and chronic homeostatic responses ultimately ending in target tissue (e.g., skeletal muscle) adaptations (e.g., increased fiber size) with continued exposure to a stimulus with training. Again, let us examine some basic overviews of the basic mechanisms, responses, and adaptations of these different systems to resistance exercise and training.

Resistance Exercise

It has become more obvious over the past decade that all resistance exercise protocols are not the same and the terms "resistance exercise" and "resistance training" are but broad umbrellas for a modality that spans many operational definitions and stimuli. As such, interpretation of research can many times send readers generalizations about a particular endocrine cybernetic that in fact requires a great deal of context to place it within a paradigm of the global nature of resistance training. So what might be a unifying principle that may help one better understand this modality?

Size Principle

When discussing responses and adaptations to resistance training, it is essential first and foremost to understand the importance of recruitment and the impact that it has on the response to resistance training—that is, if muscle fibers are not recruited, they do not adapt! Furthermore, recruitment opens up circulatory perfusion for exposure of tissues to hormonal signaling beyond normal homeostatic exposure and is involved with activation of receptors. The size principle is credited to Elwood Henneman [1], although with some debate [2], who recognized that recruitment of motor neurons is based on sizing factor (e.g., number of fibers and size of fibers). In a classic study using anaesthetized cats, small motor neurons were recruited first with the lowest levels of electrical stimulation (5 V). With increases in the intensity of the stimulation, larger motor neurons would fire, identifiable by larger responses in amplitude. At 18.7 V, further increases in shock strength did not recruit additional motor neurons. These classical findings were later confirmed in humans [3] with the use of voluntary isometric contractions. Today, this mechanism of recruitment is widely accepted and is paramount in understanding exercise demands.

As a result, if we are to study the adaptations that occur in response to resistance training, the context of the stimulus is paramount—for if the electrical charge is not sufficient, motor units will go unrecruited. This was highlighted by Campos et al. [4] who observed in untrained young men non-significant differences in the size of the cross-sectional area of type I and type II muscle fibers following 8 weeks of progressive, multi-exercise, multiple set resistance training when the intensity of the different lower body resistance exercises used in the program was light (20–28 repetition maximum (RM)). In that same study, this stood in stark contrast to the increases in type I and type II muscle fiber cross-sectional areas when the intensity was moderate to heavy (9–11 and 3–5 RMs, respectively). Later, these same findings were observed for untrained young women by the same laboratory group, demonstrating the importance of the resistance exercise intensity even over short training periods, thus underscoring the importance of intensity for optimal recruitment of motor units and associated muscle fibers for the lower body exercises used [5]. One would have speculated that in untrained individuals, even light resistances might have had a more dramatic effect, but such studies point to the importance of the hertz (Hz) level when motor units are depolarized.

Heavier resistances activate higher threshold motor units and also carry with them a higher Hz exposure to the muscle fibers recruited. These results clearly indicate that lighter loads (resistances) do not maximize recruitment and that unrecruited muscle tissue does not adapt. The voltage amplitude is the stimulus that is critical for stimulation of sarcolemma ionophores, ion channels, and receptors. Therefore, if the resistance exercise stimulus, or exercise in general, is not sufficient to recruit motor units needed to respond to the external force/power recruitment, these fibers are not exposed to increased hormonal influences and many receptors are not activated beyond resting homeostatic levels.

Up front, it is important to understand that motor unit recruitment dictates the support physiological systems need by the activated fibers to perform in response to the external stimuli and allow for homeostatic regulation both during and following exercise stress. For example, the level of physiological support would be greater for performance of 6 sets of 8–10 RM squats than for flexing one's index finger for 6 sets of 10 RM. While somewhat silly, it still brings out the concept that what is recruited with activity is what the body's physiological systems, including hormonal systems, must support. The changes made in structures and functions as a result of a specific exercise stressor are in direct relationship to their ability to gain homeostatic control and management of the stressor's challenge.

Interestingly, although unrecruited motor units do not appear to respond to anabolic signaling without stimulus (recruitment and voltage amplitude level) and increased profusion of blood with circulatory mechanisms, they may still be exposed to destructive processes, such as those that are caused by reactive oxygen species, free radicals due to invagination of immune cells proximate to other tissue damage, as well as continued higher concentrations of cortisol [6]. Chemical damage of the trilaminar membrane of the sarcolemma is seen in the long-term repair process needed after many types of resistance exercise (e.g., short-rest metabolic workouts) that are not completely mediated by the eccentric component of the exercise stress. Despite the countless positive adaptations that occur as a result of various forms of exercise, contracting skeletal muscle produces free radicals that can result in oxidative damage [7]. Although oxidative damage is typically associated with endurance activity, recent research has documented elevated reactive oxygen species in resistance training [8]. As well as an intracellular generation of superoxide and nitric oxide, reactive oxygen species are also released into the interstitial space [9–11]. As a result, it could be argued that even muscle fibers that did not produce the reactive oxygen species themselves may still be susceptible to the consequences of their presence. Such consequences include protein oxidation, due to the numerous oxidizable functional groups of amino acids, which might result in impaired biological activity and changes in the secondary and tertiary structure [12]. Furthermore, oxidative damage can lead to alterations in lipids and DNA and has the potential to impact the epigenomics of the cell [12]. How much damage is needed and can be tolerated to influence more optimal control of inflammation-related damage remains unclear [13]. How much oxidative stress and muscle fiber degradation is needed in the process of stimulating hypertrophic adaptations remains unclear albeit, higher levels of inflammatory responses do not seem to be related to optimal time courses for adaptive responses to training. The hormonal signals related to both the anabolic and catabolic functions in response to resistance exercise and training play important roles in the cell signaling process [14]. With resistance exercise, the adrenergic response (e.g., increased catecholamines) is a major signaling key vital to other endocrine glands and tissues for the level of acute physiological support needed to respond to the stress (classic fight/flight chain of events).

As mentioned, providing the muscle tissue is adequately activated, adaptation can begin to occur and is mediated by a host of different signaling mechanisms of which hormones play a major role. With activation at the very top of a cascade of complex and interacting biological events, the adaptations will ultimately be governed by the upper regulatory elements, which are a variety of factors such as nutrition, age, sex, and the exercise stimuli which impact downstream processes [14]. Although this part of the chapter will discuss endocrinology in the context of resistance training as the stimulus, it is essential that the readers appreciate that the biological processes discussed here can all be impacted by the upper regulatory elements. The processes that can occur as a result of resistance training are illustrated in Fig. 8.1.

Adrenergic Responses and Cortisol Interactions

The adrenergic response is related to the sympathetic nervous system (SNS) and the associated neural stimulation of the adrenal medulla in response to stress, including resistance exercise. High-intensity and/or high metabolic stress caused by a resistance training workout can dramatically increase the sympatho-adrenal respons-

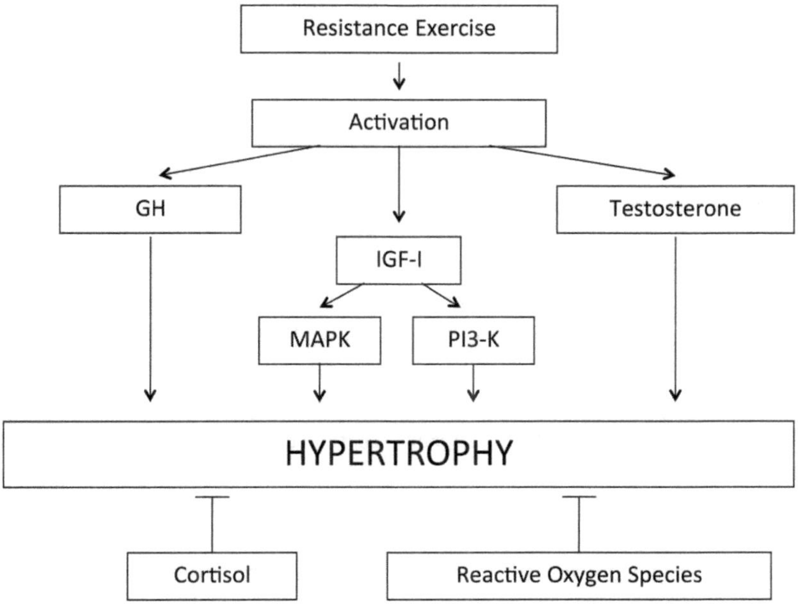

Fig. 8.1 Hormonal responses to strength training. Basic mechanisms regulating muscle hypertrophy (stimulatory, inhibitory)

es with high elevations in the concentrations of catecholamines (i.e., epinephrine, norepinephrine, and dopamine) and sympathetic stimulation (norepinephrine). The adrenal medulla releases predominately epinephrine and its response can be related to the demands of resistance exercise as to its volume and intensity of the workout protocol or the metabolic demands as represented by the changes in blood lactate. High levels of adrenergic stress as seen in extremely short rest period (1 min or less between sets and exercises) workouts using light-to-moderate resistances or higher volume and high-intensity workouts also can result in increases in cortisol concentrations in the blood [15–17] due to the influence of epinephrine on the adrenal cortex via a portal circulation. Therefore, cortisol's response may go into recovery but can be maintained for longer periods of time, thereby negatively influencing other cell and tissue recovery time courses if not mitigated to resting concentrations [13].

Muscle fibers that have not been recruited may also be susceptible to the effects of cortisol, which is released from the zona fasciculata of the adrenal cortex in response to exercise stress. Cortisol alters protein balance by inhibiting muscle protein synthesis and increasing muscle protein degradation, which has been attributed to activation of the ubiquitin pathway [18]. The impact of this glucocorticoid response is substantial as it leads to a decreased synthesis of actin and myosin heavy chains [19]. Furthermore, it is primarily type II muscle fibers that are degraded in response to increased concentrations of cortisol [20, 21], which coincidently are exactly those fibers that will not be recruited if the load lifted is not heavy enough. In addition, it can block downstream anabolic signaling of the Akt/mTOR system [22].

Resistance training programs that produce the highest blood lactate concentrations appear to produce the highest cortisol concentrations in both men and women [23–26]. As heavy resistance training that is capable of fully recruiting type II muscle fibers can significantly increase salivary cortisol concentrations over non-exercising controls, so too can resistance training programs that are not capable of full recruitment, such as 60% 1 RM [27] and 80% of 12 RM [28]. In such circumstances, where heavy resistance training is capable of inducing maximum recruitment of motor units, light resistance training will not only fail to recruit type II muscle fibers and prevent their adaptation, but again such fibers will also be exposed to the catabolic effects of cortisol that were previously discussed as part of the impairment related to prolonged chemical damage influences (e.g., free radicals and elevated cortisol).

Also, not only do heavier resistance training programs have the important benefit of inducing full activation, but a significant testosterone response has also been consistently observed in response to heavy resistance training [15, 23, 28, 29], which can mitigate the negative effects of elevations in circulating cortisol. Interestingly, although some studies have observed an elevation in cortisol in response to heavy resistance training [23], others have not [28]. As a result, at the very least, testosterone would be able to mediate the cortisol response, but may even stimulate anabolic processes with minimal opposition from catabolic processes. Interestingly, resistance-trained women (not taking oral contraceptives) showed an elevation of the glucocorticoid receptor content concentrations in the muscle after heavy squat exercise (6 sets of 10 RM with 2-min rest periods) followed by a decrease 70 min into recovery [30]. In contrast, resistance-trained men were unresponsive as to receptor content changes but exhibited significantly lower glucocorticoid receptor concentrations indicating a potential sex difference in managing increases in acute cortisol concentration signals [30].

The take-home message regarding activation is that heavy loads are required to fully recruit type II motor units. If the motor units are not recruited, they will not adapt as a primary target of resistance training and almost all changes in connective tissue are mediated via the muscle with further importance related to the exercise variables such as resistance used and metabolic stress. Furthermore, if a resistance training program is designed in such a way that light loads are lifted but rest periods are short and volume is high, a cortisol response could damage those type II motor units that were not recruited in the processes that results from exposure to reactive oxygen species. Chronic use of extreme type programs may also increase the inflammatory levels in the body along with chronically elevated cortisol if cybernetic recovery of the adrenal cortex is not allowed. Constructs of adrenal exhaustion also appear if programs are not periodized (i.e., program variation of stress) and adequate recovery days are not allowed [31].

Testosterone

Testosterone is a steroid hormone synthesized from cholesterol in the Leydig cells, which are found in the testes in men. Despite no presence of Leydig cells in women, testosterone can also be produced in the ovaries as well as the zona reticularis of the adrenal cortex, which explains the presence of testosterone in women, albeit at much lower concentrations. Despite some confusion due to the androgenic role played in male biology, androgens including testosterone play important roles in women's anabolic signaling [32]. Although it is well known for its role in secondary male sex characteristics such as beard and body hair growth (also known as androgenic effects), in muscle it is a potent stimulus of muscle hypertrophy (anabolism). These effects are so strong that they have led to the production of drugs known as anabolic-androgenic steroids, which are synthetic derivatives of testosterone designed to reduce the androgenic effects of the hormone while continuing to promote the anabolic effects [33]. Such drugs, also known simply as steroids, have been outlawed by the World Anti-Doping Agency, but continue to be used recreationally and in competitive sports. This serves to highlight the powerful effects of testosterone and its derivatives on muscle anabolism.

Anabolism is promoted by testosterone by stimulating muscle protein synthesis [34] as well as reducing protein degradation [35]. The anabolic effects of testosterone are attributed to a translocation of the androgen receptor (AR) to the nucleus in response to testosterone binding, where the now-formed AR–testosterone complex increases gene transcription [36]. In terms of its anti-catabolic effects, testosterone appears to inhibit the glucocorticoid receptor [37], thus preventing processes such as the activation of the ubiquitin pathway as discussed earlier.

As mentioned, anabolic-androgenic steroids have been used to increase circulating testosterone concentrations. However, there is also a natural stimulus for testosterone release as a part of a resistance exercise stress signaling response in both men and women, albeit at 20–30-fold lower concentrations in women [26, 38]. While an increase in testosterone is not mandatory for many resistance training adaptations, it is part of a signaling process from the Hz depolarization of the motor units to AR cascade in muscle [30, 39]. Nevertheless, the amount of testosterone released in response to resistance training is governed by age and sex as well as the manipulation of what has been termed the acute program variables. These variables include intensity, number of sets, rest period, choice of exercise, and exercise order. A full review of the impact of these variables on testosterone is available in [40]. In brief, higher intensity (defined as a percentage of 1 RM) resistance exercise, providing an adequate number of sets are reached appears to significantly induce a testosterone response. Likewise, the use of high numbers of sets induces a testosterone response, but only when a threshold for intensity is met. Furthermore, resistance exercises that recruit more overall muscle mass (such as Olympic lifts) induce a testosterone response, whereas when small muscle groups are exercised, even if vigorously, a testosterone response is not seen. However, the homeostatic signal is dependent on the binding of the hormone with a receptor. With other stimuli in existence, changes can occur without increases in testosterone (e.g., increases in strength with heavy 2–3 RM squat training loads). However, such an exercise stimulus would also increase androgen binding with existing concentrations of testosterone in circulation.

The interpretation of circulating testosterone has been one of confusion and controversy as it is only part, albeit an important part, of a large array of signaling sets of pathways. An increase might well be only one factor in the upregulation of ARs. The voltage amplitude involved in depolarization of motor units (especially heavy resistances, e.g., 90% and greater) may well be the other primary influence increasing anabolic signaling for the regulation of ARs despite no apparent elevation in the circulating concentrations of testosterone. Furthermore, nutritional intakes may be the final stimulator of ARs as protein/carbohydrate intakes result in higher upregulated AR content than fasted conditions [41]. The increase in AR content in the muscle was explained by the decrease in circulating testosterone (almost 50% of the shared variance) demonstrating the impact of ARs to modulate concentrations of testosterone [41]. This shows the difficulty of interpretation without adequate context for the circulating values (e.g., nutritional intakes and timing). Thus, the theory of how testosterone influences muscle depends on a combination or potential integration of a number of factors from the resistance exercise stimulus to provide testosterone increases, to the level of the voltage that is involved in the depolarization of motor units (intensity to number) for sarcolemma membrane preparation (e.g., electrical gating mechanisms, protein pits activated, and beta 2 receptors activated by epinephrine), to the use of nutritional intakes (e.g., amino acid and glucose availability) around the workout resulting in a decrease in testosterone concentrations due to upregulated increased androgen content available for testosterone binding in muscle. Thus, several dimensions of this appear to be operational depending on the context of the scenario. From a sex-linked characteristic, in response to the same relative resistance exercise protocol (6 sets of 10 RM with 2-min rest periods), women with lower testosterone responses stabilize, downregulate, and then upregulate their ARs in muscle at a much more rapid rate (i.e., within an hour) compared to men who might take up to 2–6 h potentially due to processing higher concentrations of testosterone in the process.

When comparing an 8-week resistance training program among young men, Kvorning et al. [42] demonstrated that young men whose endogenous testosterone concentrations were blunted by a drug (i.e., given the drug, goserelin) failed to increase strength and lean mass in contrast to a placebo group (no pharmaceutical blocking of LH pulse). The experimental group also increased body fat percentage whereas the placebo group decreased. Thus, in young men, testosterone plays a paramount role beyond other signaling systems in its natural homeostatic concentrations and as a potent signal for anabolic functions [43]. Furthermore, if strength and lean mass gains were drastically affected, then other processes that have been highlighted here (growth hormone, GH, and insulin-like factor, IGF) while fully operational are not as dominant in young men as testosterone as a major signaling effect. In young women, testosterone has been associated with the regional fat distribution in the body due to its significant role in adipocyte alterations [38]. With older men, although testosterone is an important signaling hormone, other hormonal mechanisms (e.g., GHs and IGFs) as in women may start to play an endogenously greater role in adaptive mechanisms. Nevertheless, in larger population studies, free androgen index has been associated with muscle mass and strength in men and women over 50 years of age and dehydroepiandrosterone sulfate (DHEA-s) concentrations were related to muscle size, strength, and functional outcomes such as gait speed [44].

Growth Hormone(s)

First, growth hormone (GH) is not just one single hormone, but actually a family of hormones with over 100 variants and aggregate combinations [45, 46]. In addition, the concentrations of 22 kD in blood is but a very small portion of the concentrations of the total aggregate concentrations (e.g., 4–30 ug/L for 22 kD under various conditions vs. 2000–15,000 ug/L of aggregate under various conditions) [46]. The specific role of each variant, isoform, or aggregate is yet to be determined, but resistance training has been shown to be a potent stimulant of many of these variants (e.g., aggregates of binding proteins and/or various combinations of aggregates of the 22-kD monomer as well as splice variants of the 22-kD monomer), with acute increases following single exercise bouts as well as chronic elevations from long-term resistance training programs [47]. Typically, women demonstrate higher GH concentrations than men in the limited data from the early follicular stage of the menstrual cycle compared to men at rest [46] and, therefore, the magnitude of the increase with resistance exercise appears to be less for the 22-kD response than men due to this higher starting concentration [29].

The isoform that is most common and measured in most studies using radioassay techniques is the 191 amino acid (22 kD) that is created by the cell's genetic machinery. Thus, almost all studies examining the so-called GH have studied only the 22-kD monomer, and as a result, the process of its stimulation and secretion is well understood [46]. In response to a resistance training stimulus, growth-hormone-releasing hormone (GHRH) is secreted from the hypothalamus. GHRH travels along a network of blood vessels known as the hypophyseal portal system to the anterior pituitary where it meets its receptor. GH is then released from cells known as somatotroph cells, where it is produced. The external receptors are two GH-binding proteins followed by mediation with integral membrane receptors and then secondary signaling systems that follow for influence on the DNA in the nuclei. While an increase may occur in GHBP, no differences have been seen in men as to the effects of resistance training on the acute or chronic responses [48].

Increases of the 22 kD in circulation have been observed classically if the amount of muscle mass is great enough and, more importantly, if the metabolic needs for glycolysis are great [3, 16]. The 22 kD is very sensitive to changes in pH as reflected by high concentration of lactate in the blood [49]. Thus, short rest protocols which challenge the acid-base/pH status of the body will see more dramatic 22 kD increases in circulating concentrations [25, 26]. Conversely, various aggregates and binding proteins are less responsive to acute resistance exercise but resting concentrations are more responsive as a total change in GH molecules (all forms of GH including aggregates) [47, 50]. Measurement by bioassay is needed to mark such changes [45].

With acute resistance exercise (6 sets of 10 RM, 2-min rest between sets), no differences were observed for the tibial line bioassay examining the role of oral contraceptive (OC) use on GH aggregates and the 22 kD GH isoform [51]. The use of OC (OrthoTri-Cyclen™, 0.035 mg ethinyl estradiol and 0.180–0.250 mg norgestimate) augmented immunological GH response to the resistance exercise protocol in unfractionated plasma and >60 kD molecular weight subfraction. However, OC use only increased biological activity of GH in one of the two bioassays. Thus, how the use of OC impacts the anterior pituitary release of GHs is both differential and novel, showing the future need for the effects of other OC combinations.

When in circulation, GH can exhibit its pleiotropic effects, playing important roles in fat metabolism, growth, reproduction, and immune and neural function. In the context of resistance training, GH also plays an important role in muscle development, both independent of insulin-like growth factor-I (IGF-I), such as in muscle cell fusion [52], and also as the old classic "somatomedin hypothesis" suggests, GH effects are mediated by circulating or locally produced IGF [52]. However, GH and its many variants and aggregates can influence cellular adaptations directly without help from the IGF superfamily [53].

Insulin-Like Growth Factors (IGFs)

The signal for the release of circulating IGF-I begins at the pituitary with secretion of what is believed to be the 22-kD GH monomer which is followed by a release of IGF-I from the liver [53]. Due to the structural similarity, much of the early research into IGF-I compared its metabolic effects with insulin, such as stimulation of protein metabolism, glucose transport, and glycogen and triglyceride synthesis, which explains how this group of factors acquired their name. IGFs are part of a sophisticated system sometimes referred to as the IGF axis that includes ligands such as IGF-I and IGF-II, receptors (e.g., IGF-I receptor (IGFIR) and IGF2R), many binding proteins (IGFBP1-6), as well as splice variants (IGF-

IEa and IGF-IEc, also known as mechano growth factor (MGF)).

Ligands (IGF-I and IGF-II)

IGF-I is a 7.6-kD polypeptide consisting of 70 amino acids. IGF-I may also be a very important biomarker for health, fitness, and well-being [54]. After the early comparisons with insulin, more recent research has identified IGF-I as the signal molecule for two essential intracellular cascades: mitogen-activated protein kinase (MAPK) and phosphatidylinositol 3-kinase (PI3K). IGF-II appears to play more of a role in embryogenesis [55]. Interestingly, IGF-I has shown variable responsiveness to resistance exercise, and the starting concentrations appear to be a major determinant if increases with exercise stress are observed and changes in acute recovery are variable [26, 29, 48]. With training, increases in resting concentrations occur, showing the importance of resting IGF-I cybernetics with physiological homeostasis [48].

Binding Proteins

When in circulation, IGF-I is complexed with one of the six binding proteins. These binding proteins are thought to play a role in transporting IGF-I to the target tissue [54]. There is evidence to suggest that the changes in binding proteins within the context of exercise models are a crucial aspect of modulating IGF-I bioactivity [56–58], and that it is not the amount of IGF-I that is important but the manner in which it is partitioned among its binding proteins [58]. Again, training did not appear to impact the acute response to heavy resistance exercise in men [48].

Receptors—Testosterone Versus IGF-1 Versus Cellular and Molecular Action Mechanisms Underlying the Anabolic Actions

Again, in a very similar fashion to the insulin receptor, the IGF1R contains two extracellular alpha subunits and two transmembrane beta subunits. IGF-I binds to the alpha subunits, which induces an autophosphorylation of the beta subunit. The transmission of the signal that results in the downstream signaling of the MAPK or PI3K cascades is then determined by interactions involving insulin receptor substrate 1 (IRS-I) [53]. The MAPK cascade is primarily responsible for the proliferation of muscle cells. This occurs by changes in the amount and activity of transcription factors, such as increasing the expression of cyclins D1 and D2 which accelerates cell cycle progression [59]. The mitogenic activity of this pathway occurs essentially through the phosphorylation of ERK, half of which allows cell proliferation [60].

The PI3K cascade primarily mediates cell differentiation. PI3K signaling has three crucial roles: fusion of myoblasts into myotubes, anabolic effects on protein, and glucose uptake and resistance to apoptosis [61].

Splice Variants

More recent research regarding IGF-I have shown that in response to mechanical stimuli, an alternative splicing of IGF-I occurs. It has been suggested that this splicing event results in the production of an mRNA species that is translated into a precursor that ultimately results in a peptide that is different from the typical IGF-I peptide. This peptide has been named the IGF-IEb (in rodents) or IGF-IEc (in humans) splice variant, and also MGF due to its expression after mechanical damage. Briefly, the hypothesis for the role of MGF is that after injury or mechanical stress, it activates satellite cells and plays a role in myoblast proliferation. Yet, as MGF inhibits differentiation, concentrations of MGF decrease and another splice variant, IGF-IEa, is able to potentiate differentiation. However, this is a new area of research and recent publications have questioned the amount of support for this theory [62]. Despite the fact that many questions regarding MGF remain, it is already being used as an ergogenic aid and being sold on the black market [63].

Conclusion

The impacts of resistance exercise on the reproductive hormonal axis are important beyond the aspects of reproductive biology and influence other hypopituitary and adrenal pathways as well. The many roles it plays in anabolic and catabolic signaling are just starting to be elucidated. Again, it must be remembered that hormones are only part of a very complex signaling system in the body and this system has dramatic redundancy. When considering the responses that occur as a result of resistance training, there are certain aspects of the stimulus that must first be understood, beginning with the size principle. If anabolic hormonal responses are going to occur beyond normal homeostatic maintenance of the cell, muscle fibers, they must first be recruited as part of motor unit activation in response to an exercise demand for force and power. In addition, it is possible that not only will unrecruited tissues not adapt, but may still be susceptible to damaging processes that occur as a result of reactive oxygen species or glucocorticoid exposure. If resistance training is successful in recruiting muscle fibers, hormonal responses will be governed by the upper regulatory elements as well as the manipulation of the acute program variables [14]. There are a variety of hormones and growth factors that may be secreted to induce adaptation of muscle tissue, with each doing so via its own mechanism of action of which some have been described. However, these mechanisms often impact each other, with complex interactions. This underscores the importance of an appreciation of the "big picture" when it comes to resistance training endocrinology and its interface with other physiological systems related to reproductive biology and exercise.

Endurance/Aerobic Exercise and Training

In a single endurance/aerobic exercise session, there are several components that dictate the magnitude and direction of the hormonal response. The key components of a single session are the *intensity* at which the exercise is performed and the *duration* of the exercise session [64–66]. Typically, the greater the intensity of exercise is, the greater is the degree of stress placed on the endocrine system and the more exacerbated the hormonal response becomes, that is, there are larger disturbances in the circulating hormonal concentrations [64, 65, 67]. It is important to recognize that in endurance exercises some hormones have *intensity thresholds* which need to be reached before a discernible change in the hormonal concentration of the blood can be noted. The major examples of this phenomenon are cortisol and GH, which respond once an intensity of 50–60 % VO_{2max} is reached. The direction of the responses in the circulating hormonal concentrations is varied, principally increased, but decreases can also occur [68]. Relative to duration, typically extending the length of time of an exercise session at any given intensity tends to amplify a hormone response. However, in some situations after the initial change in the hormonal concentration with exercise, there can be a plateau (i.e., steady state) of the response even as exercise duration is extended, or even possibly to some degree a decrease occurs [68, 69]

In addition to the intensity–duration components that can influence the hormonal response to an endurance exercise session, there are several other factors that can modify the response, such as environmental conditions, age, gender, nutrition status, circadian rhythms, genetics, and level of exercise training status. Space limitations do not allow for a discussion of these components here, but the readers are directed to several select references that address them in detail [66, 69].

Exercise Responses

To characterize the typical hormonal responses involving an exercise session including endurance/aerobic activities (e.g., running, road cycling, mountain biking, race walking, orienteering, or cross-country skiing), a conceptual model first presented in the 1980s by the Danish scientist Dr. Henrik Galbo which divides the endocrine responses into phases will be used [68, 70]. The model illustration discussed below assumes that the exercise is typical for participants of such activities, prolonged duration (~60 min) and submaximal in nature (50–75 % VO_{2max}).

It is important to recognize that the principal reasons for hormonal changes during exercise are for (a) meeting the needs of increased energy expenditure (via biochemical pathway activation for direct ATP production and substrate availability utilization in such pathways), (b) bringing about necessary cardiovascular-hemodynamic adjustments, (c) maintenance of euhydration—fluid conservation, (d) thermoregulation, and finally (e) to some degree of stress–reactivity reactions [67, 68].

Phase I: Onset of Exercise

The first phase is immediately at the onset of exercise, taking just seconds to occur. It consists primarily of increased SNS activation with the onset of body motion. The increased SNS activity can also be a result of anticipation to the stress of the ensuing exercise. This increased SNS activity results in catecholamine release (primarily norepinephrine) at target tissues directly, as well as elevations in circulating catecholamine from the so-called sympathetic "spill-over" effects. This effect is further amplified by the sympathetic connection to the adrenal medullary gland which secretes additional circulating catecholamine (primarily epinephrine) [71]. These catecholamine changes are critical factors in driving appropriate cardiovascular-hemodynamic adjustments with the onset of exercise. Concurrent with these sympathetic-adrenal actions, pancreatic insulin secretion begins to be inhibited while glucagon secretion becomes stimulated. The entire process to this point seems to involve central nervous system feed-forward mechanisms to drive these initial responses, although the events are modified by peripheral afferent neural input from the skeletal muscle sensory receptors [71, 72].

Phase II: Intermediate Actions

This is the intermediate or secondary phase which takes slightly longer to develop; however, this phase is still typically very fast, beginning usually in much less than a minute. In this phase, the hypothalamus begins the process of releasing its hormones, such as corticotropin-releasing *hormone* (CRH), GHRH, and thyrotropin-releasing *hormone* (TRH), in an attempt to provoke changes at the anterior pituitary to stimulate the release of select hormones (e.g., adrenocorticotropin-releasing *hormone* (ACTH), GH, and thyroid-stimulating hormone (TSH)). As the pituitary begins to respond to the hypothalamic stimulus, its "trophic hormones" act on their specific peripheral target glands to stimulate additional hormonal release [64, 73, 74]. One of the most fast-acting in this cascade of events is the hypothalamic–pituitary–adrenocortical interaction, where CRH brings about ACTH release and that, in turn, brings about cortisol release. Endocrine glands linked together in such an interacting regulatory capacity axis referred to as an "axis" in this case, the "hypothalamic–pituitary–adrenocortical axis" [75, 76]. The release of arginine vasopressin (AVP) from the posterior pituitary also begins in this phase, although typically fluid balance had not become disturbed substantially. Nonetheless, the vasoconstrictive actions of AVP aid in the hemodynamic of blood flow and selective shunting necessary during redistribution of cardiac output in this form of exercise [77].

Phase III: Prolonged Actions

As exercise continues, there is a transition beyond the intermediate phase into a third phase of response, which is a more prolonged state and dependent on the duration of the exercise session. In phase 3, the responses of the sympathetic–adrenal axis are being augmented by other hormones from the anterior-posterior pituitary and the peripheral endocrine glands subordinated to pituitary regulation [64, 78, 79]. Table 8.1

illustrates that there are a multitude of hormones that have concentrational increases by this phase. However, there are notable exceptions such as insulin, where there is a consistent opposite effect (decrease), and the gonadotrophs (FSH–LH), where there is not a universal consistent finding of responses.

In this phase, reproductive hormones such as progesterone and estradiol-β-17 (principally women) and testosterone (principally men) are consistently found to increase [80]. Some of this increase seems due to the hemoconcentration of the blood that occurs, but some increase is also attributed to catecholamine-mediated stimulation of the gonads as well as temperature-induced dis-association from binding proteins [81]. In addition, during this phase, the skeletal and cardiac muscle tissues themselves begin to release their select cytokines, hormonal-like agents (principally interleukin-6), into circulation [82–84] to modulate and augment some hormonal actions. Also, it is in this phase that the renin–angiotensin–aldosterone system (RAAS) becomes highly activated initiating a large aldosterone response that typically persists well into recovery (phase IV) [85]. These RAAS responses and the continued release of AVP assist in fluid conservation as during this phase of exercise thermoregulation demands typically utilize large amounts of water reserves in the formation of sweat in order to induce evaporative cooling (e.g., it is very likely that sweat rates can easily reach 1–2 L/h during endurance/aerobic exercise) [86]. Prolactin levels are elevated in response to such exercise and can remain so for hours after exercise, which has been associated with the refractory reductions in testosterone seen during the period several hours after exercise [87]. Interestingly, in recent years, the physiological roles of prolactin, beyond reproduction, have been identified and it is now realized that it serves as an important regulator of the immune system [88].

Neural factors have been the primary stimuli regulating the endocrine response up to this point. But now in the third phase, there is an ever-increasing influence of the humoral and hormonal factors that regulate the overall responses due to the changes in the "internal milieu." This shifting of primary regulators allows an increasing reliance upon feedback rather than feed-forward control mechanisms. The influence of humoral and hormonal stimuli types in modulating the hormonal levels is magnified as the exercise duration is extended, and energy substrate availability causes shifts in fuel usage (i.e., ↓ carbohydrate available as liver- and muscle-glycogen stores is depleted ⇒ ↑ reliance of intramuscular and adipose lipid stores), or hydration issues (i.e., hemoconcentration and/or dehydration) begin compromising the thermoregulatory ability and heat storage increases driving up core temperature [89, 90]. The latter point, core temperature increase, is a critical factor that greatly augments the hormonal and cytokine response to this form of exercise [91].

Phase IVL: Recovery

As the exercise ends, the fourth and last phase, recovery starts. In recovery, the endocrine system attempts to return hormones to levels which would allow a return to a normal resting homeostasis within the physiological systems of the body. The duration of the recovery period is totally dependent on the severity of the exercise session, that is, how much stress the body and the endocrine system were subjected to [70–72]. Opinions by various researchers exist that this phase actually deserves to be split into two distinct phases. That is, research from several investigators indicates that there is most certainly an early "rapid" recovery that occurs within the first few minutes to hours after exercise, followed by a late "delayed" recovery phase lasting many hours in length for certain hormones after exercise ends [64, 92]. For example, work from our laboratory has shown that thyroid hormones (TSH, T_4, T_3) following 90 min of endurance exercise can be suppressed up to 24 h into recovery. Furthermore, if you couple together several days of endurance training sessions involving several hours of activity per day, these thyroid suppressions can last several days [93].

During the recovery phase, these hormonal responses occur primarily as a means to facilitate energy reserves and hydration restoration, and as a means to assist/modify protein turnover which

Table 8.1 Generalized hormonal responses to exercise (endurance/aerobic types) of varying intensity and following exercise training

Hormone	Principal physiological role[a]	Exercise response			
		Short-term submaximal	High intensity	Prolonged submaximal	Endurance training
ACTH	Adrenal regulatory	↑	↑↑	↑↑	↔, ↓
AVP	Hydration, fluids	↑ >50 %VO_{2max}	↑↑	↑↑	↔
Aldosterone	Hydration, fluids	↑	↑↑	↑↑	↔
Catecholamines	Catabolic, (e.g., lipolysis, glycogenolysis), cardio-regulatory	↑	↑↑	↑↑	↔, ↓
Cortisol	Catabolic (e.g., lipolysis, gluconeogenesis), stress reactivity	↑ >60 %VO_{2max}	↑↑	↑↑	↔, ↓
Estradiol-β-17	Bone metabolism, catabolic (e.g., lipolysis), reproductive	↑	↑	↑ ↓ if excessive	↔, ↓
FSH–LH	Reproductive	↑	↑, ↔	↑, ↓, ↔	↓
Glucagon	Glucoregulatory	↑	↑	↑↑	↓
Growth hormone	Anabolic (e.g., myoplasticity)	↑	↑↑	↑↑	↔, ↑
Insulin	Glucoregulatory	↓	↓	↓	↓
Prolactin	Immune, stress reactivity	↑	↑↑	↑↑	↑, ↓
Progesterone	Reproductive	↑	↑	↑	↔, ↓
Testosterone	Anabolic (e.g., myoplasticity)	↑	↑	↑ ↓ if excessive	↔, ↓
T_4–T_3	Calorigenesis, endo-permissive	↔	↔	↑, ↓	↔, ↓
TSH	Thyroregulatory	↑	↔, ↑	↔, ↑	↔

[a] Principal role relative to exercise ↑=increase; ↓=decrease; ↔=no change

is necessary for adaptation (i.e., myoplasticity) and the revitalization process of tissues.

Exercise Training Effects

Table 8.1 also presents the impact of endurance exercise training on many hormones. Essentially, the overriding effect normally is for training to reduce the blood level of hormones at rest, and in most situations in response to performing a single endurance/aerobic exercise session—in particular of submaximal intensities. There are a few hormones that are relatively unaffected by exercise training either at rest or in response to an exercise session [94]. The reasons for these reductions in hormonal response to a single exercise session after an exercise training are illustrated in Fig. 8.2 and discussed in the following section.

Mechanism of Hormonal Reponses to Endurance/Aerobic Exercise

The mechanisms by which blood hormone levels (i.e., concentrations) change during an exercise session are associated with alterations in vascular fluid content, rate of hormonal metabolic clearance (MCR), and glandular secretion responses. Each of these is discussed briefly below.

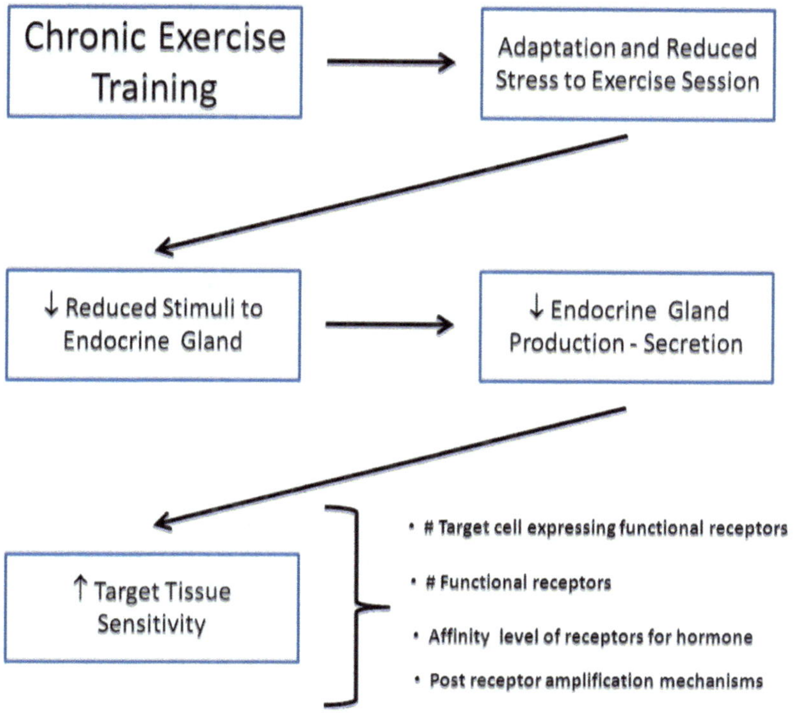

Fig. 8.2 Mechanism by which chronic exercise training induces an alteration in circulating hormonal levels and target tissue responsiveness

Vascular fluid content alterations result from plasma fluid moving into or out of the vascular bed due to osmotic gradients or as the pool of fluids used for sweat formation. During exercise, plasma volume "shifts" occur, specifically a loss of fluid, resulting in a hemoconcentration of large molecular weight hormones in the vessels. A 30–90-min exercise session can induce a 10–15 % reduction in plasma volume. This effect is magnified if the ambient environment condition creates a greater thermal load and an individual does not consume adequate fluids during the exercise. During the recovery from exercise (with ample fluids consumption), there is a rebound effect and fluid moves into the vascular space to cause a hemodilution effect on substances in the blood [64, 94].

The hormonal MCR relates to removal of substance from the blood. Hormones are "taken up" by receptor mechanisms at their target tissues which can implement physiological actions at the tissue (see discussion below). Furthermore, some clearance is done through the degradation—deactivation removal process at tissues such as the hepatocytes, or via renal filtration.

Glandular secretion involves the endocrine gland producing the hormone in response to stimuli and secreting more of the hormone into the blood, typically resulting in increases in blood levels. It is, however, possible for the increased rate of secretion and MCR removal rate to match one another. In this case, the level of the hormone in the blood does not seem to increase, but in actuality the turnover has and the target tissues are being presented with greater amounts of hormone [76, 95].

Erroneously, there is a perception that if blood hormonal levels increase, then the physiological actions of that hormone are going to be activated. This is a gross oversimplification of how endocrine actions occur. Blood hormonal concentrations are a key fundamental determinant of activation of physiological actions, but not the only one. In addition, for a hormone to initiate a physiological process, it is necessary that there must be (a) adequate numbers of target tissue cells expressing functional receptors for the hormone, (b) adequate numbers of functional receptors on the cells, (c) a high affinity level of the receptors on the cells for the hormone, and (d) sufficient post-receptor amplification mechanisms within the cells to respond [76, 95]. It is changes in many of these factors that occur with exercise training that result in the need for far less hormonal response to a single exercise session following training. These events, combined with far better fluid balance regulation and less hemoconcentration, result in less circulating hormonal release after a training program.

Maladaptation Responses: Dysregulation

If exercise training regimes are excessive in nature, or an athlete has too many additional life stresses compounding his/her situation even during appropriate training, it is possible for inappropriate hormone responses (maladaptations) to occur and conditions of endocrine dysregulation to develop. The most prevalent of the latter conditions are the *overtraining syndrome, athletic amenorrhea*, and the *exercise-hypogonadal male condition* [96–98]. The first two conditions are discussed in detail in other chapters of this book. The third, the exercise-hypogonadal male condition, is a disorder that is a male allegory to what is observed in women with athletic amenorrhea, that is, a disruption in the HPG axis that regulates reproduction function in the gender. In the male condition, the disruption is such that LH production is abnormal (typically suppressed), GnRH responsiveness is disrupted, testosterone production is suppressed, and spermatogenesis is compromised [99]. In these men, the circulating free and total testosterone levels are characteristically reduced by 30–60 % from what would be normally expected for men of their age [97, 100]. However, males are usually unaware that they have the condition (unlike women there is no outward manifestation of a problem, i.e., loss of a menstrual cycle). Interestingly, it is currently unknown whether male libido is affected by this condition; however, males with this condition have been shown to have exacerbated prolactin responses to exercise as well as drug challenges to the pituitary, and prolactin has been shown to suppress libido [101–104]. Along these lines, there is a need in the future to examine male–female couples in which both individuals are engaged in chronic endurance/aerobic exercise training to look at issues of fertility.

Conclusions

Endurance/aerobic exercise can induce large and dramatic changes (primarily increases) in circulating hormonal levels. These changes occur to bring about appropriate alterations in (a) energy expenditure, (b) cardiovascular-hemodynamic adjustments, (c) fluid conservation, (d) thermoregulation adjustments, and (e) stress–reactivity reactions [64, 98]. Exercise training when done appropriately and for a long enough period to allow adaptions results in the hormone response to a single endurance/aerobic exercise session being reduced. These reduced hormonal responses, nevertheless, allow for adequate (or enhanced) physiological responses to exercise in the tissues due to alterations in receptor characteristics and post-receptor amplification characteristics within target tissues, which results in an improved sensitivity of the tissue to hormonal influences.

An acute endurance/aerobic exercise session influences many critical hormones relative to reproductive function in both men and women (summarized in Table 8.1). Furthermore, chronic endurance/aerobic exercise training has been shown to impact the regulatory hypothalamic–pituitary–gonadal regulatory axis of both sexes. When such training becomes excessive, a maladaptation leading in some cases to a dysregulation occurs in the axis. Such dysregulation has negative consequences on the reproductive hormonal status and reproductive biology of the individual. Future research work is needed to ascertain how substantially the fertility status of exercising individuals (or couples) is influenced by these consequences and whether intervention medical steps are necessary.

References

1. Henneman E. Relation between size of neurons and their susceptibility to discharge. Science. 1957;126:1345–7.
2. Vilensky JA, Gilman S. Renaming the "Henneman size principle". Science. 1998;280:2031.
3. Milner-Brown HS, Stein RB, Yemm R. The orderly recruitment of human motor units during voluntary isometric contractions. J Physiol. 1973;230:359–70.
4. Campos GE, Luecke TJ, Wendeln HK, Toma K, Hagerman FC, Murray TF, Ragg KE, Ratamess NA, Kraemer WJ, Staron RS. Muscular adaptations in response to three different resistance-training regimens: specificity of repetition maximum training zones. Eur J Appl Physiol. 2002;88:50–60.
5. Schuenke MD, Herman J, Staron RS. Preponderance of evidence proves "big" weights optimize hypertrophic and strength adaptations. Eur J Appl Physiol. 2013;113:269–71.
6. Schakman O, Kalista S, Barbe C, Loumaye A, Thissen JP. Glucocorticoid-induced skeletal muscle atrophy. Int J Biochem Cell Biol. 2013; 45(10):2163–72.
7. Powers SK, Jackson MJ. Exercise-induced oxidative stress: cellular mechanisms and impact on muscle force production. Physiol Rev. 2008;88:1243–76.
8. Hudson MB, Hosick PA, McCaulley GO, Schrieber L, Wrieden J, McAnulty SR, Triplett NT, McBride JM, Quindry JC. The effect of resistance exercise on humoral markers of oxidative stress. Med Sci Sports Exerc. 2008;40:542–8.
9. McArdle A, Pattwell D, Vasilaki A, Griffiths RD, Jackson MJ. Contractile activity-induced oxidative stress: cellular origin and adaptive responses. Am J Physiol Cell Physiol. 2001;280:C621–7.
10. Vasilaki A, Jackson MJ, McArdle A. Attenuated HSP70 response in skeletal muscle of aged rats following contractile activity. Muscle Nerve. 2002;25:902–5.
11. Balon TW, Nadler JL. Nitric oxide release is present from incubated skeletal muscle preparations. J Appl Physiol. 1994;77:2519–21.
12. Sen CK, Packer L, Hanninen O. Handbook of oxidants and antioxidants in exercise. New York: Elsevier; 2000.
13. Pothen JJ, Poynter ME, Bates JH. The inflammatory twitch as a general strategy for controlling the host response. J Immunol. 2013;190:3510–6.
14. Spiering BA, Kraemer WJ, Anderson JM, Armstrong LE, Nindl BC, Volek JS, Maresh CM. Resistance exercise biology: manipulation of resistance exercise programme variables determines the responses of cellular and molecular signalling pathways. Sports Med. 2008;38:527–40.
15. Kraemer WJ, Noble BJ, Clark MJ, Culver BW. Physiologic responses to heavy-resistance exercise with very short rest periods. Int J Sports Med. 1987;8:247–52.
16. French DN, Kraemer WJ, Volek JS, Spiering BA, Judelson DA, Hoffman JR, Maresh CM. Anticipatory responses of catecholamines on muscle force production. J Appl Physiol. 2007;102:94–102.
17. Szivak TK, Hooper DR, Dunn-Lewis C, Comstock BA, Kupchak BR, Apicella JM, Saenz C, Maresh CM, Denegar CR, Kraemer WJ. Adrenal cortical responses to high-intensity, short rest, resistance exercise in men and women. J Strength Cond Res. 2013;27:748–60.
18. Auclair D, Garrel DR, Chaouki Zerouala A, Ferland LH. Activation of the ubiquitin pathway in rat skeletal muscle by catabolic doses of glucocorticoids. Am J Physiol. 1997;272:C1007–16.
19. Seene T. Turnover of skeletal muscle contractile proteins in glucocorticoid myopathy. J Steroid Biochem Mol Biol. 1994;50:1–4.
20. Seene T, Alev K. Effect of glucocorticoids on the turnover rate of actin and myosin heavy and light chains on different types of skeletal muscle fibres. J Steroid Biochem. 1985;22:767–71.
21. Dekhuijzen PN, Gayan-Ramirez G, Bisschop A, De Bock V, Dom R, Decramer M. Corticosteroid treatment and nutritional deprivation cause a different pattern of atrophy in rat diaphragm. J Appl Physiol. 1995;78:629–37.
22. Spiering BA, Kraemer WJ, Anderson JM, Armstrong LE, Nindl BC, Volek JS, Judelson DA, Joseph M, Vingren JL, Hatfield DL, Fragala MS, Ho JY, Maresh CM. Effects of elevated circulating hormones on resistance exercise-induced Akt signaling. Med Sci Sports Exerc. 2008;40:1039–48.
23. Ratamess NA, Kraemer WJ, Volek JS, Maresh CM, Vanheest JL, Sharman MJ, Rubin MR, French DN, Vescovi JD, Silvestre R, Hatfield DL, Fleck SJ, Deschenes MR. Androgen receptor content following heavy resistance exercise in men. J Steroid Biochem Mol Biol. 2005;93:35–42.
24. Villanueva MG, Lane CJ, Schroeder ET. Influence of rest interval length on acute testosterone and cortisol responses to volume-load-equated total body hypertrophic and strength protocols. J Strength Cond Res. 2012;26:2755–64.
25. Kraemer WJ, Fleck SJ, Dziados JE, Harman EA, Marchitelli LJ, Gordon SE, Mello R, Frykman PN, Koziris LP, Triplett NT. Changes in hormonal concentrations after different heavy-resistance exercise protocols in women. J Appl Physiol. 1993;75:594–604.
26. Kraemer WJ, Marchitelli L, Gordon SE, Harman E, Dziados JE, Mello R, Frykman P, McCurry D, Fleck SJ. Hormonal and growth factor responses to heavy resistance exercise protocols. J Appl Physiol. 1990;69:1442–50.
27. Nunes JA, Crewther BT, Ugrinowitsch C, Tricoli V, Viveiros L, de Rose D Jr, Aoki MS. Salivary hormone and immune responses to three resistance exercise schemes in elite female athletes. J Strength Cond Res. 2011;25:2322–7.

28. Leite RD, Prestes J, Rosa C, De Salles BF, Maior A, Miranda H, Simao R. Acute effect of resistance training volume on hormonal responses in trained men. J Sports Med Phys Fitness. 2011;51:322–8.
29. Kraemer WJ, Gordon SE, Fleck SJ, Marchitelli LJ, Mello R, Dziados JE, Friedl K, Harman E, Maresh C, Fry AC. Endogenous anabolic hormonal and growth factor responses to heavy resistance exercise in males and females. Int J Sports Med. 1991;12:228–35.
30. Vingren JL, Kraemer WJ, Hatfield DL, Volek JS, Ratamess NA, Anderson JM, Hakkinen K, Ahtiainen J, Fragala MS, Thomas GA, Ho JY, Maresh CM. Effect of resistance exercise on muscle steroid receptor protein content in strength-trained men and women. Steroids. 2009;74:1033–9.
31. Mazon J, Gastaldi A, Di Sacco T, Cozza I, Dutra S, Souza H. Effects of training periodization on cardiac autonomic modulation and endogenous stress markers in volleyball players. Scand J Med Sci Sports. 2013;23:114–20.
32. Enea C, Boisseau N, Fargeas-Gluck MA, Diaz V, Dugue B. Circulating androgens in women: exercise-induced changes. Sports Med. 2011;41:1–15.
33. Hoffman JR, Kraemer WJ, Bhasin S, Storer T, Ratamess NA, Haff GG, Willoughby DS, Rogol AD. Position stand on androgen and human growth hormone use. J Strength Cond Res. 2009;23:S1–59.
34. Mauras N, Hayes V, Welch S, Rini A, Helgeson K, Dokler M, Veldhuis JD, Urban RJ. Testosterone deficiency in young men: marked alterations in whole body protein kinetics, strength, and adiposity. J Clin Endocrinol Metab. 1998;83:1886–92.
35. Demling RH, Orgill DP. The anticatabolic and wound healing effects of the testosterone analog oxandrolone after severe burn injury. J Crit Care. 2000;15:12–7.
36. Dubois V, Laurent M, Boonen S, Vanderschueren D, Claessens F. Androgens and skeletal muscle: cellular and molecular action mechanisms underlying the anabolic actions. Cell Mol Life Sci. 2012;69:1651–67.
37. Mayer M, Rosen F. Interaction of glucocorticoids and androgens with skeletal muscle. Metabolism. 1977;26:937–62.
38. Nindl BC, Kraemer WJ, Gotshalk LA, Marx JO, Volek JS, Bush FA, Hakkinen K, Newton RU, Fleck SJ. Testosterone responses after resistance exercise in women: influence of regional fat distribution. Int J Sport Nutr Exerc Metab. 2001;11:451–65.
39. Spiering BA, Kraemer WJ, Vingren JL, Ratamess NA, Anderson JM, Armstrong LE, Nindl BC, Volek JS, Hakkinen K, Maresh CM. Elevated endogenous testosterone concentrations potentiate muscle androgen receptor responses to resistance exercise. J Steroid Biochem Mol Biol. 2009;114:195–9.
40. Vingren JL, Kraemer WJ, Ratamess NA, Anderson JM, Volek JS, Maresh CM. Testosterone physiology in resistance exercise and training: the up-stream regulatory elements. Sports Med. 2010;40:1037–53.
41. Kraemer WJ, Spiering BA, Volek JS, Ratamess NA, Sharman MJ, Rubin MR, French DN, Silvestre R, Hatfield DL, Van Heest JL, Vingren JL, Judelson DA, Deschenes MR, Maresh CM. Androgenic responses to resistance exercise: effects of feeding and L-carnitine. Med Sci Sports Exerc. 2006;38:1288–96.
42. Kvorning T, Andersen M, Brixen K, Madsen K. Suppression of endogenous testosterone production attenuates the response to strength training: a randomized, placebo-controlled, and blinded intervention study. Am J Physiol Endocrinol Metab. 2006;291:E1325–32.
43. Kvorning T, Andersen M, Brixen K, Schjerling P, Suetta C, Madsen K. Suppression of testosterone does not blunt mRNA expression of myoD, myogenin, IGF, myostatin or androgen receptor post strength training in humans. J Physiol. 2007;578:579–93.
44. Hwang AC, Liu LK, Lee WJ, Lin MH, Peng LN, Won CW, Chen LK. Association of androgen with skeletal muscle mass and muscle function among men and women age 50 years and older in Taiwan: results from I-Lan longitudinal aging study. Rejuvenation Res. 2013;16(6):453–9.
45. Baumann G. Growth hormone heterogeneity: genes, isohormones, variants, and binding proteins. Endocr Rev. 1991;12:424–49.
46. Kraemer WJ, Dunn-Lewis C, Comstock BA, Thomas GA, Clark JE, Nindl BC. Growth hormone, exercise, and athletic performance: a continued evolution of complexity. Curr Sports Med Rep. 2010;9:242–52.
47. Kraemer WJ, Nindl BC, Marx JO, Gotshalk LA, Bush JA, Welsch JR, Volek JS, Spiering BA, Maresh CM, Mastro AM, Hymer WC. Chronic resistance training in women potentiates growth hormone in vivo bioactivity: characterization of molecular mass variants. Am J Physiol Endocrinol Metab. 2006;291:E1177–87.
48. Rubin MR, Kraemer WJ, Maresh CM, Volek JS, Ratamess NA, Vanheest JL, Silvestre R, French DN, Sharman MJ, Judelson DA, Gomez AL, Vescovi JD, Hymer WC. High-affinity growth hormone binding protein and acute heavy resistance exercise. Med Sci Sports Exerc. 2005;37:395–403.
49. Gordon SE, Kraemer WJ, Vos NH, Lynch JM, Knuttgen HG. Effect of acid-base balance on the growth hormone response to acute high-intensity cycle exercise. J Appl Physiol. 1994;76:821–9.
50. Hymer WC, Kraemer WJ, Nindl BC, Marx JO, Benson DE, Welsch JR, Mazzetti SA, Volek JS, Deaver DR. Characteristics of circulating growth hormone in women after acute heavy resistance exercise. Am J Physiol Endocrinol Metab. 2001;281:E878–87.
51. Kraemer WJ, Nindl BC, Volek JS, Marx JO, Gotshalk LA, Bush JA, Welsch JR, Vingren JL, Spiering BA, Fragala MS, Hatfield DL, Ho JY, Maresh CM, Mastro AM, Hymer WC. Influence of oral contraceptive use on growth hormone in vivo bioactivity following resistance exercise: responses of molecular mass variants. Growth Horm IGF Res. 2008;18:238–44.
52. Sotiropoulos A, Ohanna M, Kedzia C, Menon RK, Kopchick JJ, Kelly PA, Pende M. Growth hormone promotes skeletal muscle cell fusion independent of insulin-like growth factor 1 up-regulation. Proc Natl Acad Sci U S A. 2006;103:7315–20.

53. Perrini S, Laviola L, Carreira MC, Cignarelli A, Natalicchio A, Giorgino F. The GH/IGF1 axis and signaling pathways in the muscle and bone: mechanisms underlying age-related skeletal muscle wasting and osteoporosis. J Endocrinol. 2010;205:201–10.
54. Nindl BC, Pierce JR. Insulin-like growth factor I as a biomarker of health, fitness, and training status. Med Sci Sports Exerc. 2010;42:39–49.
55. Frasca F, Pandini G, Scalia P, Sciacca L, Mineo R, Costantino A, Goldfine ID, Belfiore A, Vigneri R. Insulin receptor isoform A, a newly recognized, high-affinity insulin-like growth factor II receptor in fetal and cancer cells. Mol Cell Biol. 1999;19:3278–88.
56. Nindl BC, Alemany JA, Tuckow AP, Kellogg MD, Sharp MA, Patton JF. Effects of exercise mode and duration on 24-h IGF-I system recovery responses. Med Sci Sports Exerc. 2009;41:1261–70.
57. Nindl BC, Castellani JW, Young AJ, Patton JF, Khosravi MJ, Diamandi A, Montain SJ. Differential responses of IGF-I molecular complexes to military operational field training. J Appl Physiol. 2003;95:1083–9.
58. Nindl BC, Kraemer WJ, Marx JO, Arciero PJ, Dohi K, Kellogg MD, Loomis GA. Overnight responses of the circulating IGF-I system after acute, heavy-resistance exercise. J Appl Physiol. 2001;90:1319–26.
59. Coolican SA, Samuel DS, Ewton DZ, McWade FJ, Florini JR. The mitogenic and myogenic actions of insulin-like growth factors utilize distinct signaling pathways. J Biol Chem. 1997;272:6653–62.
60. Fuentes EN, Bjornsson BT, Valdes JA, Einarsdottir IE, Lorca B, Alvarez M, Molina A. IGF-I/PI3K/Akt and IGF-I/MAPK/ERK pathways in vivo in skeletal muscle are regulated by nutrition and contribute to somatic growth in the fine flounder. Am J Physiol Regul Integr Comp Physiol. 2011;300:R1532–42.
61. Singleton JR, Feldman EL. Insulin-like growth factor-I in muscle metabolism and myotherapies. Neurobiol Dis. 2001;8:541–54.
62. Matheny RW Jr, Nindl BC, Adamo ML. Minireview: Mechano-growth factor: a putative product of IGF-I gene expression involved in tissue repair and regeneration. Endocrinology. 2010;151:865–75.
63. Esposito S, Deventer K, Van Eenoo P. Characterization and identification of a C-terminal amidated mechano growth factor (MGF) analogue in black market products. Rapid Commun Mass Spectrom. 2012;26:686–92.
64. Borer KT. Exercise endocrinology. Champaign: Human Kinetics Publishing; 2003. p. 77–96.
65. Viru A. Hormonal ensemble in exercise—Hormones in muscular activity, Vol. 1. Boca Raton: CRC Press; 1985. p. 34–96.
66. Viru A, Viru M. Biochemical monitoring of sport training. Champaign: Human Kinetics Publishing; 2001.
67. Bunt JC. Hormonal alterations due to exercise. Sports Med. 1986;3:331–45.
68. Galbo H. Hormonal and metabolic adaptation to exercise. Stuttgart: Georg Thieme Verlag; 1983.
69. Hackney AC, Viru A. Research methodology: issues with endocrinological measurements in exercise science and sport medicine. J Athletic Training. 2008;43(6):631–9.
70. Hackney AC. Exercise as a stressor to the neuroendocrine system. Medicina. 2006;42(10):788–97.
71. Chrousos GP, Gold PW. The concept of stress systems disorders: overview of physical and behavioral homeostasis. JAMA. 1992;267:1244–52.
72. Tsigo C, Chrousos GP. Hypothalamic-pituitary-adrenal axis, neuroendocrine factors and stress. J Psychosomatic Res. 2002;53:865–71.
73. Farrell PA, Garthwaite TL, Gustafson AB. Plasma adrenocorticotropin and cortisol responses to submaximal and exhaustive exercise. J Appl Physiol. 1983;55(5):1441–4.
74. Goldstein DS. Catecholamines and stress. Endocrine Reg. 2003;37:69–80.
75. Davies CTM, Few JD. Effects of exercise on adrenocortical function. J Appl Physiol. 1973;5:887–91.
76. Widmaier EP. Metabolic feedback in mammalian endocrine systems. Hormone Metab Res. 1992;24:147–53.
77. Röcker L, Kirsch KA, Heyduck B, Altenkirch HU. Influence of prolonged physical exercise on plasma volume, plasma proteins, electrolytes, and fluid-regulating hormones. Int J Sports Med. 1989;10(4):270–4.
78. Mastorakos G, Pavlatou M, Diamanti-Kandaraki E, Chrousos GP. Exercise and the stress system. Hormones (Athens). 2005;4(2):73–89.
79. Park E, Chan O, Li Q, Kiraly M, Matthews SG, Vranic M, Riddell MC. Changes in basal hypothalamic-pituitary-adrenal activity during exercise are centrally mediated. Am J Physiol. 2005;289:R1360–71.
80. Hackney AC. Testosterone, the hypothalamo-pituitary-testicular axis and endurance exercise training: a review. Biology of Sport. 1996;13(2):85–98.
81. Fahrner CL, Hackney AC. Effects of exercise on the binding affinity of sex-hormone binding globulin for testosterone. Int J Sports Med. 1998;19(1):12–5.
82. Petersen AMW, Pedersen BK. The anti-inflammatory effect of exercise. J Appl Physiol. 2005;98:1154–62.
83. Febbraio MA, Pedersen BK. Contraction-induced myokine production and release: Is skeletal muscle an endocrine organ? Exerc Sport Sci Rev. 2005;33(3):114–9.
84. Nieman DC. Exercise effects on systemic immunity. Immunol Cell Biol. 2000;78:496–501.
85. Cody RJ. The sympathetic nervous system and the renin-angiotensin-aldosterone system in cardiovascular disease. Am J Cardiol. 1997;80(9B):9J–14J.
86. Convertino VA. Blood volume response to physical activity and inactivity. Am J Med Sci. 2007;334(1):72–9.
87. Daly W, Seegers CA, Rubin DA, Dobridge JD, Hackney AC. Relationship between stress hormones and testosterone with prolonged endurance exercise. Eur J Appl Physiol. 2005;93:375–80.

88. Ignacak A, Kasztelnik M, Sliwa T, Korbut RA, Rajda K, Guzik TJ. Prolactin—not only lactotrophin: A "new" view of the "old" hormone. J Physiol Pharmacol. 2012;63(5):435–43.
89. Dill DB, Costill DL. Calculation of percentage changes in volumes of blood, plasma, and red cells in dehydration. J Appl Physiol. 1974;2:247–8.
90. Sawka MN, Cheuvront SN, Kenefick RW. High skin temperature and hypohydration impair aerobic performance. Exp Physiol. 2012;97(3):327–32.
91. Walsh NP, Whitham M. Exercising in environmental extremes: a greater threat to immune function? Sports Med. 2006;36(11):941–76.
92. Hackney AC, Viru A. Twenty-four cortisol response to multiple daily exercise sessions of moderate and high intensity. Clin Physiol. 1999;19:178–82.
93. Hackney AC, Hodgdon JA, Hesslink R, Trygg K. Thyroid hormone responses to military winter activities in the Arctic Region. Arctic Med Res. 1995;54:82–90.
94. McMurray RG, Hackney AC. The endocrine system and exercise. In: Garrett W, editor. Exercise & sports science. New York: Lippincott Williams & Wilkins; 2000. p. 135–62.
95. Goodman HM. Endocrinology concepts for medical students. Adv Physiol Educ. 2001;25(1–4):213–24.
96. Redman LM, Loucks AB. Menstrual disorders in athletes. Sports Med. 2005;35(9):747–55
97. Hackney AC. Endurance exercise training and reproductive dysfunction in men: alterations in the hypothalamic-pituitary-testicular axis. Curr Pharm Des. 2001;7:261–73.
98. Hackney AC. Stress and the neuroendocrine system: the role of exercise as a stressor and modifier of stress. Expert Rev Endocrinol Metab. 2006;1(6):783–92.
99. Hackney AC, Szczepanowska E, Viru A. Basal testicular testosterone production in endurance-trained men is suppressed. Eur J Appl Physiol. 2003;89(2):198–201.
100. Hackney AC. The male reproductive system and endurance exercise. Med Sci Sports Exerc. 1996;28(2):180–9.
101. Hackney AC, Sharp RL, Runyan WS, Ness RJ. Relationship of resting prolactin and testosterone changes in males during intensive training. Br J Sports Med. 1989;23(3):194.
102. Hackney AC, Sinning WE, Bruot BC. Hypothalamic-pituitary-testicular axis function in endurance trained males. Int J Sports Med. 1990;11:298–303.
103. Maggi M, Buvat J, Corona G, Guay A, Torres LO. Hormonal causes of male sexual dysfunctions and their management (hyperprolactinemia, thyroid disorders, GH disorders, and DHEA). J Sex Med. 2013;10(3):661–77.
104. Simon JA. Low sexual desire—is it all in her head? Pathophysiology, diagnosis, and treatment of hypoactive sexual desire disorder. Postgrad Med. 2010;122(6):128–36.

Common Male Reproductive Tract Pathologies Associated with Physical Activity, Exercise, and Sport

9

Amy R. Lane, Alberto Da Costa Stein and Vanessa Krebs Genro

Introduction

The World Health Organization (WHO) defines health as a state of complete physical, mental, and social well-being and not merely the absence of disease or infirmity. Physical exercise has been proposed as one of the most beneficial lifestyle interventions to achieve such a state. However, exercise is a powerful stimulus to the body and it can provoke paradoxical effects on human physiology. While it can act as an important beneficial tool preventing lifestyle-related diseases such as obesity, it is also known to induce diverse stress responses in the neuroendocrine system [1]. Elite athletes are increasingly undergoing greater levels of exercise training to improve their performance. The reproductive and endocrine systems are particularly sensitive to the amount of this training stress [2]. This chapter focuses on the existing relationships between exercise training, sports practice, and their influence on the male reproductive system functionality.

A. Stein (✉)
Department of Urology and Reproduction, Insemine Human Reproduction Center, Nilo Peçanha 2825/905, Porto Alegre, Rio Grande do Sul 91330-001, Brazil
e-mail: alberto@insemine.com

A. R. Lane
Department of Allied Health Sciences, University of North Carolina, Chapel Hill, NC, USA

V. K. Genro
Department of Obstetrics and Gynecology, Universidade Federal do Rio Grande do Sul, Porto Alegre, Rio Grand do Sul, Brazil

Exercise Physiology and the Neuroendocrine System

Testosterone is one of the most potent naturally secreted androgenic-anabolic hormones, and its biological effects include promotion of muscle growth. In muscle, testosterone stimulates protein synthesis (anabolic effect) and inhibits protein degradation (anti-catabolic effect); combined, these effects account for the promotion of an increased muscular cross-sectional area (CSA; hypertrophy + hyperplasia) [3]. Testosterone is also associated with muscle strength, sports competition aggressiveness, and re-synthesis of proteins during recovery [4]. The concentration of testosterone depends on the pulsatile release of luteinizing hormone (LH) by the anterior pituitary. The majority of the circulating testosterone is transported bound to various carrier proteins, but sex hormone-binding globulin (SHBG) is the major one [5]. The concentration of testosterone is a result of the production of the hormone and the metabolic clearance by the liver. The rates of these two processes are affected by a number of changes in the physiological state [2, 5].

Testosterone production is under control of the hypothalamic–pituitary–testicular (HPT) axis. The HPT axis is definitely influenced by exercise and exercise training [2]. However, the magnitude and extent of the effect is highly variable due to

© Springer Science+Business Media New York 2016

D. Vaamonde et al. (eds.), *Exercise and Human Reproduction*, DOI 10.1007/978-1-4939-3402-7_9

the type, intensity, and duration of the exercise performed, as well as the degree of physical fitness of the individuals exercising [1, 2]. Additionally, factors such as psychological stress, sleep disturbances, and/or diet influence the HPT axis and testosterone levels [2]. Regrettably, rarely are all of these factors considered when exercise studies are conducted or reported in the literature [2].

Male Hypogonadism and Sport

The hormonal response to acute exercise is dependent on several factors including the intensity, duration, mode of exercise, and the training level of an athlete [6]. Acute exercise demands a physiological increase in testosterone. Some investigations report that total and free testosterone levels are briefly elevated following a strenuous or prolonged exercise session [7–10]. This implies high volumes of training (e.g., 10–20 h/wk) could increase levels of steroids [11], improve metabolism [12], and protect the athlete from overactivation of the immune system [13]. However, ultimately the repetitive responses of such activity could negatively affect the HPT axis as the training program progresses [14].

Tremblay et al. studied endurance-trained males and verified that with exercise, besides short-term (acute) testosterone elevation, there was an increase in dehydroepiandrosterone sulfate (DHEAS) in a dose–response manner dependent on the intensity of the acute exercise. Furthermore, it appeared that during low-intensity exercises, high exercise volumes were needed to induce a significant increase in cortisol [15]. Interestingly, in nonelite, middle-aged marathon runners, a marathon race resulted in an acute increase in blood cortisol and prolactin levels and a concomitant decline in testosterone level [16].

The HPT axis response to chronic exercise has been investigated in many retrospective studies that found lower testosterone levels in endurance-trained males [2]. In these studies, testosterone levels of athletes were found to be 60–85% of the levels of controls, not outside the clinical norm, but at the low end of the range [10, 14]. Prospective studies are more inconsistent, since some have found significant reductions in resting testosterone following endurance training regimens, and others found no association at all. Differences in the subjects (i.e., age, mass) and in their training regimens may explain these discrepancies [2].

Meanwhile, a wide population-based study involving volunteers (not athletes) found no association between total serum testosterone levels nor SHBG levels with aerobic exercise capacity or maximal power output in men [17]. These contrasting findings demonstrate that these relationships are highly complex.

Endurance-trained males also display other hormonal abnormalities such as a lack of elevation in resting LH, despite low testosterone levels and decreased prolactin, a state referred to as the *exercise-hypogonadal male condition* (EHMC) (i.e., in chronically trained men) [18]. The EHMC is associated with not only hormonal abnormalities, but also detrimental changes in semen characteristics in the spermatogenesis process (see later discussion in the article) [2, 4, 10, 18]. Interestingly, Safarinejad et al. conducted prospective work and induced similar hormonal responses but viewed this as an effect of overtraining the men (i.e, *overtraining syndrome*) and not the EHMC [19]. Luigi et al. [4], however, states that there are no evidence-based criteria that these athletes would be at risk for osteoporotic fractures, cardiovascular accidents, or sport-related anemia due to their hormonal changes, but antidotal evidence of such events has been reported [2, 19]. Unfortunately, there is no standardized definition in the literature about at which point or with what intensity of training athletes are at risk of developing these hormonal alterations.

Male Sexual Function

Male sexual function is a complex entity because it involves desire, erection, and ejaculation. It has been shown in randomized trials that balanced exercise training in healthy volunteers is beneficial to maximize erectile function and sexual health because it reduces body mass index (BMI) and influences other disorders that affect sexual function such as the metabolic syndrome and cardiovascular diseases [20, 21]. Meanwhile, as previously stated, endurance athletes are at risk for hypogonadism, and consequently, erectile dysfunction (ED) and/or decreased sexual desire occur [22] due to decreased testosterone levels.

Varicocele and Sport

Varicocele may result from abnormally dilated veins in the pampiniform plexus, and it has long been associated with male infertility according to observational studies that report an increased incidence of this pathology in infertile men [23]. Varicocele is also commonly seen in the general population—with a prevalence between 4 and 22%—but it can reach an incidence of up to 80% in men with secondary infertility [24]. Effects of varicocele in semen parameters include altered concentration, motility, and morphology. Several studies have focused on how varicocele leads to impaired spermatogenesis, most of them proposing a mechanism of altered blood flow and scrotal temperature [23]. Although debated, there is substantial evidence to support the value of varicocele repair in male infertility in order to improve semen parameters [5].

A trial, evaluating the role of sports medicine in the diagnosis of andrological diseases, found a high incidence of varicocele in athletes—29% [25]. It has been shown that sports practice does not modify the prevalence of varicocele compared to the general population [26]; however, it seems to progress from subclinical to clinical varicocele [27]. Besides, in these subjects, the effect of varicocele appears to worsen semen parameters. In an elegant study, competitive athletes presenting with varicocele were age-matched with men who engaged only in recreational activities. Although no differences were found in hormonal levels between groups, the percentages of both progressive forward motility and percentage of normal spermatozoa were significantly reduced in athletes with varicocele [28]. Therefore, diagnosis and management of varicocele in men engaging in endurance sports training are imperative to provide safety and preserve fertility.

Prostatitis

Prostatitis (inflammation of the prostate gland) is estimated to affect 2–10% of men and is the third most common diagnosis in men less than 50 years of age presenting to urologists annually [29]. According to the current medical consensus on establishing an etiology of prostatitis, the condition may be caused by multiple factors, including neuronal, inflammatory, hormonal, and psychological factors [29–31]. One potential method for diagnosing prostatitis involves testing bodily fluids for biomarkers. As prostatic secretions form a substantial proportion (25%) of the semen, seminal plasma is an excellent fluid to search for such markers of prostatic inflammation [32]. Some studies have investigated the potential of inflammatory proteins and cytokines in the seminal plasma of patients with prostatitis or chronic pelvic pain syndrome, yet none of these biomarkers appears definitive in arriving at a diagnosis [33, 34]. In fact, the most commonly used biomarker for prostate diseases, prostate-specific antigen (PSA), in wide use as a biomarker of prostate cancer, was originally found and isolated from semen [35].

Several lines of evidence indicate that physical exercise can lead to improvements in pain sensitivity and changes in immune, neuroendocrine, and autonomic function [36, 37]; hence, exercise may be an associative or causative factor and may have a role in the etiology of prostatitis [38]. Bicycle riding, for example, combines strenuous physical activity and direct pressure on the perineum and prostate. There are probable mechanisms by which cycling may influence serum PSA levels comprised of systemic factors related to the hormonal effects of strenuous physical activity [39, 40] as well as local factors including mechanical stress of the prostate caused by movement of the pelvic muscles [41], or direct perineal pressure produced by the saddle with a significant massage effect on the prostate [42]. Also, since evidence supports trained athletes may have lower basal concentration of circulating testosterone than untrained men [2, 14, 43, 44], this may result in lower risk of developing prostate diseases in athletes than in untrained subjects [45, 46]. Though studies in this area have not yielded consistent results, it seems that the interaction between physical activities and some prostate disorders may be dependent on the physiological and metabolic factors associated with exercise parameters (intensity, duration, mode of exercise, and level of the athlete) as well as factors inherent to exercise training. Further investigations are required to elucidate the relationship between physical activity and prostate disorders, and the underlying mechanisms responsible for such a relationship.

Sperm Alterations in Athletes

Alterations in motility and concentration of spermatozoa in endurance and resistance athletes were documented in a retrospective study of DeSouza et al. [47]. In a subsequent prospective study, semen volume as well as sperm motility and morphology decreased significantly over a 1-year period of marathon training, but there was no significant alteration observed in sperm count [48]. Some authors argue that exercise volume is the most important variable affecting the semen profile [49], especially for morphological characteristics [50]. Others argue that exercise intensity can be equally deleterious on reproductive function [2, 48]. While the evidence is relatively scant, it is nonetheless clear that endurance athletes may be at risk for semen alterations.

Special Situations

Steroids Abuse

Although highly prevalent in the sporting community, abuse of androgenic-anabolic steroids (AAS) received major public attention only after their use became apparent in the Olympic Games. It was not until 1967 that the International Olympic Committee released the first list of banned substances [51].

Several drugs can be used as anabolic agents such as human chorionic gonadotropin (HCG), LH (i.e., each promoters of testosterone release), as well as exogenous AAS directly, such as nandrolone and tibolone. Common areas of substance abuse include sport performance enhancement (both in strength-based [↑muscle CSA] and endurance-based [↑ recovery capacity] activities) and aging people who are seeking to abate the effects of sarcopenia [4]. AAS can exert strong effects on the human body that may be beneficial for athletic performance. Evidence supports that short-term administration of these drugs by athletes can lead to strength gains of about 5–20 % of their initial strength and increases of 2–5 kg in body mass that may be attributed to increases of the lean body mass [52].

However, AAS abuse can affect a range of organic systems and has been shown to augment mortality rates among users, especially due to cardiovascular disease [53]. Effects on the endocrine and reproductive systems include suppression of spermatogenesis, gynecomastia, and suppression of the HPT axis due to negative feedback when higher doses are used. This can subsequently lead to hypogonadism symptoms, such as ED and decreased libido [54, 55]. Furthermore, even after discontinuation of AAS use, subjects may continue to experience the effects of prolonged hypogonadism until HPT axis recovery [51].

Trauma

Traumatic injuries in sports participants are fairly common. In addition to typical musculoskeletal events, male athletes are at risk of incurring testicular injuries. Traumatic sporting injuries do not infrequently precipitate testicular torsions [56]. Testicular torsion is characterized by acute scrotal pain, and early diagnosis and definitive management are the keys to avoid testicular loss. Nevertheless, young male athletes are usually unaware of testicular pathologies and thus do not typically wear genital protection. Neither do they appreciate the difference in urgency of seeking medical treatment of painless versus painful testicular swelling [57].

Spinal trauma events also impact reproductive function as they are associated with ED and/or retrograde ejaculation. Normal ejaculatory function, a primarily sympathetic phenomenon, consists in a complex and coordinated sequence of striated and smooth muscular contractions, which results in the antegrade emission and expulsion of sperm. Spinal injury is found in participants in many adventure sports as well as a multitude of traditional sporting events [58]. Common spinal injuries that occur include muscle strains, muscle spasms, disc herniations, as well as vertebral body compression and avulsion fractures.

Cycling

Bike riding is one of the most popular sports besides being a common means of transportation. That said, it is a frequent source of significant injuries that can be classified as acute traumatic lesions or chronic overuse injuries, common in recreational riders or competitive racing riders [59]. Since there is an important association between genitourinary tract overuse injuries and cycling, the sport deserves special attention related to sexual dysfunction.

The most common problem is pudendal nerve entrapment (PNE) syndrome, presenting as genitalia numbness, reported by 50–91 % of cyclists [59]. In men attending an infertility clinic, bicycling for more than 5 h a week was associated with lower sperm concentration and motility [60]. Injurious effect of exercise on spermatogenesis can be attributed to increased scrotal temperature and HPT axis alterations, as previously discussed.

Surveys of men in Australia, England, Germany, the Netherlands, and Spain estimate the prevalence of ED to be 11–34 % in men aged 16–80 years old [61–65]. ED is also commonly seen in high-performance and/or endurance sports athletes especially in competitive cyclists [66]. The data from the Massachusetts Male Aging Study (MMAS) showed that bicycling more than 3 h per week was an independent risk factor for males (aged 40–70 years) in the development of moderate to severe ED [67]. In case-control studies, the prevalence of moderate to severe ED in bicyclists was ~4.2 % versus age-matched runners (1.1 %) and swimmers (2 %), respectively [68]. Interestingly, research on female bicyclists is very limited but indicates the same impairment as in male bicyclists [66]. The cause of ED resulting from bicycle riding is not fully understood, yet is likely a result of continuous compression and strain on the pudendal nerve as well as insufficiency of penile blood supply because of perineal arterial compression [69, 70]. The extent to which blood flow decreases while cycling in a seated position is significantly affected by seat position, saddle material, size, and geometry [66]. It has been reported that, in male cyclists aged 20–37 years old, cycling in a 90° position resulted in 40 % better penile oxygenation than cycling in a 60° position. More than 50 % better penile oxygenation was demonstrated with a wider saddle than the narrow saddle when compared using the same seat position and padding material. Finally, no significant difference in penile oxygenation was observed when cycling on a flat saddle as compared with riding on a saddle with a hole [66]. Since cyclists are at risk for ED, they should take precautionary measures to minimize the associated risk with bicycle riding: choose a wide, unpadded no-nose saddle that allows proper placement for sitting; choose a horizontal saddle position; ride in a more upright position; change their body position regularly from a seated to a standing position; and use road bicycles instead of mountain bikes.

As similar force impacts might be seen in equestrian sports, several studies have also investigated the link between chronic urogenital trauma during horse riding and sexual dysfunction in horseback riders [71–73]. While the findings have been contradictory, Turgut and associates demonstrated a significantly higher prevalence of varicocele (46 %), hydrocele (19 %), testicular cyst (4 %), epididymal cyst (35 %), testicular calcification (19 %), epididymal calcification (8 %), scrotal calculus (8 %), and inhomogeneity of parenchymal echo texture (4 %) in horseback riders than non-horse-riding men [73]. Given the above findings, additional safety measures such as frequent and sufficient rests during riding or padding of the rider's shorts to prevent injury should be considered by horseback riders. Also, to ensure penile health, sonographic examination of equestrians who have palpable mass or related symptoms has been recommended.

Conclusions

Elite athletes are increasingly undergoing greater levels of exercise training in order to maintain a higher degree of competitiveness. The magnitude of this training and the stress it induces is necessary for improvement in the cardiorespiratory and musculoskeletal systems [1]. The reproductive and endocrine systems are particularly sensitive to the amount of training stress an athlete undergoes, and regrettably these systems can develop disruption and dysfunctions if the stress is excessive. These disruptions and dysfunctions are well described in female athletes, but researchers have only recently recognized the occurrence of such events in male athletes [2]. Evidence indicates manifestation of hypogonadism, modifications in sexual function, exacerbation of existing varicocele as well as alterations in semen parameters are all possible consequences of high levels of training stress. Furthermore, aspects of sports injuries (e.g., spinal trauma) or sports practice (e.g., cycling seat parameters) can impact testicular physiology and reproductive function.

It is important that fertility clinicians who treat male athletes and chronic exercisers recognize the impact of sport-exercise training and the particulars of sporting practice as potential risk factor(s) for reproductive (sexual function) problems. Furthermore, this line of research needs additional investigations on the topic, specifically related to males, as far less work has been done than in females.

References

1. Hackney AC. Stress and the neuroendocrine system: the role of exercise as a stressor and modifier of stress. Expert Rev Endocrinol Metab. 2006;1:783–92.
2. Hackney AC. Endurance exercise training and reproductive endocrine dysfunction in men: alterations in the hypothalamic-pituitary-testicular axis. Curr Pharm Des. 2001;7:261–73.
3. Vingren JL, Kraemer WJ, Ratamess NA, Anderson JM, Volek JS, Maresh CM. Testosterone physiology in resistance exercise and training: the up-stream regulatory elements. Sports Med. 2010;40:1037–53.
4. Luigi L D, Romanelli F, Sgro P, Lenzi A. Andrological aspects of physical exercise and sport medicine. Endocrine. 2012;42:278–84.
5. Strauss JF, Barbieri RL, editors. Yen and Jaffe's reproductive endocrinology: physiology, pathophysiology, and clinical management. 7th ed. Philadelphia: Elsevier/Saunders; 2014.
6. Karkoulias K, Habeos I, Charokopos N, Tsiamita M, Mazarakis A, Pouli A, Spiropoulos K. Hormonal responses to marathon running in non-elite athletes. Eur J Intern Med. 2008;19:598–601.
7. Kraemer WJ, Ratamess NA. Hormonal responses and adaptations to resistance exercise and training. Sports Med. 2005;35:339–61.
8. Fahrner CL, Hackney AC. Effects of endurance exercise on free testosterone concentration and the binding affinity of sex hormone binding globulin (SHBG). Int J Sports Med. 1998;19:12–5.
9. Derbre F, Vincent S, Maitel B, Jacob C, Delamarche P, Delamarche A, et al. Androgen responses to sprint exercise in young men. Int J Sports Med. 2010;31:291–7.
10. Ayers JW, Komesu Y, Romani T, Ansbacher R. Anthropomorphic, hormonal, and psychologic correlates of semen quality in endurance-trained male athletes. Fertil Steril. 1985;43:917–21.
11. Duclos M, Corcuff JB, Rashedi M, Fougere V, Manier G. Trained versus untrained men: different immediate post-exercise responses of pituitary adrenal axis. A preliminary study. Eur J Appl Physiol Occup Physiol. 1997;75:343–50.
12. Duclos M, Gouarne C, Bonnemaison D. Acute and chronic effects of exercise on tissue sensitivity to glucocorticoids. J Appl Physiol (1985). 2003;94:869–75.
13. Sapolsky RM. Stress hormones: good and bad. Neurobiol Dis. 2000;7:540–2.
14. Hackney AC, Fahrner CL, Gulledge TP. Basal reproductive hormonal profiles are altered in endurance trained men. J Sports Med Phys Fit. 1998;38:138–41.
15. Tremblay MS, Copeland JL, Van Helder W. Influence of exercise duration on post-exercise steroid hormone responses in trained males. Eur J Appl Physiol. 2005;94:505–13.

16. Karkoulias K, Habeos I, Charokopos N, Tsiamita M, Mazarakis A, Pouli A, et al. Hormonal responses to marathon running in non-elite athletes. Eur J Intern Med. 2008;19:598–601.
17. Koch B, Glaser S, Schaper C, Krebs A, Nauck M, Dorr M, et al. Association between serum testosterone and sex hormone-binding globulin and exercise capacity in men: results of the Study of Health in Pomerania (SHIP). J Androl. 2011;32:135–43.
18. Hackney AC. Effects of endurance exercise on the reproductive system of men: the "exercise-hypogonadal male condition". J Endocrinol Invest. 2008;31:932–8.
19. Safarinejad MR, Azma K, Kolahi AA. The effects of intensive, long-term treadmill running on reproductive hormones, hypothalamus-pituitary-testis axis, and semen quality: a randomized controlled study. J Endocrinol. 2009;200:259–71.
20. Cheng JY, Ng EM. Body mass index, physical activity and erectile dysfunction: an U-shaped relationship from population-based study. Int J Obes (Lond). 2007;31:1571–8.
21. Esposito K, Giugliano F, Palo C D, Giugliano G, Marfella R, D'Andrea F, et al. Effect of lifestyle changes on erectile dysfunction in obese men: a randomized controlled trial. JAMA. 2004;291:2978–84.
22. Skarda ST, Burge MR. Prospective evaluation of risk factors for exercise-induced hypogonadism in male runners. West J Med. 1998;169:9–12.
23. Will MA, Swain J, Fode M, Sonksen J, Christman GM, Ohl D. The great debate: varicocele treatment and impact on fertility. Fertil Steril. 2011;95:841–52.
24. Gorelick JI, Goldstein M. Loss of fertility in men with varicocele. Fertil Steril. 1993;59:613–6.
25. Di Luigi LC A, Romanelli F. Role of sport medicine in andrological prevention. Med Sport. 1994;47:5.
26. Rigano E, Santoro G, Impellizzeri P, Antonuccio P, Fugazzotto D, Bitto L, et al. Varicocele and sport in the adolescent age. Preliminary report on the effects of physical training. J Endocrinol Invest. 2004;27:130–2.
27. Zampieri N, Dall'Agnola A. Subclinical varicocele and sports: a longitudinal study. Urology. 2011;77:1199–202.
28. Luigi L D, Gentile V, Pigozzi F, Parisi A, Giannetti D, Romanelli F. Physical activity as a possible aggravating factor for athletes with varicocele: impact on the semen profile. Hum Reprod. 2001;16:1180–4.
29. Habermacher G, Chason J, Schaeffer A. Chronic prostatitis/chronic pelvic pain syndrome. Annu Rev Med. 2006;57:195–206.
30. Potts J, Payne R. Prostatitis: infection, neuromuscular disorder, or pain syndrome? Proper patient classification is key. Cleve Clin J Med. 2007;74(3):63–71.
31. Zermann D, Ishigooka M, Doggweiler- Wiygul R, Schubert J, Schmidt RA. The male chronic pelvic pain syndrome. World J Urol. 2001;19:173–9.
32. Robert M, Gagnon C. Sperm motility inhibitor from human seminal plasma: presence of a precursor molecule in seminal vesicle fluid and its molecular processing after ejaculation. Int J Androl. 1994;17:232–40.
33. Penna G, Mondaini N, Amuchastegui S, Degli Innocenti S, Carini M, Giubelei G, Fibbi B, Colli E, Maggi M, Adorini L. Seminal plasma cytokines and chemokines in prostate inflammation: interleukin 8 as a predictive biomarker in chronic prostatitis/chronic pelvic pain syndrome and benign prostatic hyperplasia. Eur Urol. 2007;51:524–33.
34. Khadra A, Fletcher P, Luzzi G, Shattock R, Hay P. Interleukin-8 levels in seminal plasma in chronic prostatitis/chronic pelvic pain syndrome and nonspecific urethritis. BJU Int. 2006;97:1043–6.
35. Rao AR, Motiwala HG, Karim OM. The discovery of prostate-specific antigen. BJU Int. 2008;101:5–10.
36. Estabrooks PA, Glasgow RE, Dzewaltowski DA. Physical activity promotion through primary care. JAMA. 2003;289:2913.
37. Janal M, Colt E, Clark C, Glusman M. Pain Sensitivity, mood and plasma endocrine levels in man following long-distance running: effects of naloxone. Pain. 1984;19:13.
38. Pontari MA, Ruggeri MR. Mechanisms in prostatitis/chronic pelvic pain syndrome. J Urol. 2004;172:839.
39. Chicharro JL, Lopez-Calderon A, Hoyos J, Martin-Velasco AI, Villa G, Villanua MA, Lucía A. Effects of an endurance cycling competition on resting serum insulin-like growth factor I (IGF-I) and its binding proteins IGFBP-1 and IGFBP-3. Br J Sports Med. 2001;35:303–7.
40. Lucia A, Diaz B, Hoyos J, Fernandez C, Villa G, Bandres F, Chicharro J. Hormone levels of world class cyclists during the Tour of Spain stage race. Br J Sports Med. 2001;35:424–30.
41. Oremek GM, Seiffert UB. Physical activity releases prostate-specific antigen (PSA) from the prostate gland into blood and increases serum PSA concentrations. Clin Chem. 1996;42:691–5.
42. Rana A, Chisholm GD. He sold his bike for a low prostate specific antigen. J Urol. 1994;151:700.
43. Sternfeld B. Cancer and the protective effect of physical activity: the epidemiological evidence. Med Sci Sports Exerc. 1992;24:1195–209.
44. Wheeler GD, Wall SR, Belcastro AN, Cumming DC. The reduced serum testosterone and prolactin levels in male distance runners. JAMA. 1984;252:214–6.
45. LeMarchand L, Kolonel LN, Yoshizawa CN. Lifetime occupational physical activity and prostate cancer risk. Am J Epidemiol. 1991;133:103–11.
46. Lee IM, Paffenbarger RS, Hsich CC. Physical activity and risk of prostatic cancer among college alumni. Am J Epidemio. 1992;135:169–79.
47. De Souza MJ, Arce JC, Pescatello LS, Scherzer HS, Luciano AA. Gonadal hormones and semen quality in male runners. A volume threshold effect of endurance training. Int J Sports Med. 1994;15:383–91.
48. Jensen CE, Wiswedel K, McLoughlin J, van der Spuy Z. Prospective study of hormonal and semen profiles in marathon runners. Fertil Steril. 1995;64:1189–96.

49. De Souza MJ, Miller BE. The effect of endurance training on reproductive function in male runners. A 'volume threshold' hypothesis. Sports Med. 1997;23:357–74.
50. Vaamonde D, Silva-Grigoletto ME D, Garcia-Manso JM, Vaamonde-Lemos R, Swanson RJ, Oehninger SC. Response of semen parameters to three training modalities. Fertil Steril. 2009;92:1941–6.
51. Basaria S. Androgen abuse in athletes: detection and consequences. J Clin Endocrinol Metab. 2010;95:1533–43.
52. Hartgens F, Kuipers H. Effects of androgenic-anabolic steroids in athletes. Sports Med. 2004;34:513–54.
53. Parssinen M, Kujala U, Vartiainen E, Sarna S, Seppala T. Increased premature mortality of competitive powerlifters suspected to have used anabolic agents. Int J Sports Med. 2000;21:225–7.
54. MacIndoe JH, Perry PJ, Yates WR, Holman TL, Ellingrod VL, Scott SD. Testosterone suppression of the HPT axis. J Investig Med. 1997;45:441–7.
55. Lloyd FH, Powell P, Murdoch AP. Anabolic steroid abuse by body builders and male subfertility. BMJ. 1996;313:100–1.
56. Sandella B, Hartmann B, Berkson D, Hong E. Testicular conditions in athletes: torsion, tumors, and epididymitis. Curr Sports Med Rep. 2012;11:92–5.
57. Congeni J, Miller SF, Bennett CL. Awareness of genital health in young male athletes. Clin J Sport Med. 2005;15:22–6.
58. Severson EP, Sofianos DA, Powell A, Daubs M, Patel R, Patel AA. Spinal fractures in recreational bobsledders: an unexpected mechanism of injury. Evid Based Spine Care J. 2012;3:43–8.
59. Leibovitch I, Mor Y. The vicious cycling: bicycling related urogenital disorders. Eur Urol. 2005;47:277–86. (Discussion 86–7).
60. Wise LA, Cramer DW, Hornstein MD, Ashby RK, Missmer SA. Physical activity and semen quality among men attending an infertility clinic. Fertil Steril. 2011;95:1025–30.
61. Braun M, Wassmer G, Klotz T, Reifenrath B, Mathers M, Engelmann U. Epidemiology of erectile dysfunction: results of the Cologne Male Survey. Int J Impot Res. 2000;12:305–11.
62. Blanker MH, Bohnen AM, Groeneveld FP, Bernsen RM, Prins A, Thomas S, Bosch JL. Correlates for erectile and ejaculatory dysfunction in older Dutch men: a community-based study. J Am Geri Soc. 2001;49:436–42.
63. Martin-Morales A, Sanchez-Cruz JJ, Saenz de Tejada I, Rodriguez-Vela L, Jimenez-Cruz JF, Burgos-Rodriguez R. Prevalence and independent risk factors for erectile dysfunction in Spain: results of the Epidemiologia de la disfuncion erectil masculina study. J Urol. 2001;166:569–74.
64. Chew KK, Earle CM, Stuckey BG, Jamrozik K, Keogh EJ. Erectile dysfunction in general medicine practice: prevalence and clinical correlates. Int J Impot Res. 2000;12:41–5.
65. Goldmeier D, Keane FE, Carter P, Hessman A, Harris JR, Renton A. Prevalence of sexual dysfunction in heterosexual patients attending a central London genitourinary medicine clinic. Int J STD AIDS. 1997;8:303.
66. Sommer F, Goldstein I, Korda JB. Bicycle riding and erectile dysfunction: a review. J Sex Med. 2010;7:2346–58.
67. Marceau L, Kleinman K, Goldstein I, McKinlay J. Does bicycling contribute to the risk of erectile dysfunction? Results from the Massachusetts male aging study (MMAS). Int J Impot Res. 2001;13:298–302.
68. Huang V, Munarriz R, Goldstein I. Bicycle riding and erectile dysfunction: an increase in interest (and concern). J Sex Med. 2005;2:596–604.
69. Schrader SM, Breitenstein MJ, Lowe BD. Cutting off the nose to save the penis. J Sex Med. 2008;5:1932–40.
70. Sommer F. Knig D, Graft C, Schwarzer U, Bertram C, Klotz T, Engelmann U. Impotence and genital numbness in cyclists. Int J Sports Med. 2001;22:410–3.
71. Alanee S, Heiner J, Liu N, Monga M. Horseback riding: impact on sexual dysfunction and lower urinary tract symptoms in men and women. Urology. 2009;73:109–14.
72. McAleer IM, Kaplan GW, LoSasso BE. Renal and testis injuries in team sports. J Urol. 2002;168:1805–7.
73. Turgut AT, Kosar U, Kosar P, Karabulut A. Scrotal sonographic findings in equestrians. J Ultrasound Med. 2005;24:911–7.

10 Consequences of the Use of Anabolic-Androgenic Steroids for Male Athletes' Fertility

Juan Manuel García-Manso and Teresa Valverde Esteve

Introduction

Strength sports (e.g., bodybuilding, weight lifting, powerlifting, throwing) have intensely suffered the scourge of doping. In these sports, most of the athletes with known positive results in doping tests are linked to the use of anabolic agents [1, 2]. The most common substances are testosterone and its synthetic derivatives (synthetic anabolic-androgenic steroids, AAS) [3].

Hormonal Environment in Strength Sports

Most of the structural adaptations occur as a consequence of strength training, thus muscle hypertrophy is the result of a specific response of the endocrine system ensuring the right environment to increase protein synthesis [4, 5]. Many of these hormones play important roles in the male reproductive system.

The acute and chronic hormonal responses to strength training are determined by the configuration of the workload (exercise order, work intensity, number of sets and repetitions, and recovery periods), as well as the athletes' individual characteristics [6].

Hormonal changes are quite complex, and the role of these hormones in skeletal muscle continues to be the subject of intensive scientific enquiry. In addition to testosterone, more hormones pose an effect on the appropriate protein synthesis, such as anabolic (growth hormones (GH), insulin-like growth factor (IGF), and insulin), catabolic (cortisol and glucagon), or regulation (myostatin) hormones. In this chapter, we will not analyze all those hormones that, directly or indirectly, might be involved in these processes, but we will focus on the ones that have an effect on the protein synthesis and male fertility.

Testosterone

Among the anabolic agents, the hypothalamic–pituitary–gonadal (HPG) axis hormones, specifically testosterone and its derivatives, play a predominant role in strength training and male fertility (Fig. 10.1).

Natural androgens (testosterone and precursors) are synthesized from cholesterol by the organism. The secretion of gonadotropin-releasing hormone (GnRH) from the hypothalamus stimulates the biosynthesis of luteinizing hormone (LH) and follicle-stimulating hormone (FSH) that in turn initiate both intra-gonadal testosterone production and spermatogenesis, as well as

J. M. García-Manso (✉)
Department of Physical Education, Universidad de Las Palmas de GranCanaria, C/ Consuela la Maestra 29, C Santa María de Guía, Islas Canarias 35017, Spain
e-mail: jgarciamanso@gmail.com

T. Valverde Esteve
Laboratorio de Investigación de Ciencias del Deporte, Universidad Católica de Valencia San Vicente Mártir, Valencia, Spain

© Springer Science+Business Media New York 2016

D. Vaamonde et al. (eds.), *Exercise and Human Reproduction*, DOI 10.1007/978-1-4939-3402-7_10

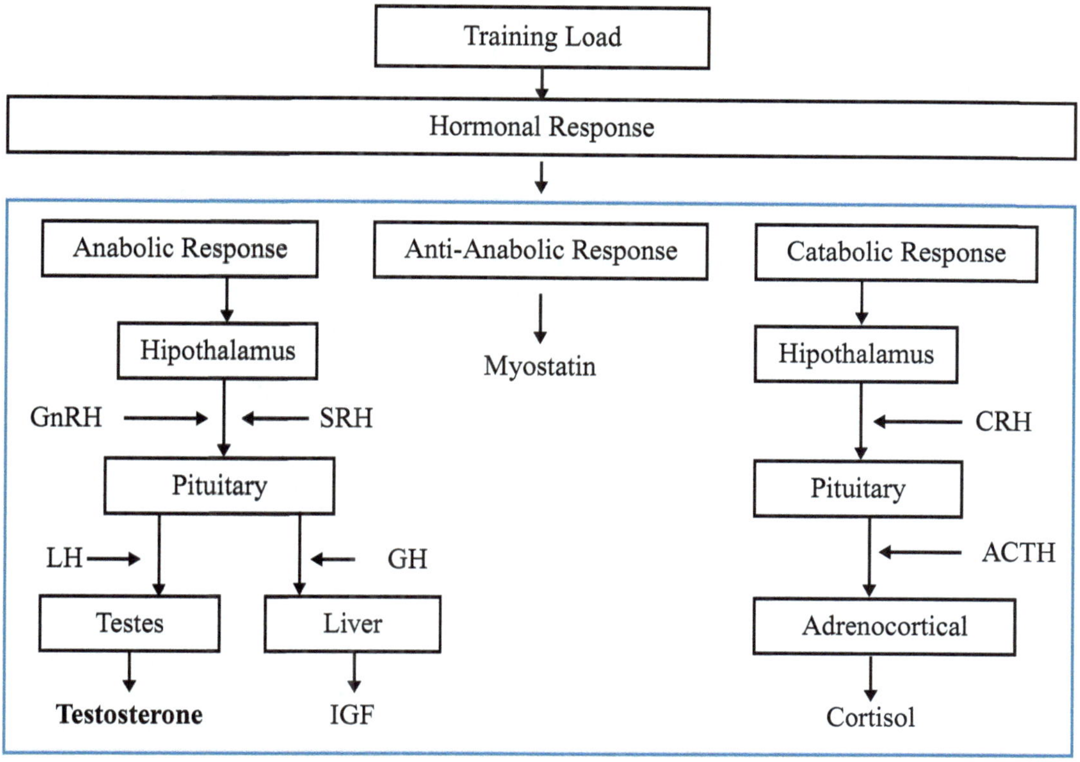

Fig. 10.1 Main hormones with an influence on the anabolic–catabolic balance in strength training. *GH* growth hormone, *GnRH* gonadotropin-releasing hormone, *SRH* somatotropin-releasing hormone, *LH* luteinizing hormone, *IGF* insulin-like growth factor, *CRH* corticotrophin-releasing hormone, *ACTH* adrenocorticotropic hormone

systemic testosterone secretion and virilization. From a chemical point of view, steroid hormones show an annular structure of four rings (cyclopentanoperhydrophenanthrene) with 19 carbon atoms, a double bond between C4 and C5, an oxygen atom at C3 position, and a hydroxyl radical (OH^-) at C17 ($C_{19}H_{28}O_2$). This structure is necessary to maintain androgenic activity.

In men, 95% of testosterone is secreted in the Leydig cells of the testes, generating approximately 2.5–12.0 mg/day of testosterone. Meanwhile, the remaining 5% (0.15–0.60 mg/day) comes from the adrenal cortex (dehydroepiandrosterone). The daily production rate varies cyclically on a circadian and pulsatile pattern (6–12 peaks every 24 h), which contributes to highest concentrations in the early morning compared with the lowest concentrations in the afternoon [7, 8]. Circulating testosterone levels in blood are maintained within a normal range as a consequence of a balance between its production and excretion by hepatic and extrahepatic metabolism [9, 10]. In adults, testosterone levels in plasma are higher in men (0.6 μg/dl) than in women (0.3 μg/dl; approximately 95–97%). The majority will be bound to the sex hormone-binding globulin (SHBG), also referred to as sex steroid-binding globulin, and testosterone–estradiol-binding globulin or to albumin, whereas a small proportion will be circulating unbound. In peripheral tissues, part of the testosterone is transformed by an enzyme from the family of HSP450 (5α-reductase) into 5α-dihydrotestosterone and joins the cellular DNA, thus having the most direct action on muscle anabolic functions and embryogenesis (process of formation of the external male genitals)). The 5α-reductase enzyme removes the C4–5 double bond of testosterone by the addition of two hydrogen atoms to its structure. It is important to note that DHT has threefold higher affinity for the androgen receptor than testosterone, thus 15–30-fold higher than adrenal androgens.

Testosterone, in supraphysiological doses (from tenfold higher than normal resting levels), is readily converted into estradiol and estrone by the enzyme aromatase and related to sexual differentiation of the brain, bone mass accretion, fusion of the epiphyses during puberty, in addition to feminizing effects [11].

The various functions performed by testosterone inside the organism can be summarized in two main points: (1) androgenic (virilizing) and (2) anabolic (myotrophic):

- The androgenic function is responsible for the changes in primary and secondary male sexual characteristics. Testosterone and a polypeptide factor (Mullerian inhibiting factor) stimulate the formation of the male genitals.
- The anabolic function stimulates nitrogen fixation and increased protein synthesis, thus provoking the growth in skeletal muscles (by increasing the synthesis of contractile proteins), collagen synthesis, and bone metabolism.

Synthetic Anabolic-Androgenic Steroids

Synthetic AAS are synthetic derivatives of testosterone, showing chemical structures similar to natural steroids. The differences artificially set condition the properties and characteristics of these substances (absorption rate, catabolism, and action). From a sports point of view, it is ideal that the substances used have moderate androgenic and virilizing effects, and elevated anabolic effects [12]. Please note this is important when selecting a steroid.

To determine the steroid's effects, we must know the *therapeutic index*, which is the relation between the anabolic (A) and virilizing (V) effect, despite the fact that complete dissociation of the *AAS's* androgenic and anabolic effects is not possible [13, 14]. When this index is equal to 1, A and V have the same values. When the index is between 1 and 2, products are strongly virilizing and anabolic, while higher values (3 and 4) are associated with anabolic products. However, values higher than 5 correspond to high anabolic products with low virilizing power.

Origin of Synthetic Anabolic-Androgenic Steroids

The development of AAS compounds was originally clinically used for treatment of delayed puberty in men and for growth promotion [15]. The road to establishing AAS's precise chemical and functional characteristics was long and full of interesting anecdotes before reaching clinical and sportive uses.

To study the origin of AAS, it becomes necessary to start with the studies performed in the nineteenth century, referencing the studies by Berthold, Brown-Séquard, Zoth, and Pregl. Berthold et al. focused their research on the study of the role of the gonads in the development of the human secondary sexual characteristics. It was in 1849 when he performed what is known as the first formal experiment in endocrinology in history. In this study, he described general rooster atrophy after castration, leading to disappearance of aggressiveness and interest in hens. Brown-Séquard presented in the Society of Biology of Paris a controversial scientific report (*Elixir of life*, 1889) in which he described how he himself had undergone a really peculiar treatment. The procedure consisted of injecting certain doses of three different preparations that he created. Initially, he administered blood doses from testicular veins, subsequently sperm, and lastly an extract from dog and/or guinea pig testes. As suggested by this author, this curious treatment assured physical and mental improvements [16]. By the end of the century, Oskar Zoth and Fritz Pregl, pioneers of exercise physiology, indicated that extracts similar to those proposed by Brown-Séquard (bull testicular extracts) might increase muscular strength in humans [17]. Zoth, some years later awarded the Nobel Prize in medicine, pointed out in his work that "the training of athletes provides an opportunity for further research in this area for a practical evaluation of our experimental results" (in the German original: "Das Training von Sportlern bietet eine Gelegenheit für weitere Forschungsarbeiten in diesem Bereich und für eine praktische Beurteilung unserer experimentellen Ergebnisse") [15, 18]. Undoubtedly, this statement represents the origin of what the use of steroids will become in the future of sports.

Eugen Steinach, three times nominated for the Nobel Prize in Physiology, performed numerous experiments on animals' sex change. He suggested a surprising surgical treatment for sperm autotransfusion into the circulatory system in order to rejuvenate male subjects [19]. The surgical manipulation of the human or animal male genitals had already been described by the scientist Voronoff in his book *Rejuvenation by Grafting* [20]. This controversial Russian researcher prepared his self-supply to use it in his patients and investigations. His first official transplant was performed in 1920 by introducing thin slices (a few-millimeters thick) of chimpanzee and baboon testes in the scrotum of a patient, with the hope that both tissues eventually merged [21].

A few years later, Pezard and Caridroit [22] and Funk and Harrow [23] focused their investigations on understanding the reasons why testicular extracts or other organs and animal anatomical structures (i.e., cockscomb) provoked functional changes in the male reproductive system and/or secondary sex organs. The authors concluded that there should be a substance carried in the blood that might regulate the functioning of these organs. Starling [24] called this substance "hormones." Subsequently, Pezard and Caridroit called it "testicular hormone." Funk and Harrow [23] located this substance in men's urine and named it *male hormone*.

Some authors designated these years as *The Golden Age of Steroid Chemistry* [25]. Adolf Butenandt, awarded the Nobel Prize in Chemistry for studying sexual hormones, furthered his studies on the analysis of more than 15,000 l of human urine, thus determining the chemical composition of *androsterone* [26]. His studies on sex hormones helped the work group of Ruzicka [27], in *Ciba laboratories*, to establish that the chemical structure of testosterone was very similar to cholesterol. His laboratory became the world reference center for organic chemistry at that time. In later decades, the Organon Company, in which Ruzicka participated from the beginning, introduced many drugs that became very popular in the sports community (Deca-Durabolin, Durabolin, Sustanon 250, and Pregnyl).

The name *testosterone* comes from the studies performed by Butenandt and Hanisch [28], Ruzicka and Wettstein [29], and David et al. [30]. The chemical structure was firmly established in previous years by David and colleagues when oxidizing testosterone to obtain androstan-4-ene-3,17-dione.

The clinical application of these substances goes back to the 1940s for the treatment of chronic debilitating illness, trauma, burns, surgery, and radiation therapy [31]. In the first scientific article published on testosterone in 1939, the author specifically described the beneficial effects of the use of sex hormones in sports performance [32]. Presumably, during this period, and even before, athletes and researchers had already been using steroids.

Brenton Huggins, an American surgical specialist in prostate cancer, showed that blocking testosterone production may decrease prostate cancer progression, thus reducing its symptoms. He was the first scientist who suggested chemotherapy as a therapy against cancer. He was awarded the Nobel Prize in 1966 [33]. On his part, the biologist Paul de Kruif promoted testosterone to reduce the symptoms of aging by claiming that this hormone increases libido, builds muscles, and sharpens intelligence. Paul de Kruif was maybe the first author to address a historical compilation of studies of testosterone by describing scientific experiences by authors such as Hammond, Werner, and Lalouche.

With the advent of World War II, works stopped or at least we do not have accurate documentation of the line of studies and objectives followed by researchers. Apparently, AAS were used by German scientists during this military confrontation to increase the soldiers' strength, courage, and aggressiveness [34, 35]. It was not until after *World War II* that studies on steroids resumed in veterinary and human medicine and sports. There is some evidence that once the conflict was over, the American and Soviet intelligence services seized steroids-relevant information from the captured Nazi scientists. These skills were quickly transferred to the sports field as one more tool in what some years later came to be named the *Cold War* between the Western and Eastern blocks.

In the mid-1950s, the study of effect of androgens on protein synthesis became accelerated. At the same time, many analogues of testosterone (synthetic steroids), nandrolone, and dihydrotestosterone were developed to obtain a purely anabolic drug. This knowledge meant at that time a topic of special interest to pharmaceutical companies, coaches, athletes, and sports physicians, especially those linked to strength sports.

Effects of AAS on Sports Performance

Despite the fact that some contradictory work reducing the sport advantages of AAS can be found in specialized bibliography, different published reviews and meta-analyses show that AAS users are clearly benefited by enhanced performance. In any case, it is a fact that research in this field is under condition of different aspects (small simple size, use of more than one drug or substance to enhance or counteract steroid effects, impossibility of carrying out double-blind placebo-controlled studies, and that dosage used in studies is often far lower than the self-administered levels for ethical reasons). These circumstances avoid the development of appropriate protocols in humans to understand the daily reality in sports [36].

It must be taken into account that performance improvements change individually (depending on sex and age) and are strongly influenced by aspects such as the dose (physiological, supraphysiological, or abuse dose) and the form of utilization (stacking or cycles of steroid administration).

Steroids became popular in the sports field since the 1950s. In that decade, American and Soviet weightlifters and sportsmen undergoing large amounts of resistance training started using these substances [37]. However, the first documented case of steroid use in sports took place in horse racing in 1941.Some sources indicate that German athletes were the first to use steroids [34].

After World War II, Soviets developed a systematic doping program by taking profit of knowledge from the German scientists who were captured after the war. The intention was to use these substances in the development of Soviet sports teams and, thus, to use their success as propaganda for their political ideology. Recall that the USSR returned to international competition at the *Olympic Games* of Helsinki (1952). In this period, androgenic steroids occupied an important place. Without doubt, the massive occurrence of steroids altered the normal evolution of the records, thus modifying the results in all the strength sports. Final implementation of steroids in sports took place in the 1960s [38].

Positive Effects

Among the most interesting benefits of AAS in sports performance (ergogenic effects), we can highlight the following: (a) It increases protein synthesis, lean body mass, lipolysis, bone mineral density, connective tissue, strength, muscular power, erythropoiesis, hemoglobin and hematocrit (aerobic endurance), pain tolerance, neural transmission, aggressiveness, and injury recovery, and (b) it reduces body fat, muscular catabolism, sensitivity to fatigue, and recovery time.

Body Mass Increase

Few argue that the use of steroids combined with specific training leads to significant gains in athletes' muscle mass [36, 39–44]. The intake of AAS transforms a negative nitrogen balance into a positive one by improving the utilization of ingested protein and increasing nitrogen retention. In addition, these substances act on the androgen receptors at the cellular level, transcribe genes, and stimulate the production of ARNm to increase protein synthesis [45]. When doses are high, steroids may compete for glucocorticosteroid receptors (anti-glucocorticoid effect of testosterone), causing an anticatabolic effect [46, 47]. Furthermore, they have an effect on other anabolic hormones belonging to GH–IGF axis by increasing the GH and IGF-1 synthesis [48].

Strength Enhancement

The evolution of different sports (i.e., weightlifting, powerlifting, throwing, etc.) and the high number of doping cases among athletes demonstrate the significant benefits of anabolic steroids on strength gains [39, 42–44, 46, 49–54]. In relation to this ability, it should be noted that AAS have effects on the athletes' behavior such as euphoria, increased aggressiveness, and reduced feelings of fatigue [55].

Endurance Enhancement

Androgens improve the volume of body fluids by increasing the renal retention of water and salt (mineralocorticoid effect), resulting in an increased blood volume and arterial pressure. Furthermore, AAS stimulate the production of red blood cells by the bone marrow (erythropoiesis). Also, hemoglobin, hematocrit, and iron incorporation into red blood cells may become elevated, thus positively influencing the delivery system of oxygen to tissues [14, 56]. Some research suggests that this substance has a positive effect on the activity of oxidative enzymes by improving the energy production via aerobic metabolism [57] and increases antioxidant capacity in selected skeletal muscles [58].

Speed of Muscle Contraction Enhancement

Some theorists of sports training highlight the importance of testosterone and AAS synthesis on muscle power enhancement and speed of muscle contraction [59]. As suggested by these authors, the athletes with better explosive strength and sprint running performances have a higher basal level of testosterone. This is due to the influence that these substances may have on certain neurotransmitters that allow faster transmission of nerve impulses.

Consequences of Continued Use of High Doses of AAS

Possibly, if athletes who use AAS knew exactly all the possible risks they face, they would avoid its use. These risks are minimized by some athletes, their coaches, and doctors, sometimes in a quite irresponsible and self-interested manner. They are more interested in the benefits than in the potential risks [60]. However, these substances have diverse adverse secondary effects, which are highly dangerous and sometimes not completely known. For this reason, the use of AAS increases the athlete's risk, especially when doses are not controlled or individualized to what each subject can tolerate without risk to their integrity.

The adverse effects are linked to behavioral changes (mood swings, aggressive behavior, depression, psychosis, addiction, withdrawal, and dependency disorders) [61, 62], thus altering numerous organs and systems [36, 48]. The latter include musculoskeletal system, endocrine system, larynx, urinary system, immune system, alopecia (male pattern baldness), liver (cholestasis, peliosis, hepatoadenoma, hepatocarcinoma), cardiovascular system (hypertension, thrombosis, decreased high-density lipoprotein (HDL) cholesterol, increased cholesterol), female reproductive system (menstrual irregularities, clitoral hypertrophy, uterine atrophy, breast atrophy, teratogenicity), and the male reproductive system.

Male Fertility

Infertility may be defined as the inability to conceive after reasonable time (12–24 months) of adequate sexual intercourse without contraceptive measures [63]. This anomaly has been associated with different genetic and nongenetic conditions (hypogonadotrophic hypogonadism, testicular maldescence, structural abnormalities of the male genital tract, genital infections, previous scrotal or inguinal surgery, varicoceles, chronic illness, medication, and exposure to chemicals) [64]. While infertility is a functional impairment that neither compromises the individual's physical integrity nor threatens his life, it may have important psychological effects.

Male Fertility and Exercise

Some studies reported the relevance and effects of physical exercise on reproductive function [65–75]. Certain sports activities (i.e., cycling and bodybuilding), their training (i.e., high volume and intensity), and associated elements (i.e., steroid issues) may also adversely affect the reproductive system, thus sometimes compromise their fertility. A prolonged and excessive training (high volume, high intensity, and low recovery) carries an overreaching/overtraining status that negatively affects the body and causes changes that affect the endocrine system at the hypothalamic–pituitary–sympathetic adrenal and the HPG axis [68, 76, 77] (discussed elsewhere in this volume Chapter 7).

Along with the training load, some collateral aspects related to sports can also be linked to male infertility: significant alterations of body mass [78], inadequate caloric intake [79], lack of appropriate intake of macro- and micronutrients in the diet [80], high physical and physiological stress [79], oxidative stress [81], alteration of the balance of energy intake [82], reproductive function [83], and possible testicular microtrauma [84]. Among these collateral aspects, we must include the use of the AAS, which, by itself, may exert the most detrimental consequences on fertility.

Male Fertility Versus Anabolic-Androgenic Steroids

The main adverse effects of the AAS on the male reproductive system include:

- Alteration of the HPG axis: reduction of the hormonal secretion and circulating rate
- Decreased spermatogenesis
- Changes in semen quality: quantitative and qualitative changes
- Apoptosis in spermatogenesis
- Testicular atrophy
- Other alterations, such as prostatic hypertrophy, prostatic carcinoma, difficulty/pain during urination, gynecomastia, priapism, and impotence

Alteration of the Hypothalamic–Pituitary–Gonadal Axis

For several decades, it has been known that the intake of AAS has powerful harmful effects on male sexual organs, particularly the testes [85]. The abusive use of some doping substances (i.e., AAS) may cause important hormonal changes that might affect the HPG and the male reproductive system as a whole. HPG axis functioning is dependent on the secretion of several hormones acting in cascade, thus providing feedback mechanisms between them. GnRH is secreted by the hypothalamus and stimulates the pituitary production of gonadotropins (FSH and LH). FSH regulates spermatogenesis in the seminiferous tubules of the testes. LH controls testosterone secretion by Leydig cells. HPG control depends on the production of inhibin, activin, and testosterone. Inhibin modulates FSH secretion, and testosterone inhibits LH secretion. Alterations of this sequence lead to changes in semen characteristics (e.g., oligozoospermia, asthenozoospermia, and teratozoospermia) that can be associated with male infertility. This problem is exacerbated by the high volume/intensity of training in athletes who use AAS or other doping substances to enhance their performance and recover from the fatigue of training more quickly [86–91]; however, apart from extreme situations, such alterations, can be reversed once AAS intake is suspended [92–97]. The recovery of the HPA axis may be accelerated using gonadotropins or gonadotropin analogues (human chorionic gonadotropin (HCG) and human menopausal gonadotropin), which help restore the functioning of the axis [44, 95, 98].

After each cycle, stopping AAS use reduces hypogonadotropic hypogonadism and reverses testicular atrophy and infertility [48, 92, 93, 95]. The time to normalize the situation is individual and depends on the type of steroid used and the dose and time of ingestion, which could sometimes be more than 12 months after stopping the drugs [99].

Sperm Quality

In males, fertility evaluation starts with a quantitative and qualitative analysis of the ejaculated semen. This fact implies the evaluation of the physical parameters (ejaculate volume, liquefaction state, pH, odor, color, absence or presence of agglutination and gelatinous bodies, viscosity, and dirt) and qualitative parameters of semen (sperm count, sperm motility, sperm morphology, sperm DNA fragmentation, and oxidative stress status). This allows us to detect possible alterations that can compromise the subject's fertility.

Our research team and other researchers through studies involving different sports modalities proved that a high training load, either volume or intensity [65, 66, 70–72, 75, 100, 101], might alter sperm quality, thus causing problems in fertility. A high training load produces alterations in mobility, vitality, morphology, and sperm DNA integrity. Other parameters linked to specific exercise modalities can be harmful, like bike saddles that impose friction [102]. Also, the use of AAS must be taken into consideration when analyzing fertility in populations of athletes. In line with this, Karila et al. [103] showed that at the end of one cycle of massive use of AAS, the sperm count decreased, but only one subject had azoospermia. Furthermore, the authors note that, despite the use of HCG, there was a significant positive correlation between the dose of HCG and the relative amount of morphologically abnormal sperm. According to data provided by this study, the use of HCG with supraphysiological doses of AAS maintains, at least to a certain extent, the spermatogenic process by preventing decrease in sperm count but not preventing morphology anomalies.

Shokri et al. [104] found alterations in sperm quantity, protamine, and DNA integrity in Wistar rats that combined exercise with the high use of AAS (nandrolone decanoate). The incidence of AAS in protamine and DNA fragmentation is a relevant topic in the study of male fertility, especially when these substances are used in high doses as in the case of some athletes. Carrell et al. [105] suggested the existence of a direct relationship between abnormal protamine expression and sperm count, motility, morphology, or fertilization.

Apoptosis in Spermatogenesis

Cellular apoptosis appears to be a constant feature in the adult testes and during early development, thus being especially important during germ cell development [106]. It has been suggested that during spermatogenesis, apoptosis plays a role in the etiology of idiopathic male infertility in light of the excessively high numbers of apoptotic germ cells observed in the testes of some infertile males [107, 108].

The influence of exercise on apoptosis of germ cells has been mainly studied in endurance sports, thus primarily impacting the effect of the oxidative stress on spermatogenesis [109–111] and testes alterations [111]. Despite the low oxygen tensions that characterize the testicular microenvironment by poor vascularization, this tissue is especially vulnerable to peroxidative injury due to the high amount of polyunsaturated fatty acids [112]. However, the abusive effect of AAS on germ cell apoptosis has not yet been analyzed enough. Shokri et al. [113] assessed germ cell apoptosis in healthy adult male albino Wistar rats that exercised and were administered steroids (nandralone decanoate). This work describes a significant increase in germ cells apoptosis compared with control animals. They also checked that the combination of nandralone decanoate and exercise increased caspase-3 enzyme activity compared with the control group. In a later study, Shokri et al. [104] checked that a combination of exercise and nandrolone decanoate (combination of running exercise and high dose of AAS) negatively influences DNA integrity and protamine content (packing). These alterations were translated into lower sperm quality and reduced pregnancy rate.

The negative effect of AAS on sperm apoptosis was also proved by Janjic et al. [114] to note that the use of testosterone enanthate stimulated the expression of inducible nitric oxide synthase 2 (NOS2) followed by increased nitric oxide production, decreased mitochondrial membrane potential, and increased prevalence of Leydig cell apoptosis.

Testicular Histology

The testes have two closely related functions to reproduction: production and storage of male germ cells and biosynthesis and secretion of male sex hormones (androgens). Some studies reported that the administration of AAS showed adverse effects on testicular function, decreasing testes mass, scrotal thickness, daily sperm production, and the numbers of Leydig cells [115–119]. After discontinuation, Leydig cells increased in number but remained below the baseline even after long periods [116].

Feinber et al. [116] proved that high doses of AAS (propionate testosterone) depleted Leydig cell number in prepubertal and adult rats but had no effect on the Leydig cell number of the peripubertal animals. The depletion of Leydig cells that occurred in the prepubertal animals was reversible after withdrawal, while the depletion of Leydig cells of the adult animals did not return to the control level, suggesting a long-lasting alteration. Squires et al. [115] reported that all the AAS treatment, in animals, reduced the number of developing germ cells. These alterations caused changes in seminiferous tubules and the thickness of the germinal epithelium. The studies by Fainber et al. [116] and Noorafshan et al. [120] also showed reduction in the length of the seminiferous tubules with a reduction in the weight and volume of the testes. Mesbah et al. [117] also reported the disruption of the seminiferous epithelium, with broad spaces between the cellular components and the testicular atrophy with shrinkage, resulting in decreased diameter of the seminiferous tubules. These authors also observed alterations in the number and cytostructure of Sertoli cells, which can have a direct influence on reducing the size of the seminiferous tubules.

In accordance with the previous authors, Hijazi et al. [119] also observed quantitative changes in the seminiferous tubules (number, diameter, and thickness) and the interstitial cells of Leydig and Sertoli cells before and after the treatment with AAS (Testoviron®). The authors pointed out that the histological sections of the testes revealed that the effects on spermatogenesis are time related, resulting in the decrease in the relative weight of the testes and the number of seminiferous tubules along with the decrease in the number and the diameter of the interstitial cell nuclei. According to the authors, these results suggest that AAS provoke adverse effects on the male reproductive tract, particularly the testicular tissues, including degenerative damage in the germ cells, Sertoli cells, and Leydig cells that can affect spermatogenesis and the male reproductive capacity. Also, Naraghy et al. [118] proved in rats that the combination of exercise (swimming) and supraphysiological doses of AAS (nandrolone decanoate) reduced the number and size of Leydig cells in the interstitial space and Sertoli cells.

Conclusion

AAS have been shown to exert clear negative effects on the male reproductive system as evidenced by hormonal alterations and damage to the reproductive tissues and accessory glands, and thus altered spermatogenic production. For this reason, it becomes necessary to educate sport doctors, technicians, and athletes on the associated risks of the massive use of these compounds on fertility.

References

1. García-Manso JM, Vitoria M. El doping en los deportes de fuerza y resistencia. Bilbao: Solar-Cubillas; 2009 (Academia Olímpica—País Vasco).
2. Mottram DR. Drugs in sports. 5th ed. New York: Taylor & Francis; 2011.
3. Yavari A. Abuse of anabolic androgenic steroids. J Stress Physiol Biochem. 2009;5(3):22–32.
4. Kumar V, Atherton P, Smith K, Rennie MJ. Human muscle protein synthesis and breakdown during and after exercise. J Appl Physiol. 2009;106(6):2026–39.
5. Arazi H, Damirchi A, Faraji H, Rahimi R. Hormonal responses to acute and chronic resistance exercise in middle-age versus young men. Sport Sci Health. 2012;8(2–3):59–65.
6. Kraemer WJ, Ratamess NA. Hormonal responses and adaptations to resistance exercise and training. Sports Med. 2005;35(4):339–61.
7. Gupta SK, Lindemulder EA, Sathyan G. Modeling of circadian testosterone in healthy men and hypogonadal men. J Clin Pharmacol. 2000;40(7):731–8.
8. Mong JA, Baker FC, Mahoney MM, Paul KN, Schwartz MD, Semba K, Silver R. Sleep, rhythms, and the endocrine brain: influence of sex and gonadal hormones. J Neurosci. 2011;31(45):16107–16.
9. Birniece V, Meinhardt UJ, Handelsman DJ, Ho KK. Testosterone stimulates extra-hepatic but not hepatic fat oxidation (Fox): comparison of oral and transdermal testosterone administration in hypopituitary men. Clin Endocrinol. 2009;71(5):715–21.
10. Kelly DM, Jones TH. Testosterone: a metabolic hormone in health and disease. J Endocrinol. 2013;217:R25–45.
11. Wu FCW. Endocrine aspects of anabolic steroids. Clin Chem. 1997;43(7):1289–92.
12. Rogozkin AV. Metabolism of anabolic androgenic steroids. Boca Raton: CRC Press; 1991.
13. Shahidi NT. A review of the chemistry, biological action, and clinical applications of anabolic-androgenic steroids. Clin Ther. 2001;23(9):1355–90.
14. Maravelias C, Dona A, Stefanidou M, Spiliopoulou C. Adverse effects of anabolic steroids in athletes: a constant threat. Toxicol Lett. 2005;158(3):167–75.
15. Tan RS, Scally MC. Anabolic steroid-induced hypogonadism. Towards a unified hypothesis of anabolic steroid action. Med Hypotheses. 2009;72(6):723–8.
16. Yesalis CE, Bahrke MS. Anabolic steroid and stimulant use in North American sport between 1850 and 1980. Sports Hist. 2005;25(3):434–51.
17. Cashmore EE. Making sense of sports. 5th ed. New York: Taylor & Francis; 2010.
18. Hoberman JM, Yesalis CE. The history of synthetic testosterone. Sci Am. 1995;272:76–81.
19. Harms E. Forty-four years of correspondence between Eugen Steinach and Harry Benjamin. Bull NY Acad Med. 1969;45:761–6.
20. Voronoff S. Rejuvenation by grafting. London: G. Allen & Unwin Ltd; 1925.
21. Gillyboeuf T. The famous doctor who inserts monkey glands in millionaires. Spring: J EE Cummings Soc. 2000;9:44–5.
22. Pezard A, Caridroit M. Le presende de l'hormone testiculaire dans le sang du coq normal, demonstration directe foundu sur la greffe autoplastique des cretillons. Compt Rend Soc Biol. 1926;95:296–8.
23. Funk C, Harrow B. The male hormone. Biochem J. 1930;24:1678–80.
24. Starling EH. On the chemical correlation of the functions of the body. The Lancet. 1905;166:339–41 (The Croonian Lectures. I.).
25. Schwarz S, Onken D, Schubert A. The steroid story of Jenapharm: from the late 1940s to the early 1970s. Steroids. 1999;64(7):439–45.
26. Butenandt A. Uber "Progynon" ein krystalliertes weibliches Sexualhormon. Naturwissenschaften. 1929;17:878.
27. Freeman ER, Bloom DA, McGuire EJ. A brief history of testosterone. J Urol. 2001;165:371–3.
28. Butenandt A, Hanisch G. Über Testosteron. Umwandlung des Dehydro-androsterons in Androstendiol und Testosteron; ein Weg zur Darstellung des Testosterons aus Cholesterin. Ber dtsch chem Ges (A and B Series). 1935;68(9):1859–62.
29. Ruzicka L, Wettstein A. Uber die kunstliche Herstellung des Testikel hormons. Testosteron (Androsten-3-on-17-ol.). Helv Chim Acta. 1935;18:1264 (Sexual hormone VII.).
30. David KG, Dingemanse E, Freud J, Laqueur E. Uber krystallinisches mannliches Hormon aus Hoden (Testosteron) wirksamer als aus harn oder aus Cholesterin bereitetes Androsteron. Hoppe Seylers Z Physiol Chem. 1935;233:281.
31. Basaria S, Wahlstrom JT, Dobs AS. Anabolic-androgenic steroid therapy in the treatment of chronic diseases. J Clin End Met. 2001;86(11):5108–17.
32. Boje O. Doping. Bul Health Organ League Nations. 1939;8:439–69.
33. Toledo-Pereyra LH. Discovery in surgical investigation: the essence of Charles Brenton Huggins. J Invest Surg. 2001;14(5):251–2.
34. Wade N. Anabolic steroids: doctors denounce them, but athletes aren't listening. Science. 1972;176(4042):1399–403.
35. Beamish R, Ritchie I. The spectre of steroids: nazi propaganda, Cold War anxiety and patriarchal paternalism. Int J Hist Sport. 2005;22(5):777–95.
36. Bonetti A, Tirelli F, Catapano A, Dazzi D, Dei Cas A, Solito F, Ceda G, Reverberi C, Monica C, Pipitone S, Elia G, Spattini M, Magnati G. Side effects of anabolic androgenic steroids abuse. Int J Sports Med. 2008;29:679–87.
37. Fair JD. Olympic weightlifting and the introduction of steroids: a statistical analysis of world championship results, 1948–72. Int J Hist Sport. 1988;5(1):96–114.
38. Silvester L. Anabolic steroids at the 1972 Olympics. Scholast Coach. 1973;43:90–2.
39. Stamford BA, Moffatt R. Anabolic steroid: effectiveness as an ergogenic aid to experienced weight trainers. J Sports Med Phys Fitness. 1974;14(3):191–7.
40. Hervey GR, Hutchinson I, Knibbs AV, Burkinshaw n, Jones PR, Norgan NG, Levell MJ. "Anabolic" effects

of methandienone in men undergoing athletic training. The Lancet. 1976;308(7988):699–702.
41. Loughton SJ, Ruhling RO. Human strength and endurance responses to anabolic steroid and training. J Sports Med Phys Fitness. 1977;17(3):285–96.
42. Hervey GR, Knibbs AV, Burkinshaw L, Morgan DB, Jones PRM, Chettle DR, Vartsky D. Effects of methandienone on the performance and body composition of men undergoing athletic training. Clin Sci. 1981;60(4):457–61.
43. Alen M, Häkkinen K, Komi PV. Changes in neuromuscular performance and muscle fiber characteristics of elite power athletes self-administering androgenic and anabolic steroids. Acta Physiol Scan. 1984;122(4):535–44.
44. Bhasin S, Storer TW, Berman N, Callegari C, Clevenger B, Phillips J, Bunnell TJ, Tricker R, Shirazi A, Casaburi R. The effects of supraphysiologic doses of testosterone on muscle size and strength in normal men. New Engl J Med. 1996;335(1):1–7.
45. Bahrke MS, Yesalis CE. Abuse of anabolic androgenic steroids and related substances in sport and exercise. Curr Opin Pharm. 2004;4(6):614–20.
46. Mottram DR, George AJ. Anabolic steroids. Best Pract Res Clin Endocrinol Metab. 2000;14(1):55–69.
47. Parkinson AB, Evans NA. Anabolic androgenic steroids: a survey of 500 users. Med Sci Sports Exerc. 2006;38(4):644.
48. Casavant MJ, Blake K, Griffith J, Yates A, Copley LM. Consequences of use of anabolic androgenic steroids. Pediatr Clin North Am. 2007;54(4):677–90.
49. O'Shea JP. The effects of an anabolic steroid on dynamic strength levels of weightlifters. Nutr Rep Int. 1971;4:363–70.
50. Johnson LC, O'shea JP. Anabolic steroid: effects on strength development. Science. 1969;164(3882):957–9.
51. Ariel G. The effect of anabolic steroid upon skeletal muscle contractile force. J Sports Med Phys Fitness. 1973;13(3):187.
52. Hickson RC, Kurowski TG. Anabolic steroids and training. Clin Sports Med. 1986;5(3):461–9.
53. Friedl KE, Dettori JR, Hannan-Jr CJ, Patience TH, Plymate SR. Comparison of the effects of high dose testosterone and 19-nortestosterone to a replacement dose of testosterone on strength and body composition in normal men. J Steroid Biochem Mol Biol. 1991;40(4):607–12.
54. Kao TC, Deuster PA, Burnett D, Stephens M. Health behaviors associated with use of body building, weight loss, and performance enhancing supplements. Annals Epedem. 2012;22(5):331–9.
55. Rosvall KA, Burns CB, Barske J, Goodson JL, Schlinger BA, Sengelaub DR, Ketterson ED. Neural sensitivity to sex steroids predicts individual differences in aggression: implications for behavioural evolution. Proc R Soc B. 2012;279(1742):3547–55.
56. Kiraly CL. Androgenic-anabolic steroid effects on serum and skin surface lipids, on red cells, and on liver enzymes. Int J Sports Med. 1988;9(4):249.
57. Saborido A, Naudí A, Portero-Otín M, Pamplona R, Megías A. Stanozolol treatment decreases the mitochondrial ROS generation and oxidative stress induced by acute exercise in rat skeletal muscle. J Appl Physiol. 2011;110(3):661–9.
58. Delgado J, Saborido A, Megías A. Prolonged treatment with the anabolic–androgenic steroid stanozolol increases antioxidant defenses in rat skeletal muscle. J Physiol Biochemistry. 2010;66(1):63–71.
59. Bosco C, Tihanyi J, Viru A. Relationships between field fitness test and basal serum testosterone and cortisol levels in soccer players. Clin Physiol. 1996;16(3):317–22.
60. Kersey RD, Elliot DL, Goldberg L, Kanayama G, Leone JE, Pavlovich M, Pope HG. National Athletic Trainers' Association position statement: anabolic-androgenic steroids. J Athl Train. 2012;47(5):567–88.
61. Clark AS, Henderson LP. Behavioral and physiological responses to anabolic-androgenic steroids. Neur Biobehavioral Rev. 2003;27(5):413–36.
62. Trenton AJ, Currier GW. Behavioral manifestations of anabolic steroid use. CNS Drugs. 2005;19(7):571–95.
63. Swerdolff R, Overstreet J, Sokol R, Raijfer J. Infertility in the male. Ann Intern Med. 1985;103(6):906–19.
64. Chemes HE, Rawe VY. Sperm pathology: a step beyond descriptive morphology. Origin, characterization and fertility potential of abnormal sperm phenotypes in infertile men. Human Reprod. 2003;9(5):405–28.
65. Arce JC, de Souza MJ. Exercise and male factor infertility. Sports Med. 1993;15(3):146–69.
66. De Souza MJ, Arce JC, Pescatello LS, Scherzer HS, Luciano AA. Gonadal hormones and semen quality in male runners. Int J Sports Med. 1994;15(07):383–91.
67. Bonifazi M, Bela E, Carli G, Lodi L, Martelli G, Zhu B, Lupo C. Influence of training on the response of androgen plasma concentrations to exercise in swimmers. Eur J Appl Physiol. 1995;70(2):109–14.
68. Lucía A, Chicharro JL, Pérez M, Serratosa L, Bandrés F, Legido JC. Reproductive function in male endurance athletes: sperm analysis and hormonal profile. J Appl Physiol. 1996;81(6):2627–36.
69. Gebreegziabher Y, Marcos E, McKinon W, Rogers G. Sperm characteristics of endurance trained cyclists. Int J Sports Med. 2004;25:247–51.
70. Vaamonde D, Silva ME D, Poblador MS, Lancho JL. Reproductive profile of physically active men after exhaustive endurance exercise. Int J Sports Med. 2006;27(9):680–9.
71. Vaamonde D, Da Silva-Grigoletto ME, García-Manso JM, Vaamonde-Lemos R, Swanson RJ, Oehninger SC. Response of semen parameters to three training modalities. Fertil Steril. 2009;92(6):1941–6.
72. Vaamonde D, Silva-Grigoletto ME, García-Manso JM, Cunha-Filho JS, Vaamonde-Lemos R. Sperm morphology normalcy is inversely correlated to

cycling kilometers in elite triathletes. Rev Andal Med Deporte. 2009;2:43–6.
73. De Souza GL, Hallak J. Anabolic steroids and male infertility: a comprehensive review. BJU Int. 2011;108(11):1860–5.
74. Vaamonde D, Da Silva-Grigoletto ME, García-Manso JM, Barrera N, Vaamonde-Lemos R. Physically active men show better semen parameters and hormone values than sedentary men. Eur J Appl Physiol. 2012;112(9):3267–73.
75. Vaamonde D, Da Silva-Grigoletto ME, García-Manso JM, Vaamonde-Lemos R. Differences in sperm DNA fragmentation between high- and low-cycling volume triathletes: preliminary results. Fertil Steril. 2012;98(3):S85.
76. Safarinejad MR, Azma K, Kolahi AA. The effects of intensive, long-term treadmill running on reproductive hormones, hypothalamus–pituitary–testis axis, and semen quality: a randomized controlled study. J Endocrinol. 2009;200(3):259–71.
77. Snyder AC, Hackney AC. The endocrine system in overtraining. In: N Constantini, AC Hackney, editors. Endocrinology of physical activity and sport. New York: Humana Press; 2013. pp. 523–534.
78. Nguyen RH, Wilcox AJ, Skjærven R, Baird DD. Men's body mass index and infertility. Human Reprod. 2007;22(9):2488–93.
79. Brant WO, Myers JB, Carrell DT, Smith JF. Male athletic activities and their effects on semen and hormonal parameters. Phys Sportsmed. 2010;38(3):114–20.
80. Du Plessis SS, Cabler S, McAlister DA, Sabanegh E, Agarwal A. The effect of obesity on sperm disorders and male infertility. Nat Rev Urol. 2010;7(3):153–61.
81. Rajesh-Kumar T, Doreswamy K, Shrilatha B. Oxidative stress associated DNA damage in testis of mice: induction of abnormal sperms and effects on fertility. Mutat Res-Gen Tox En. 2002;513(1):103–11.
82. Cameron JL. Metabolic cues for the onset of puberty. Horm Res Paed. 1991;36(3–4):97–103.
83. Zorgniotti AW. Hypothesis to explain subfertile semen. In: Adrian W Zorgniotti, editor. Temperature and environmental effects on the testis. New York: Springer US; 1991. pp. 221–223.
84. Asplund C, Barkdull T, Weiss BD. Genitourinary problems in bicyclists. Curr Sports Med Rep. 2007;6(5):333–9.
85. Heller CG, Clermont Y. Spermatogenesis in man: an estimate of its duration. Science. 1963;140(3563):184–6.
86. Bijlsma JW, Duursma SA, Thijssen JH, Huber O. Influence of nandrolon decanoate on the pituitary-gonadal axis in males. Acta Endocrinol Copenh. 1982;101:108–12.
87. Alen M, Reinila M, Vihko R. Response of serum hormones to androgen administration in power athletes. Med Sci SportsExerc. 1985;17:354–9.
88. Alen M, Hakkinen K. Androgenic steroid effects on serum hormones and on maximal force development in strength athletes. J Sports Med Phys Fitness. 1987;27:38–46.
89. Bhasin S, Storer TW, Berman N, Callegari C, Clevenger B, Phillips Bunnell TJ, Tricker R, Shirazi A, R Casaburi R. The effects of supraphysiologic doses of testosterone on muscle size and strength in normal men. N Engl J Med. 1996;335:1–7.
90. Bhasin S, Woodhouse L, Casaburi R, Singh AB, Bhasin D, Berman N, Chen X, Yarasheski KE, Magliano L, Dzekov C, Dzekov J, Bross R, Phillips J, Sinha-Hikim I, Shen R, Storer W. Testosterone dose-response relationships in healthy young men. Am J Physiol Endocrinol Metab. 2001;281:E1172–81.
91. Evans NA. Current concepts in anabolic-androgenic steroids. Am J Sports Med. 2004;32(2):534–42.
92. Turek PJ, Williams RH, Gilbaugh JH, Lipshultz LI. The reversibility of anabolic steroid-induced azoospermia. J Urol. 1995;153(5):1628–30.
93. Gazvani MR, Buckett W, Luckas MJ, Aird IA, Hipkin LJ, Lewis-Jones DI. Conservative management of azoospermia following steroid abuse. Hum Reprod. 1997;12:1706–8.
94. Boyadjiev NP, Georgieva KN, Massaldjieva R, Gueorguiev SI. Reversible hypogonadism and azoospermia as a result of anabolic-androgenic steroid use in a bodybuilder with personality disorder. A case report. J Sports Med Phys Fitness. 2000;40(3):271–74.
95. Menon DK. Successful treatment of anabolic steroid–induced azoospermia with human chorionic gonadotropin and human menopausal gonadotropin. Fertil Steril. 2003;79:1659–61.
96. Van Breda E, Keizer HA, Kuipers H, Wolffenbuttel BHR. Androgenic anabolic steroid use and severe hypothalamic-pituitary dysfunction: a case study. Int J Sports Med. 2003;24(3):195–6.
97. Zitzmann M. Exercise, training. and the hypothalamic–pituitary–gonadal axis in men. In: Hormone use and abuse by athletes. New York: Springer US; 2011. pp. 25–30.
98. Jarow JP, Lipshultz LI. Anabolic steroid-induced hypogonadotropic hypogonadism. Am J Sports Med. 1990;18(4):429–31.
99. Schürmeyer TH, Belkien, Knuth UA, Nieschlag E. Reversible azoospermia induced by the anabolic steroid 19-nortestosterone. The Lancet. 1984;323(8374):417–20.
100. De Souza MJ, Miller BE. The effect of endurance training on reproductive function in male runners. A "volume threshold" hypothesis. Sports Med. 1997;23:357–73.
101. Jensen CE, Wiswedel K, McLoughlin J, van der Spuy Z. Prospective study of hormonal and semen profiles in marathon runners. Fertil Steril. 1995;64:1189–96.
102. Brock G. Erectile function of bike patrol officers. J Androl. 2003;23:758–9.
103. Karila T, Hovatta O, Seppala T. Concomitant abuse of anabolic androgenic steroids and human chorionic gonadotrophin impairs spermatogenesis in power athletes. Int J Sports Med. 2004;25:257–63.

104. Shokri S, Hemadi M, Bayat G, Bahmanzadeh M, Jafari-Anarkooli I, Mashkani B. Combination of running exercise and high dose of anabolic androgenic steroid, nandrolone decanoate, increases protamine deficiency and DNA damage in rat spermatozoa. Andrologia. 2014;46(2):184–90.
105. Carrell DT, Emery BR, Hammoud S. Altered protamine expression and diminished spermatogenesis: what is the link? Hum Reprod Update. 2007;13(3):313–27.
106. Jeyaraj DA, Grossman G, Petrusz P. Dynamics of testicular germ cell apoptosis in normal mice and transgenic mice overexpressing rat androgen-binding protein. Reprod Biol Endoc. 2003;48:1–14.
107. Giampietri C, Petrungaro S, Coluccia P, D'Alessio A, Starace D, Riccioli A, Padula F, Palombi F, Ziparo E, Filippini A, de Cesaris P. Germ cell apoptosis control during spermatogenesis. Contraception. 2005;72:298–302.
108. Aitken RJ, Baker MA. Causes and consequences of apoptosis in spermatozoa; contributions to infertility and impacts on development. Int J Dev Biol. 2013;57:265–72.
109. Manna I, Jana K, Samanta PK. Effect of intensive exercise-induced testicular gametogenic and steroidogenic disorders in mature male Wistar strain rats: a correlative approach to oxidative stress. Acta Physiol Scand. 2003;178(1):33–40.
110. Manna I, Jana K, Samanta PK. Effect of different intensities of swimming exercise on testicular oxidative stress and reproductive dysfunction in mature male albino Wistar rats. Indian J Exp Biol. 2004;42(8):816–22.
111. Nirupama M, Devaki M, Nirupama R, Yajurvedi HN. Chronic intermittent stress-induced alterations in the spermatogenesis and antioxidant status of the testis are irreversible in albino rat. J Physiol Biochem. 2013;69(1):59–68.
112. Aitken RJ, Roman SD. Antioxidant systems and oxidative stress in the testes. Oxid Med Cell Longev. 2008;1(1):15.
113. Shokri S, Aitken RJ, Abdolvahhabi M, Ghasemi FM, Kashani I, Ejtemaeimehr S, Ahmadian S, Minaei B, Naraghi MA, Barbarestani M. Exercise and supraphysiological dose of nandrolone decanoate increase apoptosis in spermatogenic cells. Basic Clin Pharmacol Toxicol. 2010;106:324–30.
114. Janjic MM, Stojkov NJ, Andric SA, Kostic TS. Anabolic–androgenic steroids induce apoptosis and NOS2 (nitric-oxide synthase 2) in adult rat Leydig cells following in vivo exposure. Reprod Toxicol. 2012;34(4):686–93.
115. Squires EL, Todter GE, Berndtson WE, Pickett BW. Effect of anabolic steroids on reproductive function of young stallions. J Anim Sci. 1982;54(3):576.
116. Feinberg MJ, Lumia AR, McGinnis MY. The effect of anabolic-androgenic steroids on sexual behavior and reproductive tissues in male rats. Physiol Behav. 1997;62:23–30.
117. Mesbah SF, Shokri S, Karbalay-Doust S, Mirkhani H. Effects of nandrolone decanoate on ultrastructure of testis in male adult rats. Iran J Med Sci. 2008;33(2):94–100.
118. Naraghi MA, Abolhasani F, Kashani I, Anarkooli IJ, Hemadi M, Azami A, Barbarestani M, Aitken RJ, Shokri S. The effects of swimming exercise and supraphysiological doses of nandrolone decanoate on the testis in adult male rats: a transmission electron microscope study. Folia Morphol (Warsz). 2010;69(3):138–46.
119. Hijazi MM, Azmi MA, Hussain A, Naqvi SNH, Perveen R, Hijazi S. Androgenic anabolic steroidal-based effects on the morphology of testicular structures of albino rats. Pakistan J. Zool. 2012;44(6):1529–37.
120. Noorafshan A, Karbalay-Doust SAIED, Ardekani FM. High doses of nandrolone decanoate reduce volume of testis and length of seminiferous tubules in rats. Apmis. 2005;113(2):122–5.

Impact of Physical Activity and Exercise on Female Reproductive Potential

11

Rebecca J. Mallinson, Jenna C. Gibbs and Mary Jane De Souza

Abbreviations

BMD	Bone Mineral Density
EA	Energy availability
EAMD	Exercise-associated menstrual disturbances
FHA	Functional hypothalamic amenorrhea
FSH	Follicle-stimulating hormone
GnRH	Gonadotropin-releasing hormone
hCG	Human chorionic gonadotropin
HPA	Hypothalamic–pituitary–adrenal
HPO	Hypothalamic–pituitary–ovarian
LBM	Lean body mass
LH	Luteinizing hormone
LPD	Luteal phase defects
PCOS	Polycystic ovarian syndrome
PdG	Pregnanediol glucuronide
TT3	Triiodothyronine

Introduction

Regular physical activity and exercise among girls and women is beneficial for overall health and well-being; however, increases in exercise energy expenditure that are not compensated for by energy intake can lead to perturbations in the reproductive axis, resulting in infertility and numerous skeletal and cardiovascular health consequences [1–4]. Exercise-associated menstrual disturbances (EAMD) have been commonly reported in exercising women, with prevalence estimates of EAMD approaching 50 % [5]. Severe forms of EAMD such as the absence of menses (amenorrhea) or long intermenstrual intervals (oligomenorrhea) are clinically recognizable and typically identified based on menstrual history and self-report. However, other forms of EAMD such as luteal phase defects (LPD) and anovulation are not readily apparent and are often masked within cycles of regular length, yet are arguably the most prevalent [5, 6]. Therefore, these subtle menstrual disturbances in exercising women are not easily diagnosed, silently indicating an energy deficit and potentially contributing to infertility. Due to the frequency and, at times, silent nature of EAMD, awareness of the symptoms and consequences of an energy deficiency in exercising women is vital for the health and well-being of physically active girls and women.

The challenge that is imposed on physiological systems during an energy deficiency causes energy to be repartitioned toward processes that are necessary for survival, such as thermoregulation, locomotion, and cellular maintenance, and away from processes that are not critical for survival, that is, reproduction and growth [7]. As such, an energy deficiency often promotes a cascade of metabolic alterations in an effort to conserve energy, and these energy-conserving mechanisms in turn contribute to disruptions in the hypothalamic–pituitary–ovarian (HPO)

M. J. De Souza (✉) · R. J. Mallinson · J. C. Gibbs
Department of Kinesiology, Pennsylvania State University, 104 Noll Laboratory, University Park, PA 16802, USA
e-mail: mjd34@psu.edu

© Springer Science+Business Media New York 2016

D. Vaamonde et al. (eds.), *Exercise and Human Reproduction*, DOI 10.1007/978-1-4939-3402-7_11

axis [7]. Beginning with the "generator" of reproductive function in the hypothalamus and ending with ovarian steroid secretion by the follicles, alterations in the production and secretion of reproductive hormones occur at each level of the reproductive axis. As such, the purpose of this chapter is to explore the impact of physical activity and exercise on reproductive function and fertility in adolescent girls and women by examining both subtle and severe menstrual disturbances and the changes that occur within the HPO axis to induce reproductive dysfunction. The effects of exercise and, more specifically, an energy deficiency on reproductive function and fertility will be explored by assessing the presence and quality of key reproductive events such as ovulation, the normal cyclicity of reproductive hormone concentrations, and endometrial proliferation.

Normal Menstrual Cycle and HPO Axis Activity

To adequately understand the effects of exercise on reproductive function, it is imperative to begin with a description of a *normal* menstrual cycle and *optimal* reproductive function, which serve as the healthy reference point to which the changes that are observed in both subtle and severe menstrual disturbances are compared. The menstrual cycle, which is defined as the period from the onset of menses to the day before the next onset of menses, typically lasts about 28 days and is divided into two phases, the follicular phase and the luteal phase [8]. The follicular phase begins at the onset of menses and the luteal phase begins the day after ovulation occurs (Fig. 11.1). Therefore, ovulation is a mid-cycle event that separates the follicular and luteal phases.

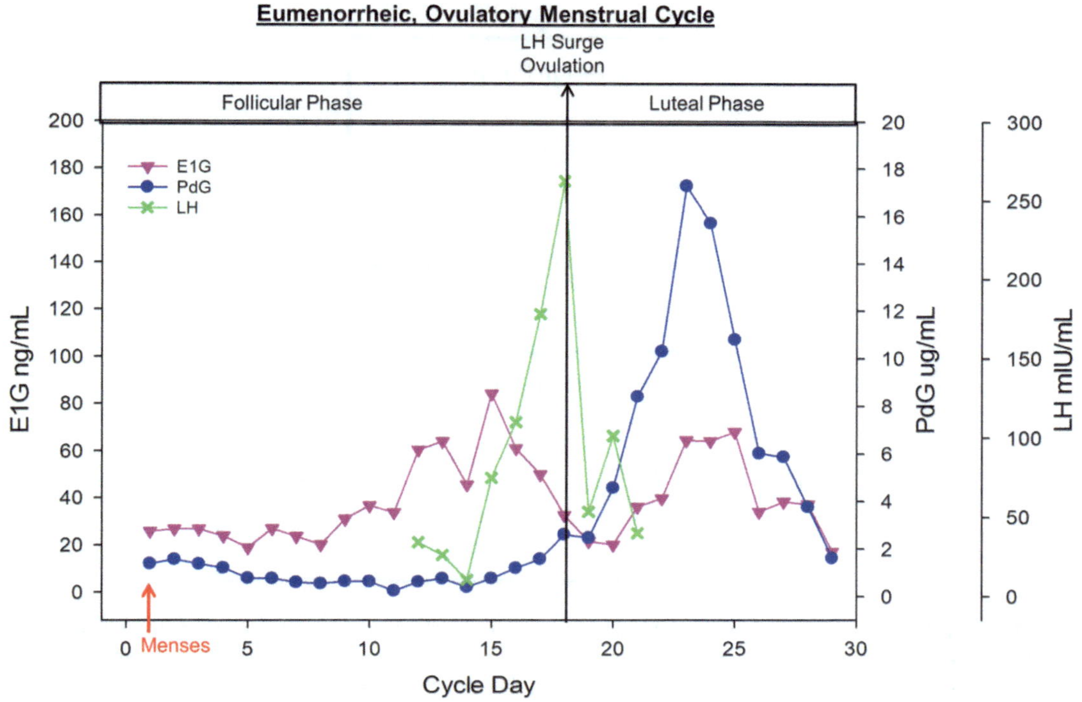

Fig. 11.1 Profile of daily urinary excretion of reproductive hormones for a representative eumenorrheic, ovulatory menstrual cycle. Classic characteristics include the E1G peak in the late follicular phase, the LH surge following the E1G peak, and rising PdG concentrations during the luteal phase. *E1G* estrone-1-glucuronide, *PdG* pregnanediol glucuronide, *LH* luteinizing hormone

The cascade of events surrounding the menstrual cycle commences with secretion of gonadotropin-releasing hormone (GnRH) from the arcuate nucleus and preoptic area of the hypothalamus which in turn stimulates the release of luteinizing hormone (LH) and follicle-stimulating hormone (FSH) from gonadotroph cells of the anterior pituitary gland, the two gonadotropins that stimulate the production of estrogen and progesterone from the ovaries [9] (Fig. 11.2).

GnRH is known as the "master hormone" of reproduction due to its role as regulator of LH and FSH pulsatility [10]. Evidence from classic experiments conducted in *rhesus* monkeys [11, 12] demonstrated the rhythmic and acute secretory actions of GnRH. Typically, GnRH release occurs every 60–90 min, and, consequently, gonadotropin secretion occurs approximately once per hour from the anterior pituitary, paralleling the release of GnRH [8, 9, 13]. During the follicular phase, GnRH pulsatility and, therefore, LH and FSH pulsatility maintain a relatively high frequency [13]. Near the end of the follicular phase, the frequency and amplitude of GnRH

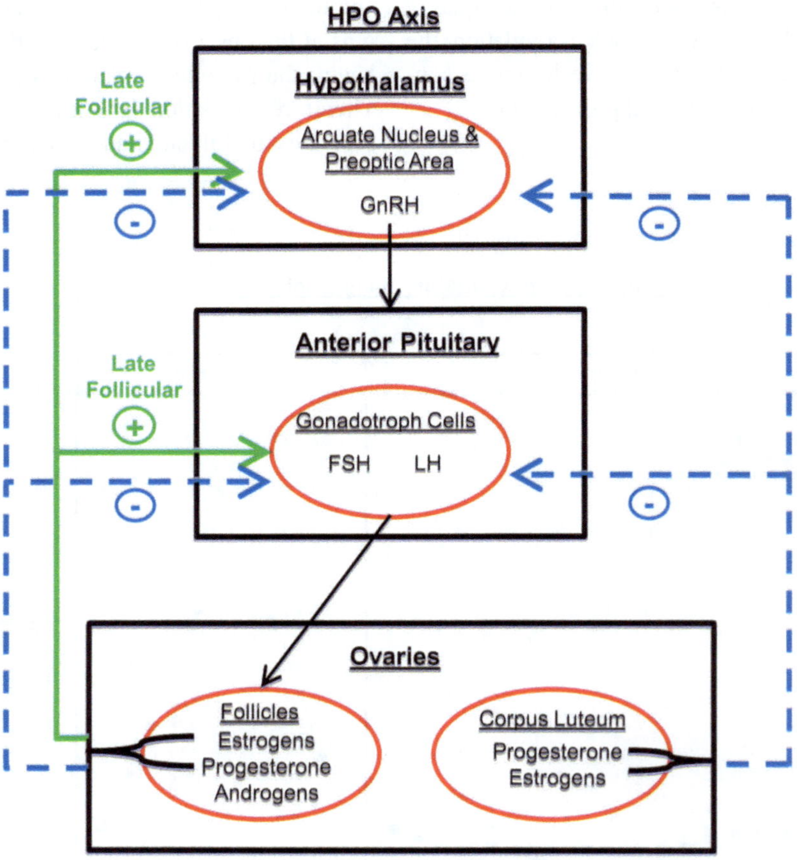

Fig. 11.2 HPO axis sequence of events related to the menstrual cycle. Neurons in the arcuate nucleus and preoptic area of the hypothalamus secrete GnRH which, in turn, stimulates the release of FSH and LH from the gonadotroph cells of the anterior pituitary gland. FSH and LH increase the production of estrogens progestins, and androgens by follicular granulosa and theca cells in the ovaries. During the luteal phase, the corpus luteum formed by the dominant follicle produces progesterone and estrogens. Typically, the ovarian hormones exert negative feedback on the anterior pituitary and hypothalamus, causing a decrease in the secretion of the gonadotropins. The negative feedback is depicted by the blue dashed lines. However, during the late follicular phase, rapidly rising estrogen concentrations exert positive feedback on the anterior pituitary and hypothalamus resulting in the LH surge. The positive feedback is depicted by the green solid lines. *HPO* hypothalamic–pituitary–ovarian, *GnRH* gonadotropin-releasing hormone, *FSH* follicle-stimulating hormone, *LH* luteinizing hormone

pulses and, subsequently, LH and FSH pulses increase in response to the positive feedback of high estradiol concentrations [13]. However, at the end of the luteal phase, GnRH and LH pulsatility declines in response to negative feedback from progesterone [9, 13]. In turn, LH and FSH bind to receptors on the granulosa and theca cells of the developing ovarian follicle during the follicular phase and luteal cells during the luteal phase to produce estrogens, androgens, and progesterone [14].

During the late luteal and early follicular phase, FSH production increases, stimulating follicular growth and recruitment of the dominant follicle within the ovaries [13]. Production of the estrogen, estradiol, by the synergistic efforts of the theca and granulosa cells of the ovarian follicles also increases [13]; thus, during the follicular phase, estradiol concentrations gradually increase, upregulating the number of FSH receptors in the mature follicles and consequently increasing the action of FSH and the production of estradiol [13, 14]. During the mid-follicular phase, negative feedback by estradiol on the anterior pituitary prevents further increases in FSH and LH [9, 15]. Near the late mid-follicular phase to the end of the follicular phase, one follicle has achieved dominance and rapidly increases its production of estradiol while the other less-dominant follicles undergo atresia [13]. The rapidly rising concentrations of estradiol exert *positive* feedback in the preoptic area of the hypothalamus and on the gonadotroph cells of the anterior pituitary, sensitizing the cells to GnRH and stimulating the release of a bolus of LH after plasma estradiol concentrations exceed a threshold for at least 36 h [9, 11, 13, 15].

Therefore, the LH surge typically occurs 24–36 h after attainment of peak estradiol secretion and lasts for approximately 24–48 h [13]. In turn, the LH surge prompts proteolytic enzymes to digest the follicular wall, allowing the release of the oocyte from the dominant follicle and initiating ovulation, the event that separates the follicular and luteal phases [13]. Under the influence of LH, luteinization of the erupted follicle occurs, resulting in the formation of a corpus luteum, consisting of theca-lutein and granulosa-lutein cells [13]. These luteinized cells produce progesterone and, to a lesser extent, estradiol, which inhibit both the release of gonadotropins from the anterior pituitary and subsequent folliculogenesis [13]. In the absence of pregnancy-induced concentrations of human chorionic gonadotropin (hCG), the corpus luteum degenerates forming the corpus albicans and progesterone production declines at the end of the luteal phase, thereby removing the negative feedback on the anterior pituitary and hypothalamus [13]. FSH concentrations begin to increase again, recruiting another cohort of follicles for the subsequent cycle [13].

Therefore, in summary, a normal menstrual cycle demonstrates slowly increasing concentrations of FSH during the luteal-follicular transition and early follicular phase. Rising estradiol concentrations during the follicular phase exert negative feedback on the anterior pituitary and hypothalamus, resulting in no further increases of FSH and LH during the mid-follicular phase [9, 13, 15]. The peak in estradiol concentration mid-cycle triggers the LH surge, leading to ovulation and commencement of the luteal phase. The luteal phase is characterized by rising progesterone concentrations that decline near the end of the cycle as the corpus luteum degenerates (Fig. 11.1).

Within the uterus, the proliferative and secretory phases of the uterine cycle coincide with the follicular and luteal phases of the ovarian cycle. The proliferative phase involves a rebuilding of the functional layer of the endometrium after it has been shed during menses [16]. The cells of the *zona basalis,* that is, basal stromal cells, proliferate in response to rising concentrations of estradiol from the developing follicles [13]. During the late proliferative phase, hyperplasia of endometrial cells results in thickening of the endometrial wall such that the endometrium may increase in thickness from 0.5 to 5 mm [13]. Stimulated by progesterone from the corpus luteum, the secretory phase involves the glandular secretion of glycogen and increased vascularization to support the implantation of an embryo in the event that fertilization occurred [13, 16].

Decidual cells formed from stromal cells produce secretions in concert with the endometrial glands and create the *zona compacta,* the dense layer of upper endometrial cells [13]. The *zona spongiosa,* that is, the mid-layer of epithelial cells which consists of prominent endometrial glands, also becomes apparent during this phase [13]. In the absence of fertilization, progesterone and estrogen concentrations decline and the endometrium is deprived of hormonal support, causing the spiral arteries to constrict and destruction of the functional layer of the endometrium, i.e., the *zona compacta* and the *zona spongiosa* [13]. Eventually, as the upper two thirds of the endometrium degenerates, the arteries relax and menses begins [16]. As such, the menstrual phase of the uterine cycle is characterized by the loss of the functional layer of the endometrium as a result of ischemia and necrosis of endometrial tissues [13]. The innermost layer of the endometrium, the *zona basalis,* is all that remains at the end of the menstrual phase [13].

Thus, it is evident that both the ovarian and uterine cycles rely on proper functioning of the HPO axis and, subsequently, adequate hormonal concentrations, for normal menstrual function. Among exercising women with reproductive disturbances, the metabolic environment alters the HPO axis, leading to disruptions in the menstrual cycle that affect both the ovarian and uterine cycles and, in turn, influence reproductive potential.

Types of EAMD

EAMD occur along a spectrum ranging from mild to severe (Fig. 11.3). The least severe presentations of menstrual dysfunction include subtle menstrual disturbances, also known as subclinical menstrual disturbances that occur without a change in cycle length and are, therefore, frequently undetected; these subtle menstrual disturbances include LPD and anovulation. Severe menstrual disturbances, also known as clinical menstrual disturbances, exist at the pathological endpoint of the continuum and are characterized by long intermenstrual intervals (oligomenorrhea) or the absence of menstruation for more than 90 days which is referred to clinically as functional hypothalamic amenorrhea (FHA).

Subtle Menstrual Disturbances: LPD

LPD are characterized by adequate ovulatory function despite poor implantation and poor endometrial quality [1, 17, 18]. More specifically, LPD cycles are characterized by ovulatory cycles with normal and repeatable intermenstrual intervals but luteal phase dysfunction; they are defined by a short luteal phase length of 10 days and/or inadequate progesterone production during the luteal phase [17, 19] (Fig. 11.4a). It has been suggested that a critical 3- or 5-day sum of mid-luteal progesterone concentrations can be used to identify inadequate progesterone exposure associated with LPD [19, 20].

As such, previous reports have used either a urinary pregnanediol glucuronide (PdG) peak of < 5 μg/ml or the sum of a 3-day mid-luteal PdG peak of < 10 μg/ml as indicators of an inadequate luteal progesterone production [5, 20]. Typically, women with LPD demonstrate a prolonged follicular phase in concert with the shortened luteal phase; thus, for example, an individual with a 28-day cycle and a 7-day luteal phase will have

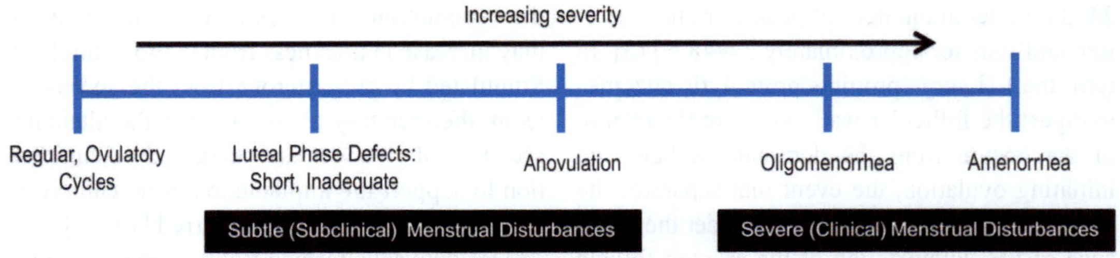

Fig. 11.3 Spectrum of exercise-associated menstrual disturbances (EAMD). The subtle menstrual disturbance, luteal phase defects (LPD), is the least severe EAMD, whereas functional hypothalamic amenorrhea (FHA), which represents a clinical menstrual disturbance, is the most severe EAMD

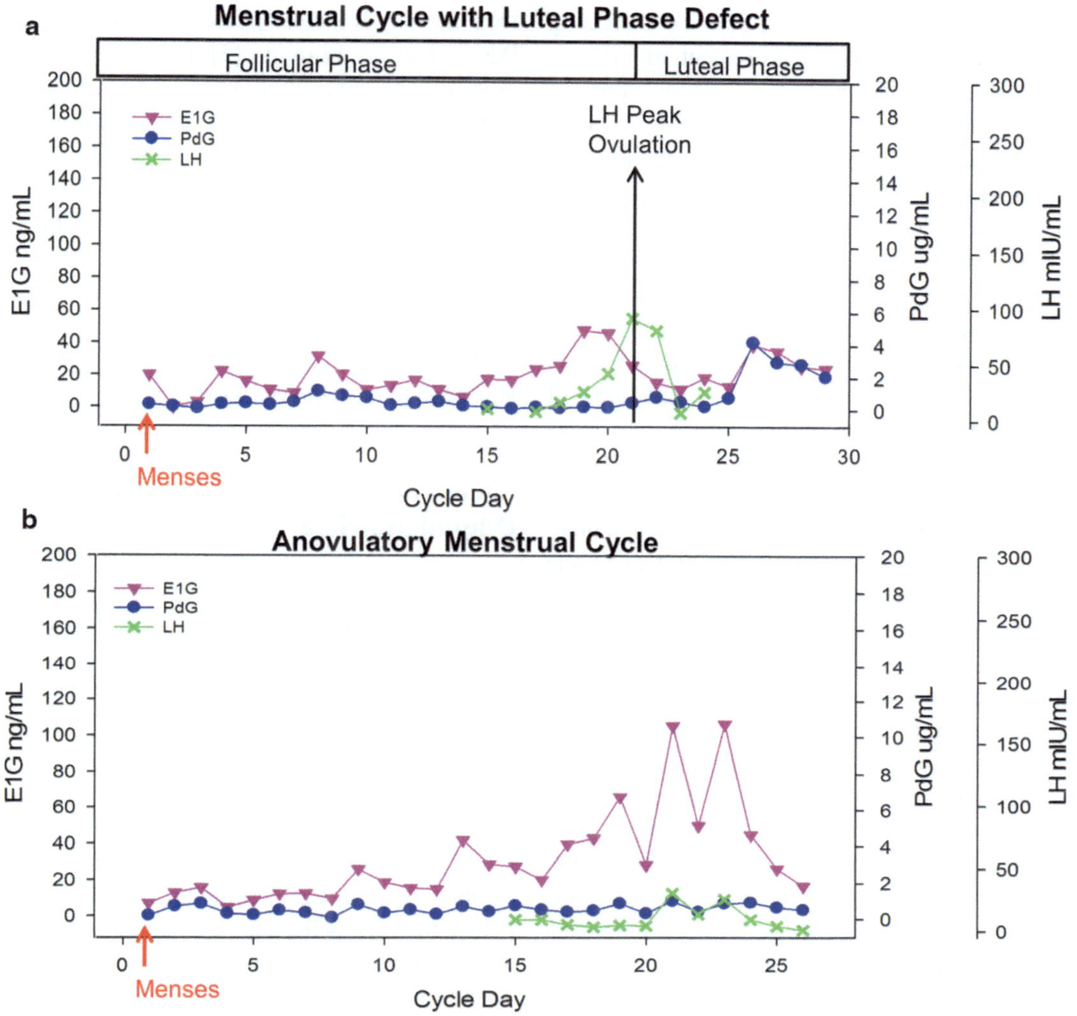

Fig. 11.4 Profile of daily urinary excretion of reproductive hormones for subtle menstrual disturbances. **a** Representative menstrual cycle with a short and inadequate luteal phase defect. Classic characteristics include a luteal phase <10 days in length and suppressed progesterone production during the luteal phase. **b** Representative anovulatory menstrual cycle. Classic characteristics include the lack of both a mid-cycle E1G peak and LH surge and the failure of PdG to rise during the latter part of the cycle, indicating the absence of ovulation. *E1G* estrone-1-glucuronide, *PdG* pregnanediol glucuronide, *LH* luteinizing hormone

a 21-day follicular phase with an LH peak occurring on day 21 compared to women with normal ovulatory cycles in whom the LH peak and presumably ovulation occurs mid-cycle (days 12–14) for a 28-day cycle [1, 19].

The etiology of LPD has been proposed to be impaired folliculogenesis and oocyte maturation that results from disruptions of the reproductive axis [1, 17, 19]. Estrogen exposure during the follicular phase is suppressed among LPD cycles of exercising women compared to ovulatory cycles with normal luteal function [6]. Likewise, there is a delayed rise in FSH concentrations during the end of the preceding luteal phase, often referred to as the luteal-follicular transition, which is a critical time period for successful follicle recruitment [6]. A reduction in the concentration of the LH peak has also been reported in LPD cycles [5, 21]. Each of these hormonal alterations may contribute to abnormal function of the corpus luteum and, subsequently, suppressed progesterone concentrations [5, 6, 17, 21].

The determination of LPD in exercising women relies on the measurement of mid-cycle LH and daily progesterone concentrations in the luteal phase via daily urine or a timed serum sample during a single cycle; however, the monitoring of multiple consecutive cycles is advised for detection of LPD due to the inconsistency with which LPD cycles are observed in exercising women [5, 6]. For example, women may present with a normal, ovulatory cycle one month followed by an LPD or anovulatory cycle the next month. Inconsistent presentations of LPD and anovulation during consecutive cycles may also occur in the same individual. In fact, it has been reported that almost half (46 %) of exercising women present with inconsistent menstrual status; therefore, monitoring only one cycle may underestimate the incidence of menstrual disturbances among exercising women by 38 % [6]. Procedures for daily urine or serum sampling are costly and often not feasible; therefore, the detection of LPD in exercising women is difficult and the majority of women with LPD are often unaware of the presence of this subclinical menstrual perturbation. Notably, self-report and/or assessment of menstrual history alone will not detect LPD, thereby further contributing to the underestimation of the prevalence of menstrual disturbances among exercising women.

Subtle Menstrual Disturbances: Anovulation

Anovulation represents a subtle menstrual disturbance that is more severe than LPD. The hallmark characteristic of anovulation is the failure of follicular estrogen to rise concomitant with the lack of the mid-cycle LH surge and the subsequent failure to ovulate [5] (Fig. 11.4b). Similar to women with LPD, women with anovulatory cycles are, for the most part, experiencing regular intermenstrual intervals, making the identification of anovulation difficult. Due to the absence of ovulation and, consequently, the failure to produce a corpus luteum, progesterone concentrations do not increase during the latter part of the cycle. Therefore, anovulation has also been defined as the lack of an increase in urinary PdG from a 5-day follicular phase baseline or a peak PdG value < 2.49 μg/ml [5]. Both estrogen and progesterone concentrations have been reported to be lower in anovulatory cycles of exercising women compared to ovulatory cycles of exercising women, suggesting that disruptions in FSH and LH pulsatility contribute to anovulation [5, 6]. Adequate estrogen concentrations, however, allow for degeneration of the functional layer of the endometrium upon withdrawal of hormonal support at the end of the luteal phase, thereby resulting in normal menses [13].

Severe Menstrual Disturbances: Oligomenorrhea

Oligomenorrhea represents cycles with long and inconsistent intermenstrual intervals of 36–90 days that are often accompanied by 3–6 menses events per year [1, 22, 23] (Fig. 11.5a). This severe menstrual disturbance is perhaps the least understood and most difficult perturbation to interpret due to its inconsistent hormonal characteristics. An oligomenorrheic cycle may be ovulatory or anovulatory, and estrogen concentrations often produce erratic profiles during the extended cycle as follicles seek dominance [1].

The etiology of oligomenorrhea in exercising women may or may not be hypothalamic in nature [22]. Oligomenorrhea can be associated with prolactin-secreting tumors, thyroidtoxicosis and other endocrinopathies, but most often, oligomenorrhea is associated with hyperandrogenism [22, 24–27]. Hyperandrogenism is often secondary to polycystic ovarian syndrome (PCOS) [28], which is causally linked to infertility in women [29].

In exercising women, oligomenorrhea has been often associated with hyperandrogenism, but may also occur secondary to an energy deficit. Investigators have observed hyperandrogenism concomitant with elevated LH/FSH ratio and free androgen index, two additional markers of PCOS, among athletes with menstrual dysfunction [24–26, 30]. Rickenlund et al. [24] identified that a distinct group of athletes with menstrual dysfunction presented with hyperandrogenism, and upon comparison of the oligo-amenorrheic athletes with hyperandrogenemia (H-OAM) to

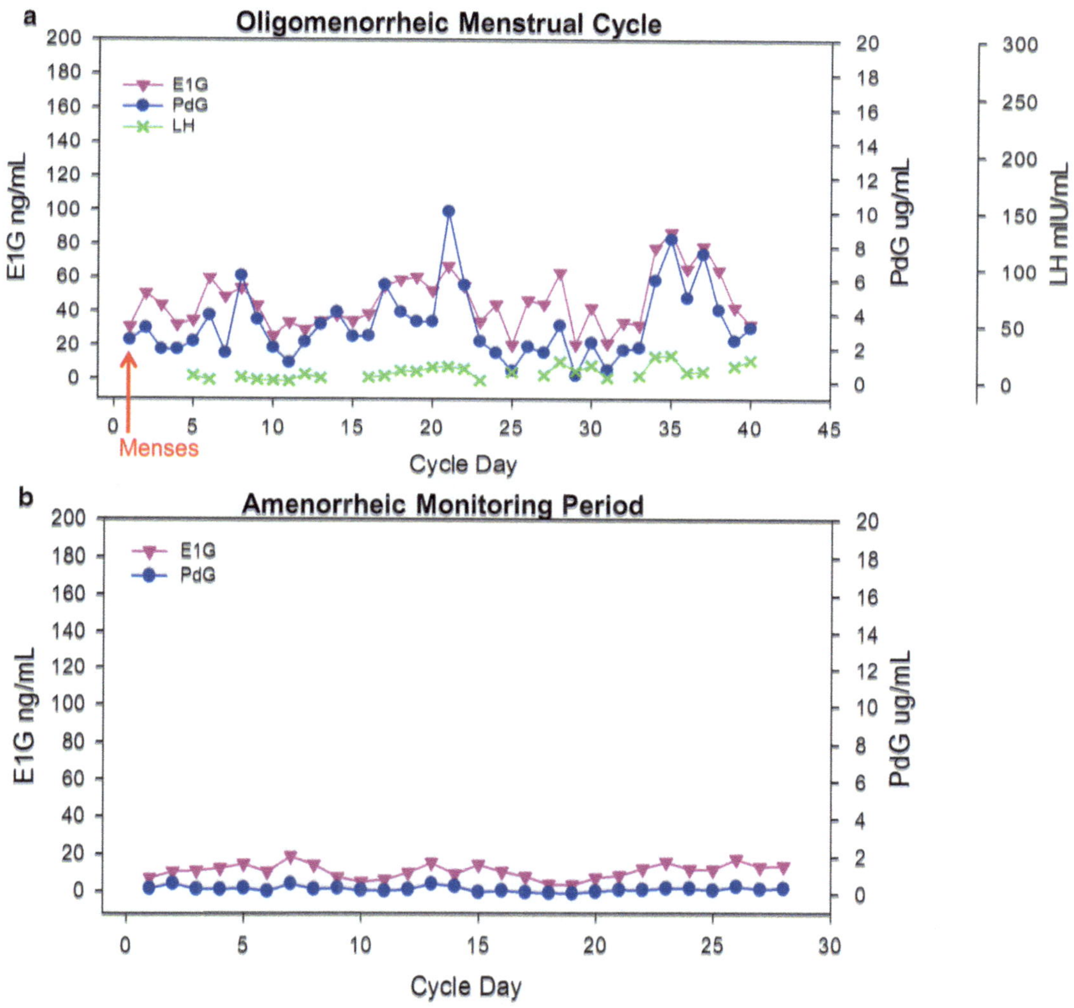

Fig. 11.5 Profile of daily urinary excretion of reproductive hormones for severe menstrual disturbances. **a** Representative oligomenorrheic, anovulatory menstrual cycle. Classic characteristics include a cycle 36–90 days in length and an erratic hormonal profile. **b** Representative amenorrheic 28-day monitoring period. Classic characteristics include chronic suppression of E1G and PdG. *E1G* estrone-1-glucuronide, *PdG* pregnanediol glucuronide, *LH* luteinizing hormone

oligo-amenorrheic athletes with normal androgen profiles (N-OAM), the H-OAM group demonstrated a higher LH/FSH ratio than the N-OAM group, indicating that the profile of reproductive hormones differed between the two groups.

Of interest, however, is that circulating concentrations of triiodothyronine (TT3), a marker of energy deficiency, were significantly lower in both the H-OAM and N-OAM groups compared to a control group of sedentary women, suggesting that both groups may have been in an energy-deficient state [24].

On the other hand, when assessing athletes based on type of menstrual disturbance, Rickenlund et al. [25] observed that 24-h diurnal secretion of testosterone was significantly elevated among oligomenorrheic athletes compared to amenorrheic and regularly menstruating athletes. In addition, amenorrheic athletes demonstrated reduced LH pulsatility, a surrogate marker of GnRH inhibition at the hypothalamus, compared to regularly-menstruating controls, whereas oligomenorrheic athletes demonstrated an LH pulse pattern similar to that observed in regularly-menstruating controls [25].

Therefore, oligomenorrheic athletes did not display the normal hormonal pattern typical of hypothalamic inhibition due to an energy deficiency as was observed in amenorrheic athletes, suggesting that other factors such as hyperandrogenism could be a mechanism underlying oligomenorrhea in athletes. As such, the etiology of oligomenorrhea among exercising women with hyperandrogenemia is ambiguous, thereby complicating the treatment of menstrual dysfunction among this subgroup of exercising women. Careful screening of oligomenorrheic exercising women is necessary to determine if the long, inconsistent cycles are due to an energy deficit or PCOS [22].

Severe Menstrual Disturbances: FHA

At the extreme end of the menstrual disturbance continuum is FHA, the most severe menstrual disturbance that is associated with severe estrogen deficiency and typically defined as the absence of menses for at least 90 days [1, 23], although definitions have varied [23, 31]. FHA is typically classified as either primary or secondary in nature [27]. Primary amenorrhea is defined as the failure to menstruate by 15 years of age in girls with secondary sex characteristics [27]; whereas, secondary amenorrhea is the abnormal cessation of the menstrual cycle after menarche [27].

FHA among exercising women refers to menstrual dysfunction that is caused by disruptions in the hypothalamus due to energy conservation and is unrelated to other causes of FHA associated with the four-compartment model [27, 32]. Exercising women with FHA present with chronically suppressed estrogen and progesterone concentrations [5, 33, 34] (Fig. 11.5b). This suppression is most likely the result of impaired GnRH, LH, and FSH pulsatility that are, therefore, inadequate to stimulate ovulation from the ovary as well as appropriate proliferation and removal of the functional layer of the endometrium.

As such, the ovaries and uterus of amenorrheic women are largely quiescent with minimal production of reproductive hormones. FHA is associated with the most severe clinical sequelae such as low bone mineral density (BMD) [35, 36], poor bone quality [37], and cardiovascular consequences, including a poor lipid profile and endothelial dysfunction [38–40].

Prevalence of EAMD

The prevalence of menstrual disturbances among exercising women has been reported to range from 0 to 60%, a large range that encompasses the prevalence of both subtle and severe menstrual disturbances [41]. The range in prevalence rates in exercising women is large because of the variations in definitions used and methods of assessment in exercising women [5, 6, 42–53]. The prevalence estimates, however, frequently exceed that observed in the general population of nonathletic women that is as low as 3–5% [5, 54–56].

Prevalence of Subtle Menstrual Disturbances

Due to the burdensome nature of investigating the presence of subtle menstrual disturbances, only a few investigators have reported their prevalence among exercising women [5, 6, 42–44] despite LPD and anovulation together representing the most common menstrual disturbances linked to exercise training [5, 6]. The prevalence of subtle menstrual disturbances is alarmingly high given that these disturbances are masked by regular intermenstrual intervals. Prevalence estimates range from 5.9 to 43.0% [5, 6, 42, 44] and 12.0 to 30.0% [5, 6, 44] for LPD and anovulation, respectively. Indeed, the ideal method of identifying subtle menstrual disturbances requires the measurement of daily urinary excretion of reproductive hormones over multiple consecutive cycles.

Based on reports from our lab which has undertaken the task of assessing multiple cycles among exercising women, we observed that 27 and 25% of exercising women with self-reported eumenorrheic cycles (i.e., 26–35 days in length) presented with an LPD or anovulatory cycle, respectively [5]. Therefore, over half of exercising women presented with a subtle menstrual disturbance, compared to only 5% of sedentary women (Fig. 11.6).

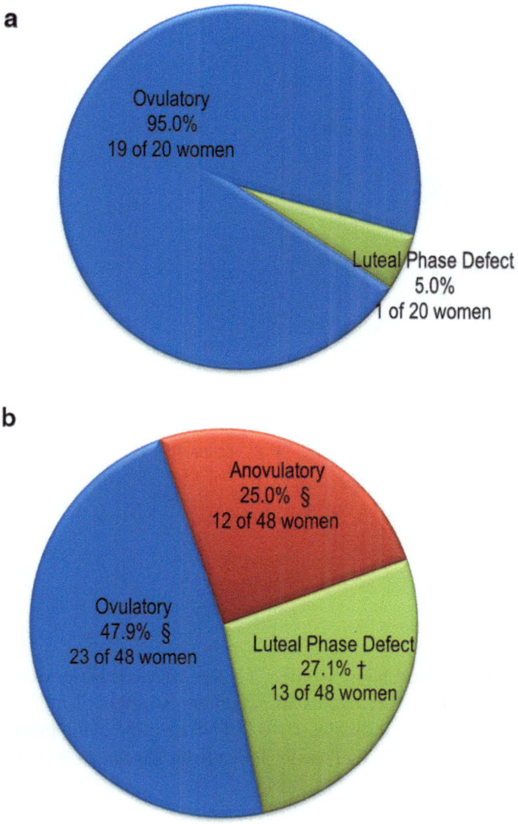

Fig. 11.6 Prevalence of subtle menstrual disturbances among sedentary and exercising women. **a** Proportion of sedentary women categorized as having ovulatory or abnormal (LPD or anovulatory) cycles. **b** Proportion of exercising women categorized as having ovulatory or abnormal (LPD or anovulatory) cycles. Exercising women compared with sedentary women: † indicates $p=0.050$; § indicates $p<0.001$. Reprinted with permission of Oxford University Press from De Souza et al. [5]

Similarly, upon evaluation of individual menstrual cycles among exercising women monitored for 1–3 menstrual cycles, 21 and 29 % of the cycles demonstrated evidence of an LPD and anovulation, respectively, representing 50 % of the 120 cycles assessed in exercising women [5]. Only 4 % of the cycles of sedentary women had a subtle menstrual disturbance, all of which were characterized by an LPD [5] (Fig. 11.7).

Therefore, these results clearly demonstrate the high prevalence with which these largely underdiagnosed menstrual disturbances occur, most often indicative of an energy-deficient state and other underlying health concerns. The strength of our study lies in the daily urinary assessment of reproductive hormones, which provides a complete picture of the hormonal fluctuation throughout the cycle. Therefore, this methodology allows for a more accurate estimate of the prevalence of EAMD than can be obtained from relying solely on self-report measures that often underestimate EAMD prevalence. The frequency at which these "hidden" menstrual disturbances present in exercising women is cause for concern due to the negative impact of an energy deficit and menstrual disturbances on health outcomes and lack of symptomatic indicators that such disturbances are present.

Prevalence of Severe Menstrual Disturbances

Several investigators have evaluated the prevalence of the severe menstrual disturbances (FHA and oligomenorrhea) in female athletes, including both high school [48, 57–59] and adult women [5, 6, 45–47, 60–65]. The earliest prevalence estimates of clinical menstrual disturbances were evaluated in long-distance runners [49–53, 66], dancers [67, 68], and gymnasts [69], and in general, severe menstrual disturbances are documented at much higher rates in premenopausal exercising women than in sedentary women [54–56].

Based on these reports in female athletes and exercising women, the prevalence of primary and secondary amenorrhea ranged from 0 to 56.0 % (determined in 13 studies) [41] and 1 to 60.0 % (determined in 35 studies) [41], respectively; whereas, the range in prevalence of oligomenorrhea was 0.9–52.5 % (determined in 23 studies) [41]. In a recent report that assessed menstrual status in recreationally active women based on daily urinary steroid excretion, investigators observed that 7 % of exercising women presented with oligomenorrhea; whereas, 37 % were amenorrheic [5]. No sedentary women in the sample, however, presented with either oligomenorrhea or amenorrhea [5]. Therefore, menstrual disturbances among exercising women are relatively

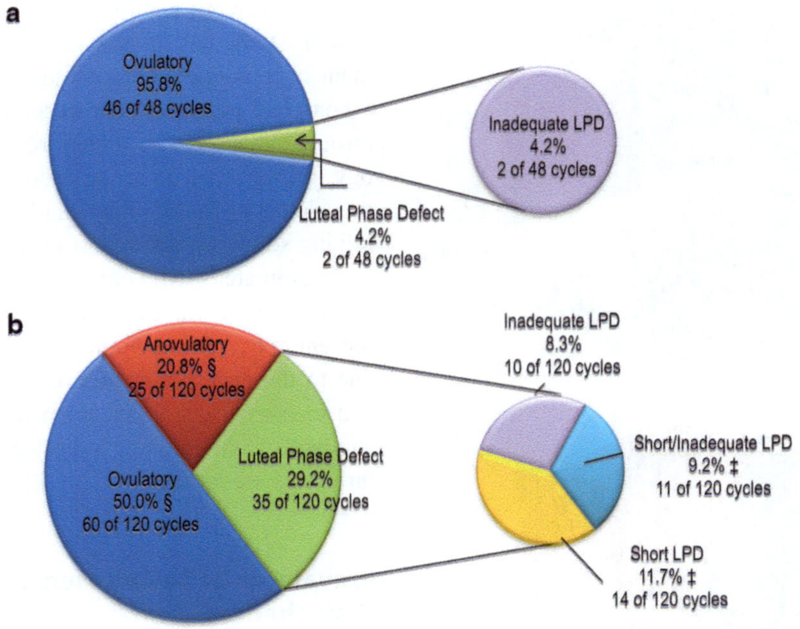

Fig. 11.7 Prevalence of subtle menstrual disturbances among individual cycles of sedentary and exercising women. **a** Proportion of cycles displaying subtle menstrual disturbances among sedentary women. **b** Proportion of cycles displaying subtle menstrual disturbances among exercising women. Cycles of exercising women compared with cycles of sedentary women: ‡ indicates $p<0.050$; § indicates $p<0.001$. Reprinted with permission of Oxford University Press from De Souza et al. [5]

frequent, highlighting the need for awareness of the problem and its associated consequences in an effort to promote healthy exercise habits.

Changes in HPO Activity Associated with EAMD

Chronic energy deficiency targets the pulsatile secretion of GnRH from the arcuate nucleus of the hypothalamus. Disruptions in GnRH pulsatility often lead to changes in the frequency and amplitude of LH and FSH pulses, longer cycle length (particularly a longer follicular phase), reductions in average and peak luteal phase progesterone concentrations, and suppressed estradiol and progesterone [70]. It is believed that GnRH pulsatility, as governed by the pulse generator located in the hypothalamus [8], is sensitive to changes in the metabolic environment that are characteristic of an energy deficiency [7, 71]. (For a detailed description of metabolic adaptations that affect reproductive function, refer to Chap. 12). Thus, an energy deficit disrupts GnRH pulsatility, beginning the cascade of alterations in FSH and LH secretion, estrogen and progesterone production, and ultimately reproductive dysfunction.

Effects of Energy Deficiency on LH Secretion

One of the characteristics of the HPO axis in response to an energy deficit that is created by either energy intake restriction or increased energy expenditure or both is the disruption of LH pulsatility. In an environment of chronic energy deficiency, a reduction in LH frequency has been observed [72, 73].

Loucks et al. [72] compared LH secretory dynamics among regularly menstruating athletes (CA), amenorrheic athletes (AA), and regularly menstruating sedentary women (CS). The frequency of LH pulses was significantly lower in the AA group compared to both CA and CS groups [72]. In addition, relative quiescence of 24-h LH pulsatility was observed in AA, as evidenced by no significant changes in the wake and sleep values of LH in AA compared to the slowing of LH pulse frequency and increase of pulse amplitude that were observed during the sleep hours versus awake hours in both CA and CS women [72].

Likewise, in a similarly designed study, Veldhuis et al. [73] also observed decreased LH pulse frequency among amenorrheic/oligomenorrheic athletes when compared with sedentary, regularly menstruating control women. In response to GnRH administration, however, the amenorrheic/oligomenorrheic athletes demonstrated greater LH secretion than the control women [73], a result that was replicated by Loucks et al. [72]. These results suggest that the reduced LH pulsatility among amenorrheic athletes is likely due to metabolically induced alterations in GnRH pulsatility rather than diminished pituitary responsiveness to GnRH [72, 73].

Causal evidence of the effect of a chronic energy deficiency derived from either dietary energy restriction or increased energy expenditure or both on LH pulsatility was demonstrated by Scheid et al. [74] in a longitudinal model and by Loucks et al. [75] and Williams et al. [76] in an acute model.

Scheid et al. [74] exposed previously sedentary women to a 3-month longitudinal model of energy deficiency that consisted of dietary restriction (−30 to−60 % of baseline energy needs) combined with regular aerobic exercise (70–80 % of maximum heart rate) performed 5 days per week. Before and after the 3-month intervention, women underwent 24-h repeated blood sampling to determine the impact of a long-term energy deficiency on LH pulsatility [74]. After completion of the intervention, a significant decline in 24-h LH pulse frequency was observed among the women exposed to the energy deficit; whereas, women in a control group who neither exercised nor restricted dietary intake demonstrated no change in LH pulse characteristics [74]. This decrease in LH pulse frequency is evident in Fig. 11.8 which depicts individual 24-h profiles of LH pulsatility pre- and post-intervention.

An acute energy deficiency has also been demonstrated to impact LH pulsatility [75, 76]. In a classic study, the induction of low energy availability (EA) (≤20 kcal/kg LBM/day) for 5 days in sedentary, regularly menstruating women resulted in suppressed LH pulse frequency and increased LH pulse amplitude compared to a replete EA (45 kcal/kg LBM/day) [75]. Similarly, restriction of energy intake by 60 % for 7 days concomitant with a short-term increase in exercise training volume for 3 days in premenopausal women resulted in a significant decrease in LH pulse frequency compared with an experimental condition characterized by a 3-day increase in exercise volume with 7 days of eucaloric intake [76]. In fact, LH pulsatility appears to rapidly respond, even within minutes, to shifts in EA in the animal model [7]. Taken together, these observations provide evidence that both chronic and acute energy deficits driven either by dietary energy restriction or increased energy expenditure or both lead to disruption of LH secretory patterns, likely due to energetically-driven alterations in GnRH pulsatility.

Energy Deficiency and FSH Secretion

Although it is well established that energy deficiency alters LH pulsatility, likely via disruptions in GnRH pulsatility, the role of FSH in menstrual disturbances has not been well characterized [75]. It appears, however, that FSH secretion is indeed impacted by an energy deficiency and contributes to menstrual disturbances.

Among exercising women with LPD and a low EA, De Souza et al. [6] observed significantly lower FSH concentrations during the luteal-follicular transition (last 5 days of the cycle) compared with cycles of sedentary ovulatory women, suggesting that a decline in FSH concentrations may contribute to the suppressed ovarian function that is observed among women with EAMD. This decrease in FSH secretion during the luteal-follicular transition is believed to impact follicular recruitment and maturation, thereby contributing to the low estrogen concentrations that were also observed in this group of

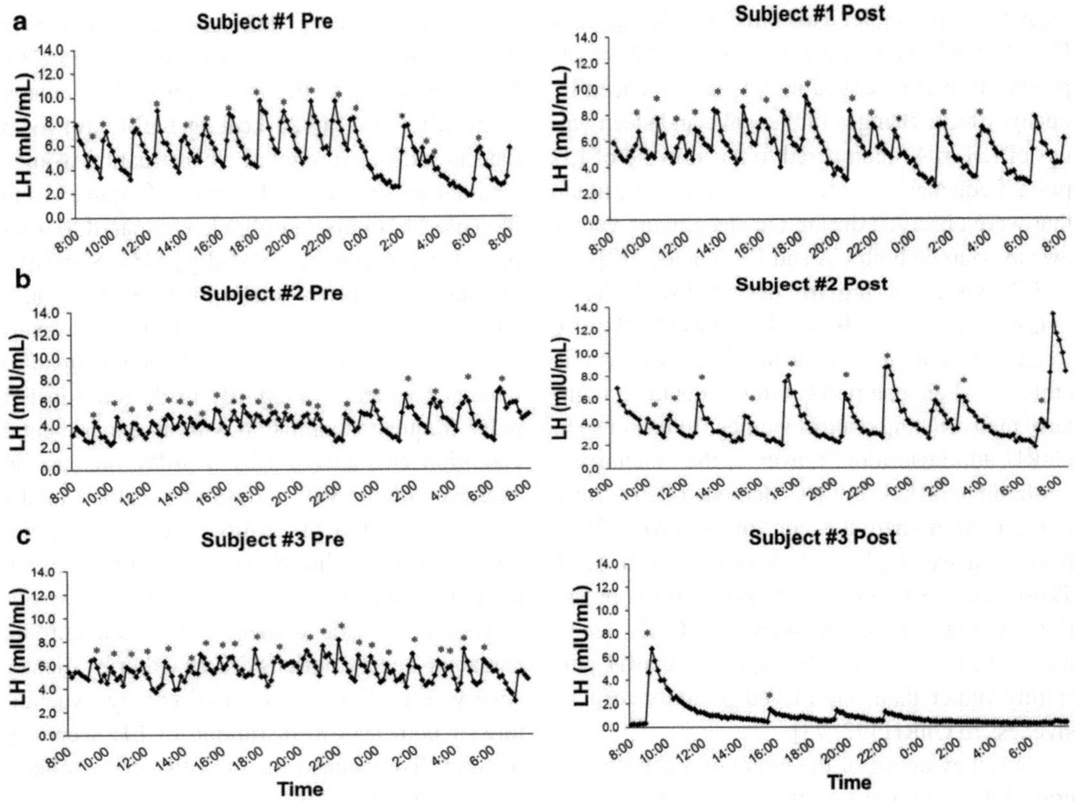

Fig. 11.8 Examples of individual 24-h profiles of LH pulsatility before (pre) and after (post) a 3-month intervention consisting of dietary restriction and aerobic exercise. **a** Subject #1 was in the Control group, lost 0.1 kg body weight, and increased LH pulse frequency by 0.02 pulses/h. **b** Subject #2 was in the Energy Deficit group, lost 3.3 kg body weight, and decreased LH pulse frequency by 0.75 pulses/h. **c** Subject #3 was in the Energy Deficit group, lost 6.3 kg body weight, and decreased LH pulse frequency by 0.89 pulses/h. * represents LH pulse determined using cluster analysis software. *LH* luteinizing hormone. Reprinted with permission of The American Physiological Society from Scheid et al. [74]

exercising women during days 6–12 of the cycle [6]. However, the imposition of low EA for 5 days among regularly menstruating women did not result in changes in FSH concentrations despite changes in LH pulsatility and estrogen concentrations compared with an adequate EA [75]. These findings suggest that FSH may respond differently to acute and chronic energy deficits.

Energy Deficiency and Ovarian Hormone Production

Disruptions in LH and FSH secretion, in turn, lead to suppression of estrogen and progesterone production from the ovaries, a hallmark characteristic of EAMD. Reductions in FSH during the luteal-follicular transition may cause delayed follicular maturation and, thus, a decrease in estrogen production from the developing follicles during the follicular phase.

Anovulatory cycles of exercising women demonstrated significantly lower estrogen excretion and area under the curve during the follicular phase compared to ovulatory cycles of both sedentary and exercising women [5]. Likewise, mean estrogen concentration and estrogen exposure during a 28-day monitoring period among amenorrheic exercising women has been observed to be significantly lower than that observed during a monitored cycle of exercising ovulatory women [34]. Disruption of LH pulsatility and the

LH surge may contribute to lower progesterone production as has been demonstrated in LPD, anovulatory, and amenorrheic cycles of exercising women compared with ovulatory cycles of sedentary and exercising women [5, 34]. As such, urinary and serum measurements of ovarian hormone concentrations in exercising women with menstrual disturbances indicating a chronic energy deficit or regularly menstruating women with an acute energy deficit have revealed declines in estrogen and progesterone concentrations [5, 33, 34, 75, 77].

The suppression in ovarian hormone concentrations varies with the severity of the menstrual disturbance, with the degree of suppression increasing from the least severe menstrual disturbance of LPD to the most severe menstrual disturbance of amenorrhea [5]. In fact, a characteristic hormonal profile of amenorrhea is a chronic suppression of estrogen and progesterone, with the normal peaks of these ovarian hormones notably absent (Fig. 11.5b). Therefore, taken together, menstrual dysfunction associated with exercise, of which the underlying etiology is an energy deficit, is the result of a sequence of reproductive hormone changes, beginning in the hypothalamus and affecting each level of the HPO axis.

Stress Hypothesis Versus EA Hypothesis

Although exercising women frequently present with menstrual dysfunction, it is imperative to highlight that it is not the exercise per se that leads to menstrual dysfunction and the cascade of subsequent health consequences; rather, it is the energy deficiency caused by inadequate caloric intake to compensate for energy expenditure that leads to the altered metabolic and hormonal environment typical of women with FHA. The "exercise stress hypothesis" postulates that the stress of exercise, defined as everything related to exercise except the energy cost, upregulates the hypothalamic–pituitary–adrenal (HPA) axis, disrupting reproductive function at the level of the hypothalamus by altering GnRH secretion [78].

On the other hand, the "energy availability hypothesis" suggests that markers of energy status alter reproductive function by influencing the GnRH pulse generator and subsequently LH pulsatility [78] (refer to Chap. 12 for a detailed description of the metabolic markers that alter reproductive function).

These hypotheses were tested by Loucks et al. [78] using a carefully designed experimental protocol that included both exercising and nonexercising treatment groups among sedentary women. For 4 days on two separate occasions, the exercising treatment group engaged in 30 kcal/kg LBM/day of exercise and were provided with either (1) a 75 kcal/kg LBM/day diet to set EA at 45 kcal/kg LBM/day (balanced) or (2) a diet of 40 kcal/kg LBM/day to set EA at 10 kcal/kg LBM/day (deprived). The nonexercising treatment group did not expend energy via exercise but were provided with either (1) a diet of 45 kcal/kg LBM/day (balanced) or (2) a diet of 10 kcal/kg LBM/day (deprived). It was previously demonstrated that an EA of 30 kcal/kg LBM/day was adequate to maintain optimal TT3 concentrations and LH pulsatility [75, 79]; whereas, at an EA below 25–30 kcal/kg LBM/day, a cascade of negative metabolic and hormonal adaptations occurred, indicating an energy-deficient state [75, 79, 80].

In the exercise treatment group, the deprived condition demonstrated a significant reduction in TT3 concentrations, a hormone that is a key marker of energy status and is typically suppressed among amenorrheic exercising women [79], as well as a reduction in LH pulse frequency compared to the balanced condition [78]. Within the nonexercise treatment group, these results were mimicked with the exception of LH pulse frequency which showed a much larger reduction in the deprived condition. However, upon comparison of the exercise treatment group with the nonexercise treatment group, the stress of exercise did not suppress TT3 concentrations or LH pulse frequency [78, 79]. Taken together, these results indicate that exercise itself, apart from its energy cost, does not disrupt the reproductive axis. On the contrary, alterations in LH pulsatility that translate to EAMD are due to the energetic cost of exercise, in particular, when energy intake is inadequate for energy expenditure, creating an energy deficit.

These findings have been supported by studies in monkeys that demonstrated that the induction of amenorrhea was associated with an increase in exercise energy expenditure that was not combined with compensatory increases in energy intake, thus creating an energy deficit [81]. Among eight monkeys that began exercise training (progressive increase to 12.3±0.9 km/d of running) without changes in energy intake, each monkey developed amenorrhea (defined as absence of menses for at least 100 days) 7–24 months into the intervention, coinciding with suppressed estrogen, progesterone, LH, and FSH concentrations [81]. Four of the monkeys were then fed supplemental calories (138–181% of energy intake during amenorrhea) without changes in exercise training [70]. These monkeys resumed normal menstrual cycles in response to the adequate energy intake, corresponding with increases in LH, FSH, and estrogen during the follicular phase and increases in progesterone during the luteal phase [70]. Accordingly, the recovery of menses correlated with energy intake during refeeding and an increase in TT3 [70]. As such, these results provide further support for the hypothesis that EA rather than the stress of exercise is primarily responsible for regulating the HPO axis in exercising women.

Reproductive Potential and Clinical Relevance

In terms of reproductive and clinical significance, the impact of menstrual dysfunction at any point along the continuum in exercising women has a profound impact on fertility. The acute effects of FHA on reproductive potential are clear in that the complete absence of the menstrual cycle precludes pregnancy. Likewise, the inconsistent presentation of oligomenorrhea with varied cycle lengths and the occurrence of both ovulatory and anovulatory cycles may create an unstable environment for both unwanted and wanted conception due to the uncertain status of the cycle at any given time. LPD are a unique menstrual disturbance in that, unlike other disturbances, the irregular cycles are masked in the presence of regular length and ovulation. However, LPD are associated with infertility and spontaneous abortion due to the inadequate progesterone environment [17]; the low progesterone production inhibits proper maturation of the endometrium, leading to poor endometrial quality that cannot support blastocyst implantation and causes embryonic loss [18–20, 82]. Therefore, in summary, women with LPD associated with inadequate progesterone production often experience disruptions in follicular growth, suppressed oocyte maturation, and endometrial dysfunction, which may lead to compromised fecundity, spontaneous abortion, and infertility [17, 19, 20].

An important consideration for reproductive potential among exercising women, particularly those presenting with apparently regular menstrual cycles, is the consistency at which ovulatory and abnormal cycles occur. De Souza et al. [5] reported that A greater proportion of sedentary women (Sed) presented with consistently ovulatory cycles compared to exercising women (Ex) (Sed: 95% vs. Ex: 32%); whereas, exercising women presented with more consistently abnormal cycles (Ex: 32% vs. Sed: 0%) and more inconsistent cycles than sedentary women (Ex: 36% vs. Sed: 6%) [5]. These findings indicate that exercising women are more likely to experience abnormal cycles over the course of several consecutive cycles [5]. The inconsistent presentations of normal and abnormal cycles in exercising women introduce challenges for exercising women with respect to fertility.

Although the impact of EAMD on reproductive potential is unfavorable, consequences of EAMD on reproductive function appear to be acute and do not cause permanent damage [83, 84]. Upon recovery of an optimal energy status, exercising women with menstrual dysfunction can recover normal menstrual function [83–86], allowing proper follicular, ovarian, and endometrial function. It is believed that as the improvement in energy status progresses, menstrual disturbances may also move along the spectrum from the most severe (i.e., amenorrhea) to the least severe (i.e., LPD) before attaining eumenorrheic, ovulatory cycles [83, 88] thus, complete restoration of energy status is essential for optimal reproductive function. For example, an amenorrheic woman who resumes normal menses may still present with anovulatory or LPD cycles, identifying that a small degree of energy deficiency may still be present. Continued improvement in energy status would be necessary to prevent infertility and spontaneous abortion.

Effective nonpharmacological treatment strategies for EAMD include an increase in caloric intake and weight gain. Dueck et al. [85] and Kopp-Woodroffe et al. [86] described case studies of five amenorrheic recreationally active women and female athletes who participated in a diet and training intervention to reverse amenorrhea. Caloric intake was increased by approximately 360 kcal/day and training was reduced by 1 day/week for 12–20 weeks, contributing to a weight gain of 1–3 kg [85, 86]. During the intervention, three of the five women resumed menses [85, 86]. Of the two that did not resume menstruation during the intervention, one woman maintained the increased caloric intake and resumed menses 3 months after completion of the intervention [85]. The other woman withdrew from the study to begin oral contraceptives; therefore, it cannot be determined if resumption of menses would have eventually occurred [86].

Other case reports in recreationally active women with amenorrhea have revealed that an increase in caloric intake of approximately 300 kcal and a weight gain of 3–4 kg contributes to resumption of menses [88]. Although the actual time to resumption of menses may vary for women depending on the severity of the energy deficiency and menstrual disturbance, the amount of weight that is typically gained leading to resumption of menses is not exorbitant, thereby alleviating some concerns that exercising women may have about weight gain.

In addition, weight gain that leads to resumption of menses is also associated with improvement of other clinical sequelae characteristic of exercise-associated amenorrhea [87]. Miller et al. [87] reported that resumption of menses occurred in anorexic women who gained 4 kg of body mass, on average, and the combined effects of weight gain and resumption of menses contributed to significant improvements in lumbar spine and hip BMD. As such, relatively small increases in body mass can lead to a cascade of beneficial health outcomes among women with menstrual dysfunction associated with an energy deficiency.

Conclusion

Adolescent girls and premenopausal women engaging in regular exercise, including both recreational and competitive physical activity, are at risk of developing a menstrual disturbance if energy intake is inadequate to compensate for energy expenditure, resulting in an energy deficit. EAMD include both clinical presentations (i.e., FHA and oligomenorrhea) and subclinical presentations (i.e., LPD and anovulation); therefore, awareness of the importance of adequate energy intake among exercising girls and women is essential. Each menstrual disturbance is linked to spontaneous abortion or infertility, thereby having a profound effect on fecundity. However, with the maintenance of a replete energy state, EAMD that is commonly observed among exercising women can be avoided. Nonpharmacological strategies to prevent and reverse EAMD include consuming adequate kilocalories on a daily basis to support healthy body weight and menstrual function. Although energy intake requirements vary among individuals, regular estimations of daily energy expenditure and energy intake and subsequent calculations of energy balance (energy intake–energy expenditure) will promote maintenance of a positive energy balance that should ultimately result in favorable outcomes for both reproductive and overall health.

References

1. De Souza MJ, Williams NI. Physiological aspects and clinical sequelae of energy deficiency and hypoestrogenism in exercising women. Hum Reprod Update. 2004;10(5):433–48.
2. O'Donnell E, De Souza MJ. The cardiovascular effects of chronic hypoestrogenism in amenorrhoeic athletes: a critical review. Sports Med. 2004;34(9):601–27.

3. O'Donnell E, Harvey PJ, De Souza MJ. Relationships between vascular resistance and energy deficiency, nutritional status and oxidative stress in oestrogen deficient physically active women. Clin Endocrinol (Oxf). 2009;70(2):294–302.
4. Keen AD, Drinkwater BL. Irreversible bone loss in former amenorrheic athletes. Osteoporos Int. 1997;7(4):311–5.
5. De Souza MJ, Toombs RJ, Scheid JL, O'Donnell E, West SL, Williams NI. High prevalence of subtle and severe menstrual disturbances in exercising women: confirmation using daily hormone measures. Hum Reprod. 2010;25(2):491–503.
6. De Souza MJ, Miller BE, Loucks AB, Luciano AA, Pescatello LS, Campbell CG, et al. High frequency of luteal phase deficiency and anovulation in recreational women runners: blunted elevation in follicle-stimulating hormone observed during luteal-follicular transition. J Clin Endocrinol Metab. 1998;83(12):4220–32.
7. Wade GN, Schneider JE, Li HY. Control of fertility by metabolic cues. Am J Physiol. 1996;270(1 Pt 1):E1–19.
8. Yen SSC. The human menstrual cycle: neuroendocrine regulation. In: Yen SSC, Jaffe RB, Barbieri RL, editors. Reproductive endocrinology: physiology, pathology, and clinical management. 4th ed. Philadelphia: Saunders; 1999. p. 191–217.
9. Knobil E. The wisdom of the body revisited. News Physiol Sci. 1999;14:1–11.
10. Tsutsumi R, Webster NJ. GnRH pulsatility, the pituitary response and reproductive dysfunction. Endocr J. 2009;56(6):729–37.
11. Knobil E, Plant TM, Wildt L, Belchetz PE, Marshall G. Control of the rhesus monkey menstrual cycle: permissive role of hypothalamic gonadotropin-releasing hormone. Science. 1980;207(4437):1371–3.
12. Plant TM, Krey LC, Moossy J, McCormack JT, Hess DL, Knobil E. The arcuate nucleus and the control of gonadotropin and prolactin secretion in the female rhesus monkey (Macaca mulatta). Endocrinology. 1978;102(1):52–62.
13. Jones EE, DeCherney AH. Chapter 54: the female reproductive system. In: Boron WF, Boulpaep EL, editors. Medical physiology. 2nd ed. Philadelphia: Elsevier Saunders; 2005. p. 1141–66.
14. Rhoades R, Pflanzer R. Chapter 30: reproductive physiology. Human physiology. 2nd ed. Philadelphia: Saunders; 1992. p. 986–98.
15. Karsch FJ, Dierschke DK, Weick RF, Yamaji T, Hotchkiss J, Knobil E. Positive and negative feedback control by estrogen of luteinizing hormone secretion in the rhesus monkey. Endocrinology. 1973;92(3):799–804.
16. Marieb EN. Chapter 27: the reproductive system. Human anatomy and physiology. 6th ed. San Francisco: Pearson Benjamin Cummings; 2004. p. 1064–108.
17. Jones GS. The luteal phase defect. Fertil Steril. 1976;27(4):351–6.
18. Jones GS. Some newer aspects of the management of infertility. JAMA. 1949;141(16):1123–9.
19. De Souza MJ. Menstrual disturbances in athletes: a focus on luteal phase defects. Med Sci Sports Exerc. 2003;35(9):1553–63.
20. McNeely MJ, Soules MR. The diagnosis of luteal phase deficiency: a critical review. Fertil Steril. 1988;50(1):1–15.
21. Ayabe T, Tsutsumi O, Momoeda M, Yano T, Mitsuhashi N, Taketani Y. Impaired follicular growth and abnormal luteinizing hormone surge in luteal phase defect. Fertil Steril. 1994;61(4):652–6.
22. Awdishu S, Williams NI, Laredo SE, De Souza MJ. Oligomenorrhoea in exercising women: a polycystic ovarian syndrome phenotype or distinct entity? Sports Med. 2009;39(12):1055–69.
23. Loucks AB, Horvath SM. Athletic amenorrhea: a review. Med Sci Sports Exerc. 1985;17(1):56–72.
24. Rickenlund A, Carlstrom K, Ekblom B, Brismar TB, von Schoultz B, Hirschberg AL. Hyperandrogenicity is an alternative mechanism underlying oligomenorrhea or amenorrhea in female athletes and may improve physical performance. Fertil Steril. 2003;79(4):947–55.
25. Rickenlund A, Thoren M, Carlstrom K, von Schoultz B, Hirschberg AL. Diurnal profiles of testosterone and pituitary hormones suggest different mechanisms for menstrual disturbances in endurance athletes. J Clin Endocrinol Metab. 2004;89(2):702–7.
26. Hagmar M, Berglund B, Brismar K, Hirschberg AL. Hyperandrogenism may explain reproductive dysfunction in Olympic athletes. Med Sci Sports Exerc. 2009;41(6):1241–8.
27. Practice Committee of the American Society for Reproductive Medicine. Current evaluation of amenorrhea. Fertil Steril. 2006;86(5 Suppl 1):148–55.
28. Rotterdam ESHRE/ASRM-Sponsored PCOS consensus workshop group. Revised 2003 consensus on diagnostic criteria and long-term health risks related to polycystic ovary syndrome (PCOS). Hum Reprod. 2004;19(1):41–7.
29. Usadi RS, Legro RS. Reproductive impact of polycystic ovary syndrome. Curr Opin Endocrinol Diabetes Obes. 2012;19(6):505–11.
30. Constantini NW, Warren MP. Menstrual dysfunction in swimmers: a distinct entity. J Clin Endocrinol Metab. 1995;80(9):2740–4.
31. Drinkwater BL, Bruemner B, Chesnut CH, 3rd. Menstrual history as a determinant of current bone density in young athletes. JAMA. 1990;263(4):545–8.
32. Berga S, Naftolin F. Neuroendocrine control of ovulation. Gynecol Endocrinol. 2012;28(Suppl 1):9–13.
33. De Souza MJ, Lee DK, VanHeest JL, Scheid JL, West SL, Williams NI. Severity of energy-related menstrual disturbances increases in proportion to indices of energy conservation in exercising women. Fertil Steril. 2007;88(4):971–5.

34. Scheid JL, Toombs RJ, Ducher G, Gibbs JC, Williams NI, De Souza MJ. Estrogen and peptide YY are associated with bone mineral density in premenopausal exercising women. Bone. 2011;49(2):194–201.
35. Christo K, Prabhakaran R, Lamparello B, Cord J, Miller KK, Goldstein MA, et al. Bone metabolism in adolescent athletes with amenorrhea, athletes with eumenorrhea, and control subjects. Pediatrics. 2008;121(6):1127–36.
36. Rencken ML, Chesnut CH, 3rd, Drinkwater BL. Bone density at multiple skeletal sites in amenorrheic athletes. JAMA. 1996;276(3):238–40.
37. Ackerman KE, Nazem T, Chapko D, Russell M, Mendes N, Taylor AP, et al. Bone microarchitecture is impaired in adolescent amenorrheic athletes compared with eumenorrheic athletes and nonathletic controls. J Clin Endocrinol Metab. 2011;96(10):3123–33.
38. Rickenlund A, Eriksson MJ, Schenck-Gustafsson K, Hirschberg AL. Amenorrhea in female athletes is associated with endothelial dysfunction and unfavorable lipid profile. J Clin Endocrinol Metab. 2005;90(3):1354–9.
39. O'Donnell E, Harvey PJ, Goodman JM, De Souza MJ. Long-term estrogen deficiency lowers regional blood flow, resting systolic blood pressure, and heart rate in exercising premenopausal women. Am J Physiol Endocrinol Metab. 2007;292(5):E1401–9.
40. O'Donnell E, Goodman JM, Harvey PJ. Clinical review: cardiovascular consequences of ovarian disruption: a focus on functional hypothalamic amenorrhea in physically active women. J Clin Endocrinol Metab. 2011;96(12):3638–48.
41. Gibbs JC, Williams NI, De Souza MJ. Prevalence of individual and combined components of the female athlete triad. Med Sci Sports Exerc. 2013;45(5):985–96.
42. Broocks A, Pirke KM, Schweiger U, Tuschl RJ, Laessle RG, Strowitzki T, et al. Cyclic ovarian function in recreational athletes. J Appl Physiol. 1990;68(5):2083–6.
43. Ellison PT, Lager C. Moderate recreational running is associated with lowered salivary progesterone profiles in women. Am J Obstet Gynecol. 1986;154(5):1000–3.
44. Winters KM, Adams WC, Meredith CN, Loan MD, Lasley BL. Bone density and cyclic ovarian function in trained runners and active controls. Med Sci Sports Exerc. 1996;28(7):776–85.
45. Beals KA, Manore MM. Disorders of the female athlete triad among collegiate athletes. Int J Sport Nutr Exerc Metab. 2002;12(3):281–93.
46. Cobb KL, Bachrach LK, Greendale G, Marcus R, Neer RM, Nieves J, et al. Disordered eating, menstrual irregularity, and bone mineral density in female runners. Med Sci Sports Exerc. 2003;35(5):711–9.
47. Beals KA, Hill AK. The prevalence of disordered eating, menstrual dysfunction, and low bone mineral density among US collegiate athletes. Int J Sport Nutr Exerc Metab. 2006;16(1):1–23.
48. Nichols JF, Rauh MJ, Barrack MT, Barkai HS, Pernick Y. Disordered eating and menstrual irregularity in high school athletes in lean-build and nonlean-build sports. Int J Sport Nutr Exerc Metab. 2007;17(4):364–77.
49. Glass AR, Deuster PA, Kyle SB, Yahiro JA, Vigersky RA, Schoomaker EB. Amenorrhea in Olympic marathon runners. Fertil Steril. 1987;48(5):740–5.
50. Shangold MM, Levine HS. The effect of marathon training upon menstrual function. Am J Obstet Gynecol. 1982;143(8):862–9.
51. Dale E, Gerlach DH, Wilhite AL. Menstrual dysfunction in distance runners. Obstet Gynecol. 1979;54(1):47–53.
52. Sanborn CF, Martin BJ, Wagner WW Jr Is athletic amenorrhea specific to runners? Am J Obstet Gynecol. 1982;143(8):859–61.
53. Feicht CB, Johnson TS, Martin BJ, Sparkes KE, Wagner WW Jr Secondary amenorrhoea in athletes. Lancet. 1978;2(8100):1145–6.
54. Pettersson F, Fries H, Nillius SJ. Epidemiology of secondary amenorrhea. I. Incidence and prevalence rates. Am J Obstet Gynecol. 1973;117(1):80–6.
55. Singh KB. Menstrual disorders in college students. Am J Obstet Gynecol. 1981;140(3):299–302.
56. Bachmann GA, Kemmann E. Prevalence of oligomenorrhea and amenorrhea in a college population. Am J Obstet Gynecol. 1982;144(1):98–102.
57. Nichols JF, Rauh MJ, Lawson MJ, Ji M, Barkai HS. Prevalence of the female athlete triad syndrome among high school athletes. Arch Pediatr Adolesc Med. 2006;160(2):137–42.
58. Hoch AZ, Pajewski NM, Moraski L, Carrera GF, Wilson CR, Hoffmann RG, et al. Prevalence of the female athlete triad in high school athletes and sedentary students. Clin J Sport Med. 2009;19(5):421–8.
59. Barrack MT, Rauh MJ, Nichols JF. Prevalence of and traits associated with low BMD among female adolescent runners. Med Sci Sports Exerc. 2008;40(12):2015–21.
60. Pollock N, Grogan C, Perry M, Pedlar C, Cooke K, Morrissey D, et al. Bone-mineral density and other features of the female athlete triad in elite endurance runners: a longitudinal and cross-sectional observational study. Int J Sport Nutr Exerc Metab. 2010;20(5):418–26.
61. Thompson SH. Characteristics of the female athlete triad in collegiate cross-country runners. J Am Coll Health. 2007;56(2):129–36.
62. Rauh MJ, Nichols JF, Barrack MT. Relationships among injury and disordered eating, menstrual dysfunction, and low bone mineral density in high school athletes: a prospective study. J Athl Train. 2010;45(3):243–52.
63. Reinking MF, Alexander LE. Prevalence of Disordered-Eating Behaviors in Undergraduate Female Collegiate Athletes and Nonathletes. J Athl Train. 2005;40(1):47–51.

64. Meyer NL, Shaw JM, Manore MM, Dolan SH, Subudhi AW, Shultz BB, et al. Bone mineral density of Olympic-level female winter sport athletes. Med Sci Sports Exerc. 2004;36(9):1594–601.
65. Vardar SA, Vardar E, Altun GD, Kurt C, Ozturk L. Prevalence of the female athlete triad in Edirne, Turkey. J Sport Sci Med. 2005;4(4):550–5.
66. Wakat DK, Sweeney KA, Rogol AD. Reproductive system function in women cross-country runners. Med Sci Sports Exerc. 1982;14(4):263–9.
67. Abraham SF, Beumont PJ, Fraser IS, Llewellyn-Jones D. Body weight, exercise and menstrual status among ballet dancers in training. Br J Obstet Gynaecol. 1982;89(7):507–10.
68. Calabrese LH, Kirkendall DT. Nutritional and medical considerations in dancers. Clin Sports Med. 1983;2(3):539–48.
69. Robinson TL, Snow-Harter C, Taaffe DR, Gillis D, Shaw J, Marcus R. Gymnasts exhibit higher bone mass than runners despite similar prevalence of amenorrhea and oligomenorrhea. J Bone Miner Res. 1995;10(1):26–35.
70. Williams NI, Helmreich DL, Parfitt DB, Caston-Balderrama A, Cameron JL. Evidence for a causal role of low energy availability in the induction of menstrual cycle disturbances during strenuous exercise training. J Clin Endocrinol Metab. 2001;86(11):5184–93.
71. De Souza MJ, Leidy HJ, O'Donnell E, Lasley B, Williams NI. Fasting ghrelin levels in physically active women: relationship with menstrual disturbances and metabolic hormones. J Clin Endocrinol Metab. 2004;89(7):3536–42.
72. Loucks AB, Mortola JF, Girton L, Yen SS. Alterations in the hypothalamic-pituitary-ovarian and the hypothalamic-pituitary-adrenal axes in athletic women. J Clin Endocrinol Metab. 1989;68(2):402–11.
73. Veldhuis JD, Evans WS, Demers LM, Thorner MO, Wakat D, Rogol AD. Altered neuroendocrine regulation of gonadotropin secretion in women distance runners. J Clin Endocrinol Metab. 1985;61(3):557–63.
74. Scheid JL, De Souza MJ, Hill BR, Leidy HJ, Williams NI. Decreased luteinizing hormone pulse frequency is associated with elevated 24-hour ghrelin after calorie restriction and exercise in premenopausal women. Am J Physiol Endocrinol Metab. 2013;304(1):E109–16.
75. Loucks AB, Thuma JR. Luteinizing hormone pulsatility is disrupted at a threshold of energy availability in regularly menstruating women. J Clin Endocrinol Metab. 2003;88(1):297–311.
76. Williams NI, Young JC, McArthur JW, Bullen B, Skrinar GS, Turnbull B. Strenuous exercise with caloric restriction: effect on luteinizing hormone secretion. Med Sci Sports Exerc. 1995;27(10):1390–8.
77. Williams NI, Reed JL, Leidy HJ, Legro RS, De Souza MJ. Estrogen and progesterone exposure is reduced in response to energy deficiency in women aged 25–40 years. Hum Reprod. 2010;25(9):2328–39.
78. Loucks AB, Verdun M, Heath EM. Low energy availability, not stress of exercise, alters LH pulsatility in exercising women. J Appl Physiol. 1998;84(1):37–46.
79. Loucks AB, Heath EM. Induction of low-T3 syndrome in exercising women occurs at a threshold of energy availability. Am J Physiol. 1994;266(3 Pt 2):R817–23.
80. Ihle R, Loucks AB. Dose-response relationships between energy availability and bone turnover in young exercising women. J Bone Miner Res. 2004;19(8):1231–40.
81. Williams NI, Caston-Balderrama AL, Helmreich DL, Parfitt DB, Nosbisch C, Cameron JL. Longitudinal changes in reproductive hormones and menstrual cyclicity in cynomolgus monkeys during strenuous exercise training: abrupt transition to exercise-induced amenorrhea. Endocrinology. 2001;142(6):2381–9.
82. Balasch J, Vanrell JA. Corpus luteum insufficiency and fertility: a matter of controversy. Hum Reprod. 1987;2(7):557–67.
83. Bullen BA, Skrinar GS, Beitins IZ, von Mering G, Turnbull BA, McArthur JW. Induction of menstrual disorders by strenuous exercise in untrained women. N Engl J Med. 1985;312(21):1349–53.
84. Beitins IZ, McArthur JW, Turnbull BA, Skrinar GS, Bullen BA. Exercise induces two types of human luteal dysfunction: confirmation by urinary free progesterone. J Clin Endocrinol Metab. 1991;72(6):1350–8.
85. Dueck CA, Matt KS, Manore MM, Skinner JS. Treatment of athletic amenorrhea with a diet and training intervention program. Int J Sport Nutr. 1996;6(1):24–40.
86. Kopp-Woodroffe SA, Manore MM, Dueck CA, Skinner JS, Matt KS. Energy and nutrient status of amenorrheic athletes participating in a diet and exercise training intervention program. Int J Sport Nutr. 1999;9(1):70–88.
87. Miller KK, Lee EE, Lawson EA, Misra M, Minihan J, Grinspoon SK, et al. Determinants of skeletal loss and recovery in anorexia nervosa. J Clin Endocrinol Metab. 2006;91(8):2931–7.
88. Mallinson RJ, Williams NI, Olmsted MP, Scheid JL, Riddle ES, De Souza MJ. A case report of recovery of menstrual function following a nutritional intervention in two exercising women with amenorrhea of varying duration. J Int Soc Sports Nutr. 2013;10:34.

Hormonal and Reproductive Changes Associated with Physical Activity and Exercise

12

Jenna C. Gibbs, Rebecca J. Mallinson and Mary Jane De Souza

Abbreviations

ACSM	American College of Sports Medicine
AgRP	Agouti-related protein
BMD	Bone mineral density
CART	Cocaine- and amphetamine-regulated transcript
DR	Cognitive dietary restraint
DT	Drive for thinness
EA	Energy availability
EAMD	Exercise-associated menstrual disturbances
E1G	Estrone-1-glucuronide
E_2	Estradiol
FFM	Fat-free mass
FHA	Functional hypothalamic amenorrhea
FSH	Follicular-stimulating hormone
GH	Growth hormone
GnRH	Gonadotropin-releasing hormone
HPO	Hypothalamic–pituitary–ovarian
IGF-1	Insulin-like growth factor 1
LH	Luteinizing hormone
LPD	Luteal phase defects
NPY	Neuropeptide Y
P_4	Free progesterone
PCOS	Polycystic ovarian syndrome
PdG	Pregnanediol glucuronide
POMC	Proopiomelanocortin
PYY	Peptide YY
REE	Resting energy expenditure
REE/pREE	Ratio of measured REE compared to predicted REE
TT_3	Total triiodothyronine

M. J. De Souza (✉) · J. C. Gibbs · R. J. Mallinson
Department of Kinesiology, Pennsylvania State University, 104 Noll Laboratory, University Park, PA 16802, USA
e-mail: mjd34@psu.edu

Introduction

Menstrual disturbances are frequently observed in exercising women participating in recreational and competitive-level training and sport [1]. The etiology of these menstrual disturbances is linked to inadequate energy intake relative to high energy expenditure, also referred to as an energy deficiency [2, 3]. Exercising women may induce an energy deficit for several reasons: (1) intentionally, that is, to improve performance by modifying body size and composition; (2) compulsively, that is, as a result of disordered eating behavior or pathological weight control; or (3) inadvertently, that is, failing to match energy intake to exercise-induced energy expenditure [4].

Exercising women often adopt restrictive eating behavior to maintain or reduce their body weight as a means to achieve optimal performance or physical attractiveness [5]. Consequently, chronic energy deficiency may develop, which is characterized by hallmark changes in resting energy expenditure (REE) and an endocrine panel of metabolic hormones (i.e., total triiodothyronine (TT_3), ghrelin, peptide YY (PYY),

© Springer Science+Business Media New York 2016

D. Vaamonde et al. (eds.), *Exercise and Human Reproduction*, DOI 10.1007/978-1-4939-3402-7_12

and leptin) that if sustained for a prolonged period, the cumulative effect of these energetic/metabolic disturbances will translate to exercise-associated menstrual disturbances (EAMD) [6].

Chronic energy deficiency promotes compensatory mechanisms to conserve metabolic fuel for vital physiological processes [7]. As already mentioned, these energy conservation mechanisms are associated with changes in energetic and metabolic signals to restore energy homeostasis [6] and to suppress growth-related functions, the least critical physiological process [7]. In the presence of a sustained energy deficiency, the next physiological process considered least vital for survival is reproduction. Consequently, reproductive function is suppressed [7] and typically, reproductive dysfunction results in subclinical (luteal phase defects (LPD) and anovulation) or clinical EAMD (functional hypothalamic amenorrhea (FHA) and oligomenorrhea) [1] (Fig. 12.1). In turn, the energy- and estrogen-deficient environment contributes to loss of bone mass or the failure to achieve peak bone mineral density (BMD) [8].

This constellation of sequelae (chronic energy deficiency, menstrual disturbances, and low BMD) is a syndrome known as the Female Athlete Triad [9]. The Female Athlete Triad was first defined in 1997 by the American College of Sports Medicine (ACSM) as a condition consisting of three components: disordered eating, FHA, and osteoporosis [10–12]. These clinical consequences are most commonly observed in exercising women participating in sports that emphasize a lean physique or low body weight, such as distance running and gymnastics [13]. As more research was completed in this area [14–17], our understanding of the etiology, pathophysiology, and clinical consequences of this syndrome was advanced. In 2007, a revision to the 1997 ACSM position stand [9] was published to present updated scientific information on this syndrome and to offer new recommendations for screening, diagnosis, prevention, and treatment. The most recent conceptual model of the Female Athlete Triad presents energy availability (EA) (with or without disordered eating), menstrual function, and BMD across a continuum of healthy (opti-

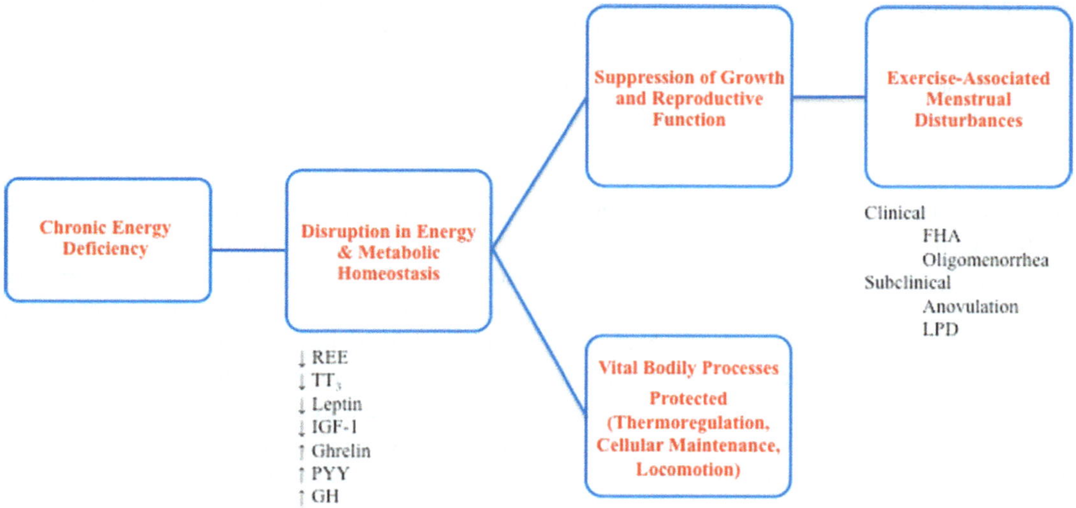

Fig. 12.1 The association between chronic energy deficiency and exercise-associated menstrual disturbances. *Chronic energy deficiency* in both humans and animals promotes a *disruption in energy and metabolic homeostasis* (suppressed resting energy expenditure, total triiodothyronine, leptin, and insulin-like growth factor-1 and increases in ghrelin, peptide YY and growth hormone) and changes in the partitioning of energy wherein the least critical physiological processes for survival are suppressed, that is, *growth and reproductive function*, in order to protect *vital bodily processes*, that is, *thermoregulation, cellular maintenance, and locomotion*. Typically, reproductive dysfunction manifests as subclinical (luteal phase defects and anovulation) or clinical *exercise-associated menstrual disturbances* (functional hypothalamic amenorrhea and oligomenorrhea) in exercising women. *REE* resting energy expenditure, TT_3 total triiodothyronine, *PYY* peptide YY, *IGF-1* insulin-like growth factor-1, *GH* growth hormone *FHA* functional hypothalamic amenorrhea, *LPD* luteal phase defects

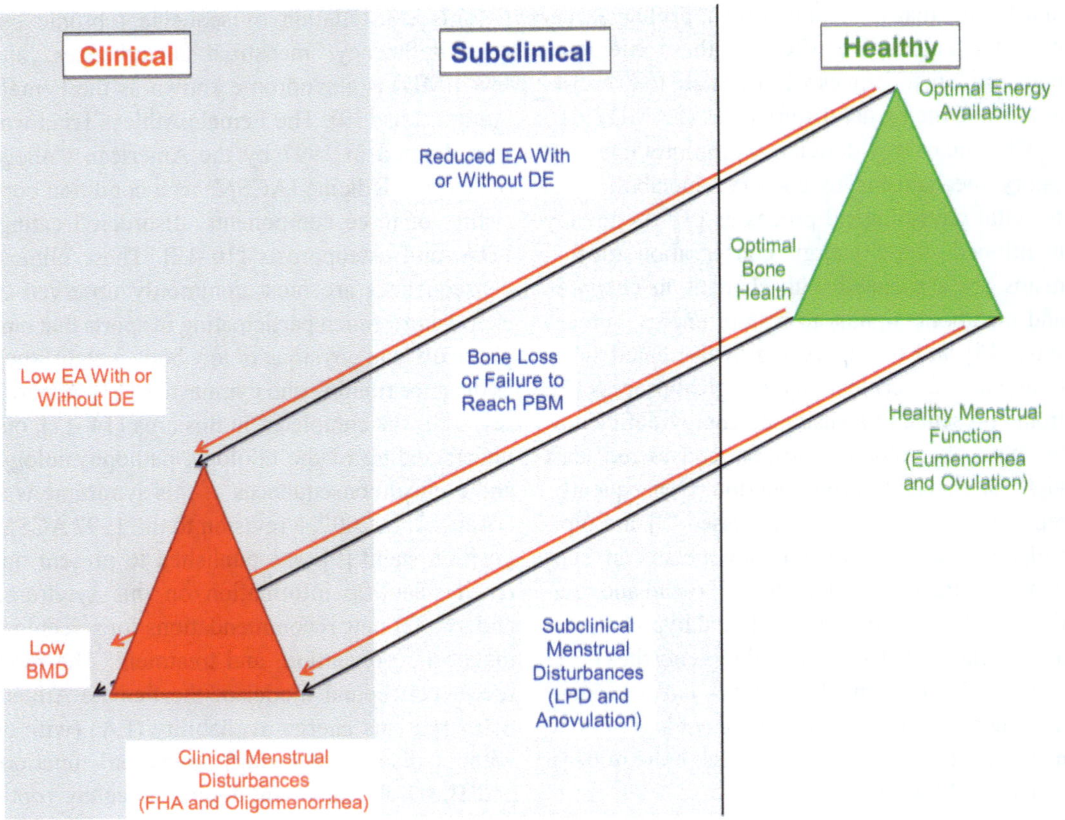

Fig. 12.2 Model of the Female Athlete Triad characterizing an interrelated syndrome of low energy availability *(EA)* with or without disordered eating *(DE)*, low bone mineral density *(BMD)*, and *clinical menstrual disturbances* (functional hypothalamic amenorrhea *(FHA)* and oligomenorrhea) across a continuum of healthy/optimal conditions to *subclinical* and *clinical* disorders. *ED* eating disorders, *LPD* luteal phase defects, *PBM* peak bone mass. (Modified from [6] with permission from Oxford University Press)

mal EA, normal menstrual cycles, and optimal BMD) to increasingly severe pathological presentations (low EA, FHA, and low BMD) [9] (Fig. 12.2).

Exercising women may exist anywhere along the continuum for any one component and can move in either direction (from health → disease and vice versa) at different rates depending on factors such as energy intake, energy expenditure, eating behavior, and type and amount of mechanical loading [9].

The Female Athlete Triad is associated with significant health risks, such as FHA, eating disorders, infertility, premature osteoporosis, and stress fractures [9]. Per se, inadequate exposure to reproductive hormones, particularly estrogen [8, 18] and metabolic hormones, such as insulin-like growth factor 1 (IGF-1), TT_3, and leptin [19, 20], impairs bone mineral accrual during adolescence [21–23] and promotes bone loss during adulthood [24]. Alternatively, healthy energy status promotes both a normal ovulatory menstrual cycle and BMD [8]. This chapter will focus primarily on the metabolic, hormonal, and reproductive changes that occur in exercising women to result in clinical consequences such as chronic energy deficiency and EAMD.

EAMD: Subclinical and Clinical Disturbances

The menstrual cycle is a repetitive process involving the interaction of the hypothalamic–pituitary–ovarian (HPO) axis with cyclic structural and hormonal changes in support of reproduction and fertilization [25]. Each cycle is defined by the interval between the first day of menstrual bleeding in consecutive cycles. The length of the menstrual cycle varies, and a regular cycle length in eumenorrheic women is generally 26–35 days [6]. As mentioned earlier, menstrual disturbances occur across a continuum of severity from subclinical to clinical perturbations [6] wherein estrogen and progesterone exposure decreases with increasing severity (See Chap. 11 for more in-depth discussion of the changes in reproductive hormones and potential associated with physical activity and exercise).

Subclinical menstrual disturbances, which include LPD and anovulation, are the least severe along the spectrum of menstrual disturbances and characterize those perturbations that occur in the presence of apparently regular cycle length [26]. LPD are characterized by a short luteal phase (< 10 days in length), an inadequate luteal phase (suppressed progesterone concentrations) or both [27]. Anovulatory cycles, which represent the more severe form of subclinical menstrual disturbances, are typically characterized by the lack of a luteinizing hormone (LH) surge, absence of an ovulatory event, and subsequently suppressed progesterone concentrations [1]. Subclinical menstrual disturbances occur in cycles of regular length and as such are not readily apparent without hormonal assessment of an entire cycle [1, 6, 27].

Clinical menstrual disturbances, which include oligomenorrhea and FHA, are easily detected by a change in cycle length and represent more severe perturbations of menstrual function [1]. Oligomenorrhea is characterized by long and inconsistent intermenstrual intervals of 36–90 days in length [1]. This severe menstrual disturbance is perhaps the least understood and most difficult perturbation to interpret due to its inconsistent hormonal characteristics. Oligomenorrhea presents with or without ovulation, and analysis of ovarian steroid profiles in oligomenorrheic women has revealed erratic yet overall suppressed estrogen production [1, 6, 28].

The etiology of oligomenorrhea may or may not be hypothalamic in nature, and moreover, oligomenorrheic cycles are often associated with hyperandrogenism [28] and polycystic ovarian syndrome (PCOS), causally linked to infertility in women [29, 30]. Recently, investigators have recommended performing rigorous screening of oligomenorrheic exercising women to rule out the presence of PCOS [28, 31, 32]. FHA, the most severe form of EAMD and the disturbance associated with the most severe health consequences, is typically defined as the absence of menses for at least 90 days [1]. FHA originates at the hypothalamus (specifically the arcuate nucleus) and is the outcome of reduced LH pulsatility, chronically suppressed ovarian steroid hormones (estrone-1-glucuronide, E1G and pregnanediol glucuronide, PdG) and unaltered pituitary responsiveness to gonadotropin-releasing hormone (GnRH) [6, 25]. FHA may be classified as either primary or secondary. Primary amenorrhea is defined as the failure to menstruate by 15 years in girls with secondary sex characteristics [33], whereas secondary amenorrhea is the abnormal cessation of menses after menarche [33]. The criteria defining FHA has varied in the literature [34, 35]; however, a conservative definition specifies no menses for at least 3 months [1, 6].

The Etiology of EAMD in Exercising Women

The etiology of EAMD in exercising women is linked to energy deficiency where dietary energy intake is inadequate relative to energy expenditure [6]. Chronic energy deficiency has been postulated as one of the key factors inducing alterations in metabolic and reproductive function [2, 3, 36–39]. In a wide variety of mammalian species, reproductive function is dependent on cellular availability of oxidizable metabolic fuel [7], and in general, any experimental model of energy deficiency (i.e., famine, eating disorders, excessive exercise, and cold exposure) can present with aberrations in reproductive status [7, 38]. Alternatively, reproduction can be resumed when an optimal energy status is restored [3, 7].

Definitive work by Wade et al. [7] in *Syrian* hamsters demonstrated experimental models in support of the EA hypothesis wherein dietary energy is oxidized to metabolic fuel that is partitioned to five major physiological processes (thermoregulation, locomotion, cellular maintenance, reproduction, and growth). In circumstances of insufficient energy intake, less critical physiological functions, such as growth and reproduction [7], may be compromised to maintain energetic partitioning to vital functions, such as thermoregulation and cellular maintenance. Furthermore, classic work by Warren [40] illustrates that an "energy drain" is incurred in those women who experience an imbalance in energy input versus output and, as such, menarche may be delayed in adolescent girls and reproductive dysfunction may occur in premenopausal women.

Chronic energy deficiency translates to metabolic and reproductive changes via a cascade of energy conservation mechanisms [6, 38, 41]. Once initiated, these compensatory responses may acutely affect energy expenditure, that is, suppression of REE [41, 42], and metabolic hormone concentrations, including reduced TT_3 [36, 41, 42], IGF-1/IGF-binding protein-1 [19, 43], leptin [44], and insulin concentrations [19, 43], and elevated cortisol [19, 45, 46], growth hormone (GH) [19, 43], PYY [47], and ghrelin [48].

In turn, these metabolic indicators of energetic and nutritional status target the HPO axis during an energy deficiency, suppressing the normal release of reproductive hormones, that is, GnRH, LH, and FSH, thereby altering the production of ovarian steroids, that is, E1G and PdG [6] (Fig. 12.3). As such, an energy deficiency ultimately leads to menstrual disturbances character-

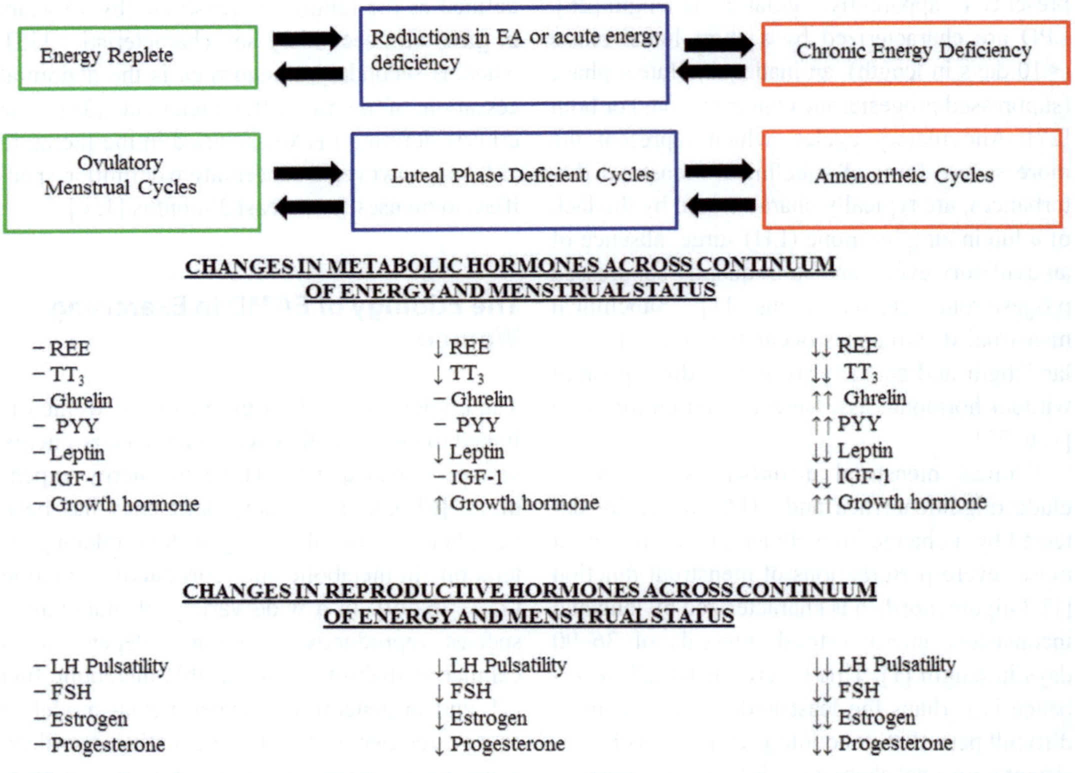

Fig. 12.3 Changes in metabolism and reproductive hormones in exercising women across the continuum of energy and menstrual status. *Reductions in energy availability (EA) or an acute energy deficiency* induce a cascade of alternations in resting energy expenditure *(REE)*, metabolic, and reproductive hormones indicative of an energy deficiency acting to restore energy homeostasis and prevent any significant deviation from a set point of body weight. When an energy deficiency is sustained for a prolonged period of time, reproductive function is suppressed and results in functional hypothalamic amenorrhea (FHA). FHA is characterized by a metabolic hormone profile of supressed REE, total triiodothyronine (*TT_3*), leptin, and insulin-like growth factor-1 (*IGF-1*) and elevated ghrelin,

ized by altered release and production of several hormones from the level of the hypothalamus to the ovaries [25, 49].

Several hypotheses have been proposed to explain the mechanism underlying the induction of menstrual disturbances in exercising women. Past notions wherein "exercise stress" was deemed the primary factor in the induction of reproductive dysfunction have been refuted [2]. A classic theory based on a study by Frisch and McArthur [50] suggested that reproductive function was compromised below a body fat percentage of 22 % and that menarche occurs once percent body fat is above 17 % in young girls. The lack of causal evidence in support of this theory infers that these findings are merely associative, and on the contrary, menstrual abnormalities have been shown to occur at various percentages of body fat above and below these proposed thresholds [51]. In spite of these early hypotheses [50], the accumulating evidence in support of the role of energy status in reproductive function has suggested that those exercising women who are in an energy deficit (also referred to as "low EA" or "energy drain") are more likely to experience metabolic alterations and menstrual disturbances [2, 36–38, 40].

Causal links between the energetic cost of exercise training and menstrual dysfunction have been provided in both human and animal studies wherein energy intake and expenditure have been manipulated. For example, in a prospective exercise training study by Bullen et al. [52], an abrupt increase in exercise training was imposed in 28 untrained, eumenorrheic women for two menstrual cycles wherein the women were randomly assigned to either a weight-loss or weight-maintenance group. Throughout the study, only four of the 28 women (three in the weight-maintenance group, one in the weight-loss group) maintained regular menses during training. Specifically, strenuous exercise combined with weight loss resulted in a higher incidence of an absent LH surge (81 % vs. 42 %) and delayed menarche (75 % vs. 8 %) in previously untrained women compared to similar exercise in women in the weight maintenance group. Alternatively, the participants in the weight-maintenance group did not demonstrate similar changes in hormonal dysfunction over the course of the study. Notably, all participants regained normal menstrual function upon completion of the study.

Taken together, Bullen et al. [52] demonstrated that women who completed strenuous exercise training and dieting for two menstrual cycles were more likely to present with menstrual disturbances than women who only exercised. In a follow-up study by Beitins et al. [53], investigators corroborated menstrual abnormalities with hormonal assessments of LH, FSH, estriol, and free progesterone (P_4) in these same 28 participants. In this sample, 18 of the 28 women demonstrated an inadequate or short luteal phase (20 out of 53 monitored cycles) among the 2 months of exercise training. To this end, these researchers provided evidence of an altered neuroendocrine regulation of key reproductive hormones associated with exercise training in previously ovulating, untrained women, specifically a delay in the LH peak and suppressed LH and P_4 in the luteal phase indicative of corpus luteum dysfunction [52].

Using an animal model, Williams et al. [3] investigated the induction and reversal of EAMD in female *cynomolgus* monkeys. The study protocol involved an increase in exercise volume (12.3 ± 0.9 km/day of running) without changes in energy intake in eight female monkeys. All eight monkeys developed amenorrhea (defined as absence of menses for at least 100 days, with consistently suppressed LH, FSH, estradiol (E_2), and P_4) within a 7–24-month period. Despite interindividual variability, abrupt decreases in LH and FSH, average and peak E_2, and average and peak P_4 occurred within one or two cycles prior to the induction of amenorrhea. Moreover, the induction of amenorrhea was preceded by a decrease in TT_3. Four of the monkeys were then fed supplemental calories (138–181 % of energy

peptide YY (*PYY*), and growth hormone profile of suppressed luteinizing hormone *(LH) pulsatility*, follicular-stimulating hormone *(FSH)*, estrone-1-glucuronide (E1G) and pregnanediol glucuronide (PdG) in comparison to an *energy replete*, regularly menstruating woman. (Modified from [6] with permission from Oxford University Press)

intake during amenorrhea) without a reduction in exercise training volume. These monkeys resumed normal menstrual cycles in response to increased energy intake, and accordingly, the recovery of menses correlated with volume of energy intake during refeeding. In other words, the monkeys that ate the most during refeeding regained menses the fastest.

To summarize, from data in human and animal models, changes in reproductive function secondary to energy deficiency in exercising women are proposed to reflect an energy-deficient environment and present with a suppression of gonadotropin (LH and FSH) release followed by an increase in follicular phase length and a corresponding reduction in luteal phase P_4, which likely precedes the development of amenorrhea [3, 39, 53].

Metabolic Considerations in Amenorrheic Exercising Women

REE

REE is a major factor influencing total daily energy expenditure [54] in premenopausal women, and comprises 60–75 % of an individual's energy losses. REE is defined as the energy necessary to maintain physiological function and homeostasis [54]. When energy intake fails to compensate for energy expenditure, mechanisms of energy conservation are initiated, including a reduction in REE, and concomitant adaptations in fasting circulating hormone concentrations, including reduced TT_3, to restore homeostasis [41, 55, 56]. As such, REE represents an indication of energy status, and previous evidence in exercising women with FHA demonstrates an association between suppressed REE and chronic energy deficiency [8, 41, 47]. Suppressed REE is also often observed concomitant with alterations in metabolic hormonal profiles indicative of energy restriction [41, 42].

De Souza et al. [41] observed decreases in REE controlled for fat-free mass (FFM) alongside changes in key metabolic hormones (TT_3, ghrelin, and leptin) reflective of an energy deficiency in exercising women with FHA versus their ovulatory counterparts (sedentary and exercising). Furthermore, exercising women with subclinical menstrual disturbances (consistently anovulatory or inconsistent presentations of ovulatory, LPD, or anovulatory cycles) also demonstrated lower REE controlled for FFM compared to sedentary, ovulatory women [41].

A ratio of measured REE compared to predicted REE (REE/pREE) has been calculated to provide an estimate of energy deficiency in amenorrheic exercise women [8, 41, 47, 55, 57]. A reduced ratio of REE/Harris–Benedict pREE in the range of 0.60–0.80 has been observed in women with anorexia nervosa during periods of low body weight and prior to refeeding [58–60]. Energy deficiency has been operationally defined as an REE/Harris-Benedict pREE of < 0.90 since this cut-off best discriminated energy status (energy deficiency vs. energy replete) and menstrual status (amenorrheic vs. ovulatory) in exercising women [8, 55, 57]. Exercising women with FHA typically demonstrate REE/pREE between 0.80 and 0.88 [8, 47] reflective of less severe undernutrition compared to women with anorexia nervosa who demonstrate REE/pREE between 0.60 and 0.80 [58–60].

TT_3

TT_3 is the most active form of thyroid hormone and is produced mostly in the peripheral tissues from thyroxine (T_4) [61]. TT_3 is involved in the regulation of several physiological processes such as growth and development, metabolism, body temperature, and heart rate [61]. TT_3 is tightly coupled with REE, oxygen consumption, and total energy expenditure [62]. As such, there is evidence in animal and human experiments that supports the influence of energy and macronutrient intake directly on thyroid hormone status and indirectly on REE [63–65].

TT_3 is frequently used as an indicator of energy deficiency because reductions in TT_3 concentrations are suggested to initiate energy conservation mechanisms to restore homeostasis in underweight individuals [63, 64] and in sedentary, regularly menstruating women exposed to low EA treatment [36, 37]. Onur et al. [66] demonstrated low plasma TT_3 concentrations in women with anorexia nervosa in conjunction with decreased REE. In addition, anorexic women who gained weight exhibited increases in TT_3 concentrations and concomitant increases in REE independent of FFM [66].

Evidence of the effect of manipulations of EA on TT_3 has been demonstrated in a series of eloquent experiments in sedentary, regularly menstruating women [36, 37]. In these studies, reductions in TT_3 were induced in response to low EA treatment and then restored to normal values alongside appropriate increases in EA [36]. Furthermore, these changes in TT_3 were independent of exercise intensity and in particular, it was the energetic cost of exercise on EA that impacted TT_3 concentrations. Loucks et al. [37] revealed in a follow-up study wherein reductions in TT_3 were induced abruptly in participants with EA values between 19 and 25 kcal/kg lean body mass. Thus, TT_3 represents a sensitive marker of changes in EA associated with energy restriction and/or exercise training in women [36, 37].

Low TT_3 has also been linked to reproductive dysfunction in women with anorexia nervosa [67] and exercising women with FHA [41, 68, 69]. Loucks et al. [69] demonstrated suppressed TT_3 concentrations in amenorrheic female athletes but not in their eumenorrheic counterparts. TT_3 concentrations, similar to REE, have been shown to be significantly lower in exercising women with FHA compared to exercising and sedentary ovulatory groups [41]. These findings support the premise that REE and TT_3 are highly correlated. Furthermore, REE and TT_3 present in a dose–response manner across the continuum of menstrual disturbances such that increases in energy conservation (reductions in REE and TT_3) occur in association with increases in the severity of EAMD [41] (Fig. 12.4).

Causal links between thyroid hormones and reproductive function have been demonstrated in both human and animal experiments. In a study by Michaud et al. [70], thyroidarche (the maturation of the thyroid axis occurring between 9–11 years) has been shown to precede menarche (the maturation of the ovarian axis) in healthy adolescents. Williams et al. [3] demonstrated that changes in circulating TT_3 were correlated with the induction and reversal of amenorrhea in female monkeys. Specifically, TT_3 concentrations dramatically decreased by 27 % during the period of restricted dietary energy intake, whereas TT_3 concentrations increased significantly by 18 % during the resumption of regular menses. Taken together, these findings [3, 41, 68, 69] are in agreement that menstrual dysfunction is linked to energy conservation mechanisms underlying an energy deficiency with TT_3 and REE representing key markers of the induction of these mechanisms. Alternatively, recovery of menstrual function is associated with restoring an adequate energy intake relative to energy expenditure [3, 39], which also may be indicated by increases in TT_3 and REE.

Gastrointestinal Peptides: Ghrelin and PYY

Ghrelin and PYY are gastrointestinal peptides that are released into the periphery and travel through blood-borne and neural pathways to influence central mechanisms regulating energy homeostasis [71] and reproductive function [72–77]. Ghrelin is an orexigenic hormone secreted from a distinct endocrine cell type, also known as X/A-like or ghrelin cells, in the stomach and gastrointestinal tract [78, 79]. PYY is an anorexigenic hormone secreted from the endocrine L cells of the intestine [71, 80]. Both ghrelin and PYY control the actions of neuropeptide Y (NPY) and agouti-related protein (AgRP) which interact with proopiomelanocortin (POMC) and cocaine- and amphetamine-regulated transcript (CART) in the arcuate nucleus of the hypothalamus [81].

Ghrelin and PYY have well-documented actions associated with the regulation of energy homeostasis and appetite in exercising and sedentary humans [82, 83]. Ghrelin is the only peripheral gut hormone known to stimulate appetite and per se, increases in ghrelin are proportional to increases in hunger and food intake [82, 84, 85]. The mechanism whereby ghrelin regulates appetite is via the activation of NPY/AgRP and

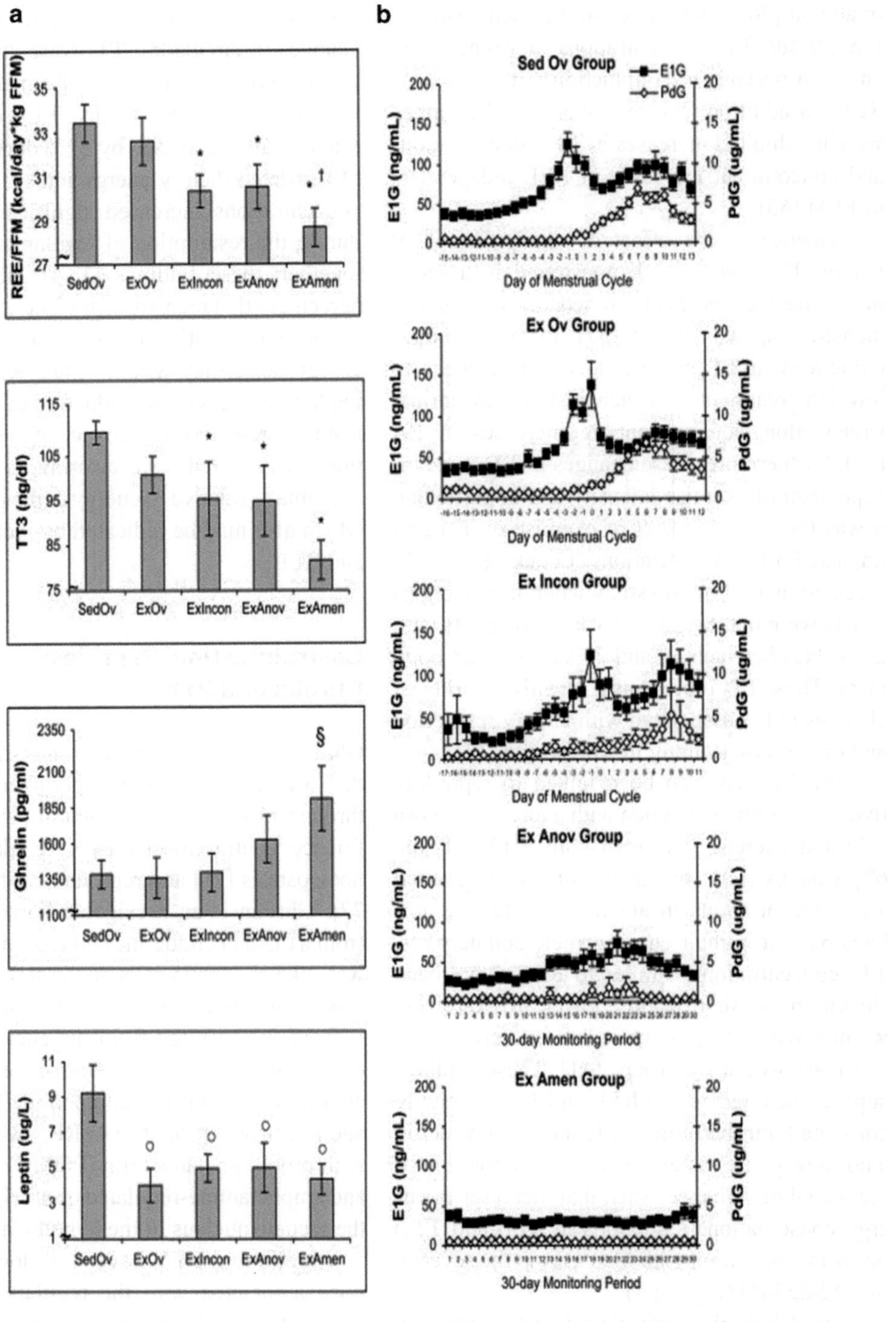

Fig. 12.4 Resting energy expenditure and metabolic hormone characteristics across the continuum of menstrual status. *Panel A* exhibits *REE* per kilogram (kg) fat-free mass *(FFM)* (kcal/day of *REE* per kg of *FFM*), total triiodothyronine *(TT$_3$)* (ng/dL), *ghrelin* (pg/mL), and *leptin* (μg/L) in sedentary and exercising women categorized by menstrual status. Values are mean ± SEM. Significant differences are denoted as follows: * *ExAmen, ExAnov, ExIncon* vs. *SedOv*; + *ExAmen* vs. *ExOv*; § *ExAmen* vs. *SedOv, ExOv, ExIncon, ExAnov*; and ° *ExAmen, ExAnov, ExIncon, ExOv* vs. *SedOv*. *Panel B* exhibits composite graphs of menstrual status depicted by daily estrone 3-glucuronide *(E1G)* (ng/mL) and pregnanediol 3-glucuronide *(PdG)* concentrations (μg/mL) in sedentary and

the suppression of POMC/CART [81]. Ghrelin concentrations increase in the fasted state, and alternatively, decrease in the fed state [84]. Consequently, changes in ghrelin act as metabolic signals for meal initiation and meal termination by rising preprandial and falling postprandial, respectively [84].

Ghrelin is also associated with 24-h energy intake [85] and when administered intravenously in nonobese men and women, ghrelin has been shown to be associated with a large increase in energy intake [86]. PYY has well-recognized actions as a satiety factor [86]. PYY converts to its active form, PYY_{3-36} [87, 88], which subsequently binds to Y2 receptors initiating the opposite actions to ghrelin on the NPY/AgRP and POMC/CART pathway [89].

This cascade of responses at the level of the hypothalamus leads to decreases in energy intake and, supposedly, decreases in body weight [89]. Changes in ghrelin and PYY are proposed to act as homeostatic feedback mechanisms involved in the regulation of energy intake and appetite to return to a predetermined set point and promote resultant changes in body weight [71, 90–92]. As such, alterations in these gut peptides are considered pivotal in weight loss and weight maintenance in healthy populations [90–92]. These hormones are also implicated as critical factors in the development of clinical outcomes associated with reproductive dysfunction [93] as observed in models of severe chronic energy deficiency, that is, women with anorexia nervosa [94–96] and as observed in models of moderate chronic energy deficiency, that is, exercising women with FHA [6, 47].

Ghrelin is a well-known marker of energy deficiency and chronic undernutrition [6, 47, 94–96]. Studies in women with anorexia nervosa [94–96] and exercise-associated FHA [47, 48] have consistently observed elevated fasting ghrelin concentrations compared to control groups. Interestingly, women with anorexia nervosa [94, 97, 98] do not demonstrate the typical meal-induced decline in ghrelin and furthermore, total ghrelin secretion over a subsequent 12-h period is in fact elevated compared to healthy controls [94].

Similarly, De Souza et al. [48] observed elevations in fasting ghrelin in exercising women with FHA, 85 % higher than exercising women with LPD/anovulation and exercising and sedentary ovulatory women. Changes in total ghrelin patterns, to include fasting, mealtime peak, and nocturnal peak, have been observed in premenopausal normal-weight women following a 3-month diet and exercise intervention resulting in a negative energy balance [91, 92]. Specifically, Leidy et al. [91] demonstrated that 24-h ghrelin is elevated after diet- and exercise-induced weight loss. Furthermore, these investigators demonstrated that circulating ghrelin is sensitive to changes in body weight. Such findings in energy-deficient populations are perplexing such that despite elevated fasting ghrelin concentrations, these women consistently report suppressed hunger, lower energy intake and/or weight loss [47, 48, 99, 100]. Thus, the mechanism whereby exercising women with FHA present with chronically low energy intake or lose body weight despite elevated ghrelin concentration is complex and involves both physiological and psychological explanations.

There is emerging interest in examining the role of PYY in the etiology of chronic energy deficiency and associated menstrual disturbances in exercising women with FHA. Notably, elevated PYY concentrations have been observed in anorexic women [101–103]. As such, a metabolic profile wherein both fasting PYY and ghrelin concentrations are elevated is proposed to have an anorexigenic effect such that PYY may restrain the orexigenic effects of ghrelin in women with anorexia nervosa [101] and exercising women with FHA [47]. In a study by Scheid et al. [47],

exercising women categorized by menstrual status. *E1G* and *PdG* data for *SedOv*, *ExOv*, and *ExIncon* groups are aligned by LH peak, defined as day 0. The *ExAnov* and *ExAmen* participants' *E1G* and *PdG* data are aligned by chronological day of daily urinary hormone collection. Number of days depicted for *ExAmen* participants is the mean cycle length of the menstruating participants. Values are mean ± SEM. *SedOv* sedentary ovulatory, *ExOv* exercising ovulatory, *ExIncon* exercising ovulatory, luteal phase defect and anovulatory inconsistent cycles, *ExAnov* exercising anovulatory, *ExAmen* exercising amenorrheic. (Reprinted from [41] with permission from Elsevier)

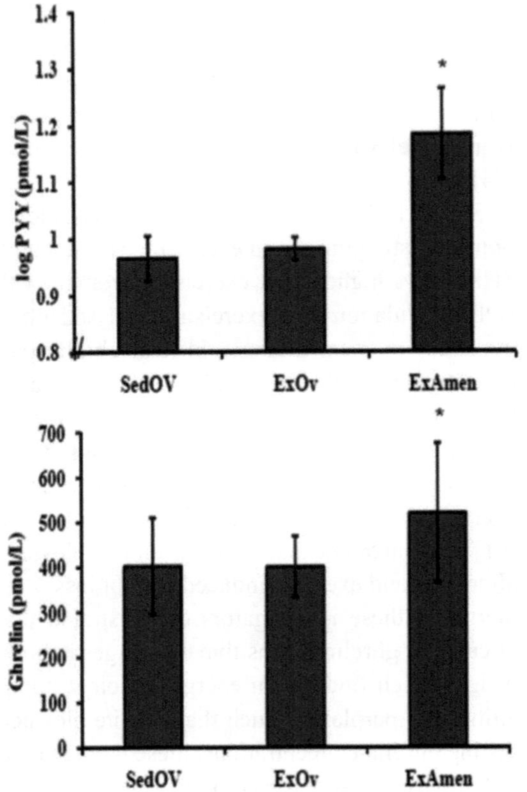

Fig. 12.5 Fasting total peptide YY *(PYY)* and *ghrelin* concentrations in sedentary *(SedOv)* ($n=8$) and exercising women with ovulatory cycles *(ExOv)* ($n=20$) compared to exercising women with amenorrhea *(ExAmen)* ($n=20$). *ExAmen* had higher fasting total log *PYY* (*Log-PYY*, pmol/L) and *ghrelin* (pmol/L) compared to *SedOv* and *ExOv* groups. *$p<0.05$ vs. *SedOv* and *ExOv*. Results are expressed as mean ± SEM. (Reprinted from [47] with permission from Elsevier)

elevated fasting ghrelin concentrations concomitant with elevated fasting PYY were shown in exercising women with FHA similar to women with anorexia nervosa (Fig. 12.5). Additionally, fasting PYY concentrations were negatively correlated with REE/FFM indicative of the association between appetite-related hormones and energy conservation mechanisms [47]. Taken together, chronically elevated fasting PYY may represent a physiological mechanism in support of energy restriction in exercising women with FHA despite elevated fasting ghrelin concentrations.

From a psychological standpoint, subclinical and clinical disordered eating behavior is another pathway to chronic energy deficiency in exercising women with FHA [55, 57]. It is hypothesized that appetite-related hormones (i.e., ghrelin and PYY) might represent underpinnings of an eating behavioral phenotype associated with a greater susceptibility to chronic energy deficiency and EAMD [47, 55]. Researchers have recently examined the relationship between gut hormones and psychometric indicators of eating behavior, such as the drive for thinness (DT) subscale [47, 55]. Evidence of a link between subclinical, and if severely elevated clinical, elevations in DT score and a metabolic profile indicative of chronic energy deficiency has been exhibited in exercising women [47, 55, 57]. Accordingly, De Souza et al. [55] demonstrated that women with high DT present with significantly higher ghrelin concentrations compared to women with normal DT. Thus, a high DT may contribute to the suppression of energy intake in the presence of elevated ghrelin concentrations. Scheid et al. [47] also found a positive correlation between fasting PYY concentrations and DT score in women categorized by exercise (exercising vs. sedentary) and menstrual status (FHA vs. ovulatory). Interestingly, despite consistently observing a positive correlation between DT and cognitive dietary restraint DR scores [55, 57, 104], DR has been notably unsuccessful at discriminating energy status (differences in REE controlled for FFM or REE/pREE and metabolic hormones such as TT_3, ghrelin, and PYY) [104]. Women with higher DR scores do not differ from women with normal DR scores with respect to ghrelin and PYY concentrations [104]. In summary, elevated PYY concentrations, with simultaneously elevated ghrelin, are suggested to prevent compensatory increases in energy intake secondary to psychological markers of subclinical disordered eating (i.e., high DT) and increased exercise energy expenditure in exercising women with FHA [47, 55].

Several researchers have explored the effect of acute exercise on ghrelin and PYY to better understand the regulation of energy balance in nonobese and obese populations [105–107]. A well-documented suppression of appetite has been consistently observed in response to an acute exercise bout [105–108] and has been suggested to promote a decrease in relative energy intake in both women and men. Experimental findings by Hubert et al. [108] demonstrated that a diet-induced energy deficit increased hunger, whereas an exercise-induced energy deficit did not. These results suggest that a lack in initiative to match energy intake to exercise energy expenditure may be biologically driven [4]. Furthermore, high carbohydrate diets, routinely prescribed in endurance athletes, may perpetuate the ad libitum energy deficit following exercise [109–111]. This mechanism, known as "exercise-induced anorexia," is complex, but appetite-related hormones have been proposed as contributing factors [106, 107]. Suppressed concentrations of acylated ghrelin have been demonstrated during aerobic exercise [105–107] and interestingly, ad libitum energy intake following an exercise bout has been shown to be similar to ad libitum energy intake following a rest condition [105]. However, exercise-induced suppression of ghrelin seems to be temporary, and it is per se elevations in circulating PYY concentrations that oppose the actions of ghrelin to promote satiety and chronic energy restriction [106, 107]. This anorexigenic hormone profile following exercise has been proposed as the mechanism whereby gut hormones suppress appetite [106] and lead to an uncoupling between energy intake and energy expenditure. If sustained for prolonged periods, this phenomenon is thought to support "inadvertent under eating" where exercising women simply do not consume enough energy to compensate for exercise energy expenditure [4]. "Inadvertent under eating" has been hypothesized to lead to the development of chronic energy deficiency in exercising women [4]. Therefore, the cumulative effect of this anorexigenic appetite-related hormone profile at rest and following exercise is advanced as an explanation for the induction of a chronic energy deficiency and EAMD in exercising women.

Ghrelin and PYY are proposed as key metabolic signals in a complex network of mechanisms underlying disruption or restoration of energy homeostasis and reproductive function in exercising women [72, 93] (Fig. 12.6). As such, energy deficiency-induced changes in ghrelin and PYY are advanced as important factors involved in the suppression of the HPO axis [89, 93] and, ultimately, the transition to FHA. Ghrelin has been linked to reproductive function by directly acting on hypothalamic neurons in the arcuate nucleus or indirectly altering GnRH pulsatility [89, 93] to result in suppressed LH secretion and pulsatility [72].

Experiments in animals [73, 74, 112] and men [75, 76] have demonstrated a direct relationship between elevated ghrelin and reproductive suppression (specifically via decreased LH secretion). A recent study by Scheid et al. [72] examined the impact of diet- and exercise-induced weight loss on LH pulsatility in premenopausal women. Scheid et al. [72] found decreases in LH pulse frequency alongside increases in 24-h mean ghrelin in the participants who underwent exercising training and lost weight. Change in LH pulse frequency was negatively associated with the change in mean 24-h ghrelin and change in peak ghrelin at lunch [72]. These findings infer that ghrelin is involved in the suppression of LH pulsatility associated with an energy deficiency in premenopausal trained women and, to this end, elevated ghrelin concentrations may have a suppressive effect on reproduction. These findings extend to menstrual cyclicity as observed in women with anorexia nervosa and exercising women with FHA, both clinical populations that typically experience reproductive suppression concomitant with elevated ghrelin concentrations [48, 99, 100]. Future prospective intervention research is necessary to determine the role of ghrelin and PYY in the induction and resumption of menstrual function in women with EAMD.

Leptin

Leptin, an adipocyte-secreted protein product of the *ob* gene, has been proposed as a factor involved in the hormonal regulation of both reproductive function and energy homeostasis in humans [113]. Leptin is implied to play a role in the coordinated response of the HPO axis to metabolic fuel availability [113]. Leptin regu-

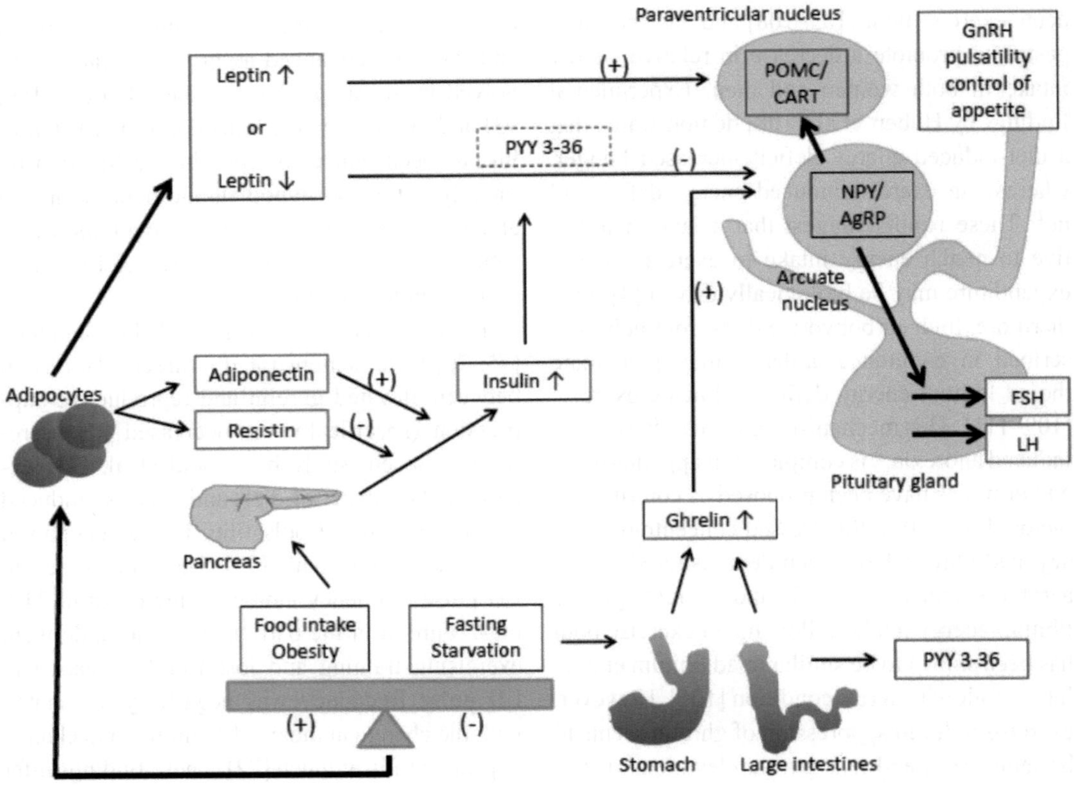

Fig. 12.6 A mechanistic overview of the actions of metabolic and gastrointestinal hormones, including *ghrelin*, peptide YY *(PYY3–36)*, and *leptin*. All of these hormones have the capacity to permeate the blood–brain barrier and regulate appetite via interactions with neuropeptide Y *(NPY)* and agouti-related protein *(AgRP)* and proopiomelanocortin *(POMC)* and cocaine- and amphetamine-regulated transcript *(CART)* located in the *arcuate nucleus*. These hormones also are proposed in the regulation of reproductive function via the hypothalamic–pituitary–ovarian axis affecting gonadotropin-releasing hormone *(GnRH) pulsatility* and downstream release of luteinizing hormone *(LH)* and follicular-stimulating hormone *(FSH)*. (Reprinted from [93] with permission from Elsevier)

lates energy homeostasis via similar pathways as ghrelin and PYY and can also cross the blood–brain barrier to activate leptin receptor-bearing cells in the arcuate nucleus in the hypothalamus [114] (Fig. 12.6). Specifically, leptin is a satiety factor and displays opposing actions to ghrelin [94]. Mechanistically, leptin inhibits NPY/AgPR neurons that subsequently activate POMC/CART to decrease food intake [114]. Experiments in animals [115] and humans [116] infer that hypoleptinemia plays a causal role in the development of obesity. Leptin resistance supposedly perpetuates an obesity-related metabolic profile characterized by a decrease in satiety alongside an increase in food intake and weight gain [117]. Alternatively, leptin is relevant in the neuroendocrine adaptation to starvation, particularly as a protective mechanism in support of restoring a eumetabolic state [118]. In the short term, fasting or severe energy restriction is associated with reduced leptin concentrations independent of declines in fat mass [118]. Diet-induced weight loss also results in a decrease in circulating leptin concentration [119, 120]. As such, leptin represents a metabolic signal controlling short-term and long-term energy homeostasis at both ends of the weight spectrum (energy deprived vs. obese).

Leptin is a well-known indicator of chronic energy status based on a tight correlation between leptin concentration and body fat [121]. Low leptin concentration acts as a metabolic signal to the hypothalamus communicating a state of energy deficiency, whereas high leptin concentration promotes subsequent leptin resistance in support of suppressing appetite and increasing energy expenditure [121]. Models of chronic energy deficiency, that is, women with anorexia nervosa and women with FHA, consistently display suppressed leptin concentrations [44, 94, 122–124]. As such, serum leptin concentrations in women with anorexia nervosa are typically lower than those of normal-weight controls [125–131]. Tolle et al. [94] observed decreased leptin concentrations in women with anorexia nervosa across a 24-h sampling period and, alternatively, exhibited that leptin returns to control values following refeeding. Women with disordered eating and low energy intake, which are less severe presentations of abnormal eating behaviors compared to clinical eating disorders, also demonstrate significantly lower leptin concentrations, with both a lower baseline value and a blunted diurnal leptin pattern [40, 44].

Investigations in animal and human studies suggest that leptin plays a role in the regulation of the reproductive function [20, 129, 130]. In vivo and in vitro experimental findings identified leptin receptors at all levels of the HPO axis [132, 133]. Furthermore, impaired GnRH pulsatility and secretion is demonstrated in leptin-deficient animals and conversely, ovulation is restored by leptin administration [134, 135]. Leptin has also been linked to the maintenance of LH pulsatility [136–138] and the preovulatory LH surge [139].

Similar to women with anorexia nervosa, women with FHA typically present with lower leptin concentrations than their ovulatory counterparts [123]. Miller et al. [122] observed suppressed leptin concentrations in women with FHA compared to age-, weight-, and body-fat-matched eumenorrheic controls. Similarly, Kaufman et al. [124] found a higher incidence of FHA in ballet dancers with suppressed leptin concentrations versus age-, weight-, and body-fat-matched controls. Thus, suppressed leptin concentrations are likely associated with chronic energy restriction in women with FHA versus controls. In exercising and non-exercising female adolescents, Ackerman et al. [140] reported a significant positive association between leptin and LH secretion. Additionally, leptin pulsatile secretion and area under the curve were significant predictors of LH pulsatile secretion and area under the curve, respectively [140]. Therefore, these results suggest that suppressed leptin concentration may act as a metabolic signal communicating nutritional inadequacy from the periphery to the hypothalamus to initiate reproductive consequences.

To date, the relationship between leptin and reproductive function in exercising women with FHA is unclear. Since FHA is a hallmark condition presenting in women with chronic energy deficiency and these women often demonstrate low leptin concentrations, a critical leptin threshold hypothesis has been postulated in the literature [129, 141, 142], which states that a specific leptin concentration (approximately 2.57 ng/mL) is necessary for regular menses to occur in underweight women. However, this hypothesis remains to be confirmed by intervention studies [129, 130, 143, 144]. On the contrary, there is evidence of variability in leptin concentrations in exercising women with FHA and these concentrations have been shown to overlap with concentrations observed in ovulatory women.

Corr et al. [123] demonstrated that the ranges in leptin were similar in exercising women with FHA (range: 0.30–16.98 ng/mL) and ovulatory cycles (range: 2.57–18.28 ng/mL), and after adjusting for adiposity, the difference in leptin concentrations were no longer significant. These results conflict with the premise of a critical leptin threshold associated with menstrual cyclicity [129, 141, 142]. As such, the regulation of menstrual function may not be associated with leptin alone and thus, other factors should also be considered in the etiology of FHA in exercising women [123].

Notably, exercising women irrespective of menstrual status have been shown to present with decreased body fat compared to sedentary controls. To this end, significant differences in leptin concentration between exercising women with FHA versus ovulatory cycles may not be captured [41, 44, 48]. De Souza et al. [41, 48] and Laughlin and Yen [44] observed similar leptin concentrations in women with exercise-associated FHA compared to their ovulatory counterparts. However, definitive work by Laughlin and Yen [44] demonstrated an absence of the diurnal leptin rhythm in only the amenorrheic athletes. This finding indicates an association between nutritional and reproductive status that is not necessarily related to leptin but the absence of a diurnal rhythm pattern in leptin.

The modulation of leptin in women with exercise-associated FHA is complex and represents a research area in need of further investigation. Certain investigators propose that other hormones and metabolic substrates may interact with leptin to promote normal cyclicity [43, 141]. Proposed modulators of leptin concentration include plasma insulin concentration [123, 145], carbohydrate intake [146], glucose availability [147], sympathetic nervous activity [148], glycerol [123], and gonadal steroid environment [149]. Laughlin and Yen [44] proposed that adaptations consistent with an energy deficiency in female athletes such as suppressed insulin and elevated cortisol concentrations may influence leptin regulation. Additionally, the modulation of leptin synthesis differs in exercising women based on menstrual status [123]. In exercising women with FHA, insulin and glycerol explained an additional significant portion of the variance in leptin [123], whereas percent body fat in both amenorrheic and ovulatory exercising women best predicted leptin. Therefore, additional research is necessary to describe the integrated control of reproductive function associated with several hormones and metabolic substrates in addition to leptin in exercising women with FHA.

Leptin has been implicated as a factor involved in the maintenance or restoration of normal menstrual cyclicity in women with FHA [20, 150]. Welt et al. [20] demonstrated that the administration of recombinant leptin restored normal ovulation in three of eight women with FHA. Additionally, leptin administration was associated with improvements in reproductive, thyroid, and GH axes [20], suggesting that leptin represents an important metabolic signal relaying the adequacy of energy stores to the hypothalamus in support of normal reproductive function.

In a study by Chou et al. [150], human recombinant leptin (metreleptin) was administered for 36 weeks in women with FHA. During the intervention, seven of the ten women receiving metreleptin resumed menses, and four of these women were considered to be ovulatory [150]. In addition, E_2 and PdG concentrations increased significantly among the women treated with metreleptin compared to the women treated with placebo [150]. Conversely, in a study by Audi et al. [130], investigators compared amenorrheic and eumenorrheic weight-recovered patients with anorexia nervosa and despite similar BMI and leptin levels in these groups, the eumenorrheic weight-recovered women presented with increased serum-free E_2 and urinary GH compared to their amenorrheic counterparts. These findings infer that leptin plays a permissive role and is not necessarily a prerequisite signal in the restoration of menses [130]. Further, it must be underscored that the other metabolic hormones associated with chronic energy deficiency also need to be fully normalized prior to the recovery of normal menstrual cyclicity [123].

Treatment studies in women with anorexia nervosa present an increase in serum leptin concentrations as weight recovers and this rise in leptin also correlates with increases in gonadotropins [125, 144, 151]. The rise in gonadotropins is indicative of the sensitivity of leptin to changes in weight gain that are associated with activation of the HPO axis [125, 144, 151]. Similar interventional research is required in women with EAMD to elucidate the effect of energy status on circulating leptin concentration and signaling patterns during the induction and resumption of EAMD in women.

Conclusion and Future Directions

In conclusion, physical activity and exercise is associated with changes in metabolic and reproductive hormones in the presence of a chronic energy deficiency and menstrual dysfunction in women. Classic work in animal and human studies have illustrated that the etiology of clinical and subclinical EAMD is linked to a cascade of alternations in REE and metabolic hormones, such as TT_3, ghrelin, PYY, and leptin, indicative of a chronic energy deficiency. Alternatively, the restoration of an optimal energetic/metabolic and reproductive environment in exercising women is associated with favorable changes in REE and the metabolic hormone profile. An interrelated network of these hormonal responses are underpinning factors involved in the mechanisms associated with the induction and recovery of EAMD in exercising women. Dietary strategies to restore menstrual function (i.e., by increasing energy intake) appear to be optimal approaches such that the focus of the treatment is on improvement of the full metabolic hormone profile (occurs within weeks) concomitant with recovery of menstrual function (occurs within months). Future research on the effectiveness of these non-pharmacological treatment strategies associated with EAMD is necessary. Additionally, the identification of metabolic biomarkers indicative of risk for or presence of EAMD in exercising women would be beneficial to prevent and manage EAMD and other Triad-related clinical sequelae.

References

1. De Souza MJ, Toombs RJ, Scheid JL, O'Donnell E, West SL, Williams NI. High prevalence of subtle and severe menstrual disturbances in exercising women: confirmation using daily hormone measures. Hum Reprod. 2010;25(2):491–503.
2. Loucks AB, Verdun M, Heath EM. Low energy availability, not stress of exercise, alters LH pulsatility in exercising women. J Appl Physiol. 1998;84(1):37–46.
3. Williams NI, Helmreich DL, Parfitt DB, Caston-Balderrama A, Cameron JL. Evidence for a causal role of low energy availability in the induction of menstrual cycle disturbances during strenuous exercise training. J Clin Endocrinol Metab. 2001;86(11):5184–93.
4. Loucks AB, Kiens B, Wright HH. Energy availability in athletes. J Sports Sci. 2011;29(Suppl 1):S 7–15.
5. Sundgot-Borgen J, Torstveit MK. Aspects of disordered eating continuum in elite high-intensity sports. Scand J Med Sci Sports. 2010;20(Suppl 2):112–21.
6. De Souza MJ, Williams NI. Physiological aspects and clinical sequelae of energy deficiency and hypoestrogenism in exercising women. Hum Reprod Update. 2004;10(5):433–48.
7. Wade GN, Schneider JE, Li HY. Control of fertility by metabolic cues. Am J Physiol. 1996;270(1 Pt 1):E1–19.
8. De Souza MJ, West SL, Jamal SA, Hawker GA, Gundberg CM, Williams NI. The presence of both an energy deficiency and estrogen deficiency exacerbate alterations of bone metabolism in exercising women. Bone. 2008;43(1):140–8.
9. Nattiv A, Loucks AB, Manore MM, Sanborn CF, Sundgot-Borgen J, Warren MP. American College of Sports Medicine position stand. The female athlete triad. Med Sci Sports Exerc. 2007;39(10):1867–82.
10. Otis CL, Drinkwater B, Johnson M, Loucks A, Wilmore J. American College of Sports Medicine position stand. The female athlete triad. Med Sci Sports Exerc. 1997;29(5):i–ix.
11. Nattiv A, Agostini R, Drinkwater B, Yeager KK. The female athlete triad. The inter-relatedness of disordered eating, amenorrhea, and osteoporosis. Clin Sports Med. 1994;13(2):405–18.
12. Yeager KK, Agostini R, Nattiv A, Drinkwater B. The female athlete triad: disordered eating, amenorrhea, osteoporosis. Med Sci Sports Exerc. 1993;25(7):775–7.
13. Sundgot-Borgen J. Prevalence of eating disorders in elite female athletes. Int J Sport Nutr. 1993;3(1):29–40.
14. Lauder TD, Williams MV, Campbell CS, Davis G, Sherman R, Pulos E. The female athlete triad: prevalence in military women. Mil Med. 1999;164(9):630–5.
15. Cobb KL, Bachrach LK, Greendale G, Marcus R, Neer RM, Nieves J, et al. Disordered eating, menstrual irregularity, and bone mineral density in female runners. Med Sci Sports Exerc. 2003;35(5):711–9.
16. Torstveit MK, Sundgot-Borgen J. The female athlete triad exists in both elite athletes and controls. Med Sci Sports Exerc. 2005;37(9):1449–59.
17. Torstveit MK, Sundgot-Borgen J. The female athlete triad: are elite athletes at increased risk? Med Sci Sports Exerc. 2005;37(2):184–93.
18. Zanker CL, Swaine IL. Relation between bone turnover, oestradiol, and energy balance in women distance runners. Br J Sports Med. 1998;32(2):167–71.
19. Laughlin GA, Yen SS. Nutritional and endocrine-metabolic aberrations in amenorrheic athletes. J Clin Endocrinol Metab. 1996;81(12):4301–9.
20. Welt CK, Chan JL, Bullen J, Murphy R, Smith P, DePaoli AM, et al. Recombinant human leptin in women with hypothalamic amenorrhea. N Engl J Med. 2004;351(10):987–97.
21. Bailey DA, McKay HA, Mirwald RL, Crocker PR, Faulkner RA. A six-year longitudinal study of the relationship of physical activity to bone mineral accrual in growing children: the university of Saskatchewan bone mineral accrual study. J Bone Miner Res. 1999;14(10):1672–9.
22. Weaver CM. Adolescence: the period of dramatic bone growth. Endocrine. 2002;17(1):43–8.
23. Bachrach LK. Acquisition of optimal bone mass in childhood and adolescence. Trends Endocrinol Metab. 2001;12(1):22–8.
24. Jonnavithula S, Warren MP, Fox RP, Lazaro MI. Bone density is compromised in amenorrheic women despite return of menses: a 2-year study. Obstet Gynecol. 1993;81(5 (Pt 1)):669–74.
25. Yen SSC. The human menstrual cycle: neuroendocrine regulation. In: Yen SSC, Jaffe RB, Barbieri RL, editors. Reproductive endocrinology, physiolo-

gy, pathophysiology, and clinical management. Philadelphia: W.B. Saunders Co; 1999. pp. 191–217.
26. De Souza MJ. Menstrual disturbances in athletes: a focus on luteal phase defects. Med Sci Sports Exerc. 2003;35(9):1553–63.
27. De Souza MJ, Miller BE, Loucks AB, Luciano AA, Pescatello LS, Campbell CG, et al. High frequency of luteal phase deficiency and anovulation in recreational women runners: blunted elevation in follicle-stimulating hormone observed during luteal-follicular transition. J Clin Endocrinol Metab. 1998;83(12):4220–32.
28. Awdishu S, Williams NI, Laredo SE, De Souza MJ. Oligomenorrhoea in exercising women a polycystic ovarian syndrome phenotype or distinct entity? Sports Med. 2009;39(12):1055–69.
29. Azziz R. Controversy in clinical endocrinology: diagnosis of polycystic ovarian syndrome: the Rotterdam criteria are premature. J Clin Endocrinol Metab. 2006;91(3):781–5.
30. Franks S. Polycystic ovary syndrome. Trends Endocrinol Metab. 1989;1(2):60–3.
31. Sum M, Warren MP. Hypothalamic amenorrhea in young women with underlying polycystic ovary syndrome. Fertil Steril. 2009;92(6):2106–8.
32. Wang JG, Lobo RA. The complex relationship between hypothalamic amenorrhea and polycystic ovary syndrome. J Clin Endocrinol Metab. 2008;93(4):1394–7.
33. American Academy of Pediatrics Committee on Sports Medicine and Fitness. Medical concerns in the female athlete. Pediatrics. 2000;106:610–3.
34. Loucks AB, Horvath SM. Athletic amenorrhea: a review. Med Sci Sports Exerc. 1985;17(1):56–72.
35. Drinkwater BL, Bruemner B, Chesnut CH 3rd. Menstrual history as a determinant of current bone density in young athletes. JAMA. 1990;263(4):545–8.
36. Loucks AB, Callister R. Induction and prevention of low-T3 syndrome in exercising women. Am J Physiol. 1993;264(5 Pt 2):R924–30.
37. Loucks AB, Heath EM. Induction of low-T3 syndrome in exercising women occurs at a threshold of energy availability. Am J Physiol. 1994;266(3 Pt 2):R817–23.
38. Loucks AB, Thuma JR. Luteinizing hormone pulsatility is disrupted at a threshold of energy availability in regularly menstruating women. J Clin Endocrinol Metab. 2003;88(1):297–311.
39. Williams NI, Caston-Balderrama AL, Helmreich DL, Parfitt DB, Nosbisch C, Cameron JL. Longitudinal changes in reproductive hormones and menstrual cyclicity in cynomolgus monkeys during strenuous exercise training: abrupt transition to exercise-induced amenorrhea. Endocrinology. 2001;142(6):2381–9.
40. Warren MP. The effects of exercise on pubertal progression and reproductive function in girls. J Clin Endocrinol Metab. 1980;51(5):1150–7.
41. De Souza MJ, Lee DK, VanHeest JL, Scheid JL, West SL, Williams NI. Severity of energy-related menstrual disturbances increases in proportion to indices of energy conservation in exercising women. Fertil Steril. 2007;88(4):971–5.
42. Myerson M, Gutin B, Warren MP, May MT, Contento I, Lee M, et al. Resting metabolic rate and energy balance in amenorrheic and eumenorrheic runners. Med Sci Sports Exerc. 1991;23(1):15–22.
43. Laughlin GA, Dominguez CE, Yen SS. Nutritional and endocrine-metabolic aberrations in women with functional hypothalamic amenorrhea. J Clin Endocrinol Metab. 1998;83(1):25–32.
44. Laughlin GA, Yen SS. Hypoleptinemia in women athletes: absence of a diurnal rhythm with amenorrhea. J Clin Endocrinol Metab. 1997;82(1):318–21.
45. Loucks AB, Mortola JF, Girton L, Yen SS. Alterations in the hypothalamic-pituitary-ovarian and the hypothalamic-pituitary-adrenal axes in athletic women. J Clin Endocrinol Metab. 1989;68(2):402–11.
46. De Souza MJ, Maguire MS, Maresh CM, Kraemer WJ, Rubin KR, Loucks AB. Adrenal activation and the prolactin response to exercise in eumenorrheic and amenorrheic runners. J Appl Physiol. 1991;70(6):2378–87.
47. Scheid JL, Williams NI, West SL, VanHeest JL, De Souza MJ. Elevated PYY is associated with energy deficiency and indices of subclinical disordered eating in exercising women with hypothalamic amenorrhea. Appetite. 2009;52(1):184–92.
48. De Souza MJ, Leidy HJ, O'Donnell E, Lasley B, Williams NI. Fasting ghrelin levels in physically active women: relationship with menstrual disturbances and metabolic hormones. J Clin Endocrinol Metab. 2004;89(7):3536–42.
49. Knobil E, Plant TM, Wildt L, Belchetz PE, Marshall G. Control of the rhesus monkey menstrual cycle: permissive role of hypothalamic gonadotropin-releasing hormone. Science. 1980;207(4437):1371–3.
50. Frisch RE, McArthur JW. Menstrual cycles: fatness as a determinant of minimum weight for height necessary for their maintenance or onset. Science. 1974;185(4155):949–51.
51. Loucks AB. Energy availability, not body fatness, regulates reproductive function in women. Exerc Sport Sci Rev. 2003;31(3):144–8.
52. Bullen BA, Skrinar GS, Beitins IZ, von Mering G, Turnbull BA, McArthur JW. Induction of menstrual disorders by strenuous exercise in untrained women. N Engl J Med. 1985;312(21):1349–53.
53. Beitins IZ, McArthur JW, Turnbull BA, Skrinar GS, Bullen BA. Exercise induces two types of human luteal dysfunction: confirmation by urinary free progesterone. J Clin Endocrinol Metab. 1991;72(6):1350–8.
54. Poehlman ET. A review: exercise and its influence on resting energy metabolism in man. Med Sci Sports Exerc. 1989;21(5):515–25.
55. De Souza MJ, Hontscharuk R, Olmsted M, Kerr G, Williams NI. Drive for thinness score is a proxy indicator of energy deficiency in exercising women. Appetite. 2007;48(3):359–67.

56. O'Brian JT, Bybee DE, Burman KD, Osburne RC, Ksiazek MR, Wartofsky L, et al. Thyroid hormone homeostasis in states of relative caloric deprivation. Metabolism. 1980;29(8):721–7.
57. Gibbs JC, Williams NI, Scheid JL, Toombs RJ, De Souza MJ. The association of a high drive for thinness with energy deficiency and severe menstrual disturbances: confirmation in a large population of exercising women. Int J Sport Nutr Exerc Metab. 2011;21(4):280–90.
58. Melchior JC, Rigaud D, Rozen R, Malon D, Apfelbaum M. Energy expenditure economy induced by decrease in lean body mass in anorexia nervosa. Eur J Clin Nutr. 1989;43(11):793–9.
59. Polito A, Fabbri A, Ferro-Luzzi A, Cuzzolaro M, Censi L, Ciarapica D, et al. Basal metabolic rate in anorexia nervosa: relation to body composition and leptin concentrations. Am J Clin Nutr. 2000;71(6):1495–502.
60. Konrad KK, Carels RA, Garner DM. Metabolic and psychological changes during refeeding in anorexia nervosa. Eat Weight Disord. 2007;12(1):20–6.
61. Silverthorn DU editor. Human physiology: an integrated approach. 4th ed. San Francisco: Pearson Education, Inc.; 2009.
62. Danforth E Jr, Burger AG. The impact of nutrition on thyroid hormone physiology and action. Annu Rev Nutr. 1989;9:201–27.
63. Wimpfheimer C, Saville E, Voirol MJ, Danforth E Jr, Burger AG. Starvation-induced decreased sensitivity of resting metabolic rate to triiodothyronine. Science. 1979;205(4412):1272–3.
64. Burger AG, Berger M, Wimpfheimer K, Danforth E. Interrelationships between energy metabolism and thyroid hormone metabolism during starvation in the rat. Acta Endocrinol (Copenh). 1980;93(3):322–31.
65. Rosenbaum M, Hirsch J, Murphy E, Leibel RL. Effects of changes in body weight on carbohydrate metabolism, catecholamine excretion, and thyroid function. Am J Clin Nutr. 2000;71(6):1421–32.
66. Onur S, Haas V, Bosy-Westphal A, Hauer M, Paul T, Nutzinger D, et al. L-tri-iodothyronine is a major determinant of resting energy expenditure in underweight patients with anorexia nervosa and during weight gain. Eur J Endocrinol. 2005;152(2):179–84.
67. Bannai C, Kuzuya N, Koide Y, Fujita T, Itakura M, Kawai K, et al. Assessment of the relationship between serum thyroid hormone levels and peripheral metabolism in patients with anorexia nervosa. Endocrinol Jpn. 1988;35(3):455–62.
68. Berga SL, Mortola JF, Girton L, Suh B, Laughlin G, Pham P, et al. Neuroendocrine aberrations in women with functional hypothalamic amenorrhea. J Clin Endocrinol Metab. 1989;68(2):301–8.
69. Loucks AB, Laughlin GA, Mortola JF, Girton L, Nelson JC, Yen SS. Hypothalamic-pituitary-thyroidal function in eumenorrheic and amenorrheic athletes. J Clin Endocrinol Metab. 1992;75(2):514–8.
70. Michaud P, Foradori A, Rodriguez-Portales JA, Arteaga E, Lopez JM, Tellez R. A prepubertal surge of thyrotropin precedes an increase in thyroxine and 3,5,3'-triiodothyronine in normal children. J Clin Endocrinol Metab. 1991;72(5):976–81.
71. Huda MS, Wilding JP, Pinkney JH. Gut peptides and the regulation of appetite. Obes Rev. 2006;7(2):163–82.
72. Scheid JL, De Souza MJ, Hill BR, Leidy HJ, Williams NI. Decreased luteinizing hormone pulse frequency is associated with elevated 24-hour ghrelin after calorie restriction and exercise in premenopausal women. Am J Physiol Endocrinol Metab. 2013;304(1):E109–16.
73. Fernandez-Fernandez R, Tena-Sempere M, Navarro VM, Barreiro ML, Castellano JM, Aguilar E, et al. Effects of ghrelin upon gonadotropin-releasing hormone and gonadotropin secretion in adult female rats: in vivo and in vitro studies. Neuroendocrinology. 2005;82(5–6): 245–55.
74. Vulliemoz NR, Xiao E, Xia-Zhang L, Germond M, Rivier J, Ferin M. Decrease in luteinizing hormone pulse frequency during a 5-hour peripheral ghrelin infusion in the ovariectomized rhesus monkey. J Clin Endocrinol Metab. 2004;89(11):5718–23.
75. Lanfranco F, Bonelli L, Baldi M, Me E, Broglio F, Ghigo E. Acylated ghrelin inhibits spontaneous luteinizing hormone pulsatility and responsiveness to naloxone but not that to gonadotropin-releasing hormone in young men: evidence for a central inhibitory action of ghrelin on the gonadal axis. J Clin Endocrinol Metab. 2008;93(9):3633–9.
76. Kluge M, Schussler P, Uhr M, Yassouridis A, Steiger A. Ghrelin suppresses secretion of luteinizing hormone in humans. J Clin Endocrinol Metab. 2007;92(8):3202–5.
77. Messini CI, Dafopoulos K, Chalvatzas N, Georgoulias P, Messinis IE. Effect of ghrelin on gonadotrophin secretion in women during the menstrual cycle. Hum Reprod. 2009;24(4):976–81.
78. Kojima M, Hosoda H, Date Y, Nakazato M, Matsuo H, Kangawa K. Ghrelin is a growth-hormone-releasing acylated peptide from stomach. Nature. 1999;402(6762):656–60.
79. Date Y, Kojima M, Hosoda H, Sawaguchi A, Mondal MS, Suganuma T, et al. Ghrelin, a novel growth hormone-releasing acylated peptide, is synthesized in a distinct endocrine cell type in the gastrointestinal tracts of rats and humans. Endocrinology. 2000;141(11):4255–61.
80. Batterham RL, Cohen MA, Ellis SM, Roux CW L, Withers DJ, Frost GS, et al. Inhibition of food intake in obese subjects by peptide YY3-36. N Engl J Med. 2003;349(10):941–8.
81. Kamegai J, Tamura H, Shimizu T, Ishii S, Sugihara H, Wakabayashi I. Chronic central infusion of ghrelin increases hypothalamic neuropeptide Y and Agouti-related protein mRNA levels and body weight in rats. Diabetes. 2001;50(11):2438–43.

82. Nakazato M, Murakami N, Date Y, Kojima M, Matsuo H, Kangawa K, et al. A role for ghrelin in the central regulation of feeding. Nature. 2001;409(6817):194–8.
83. Horvath TL, Diano S, Sotonyi P, Heiman M, Tschop M. Minireview: ghrelin and the regulation of energy balance–a hypothalamic perspective. Endocrinology. 2001;142(10):4163–9.
84. Cummings DE, Purnell JQ, Frayo RS, Schmidova K, Wisse BE, Weigle DS. A preprandial rise in plasma ghrelin levels suggests a role in meal initiation in humans. Diabetes. 2001;50(8):1714–9.
85. St-Pierre DH, Faraj M, Karelis AD, Conus F, Henry JF, St-Onge M, et al. Lifestyle behaviours and components of energy balance as independent predictors of ghrelin and adiponectin in young non-obese women. Diabetes Metab. 2006;32(2):131–9.
86. Wren AM, Bloom SR. Gut hormones and appetite control. Gastroenterology. 2007;132(6):2116–30.
87. Grandt D, Schimiczek M, Beglinger C, Layer P, Goebell H, Eysselein VE, et al. Two molecular forms of peptide YY (PYY) are abundant in human blood: characterization of a radioimmunoassay recognizing PYY 1–36 and PYY 3–36. Regul Pept. 1994;51(2):151–9.
88. Grandt D, Schimiczek M, Struk K, Shively J, Eysselein VE, Goebell H, et al. Characterization of two forms of peptide YY, PYY(1–36) and PYY(3–36), in the rabbit. Peptides. 1994;15(5):815–20.
89. Hill JW, Elmquist JK, Elias CF. Hypothalamic pathways linking energy balance and reproduction. Am J Physiol Endocrinol Metab. 2008;294(5):E827–32.
90. Scheid JL, De Souza MJ, Leidy HJ, Williams NI. Ghrelin but not peptide YY is related to change in body weight and energy availability. Med Sci Sports Exerc. 2011;43(11):2063–71.
91. Leidy HJ, Dougherty KA, Frye BR, Duke KM, Williams NI. Twenty-four-hour ghrelin is elevated after calorie restriction and exercise training in non-obese women. Obesity (Silver Spring). 2007;15(2):446–55.
92. Leidy HJ, Gardner JK, Frye BR, Snook ML, Schuchert MK, Richard EL, et al. Circulating ghrelin is sensitive to changes in body weight during a diet and exercise program in normal-weight young women. J Clin Endocrinol Metab. 2004;89(6):2659–64.
93. Budak E, Fernandez Sanchez M, Bellver J, Cervero A, Simon C, Pellicer A. Interactions of the hormones leptin, ghrelin, adiponectin, resistin, and PYY3-36 with the reproductive system. Fertil Steril. 2006;85(6):1563–81.
94. Tolle V, Kadem M, Bluet-Pajot MT, Frere D, Foulon C, Bossu C, et al. Balance in ghrelin and leptin plasma levels in anorexia nervosa patients and constitutionally thin women. J Clin Endocrinol Metab. 2003;88(1):109–16.
95. Tanaka M, Naruo T, Yasuhara D, Tatebe Y, Nagai N, Shiiya T, et al. Fasting plasma ghrelin levels in subtypes of anorexia nervosa. Psychoneuroendocrinology. 2003;28(7):829–35.
96. Misra M, Miller KK, Kuo K, Griffin K, Stewart V, Hunter E, et al. Secretory dynamics of ghrelin in adolescent girls with anorexia nervosa and healthy adolescents. Am J Physiol Endocrinol Metab. 2005;289(2):E347–56.
97. Misra M, Miller KK, Herzog DB, Ramaswamy K, Aggarwal A, Almazan C, et al. Growth hormone and ghrelin responses to an oral glucose load in adolescent girls with anorexia nervosa and controls. J Clin Endocrinol Metab. 2004;89(4):1605–12.
98. Nedvidkova J, Krykorkova I, Bartak V, Papezova H, Gold PW, Alesci S, et al. Loss of meal-induced decrease in plasma ghrelin levels in patients with anorexia nervosa. J Clin Endocrinol Metab. 2003;88(4):1678–82.
99. Schneider LF, Warren MP. Functional hypothalamic amenorrhea is associated with elevated ghrelin and disordered eating. Fertil Steril. 2006;86(6):1744–9.
100. Christo K, Cord J, Mendes N, Miller KK, Goldstein MA, Klibanski A, et al. Acylated ghrelin and leptin in adolescent athletes with amenorrhea, eumenorrheic athletes and controls: a cross-sectional study. Clin Endocrinol (Oxf). 2008;69(4):628–33.
101. Misra M, Miller KK, Tsai P, Gallagher K, Lin A, Lee N, et al. Elevated peptide YY levels in adolescent girls with anorexia nervosa. J Clin Endocrinol Metab. 2006;91(3):1027–33.
102. Nakahara T, Kojima S, Tanaka M, Yasuhara D, Harada T, Sagiyama K, et al. Incomplete restoration of the secretion of ghrelin and PYY compared to insulin after food ingestion following weight gain in anorexia nervosa. J Psychiatr Res. 2007;41(10):814–20.
103. Pfluger PT, Kampe J, Castaneda TR, Vahl T, D'Alessio DA, Kruthaupt T, et al. Effect of human body weight changes on circulating levels of peptide YY and peptide YY3-36. J Clin Endocrinol Metab. 2007;92(2):583–8.
104. Vescovi JD, Scheid JL, Hontscharuk R, De Souza MJ. Cognitive dietary restraint: impact on bone, menstrual and metabolic status in young women. Physiol Behav. 2008;95(1–2):48–55.
105. King JA, Miyashita M, Wasse LK, Stensel DJ. Influence of prolonged treadmill running on appetite, energy intake and circulating concentrations of acylated ghrelin. Appetite. 2010;54(3):492–8.
106. King NA, Caudwell PP, Hopkins M, Stubbs JR, Naslund E, Blundell JE. Dual-process action of exercise on appetite control: increase in orexigenic drive but improvement in meal-induced satiety. Am J Clin Nutr. 2009;90(4):921–7.
107. Martins C, Morgan LM, Bloom SR, Robertson MD. Effects of exercise on gut peptides, energy intake and appetite. J Endocrinol. 2007;193(2):251–8.
108. Hubert P, King NA, Blundell JE. Uncoupling the effects of energy expenditure and energy intake: appetite response to short-term energy deficit induced by meal omission and physical activity. Appetite. 1998;31(1):9–19.

109. Horvath PJ, Eagen CK, Ryer-Calvin SD, Pendergast DR. The effects of varying dietary fat on the nutrient intake in male and female runners. J Am Coll Nutr. 2000;19(1):42–51.
110. Horvath PJ, Eagen CK, Fisher NM, Leddy JJ, Pendergast DR. The effects of varying dietary fat on performance and metabolism in trained male and female runners. J Am Coll Nutr. 2000;19(1):52–60.
111. Stubbs RJ, Hughes DA, Johnstone AM, Whybrow S, Horgan GW, King N, et al. Rate and extent of compensatory changes in energy intake and expenditure in response to altered exercise and diet composition in humans. Am J Physiol Regul Integr Comp Physiol. 2004;286(2):R350–8.
112. Furuta M, Funabashi T, Kimura F. Intracerebroventricular administration of ghrelin rapidly suppresses pulsatile luteinizing hormone secretion in ovariectomized rats. Biochem Biophys Res Commun. 2001;288(4):780–5.
113. Evans JJ, Anderson GM. Balancing ovulation and anovulation: integration of the reproductive and energy balance axes by neuropeptides. Hum Reprod Update. 2012;18(3):313–32.
114. Morton GJ, Schwartz MW. The NPY/AgRP neuron and energy homeostasis. Int J Obes Relat Metab Disord. 2001;25(Suppl 5):S 56–62.
115. Pelleymounter MA, Cullen MJ, Baker MB, Hecht R, Winters D, Boone T, et al. Effects of the obese gene product on body weight regulation in ob/ob mice. Science. 1995;269(5223):540–3.
116. Montague CT, Farooqi IS, Whitehead JP, Soos MA, Rau H, Wareham NJ, et al. Congenital leptin deficiency is associated with severe early-onset obesity in humans. Nature. 1997;387(6636):903–8.
117. Scarpace PJ, Zhang Y. Leptin resistance: a predisposing factor for diet-induced obesity. Am J Physiol Regul Integr Comp Physiol. 2009;296(3):R493–500.
118. Chan JL, Heist K, DePaoli AM, Veldhuis JD, Mantzoros CS. The role of falling leptin levels in the neuroendocrine and metabolic adaptation to short-term starvation in healthy men. J Clin Invest. 2003;111(9):1409–21.
119. Maffei M, Halaas J, Ravussin E, Pratley RE, Lee GH, Zhang Y, et al. Leptin levels in human and rodent: measurement of plasma leptin and ob RNA in obese and weight-reduced subjects. Nat Med. 1995;1(11):1155–61.
120. Weigle DS, Duell PB, Connor WE, Steiner RA, Soules MR, Kuijper JL. Effect of fasting, refeeding, and dietary fat restriction on plasma leptin levels. J Clin Endocrinol Metab. 1997;82(2):561–5.
121. Chan JL, Mantzoros CS. Role of leptin in energy-deprivation states: normal human physiology and clinical implications for hypothalamic amenorrhoea and anorexia nervosa. Lancet. 2005;366(9479):74–85.
122. Miller KK, Parulekar MS, Schoenfeld E, Anderson E, Hubbard J, Klibanski A, et al. Decreased leptin levels in normal weight women with hypothalamic amenorrhea: the effects of body composition and nutritional intake. J Clin Endocrinol Metab. 1998;83(7):2309–12.
123. Corr M, De Souza MJ, Toombs RJ, Williams NI. Circulating leptin concentrations do not distinguish menstrual status in exercising women. Hum Reprod. 2011;26(3):685–94.
124. Kaufman BA, Warren MP, Dominguez JE, Wang J, Heymsfield SB, Pierson RN. Bone density and amenorrhea in ballet dancers are related to a decreased resting metabolic rate and lower leptin levels. J Clin Endocrinol Metab. 2002;87(6):2777–83.
125. Hebebrand J, Blum WF, Barth N, Coners H, Englaro P, Juul A, et al. Leptin levels in patients with anorexia nervosa are reduced in the acute stage and elevated upon short-term weight restoration. Mol Psychiatry. 1997;2(4):330–4.
126. Hebebrand J, van der Heyden J, Devos R, Kopp W, Herpertz S, Remschmidt H, et al. Plasma concentrations of obese protein in anorexia nervosa. Lancet. 1995;346(8990):1624–5.
127. Grinspoon S, Gulick T, Askari H, Landt M, Lee K, Anderson E, et al. Serum leptin levels in women with anorexia nervosa. J Clin Endocrinol Metab. 1996;81(11):3861–3.
128. Mantzoros CS. Obesity, eating disorders and restrained eating: is leptin the missing link? Mol Psychiatry. 1997;2(5):377–80.
129. Kopp W, Blum WF, Ziegler A, Mathiak K, Lubbert H, Herpertz S, et al. Serum leptin and body weight in females with anorexia and bulimia nervosa. Horm Metab Res. 1998;30(5):272–5.
130. Audi L, Mantzoros CS, Vidal-Puig A, Vargas D, Gussinye M, Carrascosa A. Leptin in relation to resumption of menses in women with anorexia nervosa. Mol Psychiatry. 1998;3(6):544–7.
131. Carlo C D, Tommaselli GA, De Filippo E, Pisano G, Nasti A, Bifulco G, et al. Menstrual status and serum leptin levels in anorectic and in menstruating women with low body mass indexes. Fertil Steril. 2002;78(2):376–82.
132. Yu WH, Kimura M, Walczewska A, Karanth S, McCann SM. Role of leptin in hypothalamic-pituitary function. Proc Natl Acad Sci U S A. 1997;94(3):1023–8.
133. Sone M, Osamura RY. Leptin and the pituitary. Pituitary. 2001;4(1–2):15–23.
134. Chehab FF, Lim ME, Lu R. Correction of the sterility defect in homozygous obese female mice by treatment with the human recombinant leptin. Nat Genet. 1996;12(3):318–20.
135. Mounzih K, Lu R, Chehab FF. Leptin treatment rescues the sterility of genetically obese ob/ob males. Endocrinology. 1997;138(3):1190–3.
136. Carro E, Pinilla L, Seoane LM, Considine RV, Aguilar E, Casanueva FF, et al. Influence of endogenous leptin tone on the estrous cycle and luteinizing hormone pulsatility in female rats. Neuroendocrinology. 1997;66(6):375–7.

137. Licinio J, Negrao AB, Mantzoros C, Kaklamani V, Wong ML, Bongiorno PB, et al. Synchronicity of frequently sampled, 24-h concentrations of circulating leptin, luteinizing hormone, and estradiol in healthy women. Proc Natl Acad Sci U S A. 1998;95(5):2541–6.
138. Fenichel RM, Dominguez JE, Mayer L, Walsh BT, Boozer C, Warren MP. Leptin levels and luteinizing hormone pulsatility in normal cycling women and their relationship to daily changes in metabolic rate. Fertil Steril. 2008;90(4):1161–8.
139. Quennell JH, Mulligan AC, Tups A, Liu X, Phipps SJ, Kemp CJ, et al. Leptin indirectly regulates gonadotropin-releasing hormone neuronal function. Endocrinology. 2009;150(6):2805–12.
140. Ackerman KE, Slusarz K, Guereca G, Pierce L, Slattery M, Mendes N, et al. Higher ghrelin and lower leptin secretion are associated with lower LH secretion in young amenorrheic athletes compared with eumenorrheic athletes and controls. Am J Physiol Endocrinol Metab. 2012;302(7):E800–6.
141. Tataranni PA, Monroe MB, Dueck CA, Traub SA, Nicolson M, Manore MM, et al. Adiposity, plasma leptin concentration and reproductive function in active and sedentary females. Int J Obes Relat Metab Disord. 1997;21(9):818–21.
142. Thong FS, McLean C, Graham TE. Plasma leptin in female athletes: relationship with body fat, reproductive, nutritional, and endocrine factors. J Appl Physiol. 2000;88(6):2037–44.
143. Ballauff A, Ziegler A, Emons G, Sturm G, Blum WF, Remschmidt H, et al. Serum leptin and gonadotropin levels in patients with anorexia nervosa during weight gain. Mol Psychiatry. 1999;4(1):71–5.
144. Holtkamp K, Hebebrand J, Mika C, Grzella I, Heer M, Heussen N, et al. The effect of therapeutically induced weight gain on plasma leptin levels in patients with anorexia nervosa. J Psychiatr Res. 2003;37(2):165–9.
145. Malmstrom R, Taskinen MR, Karonen SL, Yki-Jarvinen H. Insulin increases plasma leptin concentrations in normal subjects and patients with NIDDM. Diabetologia. 1996;39(8):993–6.
146. Jenkins AB, Markovic TP, Fleury A, Campbell LV. Carbohydrate intake and short-term regulation of leptin in humans. Diabetologia. 1997;40(3):348–51.
147. Grinspoon SK, Askari H, Landt ML, Nathan DM, Schoenfeld DA, Hayden DL, et al. Effects of fasting and glucose infusion on basal and overnight leptin concentrations in normal-weight women. Am J Clin Nutr. 1997;66(6):1352–6.
148. Rayner DV, Trayhurn P. Regulation of leptin production: sympathetic nervous system interactions. J Mol Med (Berl). 2001;79(1):8–20.
149. Wabitsch M, Blum WF, Muche R, Braun M, Hube F, Rascher W, et al. Contribution of androgens to the gender difference in leptin production in obese children and adolescents. J Clin Invest. 1997;100(4):808–13.
150. Chou SH, Chamberland JP, Liu X, Matarese G, Gao C, Stefanakis R, et al. Leptin is an effective treatment for hypothalamic amenorrhea. Proc Natl Acad Sci U S A. 2011;108(16):6585–90.

Risk Biotypes and the Female Athlete Triad

13

Kathryn E. Ackerman, Maria de Lourdes Eguiguren and Michelle Barrack

Introduction

Data support the many benefits of female competitive athletic participation. Regular exercise increases overall strength and aerobic fitness, thus improving girls' cardiovascular health and lowering their risk of chronic degenerative diseases, such as atherosclerosis and diabetes [1–4]. Sports participation enhances female athletes' self-esteem, self-efficacy, and reduces feelings of depression [5]. Various reports document higher academic performance, cognitive function, and degree completion rates among girls and young women who engage in competitive sports [6, 7]. Furthermore, female athletes partake in tobacco or illicit drug use, and sexual promiscuity to a lesser degree than nonathletes [8, 9]. Therefore, female athletic involvement promotes many positive health, cognitive, and psychogenic effects [10].

The 2012 London Olympic Games were the first Olympics to include only sports in which both females and males could participate. Every sporting event at the London Games had a women's and men's division, and every participating nation was represented by at least one female athlete. In fact, for the first time in US history, there were more female American Olympic participants than male. At the 2014 Sochi Olympics, women finally were added to ski jumping. As women have lobbied for gender equity throughout the globe, and have demonstrated what the female body can do, they have pushed their bodies to new physical limits.

It is well-established that women can safely run ultradistant marathons, swim the English Channel, and climb Mount Everest. American volleyball player, Kerri Walsh-Jennings, even showed the world that she could win an Olympic gold medal while pregnant! But in the process of women pushing their bodies and benefitting from sport, some of the negative consequences of exercise participation in the setting of underfueling have emerged. Thus, this chapter will discuss the effects of inadequate energy availability in sport, the Female Athlete Triad (Triad) , and those athletes most susceptible. Also presented will be the risk biotypes and treatment and prevention strategies to help keep girls and women safely in the game.

K. E. Ackerman (✉)
Division of Sports Medicine, Boston Children's Hospital, Sports Endocrine Research Lab, Neuroendocrine Unit, Massachusetts General Hospital Boston, 319 Longwood Avenue- 6th Floor, Boston, MA 02115, USA
e-mail: kathryn.ackerman@childrens.harvard.edu

M. de Lourdes Eguiguren
Department of Pediatric and Adolescent Medicine, Mayo Clinic, 3040 Avalon Cove Ct NW, Rochester, MN 55901, USA
e-mail: Eguiguren.Maria@mayo.edu

M. Barrack
Department of Family and Consumer Sciences, California State University, 1250 Bellflower Blvd, Long Beach, CA 90840, USA
e-mail: michelle.barrack@csulb.edu

© Springer Science+Business Media New York 2016

D. Vaamonde et al. (eds.), *Exercise and Human Reproduction*, DOI 10.1007/978-1-4939-3402-7_13

The "Female Athlete Triad" Definition

The "Female Athlete Triad," a term first coined in 1992 by the Task Force on Women's Issues of the American College of Sports Medicine (ACSM), described the interrelationships of three distinct conditions: disordered eating (DE), amenorrhea, and osteoporosis [11]. The ACSM's original position statement on the Triad, published in 1997, reported that athletes with DE or eating disorders (EDs) may develop menstrual disturbances due to an inadequate energy intake relative to the energy expended from exercise [12]. The original position proposed that low energy availability may disrupt the gonadotropin releasing hormone (GnRH) pulse generator of the hypothalamus, thus disturbing luteinizing hormone (LH) pulse frequencies from the pituitary, and therefore negatively affecting sex steroids from the gonads. The low concentrations of ovarian hormones found in amenorrheic and oligomenorrheic athletes have been associated with decreased bone mineral density (BMD) and increased rates of bone loss [12].

With more clinical experience and research performed over the subsequent 10 years, the ACSM updated the Triad position statement in 2007 [10]. In the 2007 position paper, the Triad was described as a "spectrum" of energy availability, menstrual function, and BMD. At the ideal end of the spectrum, an athlete has optimal energy availability, eumenorrhea, and optimal bone health, which may then decline to "reduced energy availability with or without DE," low BMD, and/or subclinical menstrual disorders, including oligomenorrhea, luteal deficiency, and anovulation. At the pathologic end of the spectrum are the combination of "low energy availability with or without an ED," functional hypothalamic amenorrhea [FHA; absence of menses caused by suppression of the hypothalamic–pituitary–ovarian (HPO) axis without a known anatomic or organic disease cause], and osteoporosis [10]. This position statement emphasized the concept of a continuum, clarifying that athletes are at risk for developing aspects of the Triad that could have negative consequences without being at the extreme end of the Triad spectrum.

More recently, in 2014, the Female Athlete Triad Coalition published a consensus statement on treatment and return to play for female athletes with the Triad [13]. The purpose of the consensus statement was to provide more comprehensive guidelines regarding screening, assessment, treatment, and management of the components of the Triad and to recommend an algorithm for return to play of Triad athletes at different stages of severity [13]. Additionally, in 2014, the International Olympic Committee (IOC) produced a consensus statement suggesting a change in terminology to "Relative Energy Deficiency in Sport (RED-S)," to reflect a broader scope of the syndrome, including many aspects of physiological function, health, and athletic performance [14]. Because the 2007 Triad Position Statement and the 2014 Triad Coalition Consensus Statement also mention additional potential consequences of the Triad, including increased risk of injury and consequences to endocrine, gastrointestinal, renal, and neuropsychiatric systems as well as effects on musculoskeletal and cardiovascular health [12, 15], for the purposes of this chapter, we will continue to use the term "Triad."

The Interrelationship of the Three Components of the Triad

When discussing the three main components of the Triad, it is widely accepted that maintaining an appropriate level of energy availability (30–45 kcal/kg of fat-free mass/day), by consuming an adequate level of energy relative to exercise energy expenditure, is paramount to optimize health, performance, and injury risk. An energy deficit develops when an athlete is unable to consume sufficient energy to compensate for the calories burned from exercise. Among some athletes, the energy deficit is intentional, as in those with DE/EDs. However, others develop a caloric deficit inadvertently because of a lack of education and knowledge of the nutritional needs related to their sport and exercise. Regardless of the cause of energy deficit, the results can be similar.

Studies by Loucks, De Souza, and others have clearly demonstrated a link between decreased energy availability and menstrual dysfunction [15–17]. We now know that menstrual disturbances are common in female athletes and range from subtle disturbances, such as luteal phase defects (LPD) and anovulation in asymptomatic, eumenorrheic women, to more severe menstrual dysfunction, including oligomenorrhea and amenorrhea. Exercise-associated amenorrhea, a form of FHA, is a disruption in hormone cycling that includes abnormal patterns of GnRH secretion at the hypothalamus. FHA in athletes has been causally linked to decreased energy availability, as energy is diverted away from the reproductive axis to more vital bodily processes, such as cell maintenance and immune function. Suppression of the HPO axis is coupled with energy-conserving mechanisms [10]. For example, amenorrheic athletes have consistently demonstrated lower resting energy expenditure (REE) and triiodothyronine (T3) than their eumenorrheic counterparts [18, 19].

Normal GnRH pulsatility is critical for LH and FSH release from the anterior pituitary. LH and FSH subsequently induce production of a variety of hormones including estradiol, progesterone, androstenedione, testosterone, inhibin, activin, and insulin-like growth factor I (IGF-1). In addition, many hormones and neurotransmitters can modulate GnRH secretion, illustrating the complexity of GnRH control. These include the gonadal steroids, which have positive and negative effects on GnRH pulsatility, as well as prolactin, corticotropin-releasing hormone (CRH), neuropeptide Y (NPY), catecholamines, and opiates. Some factors, including CRH and NPY, also impact areas that affect caloric consumption and appetite. Additionally, appetite regulating hormones, such as leptin, ghrelin, and peptide YY (PYY), can impact GnRH pulsatility, as can hormones such as insulin and IGF-1 [20].

Prior research suggests that many of these complex hormonal processes are disrupted in athletes with FHA. Specifically, amenorrheic athletes have a decrease in GnRH, FSH, LH, estradiol, androgens, insulin, glucose, IGF-1, T3, and leptin [21]. All of the aforementioned hormones have been implicated in bone metabolism. Estrogens have an important antiresorptive effect on bone, as do androgens such as testosterone. Estradiol levels in female athletes correlate highly with lumbar, hip, and whole body BMD in various studies [22]. While the exact mechanism is unclear, clinical and animal data suggest an anabolic role for insulin on bone metabolism [23]. IGF-1 exerts an anabolic effect on bone and the effects of growth hormone are primarily mediated through IGF-1. Hypothyroidism decreases metabolic rate, and while some studies have demonstrated increases in BMD in those with hypothyroidism, bone quality was poor, leading to a positive association between hypothyroidism and increased fracture risk [24]. T3 is important for local IGF-1 secretion in bone, which may account for poor bone quality in patients with hypothyroidism [25].

Leptin acts as a key messenger of nutritional status and influences appetite, energy balance, and reproduction [26]. It exerts centrally and peripherally mediated effects on bone. Centrally, mouse models suggest that leptin induces cortical bone formation, but also induces trabecular bone loss, acting via sympathetic signaling, the GH-IGF-1 axis, kisspeptin, and NPY [27]. Peripherally, leptin increases the expression of osteogenic genes versus adipogenic genes in bone marrow stromal cells, increases osteoblast proliferation, decreases osteoclastogenesis, and has a positive effect on the appendicular skeleton [28].

Athletes with FHA also exhibit an increase in fasting PYY, ghrelin, cortisol, and growth hormone resistance [21, 29, 30]. PYY, an anorexigenic peptide hormone secreted by neuroendocrine L cells of the distal intestine, typically increases in response to caloric intake. Utz et al. demonstrated a strong inverse relationship between mean overnight PYY levels and lumbar, hip, and radius BMD in adult women with anorexia nervosa [31]. In a study of adolescent amenorrheic and eumenorreic athletes and eumenorrheic controls, PYY negatively predicted the bone formation marker, P1NP, as well as lumbar bone mineral apparent density, a surrogate for volumetric bone density [32]. More research is needed to better understand the relationship of PYY and bone.

Ghrelin is secreted primarily by the P/D1 cells in the gastric fundus and is another hormone that reflects energy status. Levels are high in conditions of fasting and hypoglycemia and decrease after food, particularly carbohydrate intake [33]. Ghrelin negatively correlates with BMI, body fat percentage, fat mass, body weight, insulin, T3, and leptin in cross-sectional and longitudinal studies of individuals at the extremes of the weight spectrum: anorexia nervosa and obesity, as well as in athlete studies across the menstrual spectrum: amenorrhea to eumenorrhea [34–38]. De Souza et al. have reported that fasting ghrelin levels are elevated by about 85 % in amenorrheic exercising females compared with sedentary ovulatory women, exercising ovulatory women, and even luteal phase defect/anovulatory exercisers [37]. Direct effects of ghrelin on bone have yet to be fully elucidated, however. Finally, cortisol secretion is higher in amenorrheic athletes than eumenorrheic athletes and controls, and correlates negatively with BMD in those with FHA as well as other hypercortisolemic populations [39].

Interestingly, among athletes with the Triad, treatment through dietary behavioral change and increased intake of energy has been shown to successfully reverse the menstrual cycle disruption and promote normal menstruation and fertility [40–43]. However, prior research indicates that an inability to accrue optimal levels of bone mass during the adolescent years may be irreversible and consequences to bone during the adolescent years may lead to lifelong low bone mass [44, 45].

Additional Consequences of the Triad

Along with effects on menstrual function and bone mass, other negative outcomes of the Triad include increased risk of bone stress or musculoskeletal injury, hindered performance, negative effects on the cardiovascular system (e.g., endothelial dysfunction), metabolic and reproductive dysfunction, and gastrointestinal disorders [10, 46]. Additionally, the Triad, particularly among those with ED or DE, may exhibit psychological comorbidities, including anxiety disorders, depression, low self-esteem, and/or body image disturbances [10]. The following paragraphs will explore three of these additional consequences in more detail: bone and musculoskeletal injury, hindered performance, and endothelial dysfunction.

Bone and Musculoskeletal Injury

The development of a bone stress injury, ranging from a low grade stress reaction to a frank stress fracture, depends on many factors, including those related to nutritional status, biomechanics, bone mass and bone metabolism, impact attenuation, training volume, training surface, among other influences. The Triad negatively impacts several factors, including nutritional status, bone metabolism, and bone mass. Research in healthy women indicates that energy availability below a critical threshold of 30 kcal/kg of fat-free mass/day lowers leptin, estradiol, and IGF-1 [39, 47, 48]. This hormone profile parallels changes in biomarkers of bone formation and resorption consistent with reduced bone formation and enhanced bone loss. This may reduce the body's ability to form new bone and repair microdamage from repetitive exercise loading, stress, and strain. Low energy availability may also contribute to micronutrient deficiencies, which may also limit new bone formation.

In adult women, there is a strong relationship between bone density and fracture risk. Prior reports indicate that in postmenopausal women, for every 1 SD decrease in bone density T-score, fracture risk doubles [49]. However, studies that evaluated the relationship between bone density levels and rate of bone stress injury in adolescents and young adult athletes yield conflicting results. Some research among cross country runners, track and field athletes, and female adolescents report an association between lower bone mass [50, 51] or a family history of osteoporosis [51, 52] and fracture risk; however other studies report no association [53–56]. Two prospective investigations, by Bennell et al. and Kelsey et al., who followed female adult runners for 1–2 years, found a significant negative relationship between bone mass and risk of developing a stress fracture [50, 51]. In a recent study of over 250 active girls and young women, a BMD Z-score <-1.0 was one of the strongest factors associated with the development of bone stress injury. Furthermore, in a study of male and female collegiate athletes, Nattiv et al. found that low BMD negatively influenced time to full return to sport among athletes who had developed a bone stress injury [57].

In addition to low bone mass, DE and menstrual dysfunction (i.e., amenorrhea) correlate with bone stress injury. Five prior studies reported associations between DE and fracture history [53, 54, 58–60]. Runners with a history of stress fracture had higher cognitive dietary restraint [58] or restrictive eating [60], a more prevalent history of anorexia nervosa or bulimia nervosa [59], or scored higher on the EAT-40 [54] than those who never sustained a fracture. A study among ballet dancers also reported that those with stress fracture history more often reported an ED or restrictive eating [53]. FHA and oligomenorrhea have been repeatedly associated with stress fracture. Two prospective studies that evaluated track and field or cross country athletes for 2–5 years found that menstrual irregularity was a significant independent predictor of bone stress injury in their multivariate models [51, 60]. Another found that those who developed stress fractures had fewer menses in the past year [50]. Several other cross-sectional studies found an association between stress fracture history and a history of amenorrhea or oligomenorrhea [51, 52, 54, 55, 59, 61, 62]. Furthermore, a dose–response relationship between the number of Triad-related risk factors and bone stress injury incidence has been noted [63]. These findings provide strong support for the negative effect of the Triad on bone stress injury.

Additionally, the Triad has been linked to the development of soft tissue musculoskeletal injury. Rauh et al. prospectively assessed the rate of musculoskeletal injury among high school athletes participating in a variety of sport types [64]. Among the high school athletes, DE [classified using the Eating Disorder Examination Questionnaire (EDE-Q)], oligomenorrhea or amenorrhea in the past year, and low BMD (Z-score ≤ -2.0) were independently associated with the development of a soft tissue or bone-related musculoskeletal injury [64]. This study provides preliminary evidence, but further research is needed to better clarify the relationships between the Triad and soft tissue musculoskeletal injury.

Performance

While some athletes with an intentional or inadvertent energy deficit may perform well in the short term, *persistent* undereating leads to numerous physiological effects that could negatively affect performance in endurance, power, and skill-based sports. Low energy and carbohydrate intake deplete muscle glycogen stores, leading to premature fatigue. Additionally, reduced carbohydrate intake lowers blood glucose, reducing the supply of energy to the brain, which may hinder cognitive function and promote mental fatigue [65]. Inadequate energy and protein intake wastes muscle stores and further leads to weakness and fatigue, increasing risk of injury. Consistent with these findings, consuming a low-fat diet has been associated with lower calorie intake and reductions in endurance performance among runners [66]. Though few studies specifically address the effect of chronic low energy availability or the Triad on exercise performance, a recent study by Vanheest and colleagues explored this relationship in junior elite swimmers [67]. The athletes were categorized as cyclic or ovarian suppressed based on gonadal hormone status. The ovarian suppressed swimmers had lower energy intake, energy availability, total T3, and IGF-1. The ovarian suppressed swimmers had a 9.8% decline in 400-m swim velocity compared with an 8.2% improvement in the cycling group after 12 weeks of training. Ovarian steroids (progesterone and estradiol), metabolic hormones (T3 and IGF-1), and energy status markers (energy intake and energy availability) were highly correlated with swim velocity [67]. This study demonstrated that when exercise training occurs in the presence of underfueling, it can result in ovarian suppression and energy conservation, and is associated with poor sport performance [67]. Further research directly investigating the effect of low energy availability on athletic performance in athletes representing a variety of sport types is needed.

Endothelial Dysfunction

Triad has also been associated with endothelial dysfunction, a precursor in the development of cardiovascular disease [68]. Shear stress on vascular endothelium leads to nitric oxide (NO) release, which in turn promotes vascular smooth muscle cell (VSMC) dilatation. In addition, NO has anti-atherosclerotic properties including inhibiting platelet aggregation, smooth muscle proliferation, leukocyte adhesion, and LDL oxidation. Estrogen serves a cardioprotective effect by stimulating the endothelial NO synthase (eNOS) signaling system, binding to estrogen receptors of the endothelial cell caveolae, and also via a genomic mechanism, binding to estrogen receptors with a resultant increase in eNOS gene expression [69]. Flow-mediated dilation (FMD) of the brachial artery can be measured using ultrasound. Prior research has found a 95 % positive predictive value of abnormal brachial dilation in predicting coronary endothelial dysfunction [70].

Hoch et al., in their study of 32 collegiate running athletes, found significantly lower FMD in amenorrheic athletes compared with oligomenorrheic and eumenorrheic athletes [71]. Rickenlund et al. studied FMD and lipid profiles in endurance athletes with amenorrhea, oligomenorrhea, and eumenorrhea, along with sedentary eumenorrheic controls. FMD was significantly decreased in the amenorrheic athletes versus the other groups, and the amenorrheic athletes also had the worst lipid profiles (higher total cholesterol and LDL) of the three athlete groups [72]. In a study of teenage amenorrheic and eumenorrheic volleyball players and eumenorrheic non-athlete controls, FMD was again lowest in the amenorrheic athletes [73]. Serum estradiol levels were lowest in the amenorrheic athletes, and levels positively predicted vascular function. In the amenorrheic athletes who became eumenorrheic after quitting their strenuous sporting activity, restored vascular function was associated with increased serum estrogen levels [73]. In a study of 22 professional ballet dancers, 64 % had decreased FMD. The authors found that FMD correlated significantly with serum estrogen and whole body and lumbar BMD [74].

Risk Biotypes and Prevalence

All female athletes are potentially at risk of developing the Triad; however, athletes who participate in sports emphasizing leanness or low body weight may be at increased risk. In a study by Torstveit and Sundgot-Borgen, which included 669 elite female Norwegian athletes, 70.1 % of athletes competing in leanness sports were classified as being at risk for the Triad compared with 55.3 % of athletes in non-leanness sports [75].

Multiple studies have shown that athletes are more susceptible to developing EDs than nonathletes [76–79]. Besides the sociocultural demands placed on females to maintain an "ideal" body shape, elite athletes are confronted with the stress of optimizing performance, meeting the specific requirements of their sport, and being evaluated by coaches and judges on a regular basis [80]. These factors can lead to harmful dieting, the potential development of EDs, low energy availability, hormone disturbances, and low bone mass among leanness sport athletes. For instance, the age of menarche in athletes competing in activities that demand low weight is significantly later than that of nonathletes [81]. Other studies reported higher prevalence of menstrual dysfunction in athletes competing in leanness sports (24.8 %) compared with those competing in non-leanness sports (13.1 %) [82, 83]. In a study of 788 Iranian female competitive athletes (mean age 21.1 ± 4.5 years), Dadgostar et al. found that girls and young women who participated in weight class or endurance sports had a 2–3 times higher risk of developing oligomenorrhea or amenorrhea [84, 85]. Furthermore, other research has shown that females participating in leanness sports have lower BMD than non-leanness sports [86, 87] (See Table 13.1).

Table 13.1 Examples of leanness sports: sports in which leanness and/or a specific body weight are considered important for performance

Endurance sports	Cross-country skiing, cycling, rowing, running, speed skating, and swimming
Aesthetic sports	Cheerleading, dance, figure skating, gymnastics, and synchronized swimming
Weight-class sports	Boxing, judo, kickboxing, lightweight rowing, mixed martial arts, taekwondo, weightlifting, and wrestling
Anti-gravitational sports	Cycling, swimming, and synchronized swimming

Leanness sports often include those that (1) involve high volume training, (2) require revealing uniforms, (3) use weight categories, and/or (4) emphasize a prepubertal body for optimal performance or aesthetics [10]. The following paragraphs include further details about various leanness sport categories and data regarding the increased prevalence of low energy availability (with or without DE/EDs), clinical or subclinical menstrual disturbances, and/or low bone mass for each group.

Endurance Athletes

Studies suggest that endurance athletes exhibit a higher risk of developing DE or EDs, menstrual dysfunction, and low bone mass compared with those participating in other sport types. While the loading nature of endurance sports can be characterized as less osteogenic than ball or other sports involving high- and odd-impact loads, endurance athletes are also at high risk of developing an energy deficit, which negatively impacts bone.

Runners Prior research indicates a higher prevalence of DE/ED among endurance runners, particularly elite competitive runners participating at the collegiate or postcollegiate level. Thompson et al. reported that among a sample of 300 collegiate cross country runners, 19.4% either currently or previously had had an ED [88], while Hulley et al. found that 16% of their sample of elite women distance runners had a current ED [89]. These ED estimates are considerably higher than the 0.5−2% occurrence of anorexia nervosa or bulimia nervosa, respectively, among normal, healthy young adults [17]. Beals and Hill evaluated the eating attitudes and behaviors, menstrual function, and bone mass among 112 US collegiate athletes. They observed that the leanness sport group (consisting largely of endurance runners) reported a significantly higher frequency of moderate to extreme body dissatisfaction, binge eating, and trended ($P=0.08$) toward reporting a self-diagnosed ED more frequently than non-leanness athletes [83]. However, among a sample of 423 high school athletes, Nichols et al. did not find a higher prevalence of DE among girls participating in a leanness (consisting largely of runners) compared with those participating in a non-leanness sport [90]. How the questions were initially asked and the presence or absence of follow-up questioning may have contributed to the differing results.

Previous studies document higher estimates of menstrual dysfunction among endurance runners spanning various ages and levels of competition. Reports indicate that up to 66% of female competitive endurance runners exhibit menstrual disturbances [91–93], values that are approximately 3–5 times higher than the 5–15% [94, 95] prevalence reported in normal, healthy young women and girls. Gibson et al. observed a 66% prevalence of menstrual irregularity among 50 elite endurance runners, while Dusek et al., upon evaluation of 72 female athletes, found a 3 times higher prevalence of secondary amenorrhea among athletes compared with controls, with the highest prevalence of secondary amenorrhea (65%) reported among female endurance runners [93, 96].

Additionally, it is established that adolescent, collegiate, and postcollegiate runners spanning a range of levels of competition exhibit lower bone mass than athletes in other sports. In studies among endurance runners, prevalence estimates of low bone mass are as high as 40%, using a Z-score <-1.0 cutoff. This is significantly higher than the 5–10 % prevalence reported among non-endurance runner athletes, and the 16 % prevalence expected in a normal population distribution [91, 92]. Mudd et al., when comparing data from 99 collegiate athletes participating in 12 sport types, found that endurance runners had lower total body and lumbar spine BMD values when compared with gymnasts and softball players [97, 98]. Robinson et al. evaluated bone mass among a sample of collegiate gymnasts, runners, and nonathlete controls [98]. Runners exhibited significantly lower lumbar spine, femoral neck, and total body BMD compared with the other two groups [98].

Triathletes, Cyclists, and Swimmers There has been less research investigating Triad in triathletes, endurance cyclists, and swimmers. However, the current literature suggests that athletes participating in these sports also exhibit an elevated prevalence of Triad components. Studies report elevated levels of DE attitudes and behaviors, including food restriction and body image distortion, in triathletes [99, 100]. This is consistent with findings from Hoch et al., who reported a 60 % prevalence of energy deficiency and 40 % prevalence of current or previous amenorrhea among a group of club triathletes [101]. Interestingly, research assessing bone mass among triathletes has not found reduced bone mass in this group of athletes [102]. One explanation accounting for the lack of low BMD levels among the triathletes may be the fact that many club triathletes begin training and competing in the sport in adulthood, after peak bone mass is achieved. This may lessen any potential negative effects to bone that could have occurred if the athlete were exposed to the DE and subsequent energy deficits during adolescence. Most of these studies did not take into account the various weight-bearing activities the triathletes may have participated in during their childhood/adolescent periods. As individuals begin training for triathlon at a younger age, further investigations will be needed to better understand the unique risk profile among triathletes.

Little research has evaluated eating attitudes and behaviors, menstrual function, and bone mass among female endurance cyclists. Unlike other endurance sports, more has been reported in male rather than female cyclists. Among these studies, male cyclists exhibit an increased pressure to lose weight, have elevated scores on the eating attitudes test (EAT), and have a higher use of diet pills, laxatives, and self-induced vomiting, particularly during competition [102]. Additionally, studies report lower levels of bone mass among endurance cyclists, particularly among male master cyclists with an average of 20 years of participation in the sport. According to Nichols et al., male master cyclists had significantly lower lumbar spine and total hip BMD compared with age-matched controls and young adult cyclists [103]. Additionally, 15 % of the male master cyclists exhibited BMD T-scores <-2.5, the cutoff used in the diagnosis of osteoporosis in older adults [103]. Further research is needed among female cyclists to better identify the prevalence of DE, menstrual dysfunction, and low bone mass.

The few studies evaluating swimmers also identified an elevated prevalence of DE. Da Costa and colleagues assessed eating attitudes and behaviors using three surveys among adolescent swimmers and reported a 44 % prevalence of DE [104]. Anderson and Petrie utilized the Eating Disorder Diagnosis questionnaire and found that approximately 28 % of collegiate swimmers met criteria for either subclinical DE or a clinical ED [105]. Additionally, among Norwegian elite athletes, swimmers exhibited lower BMD values than athletes in ball or power sports [106]. In a systematic review of 64 studies focused on swimmers' bone mass, structure, and metabolism, most of the studies found similar BMD values in swimmers versus sedentary controls, but many showed lower BMD in swimmers versus other sport groups, including gymnasts, runners, volleyball players, soccer players, and basketball players [107]. This indicates that while swimming does not exert a weight-bearing, osteogenic effect on bone, it does not appear to be associated with a high prevalence of low BMD. There may be a lower rate of menstrual dysfunction and higher fat mass in swimmers versus athletes in leaner sports, which complicates conclusions regarding the additive effects of non-weight-bearing exercise in the setting of eumenorrhea. Future research is needed to investigate the prevalence of menstrual dysfunction among swimmers with better control for menstrual function and lean and fat mass.

Aesthetic Sports

One important concern of athletes participating in leanness activities is the focus on body appearance in their sports. For example, a high lean to fat mass ratio is important in sports such as figure skating, gymnastics, and sports dance for aesthetic reasons [80]. Aesthetic sports are associated with a negative self-perception during puberty because of body maturation, physiological, and behavioral changes [108]. Moreover, certain characteristics of some athletes such as competitiveness, concern with performance and body shape, and perfectionism, have also been associated with eating problems [109]. Therefore, all of these factors can influence athletes to start irregular eating behaviors, in order to improve performance and meet a specific body shape. Van Durme et al. showed that eating pathology is prevalent in aesthetic sports, especially in female athletes, and that eating concerns and sport-related factors such as competition anxiety could contribute to the dieting behavior of these athletes [110]. In general, studies of female skaters, dancers, and gymnasts have revealed a tendency toward energy-restricted diets, and high rates of clinical and subclinical EDs [79, 110–112]. One meta-analysis concluded that elite athletes in lean sports, especially dance, were at higher risk of developing EDs [109]. A large study of elite athletes showed that the prevalence of EDs in female athletes was as high as 42 % in aesthetic sports compared with 24 % in endurance, 17 % in technical, and 16 % in ball games sports [78]. Additionally, it is common to start aesthetic activities in early childhood. In a study of 5 and 7-year-old girls, those participating in aesthetic sports reported higher weight concerns than girls in nonaesthetic sports or no sports [113]. Over time, those who had reported high weight concerns or body dissatisfaction across ages 5 to 7 reported higher dietary restraint, poorer eating attitudes, and increased likelihood of dieting at age 9, regardless of their weight status [114]. A study in elite female synchronized skaters observed significant differences between perceived ideal and current body shape and reported a low mean energy intake of just 26 kcal/kg body weight [115], well below what would be required to fuel exercise expenditure and basic metabolic and reproductive functioning.

Menstrual dysfunction is more common in sports emphasizing thinness, with a prevalence ranging between 1.4 and 27.7 % [86]. However, some studies have reported particularly higher prevalence of menstrual disorders in aesthetic athletes. A study including 311 female athletes reported menstrual irregularities in 38.1 % of aesthetic athletes (including dance, sports, diving, and gymnastics) compared with 19 % in endurance athletes and team/anaerobic sports [116]. A meta-analysis showed that 36.5–70 % of professional ballet dancers had a lifetime history of menstrual disturbances and also reported a 4-year incidence of secondary amenorrhea as high as 85 % [117]. Similarly, studies in gymnasts have shown high prevalence of menstrual irregularities (71.4–78 %) and delayed puberty [87, 118]. Delayed puberty has also been reported in figure skaters, especially in elite and more specialized pair skaters [119].

Aesthetic sports have been variably associated with bone impairment. Some studies have suggested that despite the high prevalence of menstrual irregularities and EDs, female gymnasts and figure skaters have improved BMD in weight-bearing bone sites [120, 121]. Stress fractures in figure skaters have been linked more to the excessive forces placed on the skeleton rather than lower BMD [122]. Moreover, gymnasts have shown improved BMD compared with runners, despite menstrual status [98, 123, 124]. A possible explanation is that the mechanical loading of this sport, may counterbalance the negative effect of menstrual disorders and hypoestrogenism. Conversely, other studies of gymnasts and dancers found lower BMD than other athletes and controls, and concluded that the protective effects of exercise on bone is lost in the presence of menstrual irregularities [125, 126]. A study in retired gymnasts showed greater spinal BMC and BMD, trabecular volumetric density, and strength in gymnasts without a history of amenorrhea, but not in those with a history of primary or secondary amenorrhea [126]. It is possible that weight-bearing exercise improves BMD when athletes do not have accompanying metabolic, menstrual or eating irregularities, and that bone impairment is more pronounced later in life, when the protective effect of exercise is lost.

Weight-Class Sports

Other athletes at higher risk of developing the Triad are those competing in sports with weight categories such as wrestling, judo, karate, and rowing. In these sports, athletes wish to gain a competitive advantage by obtaining the lowest possible body weight or weight category while maximizing strength [80]. It is known that athletes competing in combat sports periodically practice short-term weight fluctuations prior to a competition season. One study reported that almost 90% of judoists participating in international tournaments had a rapid weight loss of 5–10% of their body weight over a 7-day period [127]. Although weight reduction in these athletes is motivated mainly by optimization of performance, meeting sport-specific demands, and is often seasonal [128, 129], a high proportion of weight-class athletes are using extreme weight-control methods [130]. The rules of some sports may be associated with the risk of continuous dieting, energy deficit, and/or use of extreme weight loss methods that can be detrimental to health and performance [130]. Even though high-impact-loading sports have a protective effect on bone [131, 132] and wrestlers have increased BMD at the lumbar spine [133], chronic states of low energy availability and cyclic weight lost can have negative effects on health parameters such as nutritional status, hormonal status, and immune functions [128].

For instance, one study of adolescent female athletes showed that the exercise-induced osteogenic benefits were less when rowing training was associated with low estrogen and progesterone metabolite excretion [134]. Also a small study in lightweight female rowers showed that 76% of athletes had a history of menstrual irregularities and it was associated with lower lumbar BMD [135]. There is a lack of literature regarding the specific prevalence of Triad among female athletes competing in weight class sports. However, there are several studies in which these sports are included and categorized as "leanness sports," with the prevalence of all components of the Triad and stress fractures being higher than other sports [86, 87, 136]. Finally, small studies in male wrestlers have demonstrated hormonal alterations such as lower testosterone and estradiol levels, and found that estrogen was a more important predictor of BMD than testosterone in this population [137, 138]. This evidence suggests that female and male athletes competing in these sports could be at risk of hormonal, bone, and nutritional impairment.

Other Sports

There are other sports in which body composition and weight play an important role because of mechanical and gravitational factors. This is the case with ski jumping and high jump, which require vertical movements of the body, with fat mass being considered a disadvantage [80]. A lower body weight may result in improved speed in sports that require the body to be lifted against the earth's gravitational field [139]. For this reason, most ski jumpers are underweight and can present with EDs. For instance, the mean BMI in ski jumpers has decreased from 23.6 kg/m^2 in 1970 to 19.4 kg/m^2 in 2002, with values as low as 16.4 kg/m^2 in World Cup athletes that year[139]. In an effort to prevent the myriad negative health effects on such athletes, there have been recent changes in the regulations of this sport in order to make it less attractive and even disadvantageous to be severely underweight. For instance, athletes with lower weight must have shorter skis, which represent an aerodynamic disadvantage that may compensate for the lower weight.

Weight concerns are also quite relevant in horseracing. Jockeys are required to have very low weight and strict weight control during the competitive seasons. Unfortunately, weight control measures in these athletes include saunas, smoking, excessive exercise, skipping meals, and restricting food intake in the 24 h prior to racing that certainly are detrimental to health [140, 141]. In one study of jockeys, energy intake was well below the recommendation for such athletes [142]. Furthermore, other studies have shown low BMD and disrupted hormonal activity in jockeys [143–145]. Thus, it is important to maintain a high level of suspicion to identify athletes at risk of the Triad, especially in sports with emphasis on lean appearance.

Special Populations

Adolescents Adolescents represent a unique subpopulation of athletes, since they must meet the needs and demands of their sport and the physiological demands of growth and development. Key processes occurring during the adolescent years include the development of secondary sex characteristics, initiation of the menstrual cycle (in females), and the process of bone mineral accrual. If an adolescent athlete does not consume sufficient energy to compensate for the energy expended from their sport and growth, over time, various metabolic and hormonal adaptations ensue, creating an environment that suppresses bone mineral accumulation, sexual maturation, and normal menstrual cyclicity. This is due to a disruption of a variety of growth hormones (i.e., insulin-like growth factors), metabolic and appetite-regulating hormones (i.e., leptin, ghrelin, TSH, and T3), and gonadal hormones (i.e., follicle-stimulating hormone, luteinizing hormone, estradiol, androgens, and progesterone) [48, 146–149]. Furthermore, energy deficiency and stress may increase cortisol levels, which augments the negative effects to bone development, sexual maturation, and menstruation [146].

Several investigators have evaluated the prevalence of the Triad among adolescent athletes. Based on the original definition of the Triad (from the 1993 ACSM Position Statement) [150], including DE/EDs, amenorrhea, and osteoporosis, among 170 high school athletes participating in a range of interscholastic sports, there was an 18 % prevalence of DE/EDs based on the EDE-Q, 24 % prevalence of menstrual irregularity (amenorrhea or oligomenorrhea), and a 22 % prevalence of low bone mass (Z-score ≤ -1) [90]. In another study, by Hoch et al., using the updated definition of the Triad (the 2007 ACSM Position Statement) [10], which includes low energy availability as the first component, there was a 36 % prevalence of low energy availability (defined as 45 kcal/kg/lean body mass), a 54 % prevalence of menstrual abnormalities, and a 16 % prevalence of low bone mass (Z-score ≤ -2.0) [151]. In this latter study, the athletes exhibited a higher prevalence of menstrual abnormalities, but a lower prevalence of low bone mass compared with sedentary controls [151].

Barrack et al. identified female adolescent endurance runners as an athlete population with an elevated prevalence of low BMD and reported a 40 versus 10 % prevalence of BMD Z-scores ≤ -1.0, among runners compared with adolescent non-runner athletes [152]. In a subsequent investigation, risk factors associated with low bone mass among the adolescent runners included elevated dietary restraint, amenorrhea, and participating in five or more seasons of an endurance running sport [92]. In a 3-year follow-up among the high school runner sample (mean age of 16 years at baseline and age 19 years at follow-up) the authors found that despite an average approximate 10 pound weight gain during the 3 years, about 90 % of runners with low BMD at baseline continued to exhibit low bone mass at the follow-up assessment [153]. These findings underscore the importance of accruing sufficient bone mass during the adolescent years, since it may be difficult to significantly increase bone mass during and after the third decade of life [44].

Male Athletes While research efforts center on female athletes in the study of the Triad, the occurrence of a similar male athlete Triad, consisting of (1) low energy availability, (2) disruptions in the hypothalamic pituitary gonadal, growth hormone, thyroid, and adrenal axes, and (3) insults to bone mass, has not been thoroughly evaluated. Currently, little research exists on male athlete groups at risk and the few studies that have evaluated adolescent and young adult male athletes are limited by a small sample size.

Current literature indicates that males participating in certain weight class sports are at risk of developing DE behaviors to cut weight. Wrestling stands as one of the highest profile sports associated with DE, as it is not uncommon for wrestlers to attempt competition in a weight class below their natural weight, as mentioned previously [102]. Behaviors reported among wrestlers to lose weight include self-induced vomiting, sauna use, excessive exercise, use of laxatives, diuretics, and wearing heavy clothing [102]. Misuse of these weight-cutting techniques has been associated with the death of at least three collegiate wrestlers [154]. As a result, new regulations have been implemented to promote the health and safety of the athletes, which included banning pathogenic behaviors and changing the timing of weigh-ins [102].

Other male athlete groups at risk of developing DE, altered hormone levels, and reduced bone mass include endurance runners and cyclists. As mentioned previously, male young adult endurance cyclists report increased pressure to lose weight, use of pathogenic behaviors, and DE, while male master cyclists exhibit reduced bone mass [102]. Several studies report significantly lower testosterone levels among male endurance runners compared with nonathlete controls [155–159], while other investigators identified lower lumbar spine BMD levels in male endurance runners compared with non-runner athletes [160] or nonathlete controls ([161]).

Interestingly, investigators report negative associations between running training volume and bone mass or sex hormones among male endurance runners [162, 163]. In these instances, running training volume may serve as a proxy for exercise energy expenditure, which may suggest that the insults to bone and reductions in the sex hormone levels may be due to an energy deficit, much like the effect of an energy drain on sex hormone levels and bone in the Female Athlete Triad. This is a notable finding since short-bout, explosive exercise movements are associated with increased testosterone levels [164]. These studies suggest that male, like female, endurance runners may be subject to similar hormone disruptions and bone-related risks.

While traditionally testosterone was thought to be the critical hormone in males for bone health, more recent research suggests that it is the conversion of androgens to estradiol that makes it beneficial to bone. In fact, in a study by Ackerman et al., estradiol levels, BMI, and resistance training were found to be more important determinants of BMD in male collegiate athletes (wrestlers, runners, and golfers) than testosterone [137]. Other male athlete sport groups with preliminary data potentially implicating them as an at-risk sport associated with behaviors and outcomes consistent with the Triad include ski jumping, sport climbing, sprint football, bodybuilding, weight lifting, rowing, and horseracing [102]. Future research is needed to more comprehensively outline male athletes′ risk profile and potential negative short- and long-term effects.

Treatment

A multidisciplinary approach is required to treat and prevent further complications of Triad. Involvement of a primary care physician and/or sport physician, dietician, psychiatrist or therapist, team coaches, and family members is necessary during recovery of athletes. There are non-pharmacological and pharmacological therapies for treating the Triad; however, there is still some controversy about which is the best approach.

In general, the primary goal of treatment is to normalize body weight and energy balance with lifestyle and dietary modifications. Diet and exercise regimen modifications should be the main focus to increase daily energy availability. When addressing these issues with athletes, a restrained and stepwise manner is advisable. For instance, modest exercise reduction (10–20 %) and an increase of energy availability to at least

30–45 kcal/kg of fat-free mass per day are reasonable goals [10]. Caloric intake should be increased slowly to avoid raising the patient's fear of becoming fat and to avoid the negative sequelae of "refeeding syndrome." Referral to a sports nutritionist/dietitian will also promote a gradual increase in energy intake and optimize overall nutrient intake. Restoration of menstrual cycles and increases in BMD have been seen with weight gain in several studies [10, 165]. Though getting BMD to an optimal range is sometimes not possible, an improvement in BMD may be seen depending on the timing, severity, and duration of energy restriction [166]. Athletes should be advised to achieve a BMI ≥ 18.5 kg/m^2 or 90 % of ideal body weight [13]. However, these weight goals may be difficult to attain and are not always sustained over time. It is also important to remember that some athletes may need to achieve even higher weight goals to restore normal menstrual function, because they may have a higher amount of lean muscle mass and a relatively lower amount of adipose tissue.

Another challenge for the physician is that many athletes are reluctant to follow activity and dietary recommendations. Therefore, pharmacological therapy may need to be considered in conjunction with behavior modifications. Oral contraceptive pills (OCPs) containing estrogen and progestin are commonly used in athletes suffering amenorrhea, although evidence regarding the effects on bone density is inconclusive [13, 167, 168]. Recently, research has focused on alternative ways of delivering hormonal therapy. Transdermal estrogen may have a better impact on bone than OCPs because of minimal effects on IGF-1, which is a bone trophic hormone essential for bone formation and remodeling [169]. Studies on postmenopausal women have shown that transdermal estrogens (alone or plus progesterone) are more effective than OCPs in increasing BMD and decreasing fracture risks [170, 171]. Spine and hip BMD improvement was also seen with transdermal estrogen and oral progesterone therapy in adolescent anorexia patients [172]. However, further studies proving the efficacy of transdermal estrogen in treating Triad are needed. Some small studies have also tested the subcutaneous analog leptin therapy for recovering menstrual cycles and improving BMD in those with FHA, but with its side effect of weight loss, adjusting dosing and confirmation of an overall benefit of leptin therapy through larger studies is absolutely required [173, 174].

Additionally, calcium, vitamin D, and sometimes potassium supplementation is recommended in athletes, especially those with restrictive eating behaviors. The daily doses suggested are 1300 mg/day of elemental calcium in divided doses in adolescents (1000 mg in women ≥ 19 years old), 400–800 IU of vitamin D, and 60–90 mg of potassium [169, 175]. In general, bisphosphonates are not recommended for BMD treatment in premenopausal populations, except in extreme circumstances and under the guidance of a bone metabolism specialist, such as an endocrinologist [13]. Antidepressant medications, specifically selective serotonin reuptake inhibitors (SSRIs), may be useful in certain cases. Several studies have shown SSRIs to be effective in the treatment of bulimia nervosa, significantly reducing the frequency of binge eating and purging; however, the evidence is less clear in the case of anorexia nervosa [176, 177]. Another advantage of using antidepressants is the treatment of comorbid conditions such as anxiety, depression, and obsessive compulsive disorder [13]. The main drawback of SSRIs is that they have been linked with weight loss in some individuals with negative effects on BMD [13, 178, 179].

The Triad is a challenging diagnosis and the management has several difficulties. Therefore, education and prevention are fundamental in reducing morbidity and mortality. Prevention and early detection are more effective strategies to reduce symptoms and decrease the risk of serious long-term complications.

Early Detection and Prevention

Awareness of the Triad is the first step. When 180 Australian female exercisers (ages 18–40 years) were surveyed about the Triad, only 10 % could name all three components and 45 % did not think amenorrhea could affect bone health. A total of

22 % of those in lean-build sports answered that they would do nothing if they were amenorrheic [180]. Of 103 American female high school track athletes, more than 90 % provided incorrect answers about the consequences of bone loss and the link to menstrual irregularity [181]. In a survey of 240 health care professionals and coaches, fewer than half the physicians could identify the three Triad components and only 8 % of the coaches answered correctly [182]. Thus, more information needs to be disseminated to health professionals, coaches, and athletes, alike.

The preparticipation evaluation (PPE) is an excellent time to screen athletes for the Triad. The majority of the US National Collegiate Athletic Association (NCAA) Division 1 universities require a PPE, including a history and physical, prior to sports participation. However, only about a third require an annual update [183]. The Female Athlete Triad Coalition developed 12 questions for inclusion in the PPE [184]. However, only 9 % of the NCAA Division 1 schools had ≥ 9 of the 12 recommended Triad-related questions as part of their PPEs, with 44 % of the universities including ≤ 4 items [183, 184]. The most recent edition of the PPE history and physical examination form endorsed by the American Academy of Family Physicians, American Academy of Pediatrics, ACSM, and others, is the most commonly recommended tool for use with PPEs for middle school through college-aged athletes. It includes 7 of the 12 items recommended by the Female Athlete Triad Coalition, omitting some DE-related questions [185].

Recently, athlete-focused DE prevention programs have been evaluated. In an 8-week program called Athletes Targeting Healthy Exercise and Nutrition Alternatives (ATHENA), coaches and peers led sessions with high school athletes. Topics in the sessions included depression, self-esteem, healthy norms, societal pressures to be thin, and steroid use. Student athletes who participated in the ATHENA program reported less diet pill use and positive improvements in diet habits and exercise self-efficacy versus those who only received informational pamphlets on the topics. When followed for up to 3 years, athletes in ATHENA showed decreases in marijuana and alcohol use, but unfortunately not in eating pathology [186].

In cognitive dissonance-based prevention (DBP), participants confront the thin-ideal standard of female beauty through various activities and discussions in order to create cognitive dissonance. In a healthy weight intervention (HWI), participants learn to make small lifestyle changes to their dietary and exercise habits in order to maintain a healthy weight. Becker et al. compared an athlete-modified DBP (AM-DBP) and an athlete-modified HWI (AM-HWI) approach in a study of 157 female collegiate athletes [187]. Both interventions reduced thin-ideal internalization, dietary restraint, bulimic pathology, shape and weight concern, and negative affect at the 6-week follow-up, with sustained reductions in bulimic pathology, shape concern, and negative affect at 1 year. In addition, there was an increase in students spontaneously seeking medical consultation for the Triad [187].

In a small study of college athletes who had achieved recovery from EDs, participants were asked what advice they would give to coaches, parents, and other athletes at risk for EDs [188]. Coaches were advised to (1) become educated on EDs to increase awareness, (2) emphasize proper athlete nutrition, (3) focus on sport skill rather than body weight to achieve performance goals, (4) refrain from singling out athletes for their body weight or shape, (5) confront an athlete with an ED if even suspected, (6) provide emotional support, (7) refer the athlete to professional care (e.g., physician, psychologist, and/or nutritionist), (8) prohibit sports participation if health risks are evident, (9) try to pair the athlete up with another athlete who has recovered from an ED, and (10) notify the athlete's family. Advice to parents also involved providing emotional support, encouraging professional treatment, and becoming educated about EDs. Suggestions for other athletes with EDs included (1) keeping optimistic about recovery, (2) determining the underlying cause of and triggers for the ED, (3) getting professional treatment, (4) seeking out emotional support from others, (5) focusing on the benefits of recovery, (6) putting the ED in perspective in terms of how it is skewing life values, and (7) focusing on what has been learned from the ED experiences [188]. Certainly enhancing awareness and taking the advice of those who have experienced aspects of the Triad are future directions in which we need to head.

Conclusion

The Triad and its individual components can occur in female athletes at any age and in any sport. Early awareness and education can help prevent struggles ranging from unsatisfying sports performances to lifelong emotional and physical health problems. Because we know there are certain sport populations at increased risk for the Triad, increased efforts need to be made to improve detection and care in these groups. Following suggestions provided by the IOC, the Female Athlete Triad Coalition, ACSM and other groups of professionals with expertise on this topic is important. In the past decade, researchers have gained a better understanding of the complexity of the Triad and the interrelationship of its components. This understanding needs to be more widely disseminated and further research needs to be conducted to enhance the care of those afflicted by the Triad.

References

1. Kemper HC, et al. Lifestyle and obesity in adolescence and young adulthood: results from the Amsterdam Growth and Health Longitudinal Study (AGAHLS). Int J Obes Relat Metab Disord. 1999;23 Suppl 3:S34–40.
2. Haskell WL, et al. Physical activity and public health: updated recommendation for adults from the American College of Sports Medicine and the American Heart Association. Med Sci Sports Exerc. 2007;39(8):1423–34.
3. Boreham C, et al. Associations between physical fitness and activity patterns during adolescence and cardiovascular risk factors in young adulthood: the Northern Ireland Young Hearts Project. Int J Sports Med. 2002;23 Suppl 1:S22–6.
4. Hasselstrom H, et al. Physical fitness and physical activity during adolescence as predictors of cardiovascular disease risk in young adulthood. Danish Youth and Sports Study. An eight-year follow-up study. Int J Sports Med. 2002;23 Suppl 1:S27–31.
5. Babiss LA, Gangwisch JE. Sports participation as a protective factor against depression and suicidal ideation in adolescents as mediated by self-esteem and social support. J Dev Behav Pediatr. 2009;30(5):376–84
6. Women's Sports Foundation editor. Play fair, a title IX playbook for victory. East Meadow: Women's Sports Foundation; 2009.
7. National Coalition for Women and Girls in Education. Beyond the headlines: a report of the National Coalition for Women and Girls in Education. National Coalition for Women and Girls in Education. Washington, DC.; 2008.
8. Kulig K, Brener ND, McManus T. Sexual activity and substance use among adolescents by category of physical activity plus team sports participation. Arch Pediatr Adolesc Med. 2003;157(9):905–12.
9. Miller KE, et al. Sports, sexual behavior, contraceptive use, and pregnancy among female and male high school students: testing cultural resource theory. Sociol Sport J. 1999;16(4):366–87.
10. Nattiv A, et al. American College of Sports Medicine position stand. The female athlete triad. Med Sci Sports Exerc. 2007;39(10):1867–82.
11. Yeager KK, et al. The female athlete triad: disordered eating, amenorrhea, osteoporosis. Med Sci Sports Exerc. 1993;25(7):775–7.
12. Otis CL, et al. American College of Sports Medicine position stand. The female athlete triad. Med Sci Sports Exerc. 1997;29(5):i–ix.
13. De Souza MJ, et al. 2014 female athlete triad coalition consensus statement on treatment and return to play of the female athlete triad: 1st International Conference held in San Francisco, California, May 2012 and 2nd International Conference held in Indianapolis, Indiana, May 2013. Br J Sports Med. 2014;48(4):289.
14. Mountjoy M, et al. The IOC consensus statement: beyond the Female Athlete Triad–Relative Energy Deficiency in Sport (RED-S). Br J Sports Med. 2014;48(7):491–7.
15. Loucks AB, Verdun M, Heath EM. Low energy availability, not stress of exercise, alters LH pulsatility in exercising women. J Appl Physiol (1985). 1998;84(1):37–46.
16. Loucks AB, et al. Alterations in the hypothalamic-pituitary-ovarian and the hypothalamic-pituitary-adrenal axes in athletic women. J Clin Endocrinol Metab. 1989;68(2):402–11.
17. De Souza MJ, et al. High prevalence of subtle and severe menstrual disturbances in exercising women: confirmation using daily hormone measures. Hum Reprod. 2010;25(2):491–503.
18. Scheid JL, et al. Elevated PYY is associated with energy deficiency and indices of subclinical disordered eating in exercising women with hypothalamic amenorrhea. Appetite. 2009;52(1):184–92.
19. Doyle-Lucas AF, Akers JD, Davy BM. Energetic efficiency, menstrual irregularity, and bone mineral density in elite professional female ballet dancers. J

Dance Med Sci. 2010;14(4):146–54.
20. Fuqua JS, Rogol AD. Neuroendocrine alterations in the exercising human: implications for energy homeostasis. Metabolism. 2013;62(7):911–21.
21. Gordon CM. Clinical practice. Functional hypothalamic amenorrhea. N Engl J Med. 2010;363(4):365–71.
22. Gruodyte R, et al. The relationships among bone health, insulin-like growth factor-1 and sex hormones in adolescent female athletes. J Bone Miner Metab. 2010;28(3):306–13.
23. Thrailkill KM, et al. Is insulin an anabolic agent in bone? Dissecting the diabetic bone for clues. Am J Physiol Endocrinol Metab. 2005;289(5):E735–45.
24. Dhanwal DK. Thyroid disorders and bone mineral metabolism. Indian J Endocrinol Metab. 2011;15 Suppl 2:S107–12.
25. Harvey CB, et al. Molecular mechanisms of thyroid hormone effects on bone growth and function. Mol Genet Metab. 2002;75(1):17–30.
26. Corr M, et al. Circulating leptin concentrations do not distinguish menstrual status in exercising women. Hum Reprod. 2011;26(3):685–94.
27. Hamrick MW, Ferrari SL. Leptin and the sympathetic connection of fat to bone. Osteoporos Int. 2008;19(7):905–12.
28. Dalamaga M, et al. Leptin at the intersection of neuroendocrinology and metabolism: current evidence and therapeutic perspectives. Cell Metab. 2013;18(1):29–42.
29. Laughlin GA, Yen SS. Nutritional and endocrine-metabolic aberrations in amenorrheic athletes. J Clin Endocrinol Metab. 1996;81(12):4301–9.
30. Scheid JL, De Souza MJ. Menstrual irregularities and energy deficiency in physically active women: the role of ghrelin, PYY and adipocytokines. Med Sport Sci. 2010;55:82–102.
31. Utz AL, et al. Peptide YY (PYY) levels and bone mineral density (BMD) in women with anorexia nervosa. Bone. 2008;43(1):135–9.
32. Russell M, et al. Peptide YY in adolescent athletes with amenorrhea, eumenorrheic athletes and non-athletic controls. Bone. 2009;45(1):104–9.
33. Erdmann J, et al. Postprandial response of plasma ghrelin levels to various test meals in relation to food intake, plasma insulin, and glucose. J Clin Endocrinol Metab. 2004;89(6):3048–54.
34. Leidy HJ, et al. Circulating ghrelin is sensitive to changes in body weight during a diet and exercise program in normal-weight young women. J Clin Endocrinol Metab. 2004;89(6):2659–64.
35. Tschop M, et al. Circulating ghrelin levels are decreased in human obesity. Diabetes. 2001;50(4):707–9.
36. Tolle V, et al. Balance in ghrelin and leptin plasma levels in anorexia nervosa patients and constitutionally thin women. J Clin Endocrinol Metab. 2003;88(1):109–16.
37. De Souza MJ, et al. Fasting ghrelin levels in physically active women: relationship with menstrual disturbances and metabolic hormones. J Clin Endocrinol Metab. 2004;89(7):3536–42.
38. Ackerman KE, et al. Higher ghrelin and lower leptin secretion are associated with lower LH secretion in young amenorrheic athletes compared with eumenorrheic athletes and controls. Am J Physiol Endocrinol Metab. 2012;302(7):E800–6.
39. Lawson EA, et al. Hypercortisolemia is associated with severity of bone loss and depression in hypothalamic amenorrhea and anorexia nervosa. J Clin Endocrinol Metab. 2009;94(12):4710–6.
40. Dueck CA, et al. Treatment of athletic amenorrhea with a diet and training intervention program. Int J Sport Nutr. 1996;6(1):24–40.
41. Kopp-Woodroffe SA, et al. Energy and nutrient status of amenorrheic athletes participating in a diet and exercise training intervention program. Int J Sport Nutr. 1999;9(1):70–88.
42. Mallinson RJ, et al. A case report of recovery of menstrual function following a nutritional intervention in two exercising women with amenorrhea of varying duration. J Int Soc Sports Nutr. 2013;10(1):34.
43. Loucks AB, Verdun M. Slow restoration of LH pulsatility by refeeding in energetically disrupted women. Am J Physiol. 1998;275(4 Pt 2):R1218–26.
44. Heaney RP, et al. Peak bone mass. Osteoporos Int. 2000;11(12):985–1009.
45. Barrack MT, et al. Body mass, training, menses, and bone in adolescent runners: a 3-yr follow-up. Med Sci Sports Exerc. 2011;43(6):959–66.
46. Barrack MT, Ackerman KE, Gibbs JC. Update on the female athlete triad. Curr Rev Musculoskelet Med. 2013;6(2):195–204.
47. Hilton LK, Loucks AB. Low energy availability, not exercise stress, suppresses the diurnal rhythm of leptin in healthy young women. Am J Physiol Endocrinol Metab. 2000;278(1):E43–9.
48. Ihle R, Loucks AB. Dose-response relationships between energy availability and bone turnover in young exercising women. J Bone Miner Res. 2004;19(8):1231–40.
49. Jackson RD, Donepudi S, Mysiw WJ. Epidemiology of fracture risk in the women's health initiative. Curr Osteoporos Rep. 2008;6(4):155–61.
50. Bennell KL, et al. Risk factors for stress fractures in track and field athletes. A twelve-month prospective study. Am J Sports Med. 1996;24(6):810–8.
51. Kelsey JL, et al. Risk factors for stress fracture among young female cross-country runners. Med Sci Sports Exerc. 2007;39(9):1457–63.
52. Loud KJ, et al. Family history predicts stress fracture in active female adolescents. Pediatrics. 2007;120(2):e364–72.
53. Frusztajer NT, et al. Nutrition and the incidence of stress fractures in ballet dancers. Am J Clin Nutr. 1990;51(5):779–83.
54. Bennell KL, et al. Risk factors for stress fractures in female track-and-field athletes: a retrospective analysis. Clin J Sport Med. 1995;5(4):229–35.
55. Korpelainen R, et al. Risk factors for recurrent stress fractures in athletes. Am J Sports Med.

2001;29(3):304–10.
56. Popp KL, et al. Bone geometry, strength, and muscle size in runners with a history of stress fracture. Med Sci Sports Exerc. 2009;41(12):2145–50.
57. Nattiv A, et al. Correlation of MRI grading of bone stress injuries with clinical risk factors and return to play: a 5-year prospective study in collegiate track and field athletes. Am J Sports Med. 2013;41(8):1930–41.
58. Guest NS, Barr SI. Cognitive dietary restraint is associated with stress fractures in women runners. Int J Sport Nutr Exerc Metab. 2005;15(2):147–59.
59. Barrow GW, Saha S. Menstrual irregularity and stress fractures in collegiate female distance runners. Am J Sports Med. 1988;16(3):209–16.
60. Goolsby MA NA, Casper J. Predictors for stress fracture and stress fracture rate in male and female collegiate track athletes: a prospective analysis. American Medical Society for Sports Medicine Annual Meeting, 2008.
61. Lloyd T, et al. Women athletes with menstrual irregularity have increased musculoskeletal injuries. Med Sci Sports Exerc. 1986;18(4):374–9.
62. Kadel NJ, Teitz CC, Kronmal RA. Stress fractures in ballet dancers. Am J Sports Med. 1992;20(4):445–9.
63. Barrack MT, et al. Higher incidence of bone stress injuries with increasing female athlete triad-related risk factors: a prospective multisite study of exercising girls and women. American Medical Society for Sports Medicine Annual Meeting, 2014.
64. Rauh MJ, Nichols JF, Barrack MT. Relationships among injury and disordered eating, menstrual dysfunction, and low bone mineral density in high school athletes: a prospective study. J Athl Train. 45(3):243–52.
65. Benton D, Parker PY. Breakfast, blood glucose, and cognition. Am J Clin Nutr. 1998;67(4):S772–8.
66. Horvath PJ, et al. The effects of varying dietary fat on performance and metabolism in trained male and female runners. J Am Coll Nutr. 2000;19(1):52–60.
67. Vanheest JL, et al. Ovarian suppression impairs sport performance in junior elite female swimmers. Med Sci Sports Exerc. 2014;46(1):156–66.
68. Zach KN, Smith Machin AL, Hoch AZ. Advances in management of the female athlete triad and eating disorders. Clin Sports Med. 2011;30(3):551–73.
69. Mendelsohn ME. Estrogen actions in the cardiovascular system. Climacteric. 2009;12 Suppl 1:18–21.
70. Anderson TJ, et al. Systemic nature of endothelial dysfunction in atherosclerosis. Am J Cardiol. 1995;75(6):71B–4B.
71. Zeni Hoch A, et al. Is there an association between athletic amenorrhea and endothelial cell dysfunction? Med Sci Sports Exerc. 2003;35(3):377–83.
72. Rickenlund A, et al. Amenorrhea in female athletes is associated with endothelial dysfunction and unfavorable lipid profile. J Clin Endocrinol Metab. 2005;90(3):1354–9.
73. Yoshida N, et al. Impaired endothelium-dependent and -independent vasodilation in young female athletes with exercise-associated amenorrhea. Arterioscler Thromb Vasc Biol. 2006;26(1):231–2.
74. Hoch AZ, et al. Association between the female athlete triad and endothelial dysfunction in dancers. Clin J Sport Med. 2011;21(2):119–25.
75. Torstveit MK, Sundgot-Borgen J. The female athlete triad: are elite athletes at increased risk? Med Sci Sports Exerc. 2005;37(2):184–93.
76. Martinsen M, Sundgot-Borgen J. Higher prevalence of eating disorders among adolescent elite athletes than controls. Med Sci Sports Exerc. 2013;45(6):1188–97.
77. Reinking MF, Alexander LE. Prevalence of disordered-eating behaviors in undergraduate female collegiate athletes and nonathletes. J Athl Train. 2005;40(1):47–51.
78. Sundgot-Borgen J, Torstveit MK. Prevalence of eating disorders in elite athletes is higher than in the general population. Clin J Sport Med. 2004;14(1):25–32.
79. Torstveit MK, Rosenvinge JH, Sundgot-Borgen J. Prevalence of eating disorders and the predictive power of risk models in female elite athletes: a controlled study. Scand J Med Sci Sports. 2008;18(1):108–18.
80. Sundgot-Borgen J, Torstveit MK. Aspects of disordered eating continuum in elite high-intensity sports. Scand J Med Sci Sports. 2010;20 Suppl 2:112–21.
81. Constantini NW, Warren MP. Special problems of the female athlete. Baillieres Clin Rheumatol. 1994;8(1):199–219.
82. Torstveit MK, Sundgot-Borgen J. Participation in leanness sports but not training volume is associated with menstrual dysfunction: a national survey of 1276 elite athletes and controls. Br J Sports Med. 2005;39(3):141–7.
83. Beals KA, Hill AK. The prevalence of disordered eating, menstrual dysfunction, and low bone mineral density among US collegiate athletes. Int J Sport Nutr Exerc Metab. 2006;16(1):1–23.
84. Dadgostar H, et al. The relation between athletic sports and prevalence of amenorrhea and oligomenorrhea in Iranian female athletes. Sports Med Arthrosc Rehabil Ther Technol. 2009;1(1):16.
85. Nichols JF, et al. Disordered eating and menstrual irregularity in high school athletes in lean-build and nonlean-build sports. Int J Sport Nutr Exerc Metab. 2007;17(4):364–77.
86. Gibbs JC, Williams NI, De Souza MJ. Prevalence of individual and combined components of the female athlete triad. Med Sci Sports Exerc. 2013;45(5):985–96.
87. Quah YV, et al. The female athlete triad among elite Malaysian athletes: prevalence and associated factors. Asia Pac J Clin Nutr. 2009;18(2):200–8.
88. Thompson SH. Characteristics of the female athlete triad in collegiate cross-country runners. J Am Coll Health. 2007;56(2):129–36.
89. Hulley AJH, Hill AJ. Eating disorders and health in elite women distance runners. Int J Eat Disord.

2001;30:312–17.
90. Nichols JF, et al. Prevalence of the female athlete triad syndrome among high school athletes. Arch Pediatr Adolesc Med. 2006;160(2):137–42.
91. Cobb KL, et al. Disordered eating, menstrual irregularity, and bone mineral density in female runners. Med Sci Sports Exerc. 2003;35(5):711–9.
92. Barrack MT, Rauh MJ, Nichols JF. Prevalence of and traits associated with low BMD among female adolescent runners. Med Sci Sports Exerc. 2008;40(12):2015–21.
93. Gibson JH, et al. Nutritional and exercise-related determinants of bone density in elite female runners. Osteoporos Int. 2004;15(8):611–8.
94. van Hooff MH, et al. The use of oral contraceptives by adolescents for contraception, menstrual cycle problems or acne. Acta Obstet Gynecol Scand. 1998;77(9):898–904.
95. Warren MP, Chua AT. Exercise-induced amenorrhea and bone health in the adolescent athlete. Ann N Y Acad Sci. 2008;1135:244–52.
96. Dusek T. Influence of high intensity training on menstrual cycle disorders in athletes. Croat Med J. 2001;42(1):79–82.
97. Mudd LM, Fornetti W, Pivarnik JM. Bone mineral density in collegiate female athletes: comparisons among sports. J Athl Train. 2007;42(3):403–8.
98. Robinson TL, et al. Gymnasts exhibit higher bone mass than runners despite similar prevalence of amenorrhea and oligomenorrhea. J Bone Miner Res. 1995;10(1):26–35.
99. DiGioacchino DeBate R, Wethington H, Sargent R. Sub-clinical eating disorder characteristics among male and female triathletes. Eat Weight Disord. 2002;7(3):210–20.
100. DiGioacchino DeBate R, Wethington H, Sargent R. Body size dissatisfaction among male and female triathletes. Eat Weight Disord. 2002;7(4):316–23.
101. Hoch AZ, Stavrakos JE, Schimke JE. Prevalence of female athlete triad characteristics in a club triathlon team. Arch Phys Med Rehabil. 2007;88(5):681–2.
102. Thompson RA, Sherman RT. Eating disorders in sport. New York: Routledge; 2010.
103. Nichols JF, Palmer JE, Levy SS. Low bone mineral density in highly trained male master cyclists. Osteoporos Int. 2003;14(8):644–9.
104. da Costa NF, et al. Disordered eating among adolescent female swimmers: dietary, biochemical, and body composition factors. Nutrition. 2013; 29(1):172–7.
105. Anderson C, Petrie TA. Prevalence of disordered eating and pathogenic weight control behaviors among NCAA division I female collegiate gymnasts and swimmers. Res Q Exerc Sport. 83(1):120–4.
106. Torstveit MK, Sundgot-Borgen J. Low bone mineral density is two to three times more prevalent in non-athletic premenopausal women than in elite athletes: a comprehensive controlled study. Br J Sports Med. 2005;39(5):282–7; discussion 282–7.
107. Gomez-Bruton A, et al. Is bone tissue really affected by swimming? A systematic review. PLoS ONE. 2013;8(8):e70119.
108. Monsma EV, Malina RM, Feltz DL. Puberty and physical self-perceptions of competitive female figure skaters: an interdisciplinary approach. Res Q Exerc Sport. 2006;77(2):158–66.
109. Smolak L, Murnen SK, Ruble AE. Female athletes and eating problems: a meta-analysis. Int J Eat Disord. 2000;27(4):371–80.
110. Van Durme K, Goossens L, Braet C. Adolescent aesthetic athletes: a group at risk for eating pathology? Eat Behav. 2012;13(2):119–22.
111. Ziegler P, et al. Energy and macronutrient intakes of elite figure skaters. J Am Diet Assoc. 2001;101(3):319–25.
112. Sundgot-Borgen J. Eating disorders in female athletes. Sports Med. 1994;17(3):176–88.
113. Davison KK, Earnest MB, Birch LL. Participation in aesthetic sports and girls' weight concerns at ages 5 and 7 years. Int J Eat Disord. 2002;31(3):312–7.
114. Davison KK, Markey CN, Birch LL. A longitudinal examination of patterns in girls' weight concerns and body dissatisfaction from ages 5 to 9 years. Int J Eat Disord. 2003;33(3):320–32.
115. Ziegler PJ, et al. Dietary intake, body image perceptions, and weight concerns of female US international synchronized figure skating teams. Int J Sport Nutr Exerc Metab. 2005;15(5):550–66.
116. Thein-Nissenbaum JM, et al. Menstrual irregularity and musculoskeletal injury in female high school athletes. J Athl Train. 2012;47(1):74–82.
117. Hincapie CA, Cassidy JD. Disordered eating, menstrual disturbances, and low bone mineral density in dancers: a systematic review. Arch Phys Med Rehabil. 2010;91(11):1777–1789.e1.
118. Klentrou P, Plyley M. Onset of puberty, menstrual frequency, and body fat in elite rhythmic gymnasts compared with normal controls. Br J Sports Med. 2003;37(6):490–4.
119. Vadocz EA, Siegel SR, Malina RM. Age at menarche in competitive figure skaters: variation by competency and discipline. J Sports Sci. 2002;20(2):93–100.
120. Helge EW, Kanstrup IL. Bone density in female elite gymnasts: impact of muscle strength and sex hormones. Med Sci Sports Exerc. 2002;34(1):174–80.
121. Smith AD. The young skater. Clin Sports Med. 2000;19(4):741–55.
122. Oleson CV, Busconi BD, Baran DT. Bone density in competitive figure skaters. Arch Phys Med Rehabil. 2002;83(1):122–8.
123. Bemben DA, et al. Influence of type of mechanical loading, menstrual status, and training season on bone density in young women athletes. J Strength Cond Res. 2004;18(2):220–6.
124. Maimoun L, et al. Despite a high prevalence of menstrual disorders, bone health is improved at a weight-bearing bone site in world-class female

rhythmic gymnasts. J Clin Endocrinol Metab. 2013;98(12):4961–9.
125. Munoz MT, et al. Changes in bone density and bone markers in rhythmic gymnasts and ballet dancers: implications for puberty and leptin levels. Eur J Endocrinol. 2004;151(4):491–6.
126. Ducher G, et al. History of amenorrhoea compromises some of the exercise-induced benefits in cortical and trabecular bone in the peripheral and axial skeleton: a study in retired elite gymnasts. Bone. 2009;45(4):760–7.
127. Artioli GG, et al. Prevalence, magnitude, and methods of rapid weight loss among judo competitors. Med Sci Sports Exerc. 2010;42(3):436–42.
128. Pettersson S, Pipping Ekstrom M, Berg CM. The food and weight combat. A problematic fight for the elite combat sports athlete. Appetite. 2012;59(2):234–42.
129. Dale KS, Landers DM. Weight control in wrestling: eating disorders or disordered eating? Med Sci Sports Exerc. 1999;31(10):1382–9.
130. Sundgot-Borgen J, Garthe I. Elite athletes in aesthetic and Olympic weight-class sports and the challenge of body weight and body compositions. J Sports Sci. 2011;29 Suppl 1:S101–14.
131. Tenforde AS, Fredericson M. Influence of sports participation on bone health in the young athlete: a review of the literature. PM R. 2011;3(9):861–7.
132. Prouteau S, et al. Bone density in elite judoists and effects of weight cycling on bone metabolic balance. Med Sci Sports Exerc. 2006;38(4):694–700.
133. Cohen B, et al. Effect of exercise training programme on bone mineral density in novice college rowers. Br J Sports Med. 1995;29(2):85–8.
134. Morris FL, Payne WR, Wark JD. The impact of intense training on endogenous estrogen and progesterone concentrations and bone mineral acquisition in adolescent rowers. Osteoporos Int. 1999;10(5):361–8.
135. Dimitriou L, et al. Bone mineral density, rib pain and other features of the female athlete triad in elite lightweight rowers. BMJ Open. 2014;4(2):e004369.
136. Movaseghi S, et al. Clinical manifestations of the female athlete triad among some Iranian athletes. Med Sci Sports Exerc. 2012;44(5):958–65.
137. Ackerman KE, et al. Estradiol levels predict bone mineral density in male collegiate athletes: a pilot study. Clin Endocrinol (Oxf). 2012;76(3):339–45.
138. Karila TA, et al. Rapid weight loss decreases serum testosterone. Int J Sports Med. 2008;29(11):872–7.
139. Muller W. Towards research-based approaches for solving body composition problems in sports: ski jumping as a heuristic example. Br J Sports Med. 2009;43(13):1013–9.
140. Moore JM, et al. Weight management and weight loss strategies of professional jockeys. Int J Sport Nutr Exerc Metab. 2002;12(1):1–13.
141. Dolan E, et al. Nutritional, lifestyle, and weight control practices of professional jockeys. J Sports Sci. 2011;29(8):791–9.
142. Leydon MA, Wall C. New Zealand jockeys' dietary habits and their potential impact on health. Int J Sport Nutr Exerc Metab. 2002;12(2):220–37.
143. Dolan E, et al. Weight regulation and bone mass: a comparison between professional jockeys, elite amateur boxers, and age, gender and BMI matched controls. J Bone Miner Metab. 2012;30(2):164–70.
144. Dolan E, et al. An altered hormonal profile and elevated rate of bone loss are associated with low bone mass in professional horse-racing jockeys. J Bone Miner Metab. 2012;30(5):534–42.
145. Warrington G, et al. Chronic weight control impacts on physiological function and bone health in elite jockeys. J Sports Sci. 2009;27(6):543–50.
146. Chan JL, Mantzoros CS. Role of leptin in energy-deprivation states: normal human physiology and clinical implications for hypothalamic amenorrhoea and anorexia nervosa. Lancet. 2005;366(9479):74–85.
147. Ackerman KE, et al. Higher ghrelin and lower leptin secretion are associated with lower LH secretion in young amenorrheic athletes compared with eumenorrheic athletes and controls. Am J Physiol Endocrinol Metab. 2012;302(7):E800–6.
148. Loucks AB, Heath EM. Induction of low-T3 syndrome in exercising women occurs at a threshold of energy availability. Am J Physiol. 1994;266(3 Pt 2):R817–23.
149. Loucks AB, Thuma JR. Luteinizing hormone pulsatility is disrupted at a threshold of energy availability in regularly menstruating women. J Clin Endocrinol Metab. 2003;88(1):297–311.
150. Yeager KK AR, Nattiv A, Drinkwater B. The female athlete triad: disordered eating, amenorrhea, osteoporosis. Med Sci Sports Exerc. 1993;25:775–77.
151. Hoch AZ, et al. Prevalence of the female athlete triad in high school athletes and sedentary students. Clin J Sport Med. 2009;19(5):421–8.
152. Barrack MT, Rauh MJ, Nichols JF. Cross-sectional evidence of suppressed bone mineral accrual among female adolescent runners. J Bone Miner Res. 2010;(8):1850–7.
153. Barrack MT, et al. Body mass, training, menses, and bone in adolescent runners: a three-year follow-up. Med Sci Sports Exerc. 2011;4(6):959–66.
154. Litsky F. Wrestling; collegiate wrestling deaths raise fears about training. The New York Times. Dec. 19th, New York, NY; 1997.
155. Hackney AC, Fahrner CL, Stupnicki R. Reproductive hormonal responses to maximal exercise in endurance-trained men with low resting testosterone levels. Exp Clin Endocrinol Diabetes. 1997;105(5):291–5.
156. Hackney AC. The male reproductive system and endurance exercise. Med Sci Sports Exerc. 1996;28(2):180–9.
157. Hackney AC. Endurance training and testosterone levels. Sports Med. 1989;8(2):117–27.
158. Hackney AC, Sinning WE, Bruot BC. Reproductive hormonal profiles of endurance-trained

and untrained males. Med Sci Sports Exerc. 1988;20(1):60–5.
159. Arce JC, et al. Subclinical alterations in hormone and semen profile in athletes. Fertil Steril. 1993;59(2):398–404.
160. Fredericson M, et al. Regional bone mineral density in male athletes: a comparison of soccer players, runners and controls. Br J Sports Med. 2007;41(10):664–8; discussion 668.
161. Bilanin JE, Blanchard MS, Russek-Cohen E. Lower vertebral bone density in male long distance runners. Med Sci Sports Exerc. 1989;21(1):66–70.
162. Kemmler W, et al. Bone status in elite male runners. Eur J Appl Physiol. 2006;96(1):78–85.
163. Hind K, Truscott JG, Evans JA. Low lumbar spine bone mineral density in both male and female endurance runners. Bone. 2006;39(4):880–5.
164. Bennell KL, Brukner PD, Malcolm SA. Effect of altered reproductive function and lowered testosterone levels on bone density in male endurance athletes. Br J Sports Med. 1996;30(3):205–8.
165. Arends JC, et al. Restoration of menses with nonpharmacologic therapy in college athletes with menstrual disturbances: a 5-year retrospective study. Int J Sport Nutr Exerc Metab. 2012;22(2):98–108.
166. Fredericson M, Kent K. Normalization of bone density in a previously amenorrheic runner with osteoporosis. Med Sci Sports Exerc. 2005;37(9):1481–6.
167. Miller BE, et al. Sublingual administration of micronized estradiol and progesterone, with and without micronized testosterone: effect on biochemical markers of bone metabolism and bone mineral density. Menopause. 2000;7(5):318–26.
168. Vescovi JD, Jamal SA, De Souza MJ. Strategies to reverse bone loss in women with functional hypothalamic amenorrhea: a systematic review of the literature. Osteoporos Int. 2008;19(4):465–78.
169. Nazem TG, Ackerman KE. The female athlete triad. Sports Health. 2012;4(4):302–11.
170. Ettinger B, et al. Effects of ultralow-dose transdermal estradiol on bone mineral density: a randomized clinical trial. Obstet Gynecol. 2004;104(3):443–51.
171. Warming L, Ravn P, Christiansen C. Levonorgestrel and 17beta-estradiol given transdermally for the prevention of postmenopausal osteoporosis. Maturitas. 2005;50(2):78–85.
172. Misra M, et al. Physiologic estrogen replacement increases bone density in adolescent girls with anorexia nervosa. J Bone Miner Res. 2011;26(10):2430–8.
173. Chou SH, et al. Leptin is an effective treatment for hypothalamic amenorrhea. Proc Natl Acad Sci U S A. 2011;108(16):6585–90.
174. Welt CK, et al. Recombinant human leptin in women with hypothalamic amenorrhea. N Engl J Med. 2004;351(10):987–97.
175. Institute of Medicine. 2010, November 30. Institute of Medicine of The National Academies. Dietary reference intakes tables and application. http://www.iom.edu/Activities/Nutrition/SummaryDRIs/DRI-Tables.aspx. Accessed 27 March 2014.
176. Thiel A. Are psychotropic drugs necessary for the treatment of anorexia and bulimia nervosa? Psychother Psychosom Med Psychol. 1997;47(9–10):332–45.
177. Zhu AJ, Walsh BT. Pharmacologic treatment of eating disorders. Can J Psychiatry. 2002;47(3):227–34.
178. Couturier J, et al. Bone mineral density in adolescents with eating disorders exposed to selective serotonin reuptake inhibitors. Eat Disord. 2013;21(3):238–48.
179. Tsapakis EM, et al. The adverse skeletal effects of selective serotonin reuptake inhibitors. Eur Psychiatry. 2012;27(3):156–69.
180. Miller SM, et al. Energy deficiency, menstrual disturbances, and low bone mass: what do exercising Australian women know about the female athlete triad? Int J Sport Nutr Exerc Metab. 2012;22(2):131–8.
181. Feldmann JM, et al. Female adolescent athletes' awareness of the connection between menstrual status and bone health. J Pediatr Adolesc Gynecol. 2011;24(5):311–4.
182. Troy K, Hoch AZ, Stavrakos JE. Awareness and comfort in treating the female athlete triad: are we failing our athletes? WMJ. 2006;105(7):21–4.
183. Mencias T, Noon M, Hoch AZ. Female athlete triad screening in National Collegiate Athletic Association Division I athletes: is the preparticipation evaluation form effective? Clin J Sport Med. 2012;22(2):122–5.
184. Mountjoy M, et al. Female Athlete Triad Pre Participation Evaluation. Female Athlete Triad Coalition; 2008.
185. American Academy of Family Physicians eds. Preparticipation Physical Evaluation. 4th ed., ed. D.T. Berhardt and W.O. Roberts. American Academy of Pediatrics: Elk Grove Village, IL; 2010.
186. Elliot DL, et al. Long-term outcomes of the ATHENA (Athletes Targeting Healthy Exercise & Nutrition Alternatives) Program for Female High School Athletes. J Alcohol Drug Educ. 2008;52(2):73–92.
187. Becker CB, et al. Can we reduce eating disorder risk factors in female college athletes? A randomized exploratory investigation of two peer-led interventions. Body Image. 2012;9(1):31–42.
188. Arthur-Cameselle JN, Baltzell A. Learning from collegiate athletes who have recovered from eating disorders: advice to coaches, parents, and other athletes with eating disorders. J Appl Sport Psychol. 2012;24(1):1–9.

Consequences of the Use of Anabolic-Androgenic Steroids on Female Athletes' Fertility

14

Juan Manuel García-Manso and
Teresa Valverde Esteve

Introduction

Anabolic-androgenic steroids (AAS) are frequently used by athletes, especially by weightlifters [1]. Presently, the use of AAS is becoming more popular among a large number of competing and amateur athletes [2–6]. Instead of decreasing, this practice seems to be gaining adherents not only among male but also female [7–9] and adolescent athletes [10–12].

Side Effects Associated with Anabolic-Androgenic Steroids

The use of AAS is not a practice without risk for the athletes' physical and psychological health regardless of gender or age. Androgen receptors are located in all major tissues, including the brain. Thus, the androgenic and anabolic properties and influence of AAS is widespread throughout the body.

One would hope that most athletes would think about it twice if they knew the risks that they face by using high doses of AAS. Usually, and regrettably, the potential risks are minimized by athletes, coaches, and many times by doctors. However, this attitude is dangerous and reveals irresponsibility and selfishness, especially when athletes and coaches believe that there are more benefits than potential risks associated with AAS use. Several key studies have shown the potential risks for these athletes [13–16]. For example, Pärssinen et al. [13] found that, among a sample of 62 Finnish weightlifters, the percentage of deaths was almost five times more than for the population of a similar age, sex, and origin. The average age of death for the weightlifters was 43 years, and the causes of death often appeared to involve the use of AAS or other endogenously administered hormones.

The health and quality of life risks for athletes using AAS depend on diverse factors such as the steroid chemical structure, its quality, dose, time of application, age of use by the athlete, and the athlete's individual characteristics [17]. However, the risk increases when there is no medical control or supervision of AAS use. Even so, there is no evidence that the threat is resolved with an important and direct collaboration of a healthcare professional.

The most common adverse effects include the following: appearance of acne, hair loss, water retention, headaches, strokes, morphological changes in the myocardium, cardiovascular problems and hypertension, adverse changes in plasma lipids (cholesterol), hepatic peliosis and

J. M. García-Manso (✉)
Department of Physical Education, Universidad de Las Palmas de GranCanaria, C/ Consuela la Maestra 29, C Santa María de Guía, Islas Canarias 35017, Spain
e-mail: jgarciamanso@gmail.com

T. Valverde Esteve
Laboratorio de Investigación de Ciencias del Deporte, Universidad Católica de Valencia San Vicente Mártir, Valencia, Spain

© Springer Science+Business Media New York 2016

D. Vaamonde et al. (eds.), *Exercise and Human Reproduction*, DOI 10.1007/978-1-4939-3402-7_14

cholestasis, liver tumors, abnormal liver enzymes with increases in blood levels of glutamic-oxaloacetic transaminase (GOT), glutamic pyruvic transaminase (GPT), and lactate dehydrogenase (LDH) especially with the 17α-alkylated, alterations in the male reproductive system (oligospermia, decreased testosterone, and infertility), prostate problems (significant increase in prostate-specific antigen or cancer), gynecomastia (enlarged mammary glands in males), changes in behavior (euphoria, aggressiveness, impaired libido, etc.), advanced closure of the epiphyseal lines of ossification, ataxias, and decrease of immunoglobulins (IgA and IgM).

Effects of Anabolic-Androgenic Steroid Use in Women

Synthetic AAS are derived from testosterone and commonly used by men and women to increase the muscle mass or improve performance. Consequently, its use increases artificially the rate of circulating testosterone with positive and negative effects for these athletes' organisms. Diverse studies have assessed and analyzed the side effects of AAS on male athletes [1, 18, 19]. Despite its effect on women not having been deeply evaluated, some studies have reported hirsutism, acne, changes in libido, virilization (dysphonia, cliteromegaly, male-pattern baldness) [7, 18, 20], alterations in the hypothalamic–pituitary–gonadal (HPG) system [21], and changes in the female reproductive system morphology and function (amenorrhea, oligoamenorrhea, vaginal and uterine atrophy, etc.) [7, 18, 21, 22]. Some of these androgenic effects may be irreversible [23].

To partially cushion these effects, athletes often use low-potential androgenic AAS, such as boldenone undecylenate (Equipoise, Equilon 100 or Equigan), bolazine caproate (Roxilon Inject), drostanolone propionate (Masteron), methyldrostanolone (Superdrol), nandrolone decanoate (ND; Decadurabolin), nandrolone phenylpropionate (Durabolin), norclostebol acetate (Anabol 4–19), stananozolol (Winstrol), methenolone acetate (Primobolan), oxandralone (Anavar), or quinbolone (Anabolicum Vister). However, because the drug has low androgenic effects does not mean that it no longer produces adverse effects among user athletes.

Effect of Steroids in Female Reproductive System and Female Fertility

High rates of testosterone may cause a negative effect on the female reproductive system and fertility. In healthy women, the circulating rate of testosterone is much less than in men. In normal conditions, a female produces about 0.1–0.4 mg/day [24–26]. In women, testosterone is secreted by the ovaries (ovarian stroma: 25 %), adrenal glands (fasciculate zone: ≈25 %), and circulating androstenedione [27], modulated by adrenocorticotropic hormone (ACTH) (adrenal) and luteinizing hormone (LH; ovary) hormones, together with intraglandular paracrine and autocrine mechanisms [24]. The majority of testosterone produced in women is converted to E2 in adipocytes by the enzyme aromatase.

In female reproductive organs, the use of AAS may cause atrophy of ovary and uterus [28–35] and alterations in ovarian cyclical activity [7, 36–39]. The administration of AAS suppresses gonadotropin secretion by the negative feedback loop of the HPG axis in both men and women and can result in infertility, testicular atrophy, disturbances of the menstrual cycle, and secondary amenorrhea [40]. The use of AAS leads to impaired function of the HPG axis by increasing the circulating androgen levels, thus reducing the release of gonadotropins through negative feedback, which decreases the secretion of estrogen in females [41–42]. The study by Penatti et al. [43] suggests that AAS treatment imposes a diestrous-like pattern of activity in gonadotropin-releasing hormone (GnRH) neurons. Therefore, these authors suggest that this effect may arise from suppression of presynaptic kisspeptin-mediated excitatory drive arising from the neurons of the anteroventral periventricular nucleus. Such hormonal changes affect the menstrual cycle negatively and potentially reduce the woman's reproductive capacity.

Also, the reproductive tissues are indirectly affected by the use of synthetic steroids as these substances alter the function of the HPG axis by artificially increasing androgen levels. Such alterations suppress estrous cyclicity, leading to follicular atresia and absence of corpora lutea [30–32]. Some vacuolated epithelial cells and stromal fibrosis have also been observed. The administration of AAS to cynomolgus macaques *(Macaca fascicularis)* revealed changes in weight and endometrial thickness of the uterine structure [33]. In addition, adenomyosis-like alterations and the incidence of mucometra have been documented [28]. It has also been reported that the bioconversion of AAS to estrogens may influence the estrous cyclicity by altering the aromatase activity [44]. De Almeida-Chuffa et al. [33] suggested that these enhanced estrogenic/antiestrogenic effects may explain the changes in cyclicity and uterine morphology with AAS use.

In the ovary, the cellular contribution to steroidogenesis is very different from that in the testis, and both granulosa cells and theca cells contribute to this process [45]. Anderson [46] proposes that high concentrations of androgens in cultured granulosa cells contribute to their degeneration through altered structure, which is associated with functional change. The filamentous actin of granulosa cells cultured in the presence of dehydroepiandrosterone was found to be deficient when compared with that of controls [47]. As suggested by this author, this lack of filamentous actin coupled with other organelle degeneration is believed to lead to early atresia of granulosa cells in vitro in the presence of high concentrations of androgens.

Animal Research

In general, biomedical research begins with the most basic aspects: in vitro effect at cellular levels, evidence of toxicity, dose-response curves, determination of reference dose, etc. However, so far, the most sophisticated simulations have not always managed to reproduce the interactions to tissue and systemic level. For this reason, it becomes necessary to use the in vitro procedure. The use of animals for experimentation has allowed significant scientific advances without submitting humans to too invasive, aggressive, or dangerous practices. The use of AAS is no stranger to this situation, and the risk involved in supraphysiological doses leads to the fact that most mechanistic studies are performed in animals.

Some of the studies performed on the effect of AAS have used ND. In the first study, Obasanjo et al. [28] evaluated the long-term ND effects (25 mg every 3 weeks for 24 months) on uterine endometrium and myometrium and on the mammary gland of female cynomolgus macaques randomized into four treatment groups: (a) intact sham ovariectomized + placebo for 2 years (sham), (b) ovariectomized, (c) ovariectomized+ND for 2 years, and (d) ovariectomized + ND + nandrolone treatment beginning 1 year after ovariectomy. The results showed ND-induced pathologic changes in ovariectomized monkeys similar to adenomyosis in the uterus. Changes induced were an increase in uterine weight, endometrial thickness, and glandular area, and a high incidence of mucometra. Glandular architecture was also altered in such manner that glands extended into the myometrium (producing an adenomyosis-like lesion).

Rubiera-Gerez et al. [30] analyzed the effects after 1, 2, or 3 weeks of administering ND intraperitoneally (one, two, or three doses of 3 mg/kg of body weight) on the ovaries and uterus of adult female rats. The data indicated that ND affects the sexual cycle and promotes histological alterations in the ovaries and uterus. These rats showed estral acyclicity, and there was destruction of follicular units and an absence of corpus luteum in the ovaries. In the uterus, ND promoted morphological changes, characterized by vacuolated epithelium and endometrial stroma fibrosis. However, ovary, uterus, and pituitary weights were not affected by the steroid treatment.

Mobini-Far et al. [48] also propose that supraphysiological doses of ND (15 mg/kg once daily during a 2-week treatment) cause morphological and physiological alterations in the uterus of female rats, such as endometrial atrophy and glands with tortuous and irregular branching. These changes were associated with a suppression of their reproductive capacity. The rats showed an enhanced rate of weight gain and myometrium thickness, while the endometrium was significantly thinner. Furthermore, these authors found that ND caused a significant proportion of the treated animals to display tortuous and irregularly branching endometrial glands, as well as a lack of the physiologically normal infiltration of eosinophilic leukocytes into the endometrium (endometrial eosinophilic homing). The weight of ovaries and hypophysis, the number of antral and atretic follicles, and the area of corpus luteum were all affected by the steroids.

Cherici-Camargo et al. [31] found that in adult rats ND (6 mg/kg of body weight, 4 consecutive weeks), whether it is associated with physical effort (swimming 20 min daily, 5 days/week, for the 4 weeks of treatment) or not, affected the morphological pattern of the ovaries (weight, number of antral and atretic follicles, and the area of corpus luteum) and the weight of the hypophysis. Conversely, in the ovaries of the control groups, a well-developed corpus luteum was observed. In the treated groups, the cortical stroma was occupied by ovarian interstitial tissue. Thus, the females treated with steroids presented estral acyclicity.

De Almeida-Chuffa et al. [33] suggested that in female Wistar rats ND has a different pattern of response and effect independent of exercise. These authors investigated the effect of ND (5 mg/kg body weight for 4 weeks), whether associated with physical effort or not (swimming 20 min/day), and observed histomorphometric changes of the uterus, estrus acyclicity, and decreased thickness of both the epithelium and endometrial stroma. In the ND-treated rats submitted to exercise, a reduction in the number and size of blood vessels was observed, in comparison to the ND sedentary rats. ND-treated rats, regardless of exercise, exhibited stromal fibrosis and reduced gland ducts that displayed high mitotic activity. It should be taken into consideration that androgenic receptors are expressed in both endometrium and myometrium and regulate the proliferative response to ND. The authors suggest that this atrophy was promoted by the maintenance of metestrus phase (depletion of estrogen levels) induced by AAS use.

The study by Karbalay-Doust and Noorafsham [34] aimed to assess the way that changes in the number and size of oocytes can lead to fertilization problems. The study's purpose was to evaluate the number, volume, and surface area of oocytes in healthy and ND-treated (one, two, and three doses of 3 mg/kg body weight in the 1st, 2nd, and 3rd weeks) mice using stereological methods. The volumes of the ovary, cortex, and medulla decreased (~50%) in the ND-treated mice and caused the reduction in the number of oocytes but not in the volume or the surface area. More recently, Bordbar et al. [35] reported the negative effect of the administration of intraperitoneal ND (3 to 19 mg/kg) over a 1-month period on the reproductive system of adult rats (Sprague-Dawley). ND was administered with and without concurrent human menopausal gonadotropin. In this regard, the authors observed that ND had a negative effect on the reproductive system as evidenced by decreased ovarian volume, number of primordial follicles, and gonadotropin levels. Human menopausal gonadotropin used along with ND was observed to have a protective effect for the low dose of ND (Table 14.1).

Other studies have compared the effects of using ND and other AAS. In this line of work, Blasberg et al. [39] observed that the treatment with 17 α-methyltestosterone, methandrostenolone, and ND, at doses that mimic those used by human athletes, produced reversible and a dose-dependent sexual receptivity conduct and estrous vaginal cytology in rats over a 2-week period. During the intervening period, the effects of the treatment with ND at a dose of 7.5 mg/kg on the estrous cycle of these animals were longer while vaginal estrous resumed within 2 months of treatment completion. Another study [32] analyzed the effects of using ND (7.5 mg/kg of body weight), testosterone esters (7.5 mg/kg of body weight), or both steroids at once during 8 weeks. The results showed that the steroidal treatment did not affect the uterine weight. In this study, all the androgenized females presented estral acyclicity and endometrium characterized by papilliferous luminal lining, edematous stroma with hemorrhagic areas, and secretory activity. Changes were observed in the morphometrical thickness parameters of the luminal epithelium, myometrium, and perimetrium in the androgenized groups. In addition, none of the female rats got pregnant when treated with steroids in the pre-gestational period. Thus, the treatment dur-

Table 14.1 Effect of the use of decanoate nandrolone in female reproductive system and reproductive capacity in animals

Research	Steroid	Dose	Effect
Obasanjo et al. [28]	Nandrolone decanoate	25 mg/3 weeks for 24 months	Increase in uterine weight Increased endometrial thickness Increased glandular area Altered glandular architecture
Rubiera-Gerez et al. [30]	Nandrolone decanoate	One, two, and three doses of 3 mg/kg BW in the 1st, 2nd, and 3rd weeks	Estral acyclicity Destruction of follicular units Absence of corpus luteum Morphological changes in uterus
Mobini-Far et al. [48]	Nandrolone decanoate	15 mg/kg once daily during 2 weeks	Endometrial atrophy Glands with tortuous and irregular branching Lack of normal infiltration of eosinophilic leukocytes into the endometrium
Cherici-Camargo et al. [31, 32]	Nandrolone decanoate	6 mg/kg BW for 4 weeks and exercise	Changes in weight of ovaries and hypophysis, number of antral and atretic follicles, and the area of corpus luteum Estral acyclicity
De Almeida-Chuffa et al. [33]	Nandrolone decanoate	5 mg/kg BW for 4 weeks and exercise	Histomorphometric changes to the uterus Estrus acyclicity Decreased thickness of the epithelium and endometrial stroma
Karbalay-Doust and Noorafsham [49]	Nandrolone decanoate	One, two, and three doses of 3 mg/kg BW in the 1st, 2nd, and 3rd weeks	Decrease in the volume of the ovary, cortex, and medulla Reduction of oocytes
Bordbar et al. [35]	Nandrolone decanoate	3–19 mg/kg for 1 month	Changes in dimension of the ovaries, number of follicles, and sex hormone levels

BW body weight

ing organogenesis affected negatively the reproductive parameters. Collectively, these findings are summarized in Table 14.1.

Some other AAS have also been used in the investigation of the effects caused by these substances on the female reproductive system, such as testosterone undecanoate [50] or testosterone [51] (summarized in Table 14.2). Bento-Silva et al. [50] observed that testosterone undecanoate (5 mg/kg, 3 days/week for 4 weeks) combined with moderate physical training (50 min/day swim, 5 days/week for 4 weeks) altered the reproductive system of rats through interruption of the estrous cycle and ovarian atrophy. Triemstra and Wood [51] observed inhibitory effects on female reproduction by administering testosterone (1.0 μg/μl) to female hamsters ($n=12$). Bronson et al. [37] investigated (9 weeks) adult female mice exposed to a combination of four AAS (testosterone, testosterone cypionate, methyltestosterone, and norethandrolone) at doses that were either one or five times the androgenic maintenance level (silastic capsule implanted under the skin on the back of a mouse). These authors suggest that chronic treatment with AAS resulted in suppression of LH, follicle-stimulating hormone (FSH), and estradiol and cessation of the vaginal cycle.

Research in Humans

Strauss et al. [7] examined the effects of high use of AAS in ten weight-trained women athletes in a pioneer study in the field of sports research and observed modifications in several body features: voice changes (ten cases); increased facial hair (nine cases); clitoral enlargement (eight cases); aggressiveness (eight cases); menstrual abnormalities (seven cases); increased libido (six cases); acne (six cases); decrease in breast size (five cases); body weight gain (five cases), and hair loss (two cases). Almost all these athletes were specialized in strength modalities but none

Table 14.2 Effect of using different anabolic-androgenic steroids in the female reproductive system and reproductive performance in animals

Research	Steroid	Dose	Effect
Bronson et al. [37]	Testosterone, testosterone cypionate, Methyltestosterone Norethandrolone	Implanted silastic capsule under the skin on the back of a mouse	Suppression of LH, FSH, and estradiol Cessation of vaginal cycle
Blasberg et al. [39]	17 α-methyltestosterone, methandrostenolone Nandrolone decanoate	7.5 mg/kg BW 5.6 mg/kg BW	Disrupts female neuroendocrine function
Cherici-Camargo et al. [31, 32]	Nandrolone decanoate Testosterone esters	7.5 mg/kg BW 7.5 mg/kg BW	Estral acyclicity Papilliferous luminal lining Edematous stroma Changes in morphometrical thickness parameters of luminal epithelium, myometrium, and perimetrium
Bento-Silva et al. [52]	Testosterone undecanoate and exercise	5 mg/kg BW 3 days/week 4 weeks	Interruption of estrous cycle Ovarian atrophy
Triemstra and Wood [51]	Testosterone	1.0 µg/µl	Inhibited female reproduction

BW body weight, *LH* luteinizing hormone, *FSH* follicle-stimulating hormone

of them practiced the most affected activities for the use of anabolic substances, such as bodybuilding, powerlifting, or weightlifting.

Considering the frequent use of AAS and their potential health risks, several studies were performed assessing the effect of these drugs in females. Studies propose the use of AAS relationship with suppression of gonadal steroidogenesis [53], menstrual irregularity [53, 54], and uterine atrophy [18]. Clark et al. [55] suggested that the existence of different routes of the steroid metabolism and its relationship with the reproductive function may be the cause of the decrease in time of vaginal estrus during 2 weeks of treatment with AAS. Also, the absence of estrus (i.e., persistent diestrus) during the recovery period, pronounced with testosterone use, may be related to the existence of different routes of metabolism of the steroid and its relationship to the reproductive function.

Malarkey et al. [56] compared nine female weightlifters using steroids with seven non-user weightlifters. Thirty-fold elevations of serum testosterone were detected in the women that used AAS. The authors observed that serum testosterone levels exceeded the upper limits for normal male testosterone concentrations in three of these women. Moreover, significant compensatory decrease in sex-hormone-binding globulin and decreased thyroid-binding proteins were noted in these athletes. High-density lipoprotein cholesterol decreased by 39% in the female weightlifters using AAS.

Example of Abuse of Anabolic-Androgenic Steroids in Sport: The Case of the German Democratic Republic

The German government awards the prestigious *Heidi-Krieger-Medaille* to individuals who have a significant career in the fight against one of the main scourges in modern sport: doping. This award is named in the honor of Andreas Krieger (ex-athlete from the German Democratic Republic (GDR), born as Heidi Krieger).

The case of Heidi (Andreas) Krieger, European shot put champion in 1986, who retired in 1990, is perhaps one of the most dramatic documented cases regarding the use and abuse of AAS. During the trial against Ewal and Höeppner, Krieger reported the psychological and physiological effects of the massive use of steroids during youth that made her look like a man, and drove her to serious psychological disorders and attempted suicide. Krieger underwent sex reassignment surgery and changed her name to Andreas Krieger. Nowadays, he lives in Germany, married to former East German swimmer Ute Krause, who was also a victim of massive doping.

Heidi Krieger was born in East Berlin (GDR) in July 1966. At the age of 14, she was recruited for her athletic talent to be part of the *Dynamo Berlin* elite sports club. Two years later, she entered into a massive doping project organized by the communist GDR government. To start the program, numerous scientists from the GDR developed a highly sophisticated and methodological plan, backed by the government itself and under the control of the *Ministerium für Staatssicherheit (STASI)* [57]. The program managers and key players were Manfred Ewald (minister of sports, 1961–1988, and president of the National Olympic Committee, 1973–1990) and the doctor Manfred Höeppner. They did not act alone, and certainly several official institutions and many researchers were involved, among them Rüdiger Häcker, director of the *Institute of Leipzig* and responsible for a program to improve the effectiveness of steroids and avoid its detection. Also, different researchers from *Jenapharm* pharmaceutical laboratories participated.

The secret doping program developed in the GDR was successful in the field of sports and allowed the country to reach leading positions in many international sporting areas, such as swimming, athletics, rowing, canoeing, and weightlifting. However, there were many side effects, especially regarding the athletes' physiological and psychological well-being, with an average of 30 annual victims as a consequence of the biological manipulation of their athletes.

To implement the project, various work programs were created, including the development of steroids and their use. Their massive use started from the early 1970s and was formalized as state plan 14.25 in 1974 [57–59]. To optimize the systematic doping, the aim of one of the projects was to develop different steroids for their athletes. The main steroid used was a variant of Dianabol (17α-methyl-17β hydroxy-1.4-androstandiene-3-one) which they named Oral-Turinabol (4-chlor-1-dehydro-17α-methyltestosterone). However, they used and performed researches with other oral anabolic substances (17α-methyl-17β-hydroxy-5α-androstane-3-on; 11-β-hydroxy-OT; 4-chlor-17α-methyl-17β-hydroxy-5α-androst-4-en-3-one; 4-chlor-17α-methyl-17β-hydroxy-5α-androst-4-en-3-one; 17α-methyl-17β hydroxy-1.4-androstandiene-3-one), Testosteron-Ampullen injectables, Testosteron-Depot-Ampullen, Testo-Tropin-Ampullen, Turinabol-Ampullen (phenylpropionate ester of 17β hydroxy-19-norandrost-4-en-3-one) or Turinabol-Depot-Ampullen (decanoate ester of phenylpropionate ester of 17β hydroxy-19-norandrost-4-en-3-one), nasal spray (testosterone esters and androstenedione), and stimulating testosterone synthesizing substances (Gonabion-Ampullen and Clomiphen).

The accuracy of the programs was surprising from a sporting point of view. However, its consequences should have been taken into consideration. After the fall of the wall, numerous athletes recognized the use of hormone treatments at an early age. In this sense, Werner Franke provided the strongest information about this topic. Franke, a molecular biologist at the *Research Center of Cancer* at Heidelberg, discovered many of the secret documents and provided more information about the studies performed in East Germany. Furthermore, he uncovered the plot on which the sport miracle of this little Central European Republic was based.

During the project, specific protocols for the different sports modalities and athletes were designed. From the documents found, we know that the initially recommended steroids dose in RDA corresponded to 0.125 mg/kg of lean mass. Furthermore, doses increased and improved with time. They also perfected the concept of intake and rest cycles to ensure the steroid affinity with its receptor. Doses varied depending on variables such as gender, type of sport, and individual characteristics. In addition, the use of Oral-Turinabol was supplemented with other steroids and hormones.

The effects of systematic and prolonged use of AAS among most of the treated women resulted in high levels of virilization. In former East Germany, some gynecological disorders were observed as a consequence of androgenization in sportswomen, such as long-term amenorrhea and ovarian cysts [60].

Conclusion

Real-life and experimental data show that the use of steroids can negatively influence athletes' health. Among the numerous negative effects, steroid abuse may adversely affect female fertility and reproductive organs. It is imperative that athletes, coaches, and sports medicine doctors be aware of these severe consequences and that steps be taken to prevent athletes from the abuse of such drugs.

References

1. Büttner A, Thieme D. Side effects of anabolic androgenic steroids: pathological findings and structure–activity relationships. In: Thieme D, Hemmersbach P, editors. Doping in sports: biochemical principles, effects and analysis. Berlin: Springer; 2010. p. 459–84.
2. Hartgens F, Kuipers H. Effects of androgenic-anabolic steroids in athletes. Sports Med. 2004;34(8):513–54.
3. Sjöqvist F, Garle M, Rane A. Use of doping agents, particularly anabolic steroids, in sports and society. Lancet. 2008;371(9627):1872–82.
4. Christakopoulos A, Ericsson M, Garle M, Villén T, Beck O. Anabolic androgenic steroids are more common in society than in sports. Lakartidningen. 2013;110(39–40):1732–4.
5. Abrahin OSC, de Sousa EC, Santos AM. Prevalence of the use of anabolic-androgenic steroids in Brazil: a systematic review. Subst Use misuse. 2014;49(9):1156–62.
6. Stubbe JH, Chorus AM, Frank LE, Hon O, Heijden PG. Prevalence of use of performance enhancing drugs by fitness centre members. Drug Test Anal. 2014;6(5):434–8.
7. Strauss RH, Liggett MT, Lanese RR. Anabolic steroid use and perceived effects in ten weight-trained women athletes. J Am Med Assoc. 1985;253(19):2871–3.
8. Yesalis CE, Kennedy NJ, Kopstein AN, Bahrke MS. Anabolic-androgenic steroid use in the United States. JAMA. 1993;270(10):1217–21.
9. Pereira HMG, Sardela VF. Stimulant doping agents used in Brazil: prevalence, detectability, analytical implications, and challenges. Subst Use Misuse. 2014;49(9):1098–114.
10. Thorlindsson T, Halldorsson V. Sport, and use of anabolic androgenic steroids among Icelandic high school students: a critical test of three perspectives. Subst Abuse Treat Prev Policy. 2010;5:32.
11. Dunn M, White V. The epidemiology of anabolic–androgenic steroid use among Australian secondary school students. J Sci Med Sport. 2011;14(1):10–4.
12. Johnston L, O'Malley PM, Bachman JG, Schulenberg JE. Monitoring the Future national survey results on drug use, 1975–2011. Volume I: secondary school students. Ann Arbor: Institute for Social Research, The University of Michigan; 2012.
13. Pärssinen M, Kujala U, Vartiainen E, Sarna S, Seppala T. Increased premature mortality of competitive powerlifters suspected to have used anabolic agents. Int J Sports Med. 2000;21(3):225–7.
14. Petersson A, Garle M, Granath F, Thiblin I. Morbidity and mortality in patients testing positively for the presence of anabolic androgenic steroids in connection with receiving medical care: a controlled retrospective cohort study. Drug Alcohol Depend. 2006;81(3):215–20.
15. Santora LJ, Marin J, Vangrow J, Minegar C, Robinson M, Mora J, Frieds G. Coronary calcification in body builders using anabolic steroids. Prev Card. 2006;9(4):198–201.
16. Paolo M D, Agozzino M, Toni C, Luciani AB, Molendini L, Scaglione M, Arbustini E. Sudden anabolic steroid abuse-related death in athletes. Int J Cardiol. 2007;114(1):114–7.
17. Yesalis CE, Bahrke MS. Anabolic-androgenic steroids. Sports Med. 1995;19(5):326–40.
18. Maravelias C, Dona A, Stefanidou M, Spiliopoulou C. Adverse effects of anabolic steroids in athletes. A constant threat. Toxic Lett. 2005;158(3):167–75.
19. Melnik B, Jansen T, Grabbe S. Abuse of anabolic-androgenic steroids and bodybuilding acne: an underestimated health problem. J Deut Dermat Gesell. 2007;5(2):110–7.
20. Casavant MJ, Blake K, Griffith J, Yates A, Copley LM. Consequences of use of anabolic androgenic steroids. Ped Clin N Am. 2007;54(4):677–90.
21. Wu FCW. Endocrine aspects of anabolic steroids. Clin Chem. 1997;43(7):1289–92.
22. Clark AS, Costine BA, Jones BL, Kelton-Rehkopf MC, Meerts SH, Nutbrown-Greene LL, Henderson LP. Sex-and age-specific effects of anabolic androgenic steroids on reproductive behaviors and on GABAergic transmission in neuroendocrine control regions. Brain Res. 2006;1126(1):122–38.
23. Elliot DL, Goldberg L. Women and anabolic steroids. Anab Steroids Sport Exerc. 2000;2:225–46.
24. Burger HG. Androgen production in women. Fertil Steril. 2002;77(4):3–5.
25. Basaria S, Wahlstrom JT, Dobs AS. Anabolic-androgenic steroid therapy in the treatment of chronic diseases. J Clin Endocrinol Metab. 2001;86(11):5108–17.
26. Burger HG. Androgen production in women. Fertil Steril. 2002;77(4):3–5.
27. Judd HL, Lucas WE, Yen SS. Effect of oophorectomy on circulating testosterone and androstenedione levels in patients with endometrial cancer. Am J Obs Gynecol. 1974;118(6):793–8.

28. Obasanjo IO, Cline JM, Schmotzer S, Weaver DS. Nandrolone decanoate causes pathologic changes in the uterus of surgically postmenopausal female cynomolgus macaques. Menopause. 1998;5(3):163–8.
29. Sprando RL, Collins TF, Black TN, Olejnik N, Grundel E, Ruggles DI. Effects of androstenedione on in utero development in rats. Food Chem Toxicol. 2004;42(6):917–24.
30. Rubiera-Gerez JR, Frei F, Camargo IC. Histological assessment of ovaries and uterus of rats subjected to nandrolone decanoate treatment. Contraception. 2005;72:77–80.
31. Cherici-Camargo IC, Barreiros-De Souza R, Mesquita S, Chuffa LG, Frei F. Ovarian histology and follicular score in female rats treated with nandrolone decanoate and submitted to physical effort. Acta Biol Hung. 2009;60(3):253–61.
32. Cherici-Camargo IC, Gaspar ALC, Frei F, Mesquita SD. Effects of androgenic anabolic steroids on the uterus and reproductive parameters of adult female rats. Rev Bras Ginecol Obs. 2009;31(9):453–60.
33. De Almeida-Chuffa LG, de Souza RB, Frei F, Mesquita S, Cherici-Camargo IC. Nandrolone decanoate and physical effort: histological and morphometrical assessment in adult rat uterus. Anatom Record. 2011;294(2):335–41.
34. Karbalay-Doust S, Noorafshan A, Ardekani FM, Mirkhani H. The reversibility of sperm quality after discontinuing nandrolonendecanoate in adult male rats. Asian J Androl. 2007;9:235–9.
35. Bordbar H, Mesbah F, Talaei T, Dehghani F, Mirkhani H. Modulatory effect of gonadotropins on rats' ovaries after nandrolone decanoate administration: a stereological study. Iran J Med Sci. 2014;39(1):44–50.
36. Howe GR, Morello CJ. Effects of an anabolic steroid on reproduction in female rats. Steroid. 1985;45(6):495–501.
37. Bronson FH, Nguyen KQ, Delarosa J. Effect of anabolic steroid on physiological characteristics of female mice. Physiol Behav. 1996;59:49–55.
38. Korkia P, Stimson GV. Indications of prevalence, practice and effects of anabolic steroid use in Great Britain. Int J Sports Med. 1997;18(7):557–62.
39. Blasberg ME, Langan CJ, Clark AS. The effects of alphathyltestosterone, methandrostenolone and nandrolone decanoate on the rat estrous cycle. Physiol Behav. 1997;61:265–72.
40. Graham S, Kennedy M. Recent developments in the toxicology of anabolic steroids. Drug safety. 1990;5(6):458–76.
41. Kao LW, Weisz J. Direct effect of testosterone and its 5alpha-reduced metabolites on pituitary LH and FSH release in vitro: change in pituitary responsiveness to hypothalamic extract. Endocrinology. 1975;96(2):253–60.
42. Strauss JF, Martinez F, Kiriakidou M. Placental steroid hormone synthesis: unique features and unanswered questions. Biol Reprod. 1996;54(2): 303–11.
43. Penatti CA, Oberlander JG, Davis MC, Porter DM, Henderson LP. Chronic exposure to anabolic androgenic steroids alters activity and synaptic function in neuroendocrine control regions of the female mouse. Neuropharmacology. 2011;61(4):653–64.
44. Friedl KE, Yesalis CE. Self-Treatment of Gynecomastia in Bodybuilders Who Use Anabolic Steroids. Case Reports. Phys Sportsmed. 1989;17(3):67–71.
45. Ruiz-Cortés ZT. Gonadal sex steroids: production, action and interactions in mammals. In: Ostojic SM, editor. Steroids—from physiology to clinical medicine. Rijeka: Intech; 2012. doi:10.5772/46119.
46. Anderson E. In vivo and in vitro effects of androgens on rat ovarian granulosa cells. Am J Obstet Gynecol. 1989;160(4):782–8.
47. Anderson E, Little B, Lee GS. Androgen-induced changes in rat ovarian granulosa cells in vitro. Tiss Cell. 1987;19(2):217–34.
48. Mobini-Far HR, Ågren G, Lindqvist AS, Marmendal M, Fahlke C, Thiblin I. Administration of the anabolic androgenic steroid nandrolone decanoate to female rats causes alterations in the morphology of their uterus and a reduction in reproductive capacity. Eur J Obs Gynec Repr Biol. 2007;131(2):189–97.
49. Karbalay-Doust S, Noorafshan A. Stereological estimation of ovarian oocyte volume, surface area and number: application on mice treated with nandrolone decanoate. Folia Histochem et Cytobiol. 2012;50(2):275–9.
50. Bassindale T, Cowan DA, Dale S, Hutt AJ, Leeds AR, Wheeler MJ, Kicmna AT. Effects of oral administration of androstenedione on plasma androgens in young women using hormonal contraception. J Clin Endoc Met. 2004;89:6030–8.
51. Triemstra JL, Wood RI. Testosterone self-administration in female hamsters. Behav Brain Res. 2004;154(1):221–9.
52. Bento-Silva MT, Martins MDCDC, Torres-Leal FL, Barros TL, Carvalho ILDNF, Carvalho Filho HA, Almeida FRDC. Effects of administering testosterone undecanoate in rats subjected to physical exercise: effects on the estrous cycle, motor behavior and morphology of the liver and kidney. Braz J Pharm Sci. 1985;46(1):79–89.
53. Kicman AT. Pharmacology of anabolic steroids. BJ Pharm. 2008;154(3):502–21.
54. Hoffman JR, Ratamess NA. Medical issues associated with anabolic steroid use: are they exaggerated? J Sports Sci Med. 2006;5(2):182–93.
55. Clark AS, Blasberg ME, Brandling-Bennett EM. Stanozolol, oxymetholone, and testosterone cypionate effects on the rat estrous cycle. Physiol Behav. 1998;63(2):287–95.
56. Malarkey WB, Strauss RH, Leizman DJ, Liggett M, Demers LM. Endocrine effects in female weight lifters who self-administer testosterone and anabolic steroids. Am J Obs Gynec. 1991;165(5):1385–90.
57. Franke WW, Berendonk B. Hormonal doping and androgenization of athletes: a secret program of

the German democratic republic government. Clin Chem. 1997;43(7):1262–79.
58. Ungerleider S. Faust's gold: inside the East German doping machine. New York: Macmillan; 2001.
59. Spitzer G. Ranking number 3 in the world: how the addiction to doping changed sport in the GDR. In: Spitzer G, editor. Doping and doping control in Europe. Aachen: Meyer & Meyer Sport; 2006. p. 57–77.
60. Prendergast HM, Bannen T, Erickson TB, Honore KR. The toxic torch of the modern olympic games. Veter Hum Toxic. 2003;45(2):97–102.

Impact of Intense Physical Activity on Puberty and Reproductive Potential of Young Athletes

15

Neoklis A. Georgopoulos and Nikolaos D. Roupas

Introduction

Over the past decades, major social changes allowed the development of a positive attitude towards physical activity, highlighting the beneficial role of exercise on mental and physical health. Thus, individuals are becoming increasingly involved in physical activities, ranging from regular mild exercise to highly competitive performance requiring intensive and strenuous training. However, as the duration, frequency, and intensity of exercise increases, great concern and major reactions arouse regarding the deleterious effects of intensive physical activity on somatic growth, pubertal development, and biological maturation.

Individual sports exert unique impacts on body composition and development, depending on the sport-related specific features, technical skills and training methods, and the state of growth and maturation of the athlete. Beginning at an early age, athletes performing at a high competitive level are exposed to high levels of physical and psychological stress resulting from many hours of intense training and competitions. The damaging effects of these factors on somatic growth, skeletal and pubertal maturation have been described in individuals performing a variety of sports. Therefore, the whole picture is extremely complex and should be approached with extreme caution and responsibility.

The aim of this chapter is to provide an overview of our current understanding and recent development in the field of exercise-induced disorders of pubertal development and reproductive function.

Exercise and Pubertal Development

Puberty is the period of transition from childhood to adolescence and is marked by the development of secondary sexual characteristics, accelerated growth, behavioral changes, and eventual attainment of reproductive capacity [1]. Moreover, puberty is a dynamic period of development with rapid changes in body size, shape, and composition.

Available approaches for the assessment of pubertal onset and progression include the use of Tanner stages for female breast and pubic hair development and male gonadal and pubic hair development, while menarche is also an important marker used for assessing puberty in girls [1]. More specifically, the onset of puberty corresponds to a specific biological age, as determined by skeletal maturation and namely, a bone age of 13 years for boys and 11 years for girls [2]. Prolonged intensive physical training has great impact on skeletal maturation, leading to a significant delay in bone age compared to chron-

N. A. Georgopoulos (✉) · N. D. Roupas
Department of Obstetrics and Gynecology,
Division of Reproductive Endocrinology,
University of Patras, Medical School,
University Hospital, Patras 26500, Greece
e-mail: neoklisg@hol.gr

© Springer Science+Business Media New York 2016

D. Vaamonde et al. (eds.), *Exercise and Human Reproduction*, DOI 10.1007/978-1-4939-3402-7_15

ological age. As in the general population, pubertal development in highly trained athletes seems to follow bone age rather than chronological age [3]. However, genetic predisposition and variation among individuals should always be considered. Specific sports favor the early matures, while others, like gymnastics, offer advantage to the later-developing individuals. Therefore, any assessment of sexual maturation must take into account the biological indicators of bone age and peak height velocity.

It should be noted that the vast majority of the published data involve the influence of physical activity on sexual maturation of female athletes. This inconsistency possibly reflects the sensitivity of the female reproductive system, which is been shown to be highly vulnerable to changes regarding intrinsic and extrinsic factors.

Delayed pubertal development in female athletes has been observed in a variety of sports, mainly gymnasts, dancers, and long-distance runners [4]. The documented delay is determined by the type, the frequency, the intensity, and the duration of exercise and is more pronounced in sports requiring strict dietary restrictions that result in higher energy expenditure in the presence of inadequate energy input.

In the case of gymnasts performing in the high competitive level of the Olympic Games, delayed menarche has been noted, compared to high school, college, and club-level athletes [5]. On the other hand, young girls or adolescents engaged in sports requiring training less than 15 h/week do not show menstrual disturbances or delay in sexual maturation [6].

In elite rhythmic (RG) and artistic (AG) gymnasts, the prepubertal stage was prolonged and pubertal development was shifted to a later age, retaining a normal progression rate [7–10]. Expectedly, the progression of puberty followed the bone age rather than the chronological age [8, 9]. It should be underlined that, for both RG and AG, pubertal progression, although delayed, was not prolonged. Normal girls require an average of 1.96 ± 0.93 years (mean ± SD) for their breast development to progress from Tanner stage II to Tanner stage IV [11]. A comparable period of time was observed for both RG and AG in our study. Therefore, pubertal maturation was entirely shifted to a later age, maintaining a normal rate of progression.

The major factor responsible for the delay in the onset of breast and pubic hair development in both sports was low body weight. Low body weight reflects an energy deficit, prominent in both sports, as a result of intensive physical training (high energy expenditure) on the one side and inadequate caloric consumption (low energy input) on the other. Gymnasts indeed are subjected to a significant energy drain, occurring early in prepubertal age, and are highly motivated to achieve low body weights consistent with their sports requirements for a lean somatotype.

On the other hand, in ballet dancers under high energy drain and low energy intake, a delayed thelarche and a normal pubarche were documented [12]. These findings suggest the existence of independent central mechanisms involved in triggering these aspects of pubertal development. Indeed, breast development and subsequently menarche are related to estrogen levels, while pubarche is mainly related to adrenal androgen production [13]. In conditions of energy imbalance and consequent reduction in adipose tissue mass, estrogen production is decreased and breast development and menarche are delayed. It is the onset, the duration, and the extent of energy deficit that determines the degree of involvement of all aspects of pubertal development. Indeed, ballet dancers with a normal pubarche start their training at the age of 8–9 years of age with only 3.5–7.3 h of training per week [12], while our examined RG and AG started their training at the age of 6.4–7.7 years with more than 30 h of training per week.

With regard to age of menarche, athletes involved in a large variety of sports, including runners, swimmers, tennis players, ballet dancers, and gymnasts, present a well-documented delayed menarche [12–20]. Although similar trends depending on type of sport are apparent, menarche is more delayed in gymnasts than in swimmers or tennis players who began training at a comparable age [3]. In RG, menarche was significantly delayed compared to their mothers and not trained sisters, an observation arguing against a genetic predisposition towards delayed menarche [10]. These adjustments reflect a natural adaptation of the body to high energy demands. In AG and RG, low body fat, low body weight (low energy input) and prolonged intensive physical training (high energy output) were the major factors influencing menarche. Low body weight, however, remained the most significant factor in delaying the onset of puberty. In addition, it is to be noted that in both RG and AG, older athletes without menarche presented lower height, weight, and body mass index (BMI) compared to their contemporaries with menarche.

Finally, with regard to the effect of physical activity on pubertal development and sexual maturation of male athletes, the data are scarce. In general, boys who participate in sports are normal or advanced for their state of skeletal and sexual maturation, and the advanced states of maturation may be attributed to the power and performance advantages associated with maturation or the existence of preselection bias in terms of sports that favor athletes who are more physically mature than other athletes of the same age [3, 21]. More specifically, in sports where large physiques were necessary for performance success (i.e., swimming and tennis), these athletes tended to have advanced sexual maturation [22]. However, for sports that may create an energy drain, the effects on pubertal development remain inconclusive. In the case of male gymnasts, a sport in which the prepubertal physique confers a performance advantage, there are studies suggestive of a late maturation status [22], while other studies reported no significant influence of intense exercise on pubertal development [21]. These discrepancies should be attributed to methodological differences, mainly regarding the competition level of the studied athletes and the pubertal development assessment methods.

Energy Homeostasis and Pubertal Development

The hallmark of puberty is the reactivation of the hypothalamic pulsatile secretion of gonadotropin-releasing hormone (GnRH), which activates the hypothalamic–pituitary–gonadal (HPG) axis and establishes the production of sex steroids. This reactivation of GnRH production, known to characterize the fetal and neonatal stages, takes place under the influence of several stimuli that are yet to be fully elucidated.

It is well known that a minimum weight-to-height and a critical lean-to-fat-mass ratio are required for menarche. According to Frisch theory, the attainment of a critical percentage of body fat lowers the metabolic rate and induces a sensitization of the hypothalamus to gonadal steroids [23, 24]. Although the principle of a critical percentage of body fat is no longer considered valid, the issue of energy balance and the status of metabolic fuel and energy stores is one of the cornerstones in the control of pubertal onset and progression [25]. Subsequently, several peripherally produced hormones related to energy homeostasis control have been shown to mediate the regulatory role of neural circuits involved in the control of pubertal development.

Among the numerous peripherally produced hormones, leptin has the most prominent and well-studied role connecting energy status with the initiation of puberty and the maintenance of the reproductive function [25]. Although leptin has been considered to play a pivotal role in signaling a metabolic interaction between body composition and reproductive function [26], the available data are inconclusive as to whether leptin is a signal for the initiation of pubertal development or if a critical leptin level is a condition for pubertal onset, acting as a permissive factor so that other critical processes of sexual maturation can occur [25]. With regard to other adipokines, there are conflicting data regarding a possible role of resistin and adiponectin in connecting energy homeostasis and sexual maturation [25].

Furthermore, the gut-derived hormone ghrelin has a well-established role in the regulation of appetite and energy balance, while there are sufficient data to support the possible involvement of ghrelin in the regulation of puberty and sexual function [25]. More specifically, it has been suggested that ghrelin signals energy availability and determines the onset and the progression of pubertal development, and this effect is predominant in males and dependent on the pubertal stage.

Exercise and Reproductive Dysfunction in Females

It is well documented that the female reproductive system is highly sensitive to changes regarding intrinsic and extrinsic factors. Thus, female athletes exposed to intensive training, psychological stress, and strict dietary restrains are vulnerable to developing reproductive dysfunction.

Prevalence

Reproductive abnormalities are present in 6–79% of females involved in sports activities [27]. Female athletes involved in a large variety of sports, including runners, swimmers, tennis players, ballet dancers, and gymnasts, present a well-documented delayed menarche [12–20]. The prevalence of menstrual dysfunction has been studied widely and varies with the specific sport and the level of competition [27].

Considering the sport-related specific features, the training methods and the technical skills, the sports could be divided into technical, endurance, aesthetics, weight class, ball game, power, and antigravitation sports. Moreover, taking into account the optimal for the specific sport somatotype, the athletic events can be divided into leanness and non-leanness sports [28].

Clinical Patterns of Exercise-Related Menstrual Abnormalities

Menstruation represents a particularly delicate function, indicating normal reproductive activity. Interrelated functions of the hypothalamus, pituitary, ovaries, and endometrium give rise to predictable, cyclic menses that indicate regular ovulation. Ovarian function and menstrual regularity depend on normal cyclic pituitary gonadotropin stimulation. The secretion of gonadotropins occurs in response to pulsatile GnRH release from the hypothalamus. The secretion of GnRH is regulated by various neurotransmitter and neuropeptide pathways.

Female athletic performance has been associated with a broad spectrum of menstrual dysfunction. The dysfunction ranges from primary amenorrhea or delayed menarche to luteal phase deficiency, oligomenorrhea, anovulation, and secondary amenorrhea.

The term amenorrhea refers to the absence or abnormal cessation of the menses. The reproductive dysfunction in amenorrhea is characterized of deranged, abnormal, infrequent or absent luteinizing hormone (LH) pulses, suppressed follicular development, ovulation and luteal activity, leading to persistently low levels of estrogens and progesterone and absence of endometrial proliferation [29]. Primary amenorrhea is indicated when there has been a failure to menstruate by the age of 15 years, in the presence of normal secondary sexual development (two standard deviations above the mean of 13 years) or within 5 years after breast development if that occurs before the age of 10 [30]. Secondary amenorrhea is defined as the absence of three or more consecutive menstrual cycles after menarche (given that pregnancy is excluded), while oligomenorrhea describes menstrual cycles of 35 days or more (alternatively, menstrual intervals of 45–90 days).

Luteal phase deficiency denotes asymptomatic subclinical menstrual disturbances, resulting in low estradiol levels in the early follicular phase, decreased but normal LH pulse frequency with increased pulse amplitude. Ovulation occurs, but the developed corpus luteum produces reduced progesterone support for proper endometrial development in the secretory phase. Thus, successful implantation of fertilized egg is prevented and infertility ensues.

Anovulation is a more severe asymptomatic reproductive dysfunction, characterized by suppressed follicular maturation leading to lack of ovulation. Both estrogen and progesterone levels are low, but some proliferation of endometrium is achieved, resulting in profuse bleeding at unexpected times.

Pathophysiology of Exercise-Related Menstrual Abnormalities

During the past decades, many studies have been conducted regarding sports activities and athletic performance, focusing on the influence of physical activity on reproductive function. The main factors etiologically correlated with menstrual disturbances in athletes are energy balance (energy availability) and body composition, stress (physical exercise and psychological stress), diet, training methods (sports character), and reproductive maturity.

Weight and Body Composition and Energy Availability

One of the earliest and most interesting approaches to menstrual dysfunction in athletes was made by Frisch et al., who theorized that the onset of menarche is achieved when body fat reaches a "critical threshold" of 17% of body weight and that menstruation is disrupted when body fat falls below a "critical threshold" of 22% of body weight. According to Frisch theory, the attainment of a critical percentage of body fat lowers the metabolic rate and induces a sensitization of the hypothalamus to gonadal steroids [24]. Since then, weight and body composition have been considered the most common and most convincing explanation of female reproductive dysfunction in athletes.

Recent studies, however, argue the existence of a critical body weight or fat percentage in order to achieve menstruation, introducing dispute over theoretical and statistical issues [31–33]. Furthermore, available data suggest a central role for energy availability (defined as dietary energy input, minus exercise-induced energy expenditure), rather than body weight, in the pathogenesis of reproductive dysfunction in female athletes [33]. It has been proposed that negative energy balance (failure to meet the metabolic requirements) causes an alteration in brain function that disrupts the GnRH pulse generator.

Researchers studying monkeys concluded that exercise-induced amenorrhea was reversed by diet and caloric supplementation, without any modification of their exercise regimen [34]. It appears that energy deprivation leads to a disruption in LH pulsatility, in contrast to exercise stress, while LH pulsatility is suppressed in the presence of energy depletion, regardless of the cause. In addition, caloric imbalance prevents the normal pulsatile secretion of LH in exercising women [35]. Thus, it is proposed that exercise has no detrimental effects on female reproductive regulation, apart from the cost on energy balance.

The emerging role of adipose tissue as an active endocrine organ has attracted the scientific concern and revealed a number of adipose-secreted factors (known as adipokines) involved in signaling and regulating homeostasis, energy balance, insulin action, reproductive function, and inflammation process. For instance, leptin has an established role in energy homeostasis, metabolism, and reproductive function, while adiponectin attracts growing interest as a mediator in metabolism and reproduction.

The discovery of leptin boosted the interest on the body composition hypothesis and provided the missing link with the energy availability hypothesis. Leptin has been investigated as a mediator between the adipose and the reproduction system [26] and has been considered to play a pivotal role in signaling a metabolic interaction between body composition and reproductive function. Serum leptin levels reflect the dietary status and caloric balance: Rapid and profound declines in leptin levels were documented in response to fasting and dietary restrictions, while extreme increases were noted in response to overfeeding and refeeding after caloric deprivation [33]. Furthermore, in severely undernourished women, the preservation of neuroendocrine control of reproductive function is mediated by leptin [36]. In addition, a critical level of leptin is required for the maturation and maintenance of menstruation [37]. Moreover, it has been reported that serum leptin levels were reduced in highly trained athletes and the diurnal pattern of leptin secretion was lost in amenorrheic, compared to menstruating athletes [38]. Finally, exogenous leptin (recombinant r-metHuLeptin) administration managed to improve the reproductive function of a small cohort of women with hypothalamic amenorrhea, due to strenuous exercise or low body weight [39].

In contrast with leptin, adiponectin is markedly reduced in obesity and rises with prolonged fasting and severe weight reduction. Despite a well-described role in metabolism, cardiovascular protection, and inflammatory process, recent studies suggest a potential role in the regulation of neuroendocrine reproductive processes. More specifically, it has been reported that adiponectin inhibits both basal and GnRH-stimulated LH secretion in short-term treated rat pituitary cells [40]. Furthermore, Lu et al. reported that adiponectin acutely reduced basal and GnRH-stimulated LH secretion but had no impact on follicle-stimulating hormone (FSH) levels [41]. Consequently, high levels of adiponectin (as found in lean and energy-restrained female athletes) may contribute to suppression of LH levels and chronic anovulation. Thus, adiponectin could be considered as a link between adiposity and reproduction.

In addition to the role of the aforementioned adipokines, there are gut-derived hormones signaling energy homeostasis implicated in normal reproductive function [25]. Among them, ghrelin has a well-studied role in the regulation of puberty and sexual function. Studies in rodents and humans have shown that ghrelin reduces baseline LH secretion, with reductions in both pulse amplitude and frequency [25].

Physical Stress

The hypothesis that menstrual disturbances in athletes might be caused by the stress of exercise was originally based on animal experiments and recently on studies of amenorrheic athletes. The interaction between HPA axis and reproductive system was studied in rats and monkeys [42, 43], demonstrating that the hormones of the HPA axis could disrupt the reproductive function by both central and peripheral mechanisms [44].

A few decades ago, Bullen et al. reported the induction of menstrual disorders in regularly menstruating women, by imposing strenuous exercise [45]. Regularly menstruating, untrained women were exposed to high-volume aerobic exercise, which leads to a large prevalence of luteal phase deficiency and anovulation. Since then, a mild degree of elevated cortisol levels has been documented in amenorrheic athletes [29, 45, 46].

HPA axis activation provides a hormonal mechanism of reproductive dysfunction in female athletes. Cortisol can suppress gonadotropin secretion from the pituitary [47] and corticotropin-releasing hormone (CRH) can suppress GnRH secretion from the hypothalamus by increasing the hypothalamic opiate inhibition [48]. Furthermore, it has been suggested that athletes presenting more profound menstrual disorders exhibit a greater activation of the HPA axis [29].

Psychological Stress

Psychological stress is another factor commonly implicated in the etiology and pathogenesis of exercise-induced menstrual disturbances. Although there are studies correlating behavioral and psychological parameters in women with functional hypothalamic amenorrhea, few data exist to support this hypothesis in athletes [49]. Amenorrheic athletes exhibit similar psychological profile compared with menstruating athletes [50], while studies regarding musicians, with a competitive lifestyle similar to that of athletes, concluded that the psychological stress of competitions has no causative role in reproductive dysfunction of most individuals [12].

Diet

Few data exist regarding a possible role of diet composition on the pathogenesis of menstrual disorders in athletes. Apart from the influence of inadequate caloric intake (insufficient to compensate the increased energy expenditure), the diet composition has been studied separately regarding a possible correlation with reproductive dysfunction in female athletes. Protein and fat intake appears to be decreased in amenorrheic athletes. The controversial data resulting from studies attempting to correlate the incidence of menstrual disorders with vegetarian diets—favored by some athletes—might imply the synergic effect of other factors (such as energy balance, training intensity, or emotional stress) in the development of reproductive dysfunction [51, 52].

Training Methods/Sports Characteristic Features

It is well known that the unique character of each sport consists of specific skills requirements, favorable somatotype, and special training methods. The age of training onset, the optimal somatotype, the specific sports demands as well as the intensity, frequency, and duration of training determine dietary restrictions and certain energy and metabolic profile, influencing the menstrual status of female athletes.

Heavy training load appears to exert more harmful effect on menstrual function when initiated abruptly, compared with a gradual acceleration [53]. Moreover, long-term training at levels of energy expenditure above the lactate threshold affects menstrual function more than long-term training at or below the lactate threshold [54]. Furthermore, exercise-induced menstrual disorders are more common in endurance runners and ballet dancers than in swimmers and cyclists [17, 55, 56]. This observation could be interpreted considering the optimal somatotype demands, attracting individuals of certain body characteristics to different types of elite competitive sports (e.g., thinness in ballet dancers and long-distance runners), combined with dietary adaptations and restrictions.

Reproductive Maturity

It has been suggested that intense training has less effect on menstrual function of previously sedentary menstruating individuals, compared with premenarcheal adolescents [57]. This might be due either to a sensitivity of reproductively immature females to the influence of intense exercise or as a predisposition of young individuals to exercise-mediated reproductive disorders [58]. Nevertheless, it seems very difficult to isolate and evaluate reproductive maturity as a factor interfering in the pathogenesis of exercise-induced reproductive dysfunction, separated from energy availability, body fat, and body weight [33].

Menstrual Disorders in Specific Sports

Somatic growth and biological maturation in runners have been well studied and described. Although in the same sport field, runners are divided in recreational, small distance, and long distance, considering the training methods, the technical skills, the favorable somatotype, and the specific requirements of each event. Athletes participating in power events (e.g., sprints, hurdles) train at maximal or near-maximal intensity in short bursts. Conversely, athletes participating in endurance events (e.g., middle-distance and long-distance running) train at lower intensity levels for extended periods. Power athletes are heavier and have more total lean mass than their endurance counterparts [59].

Menstrual disorders characterize as much as 24–26% of female runners [60, 61]. Within distance runners, prevalence of amenorrhea increased from 3 to 60% as training distance increased from <13 to >113 km/week, while their body weights decreased from >60 to <50 kg [56]. Furthermore, subclinical menstrual disorders are present in both highly trained [29] and recreational [62] eumenorrheic athletes; luteal deficiency or anovulation was found in 78% of eumenorrheic recreational runners in at least one menstrual cycle out of three [62]. On the other hand, in sub-elite moderately exercising female runners, no effect on pubertal development was demonstrated [63].

Dance training has been shown to be associated with a high incidence of menstrual dysfunction, particularly in disciplines such as ballet [55]. Ballet dancers begin strenuous training at an early age, undergo intensive exercise and heavy caloric restrictions leading to energy deficit, in order to perform at a competitive level and retain a lean physique. Teenage ballet dancers are lighter, with less body fat and higher incidence of delayed puberty and primary and secondary amenorrhea, compared with less physically active girls [53, 55].

Swimmers present normal weight, less fat, and more muscle mass than nonathletic girls but a greater percentage of fat than that of amenorrheic athletes in other sports [12]. The latter reflects an adjustment to the sport-specific requirements, as in aquatic sports, subcutaneous fat helps floatation, reducing energy expenditure for water surface maintenance. Constantini et al. studied swimmers of competitive level and demonstrated that menstrual cycles were more irregular or anovulatory rather than absent. Considering the greater amount of fat in swimmers, functioning as an estrogen producer and reservoir, the observed menstrual disturbances could not be attributed to hypoestrogenism and might be due to mild hyperandrogenism [64].

In gymnastics, in the case of gymnasts performing in the high competitive level of the Olympic Games, a delayed menarche has been noted, compared to high school, college, and club-level athletes [5]. Furthermore, young girls or adolescents engaged in sports requiring training less than 15 h/week less frequently have menstrual disturbances or delayed sexual maturation [6]. In addition, elite RG menarche was significantly delayed compared to their mothers and not trained sisters, a finding arguing against a genetic predisposition towards delayed menarche [65].

Skeletal Implications

Exercise-induced menstrual dysfunction and the consistent estrogen deficiency have profound impacts on the skeleton. Failure to reach peak bone mass, bone loss, and inadequate bone mineralization predispose hypoestrogenic athletes to osteopenia and osteoporosis and increase the risk of bone fracture [27]. Although genetic factors considerably influence bone mass, other factors such as nutrition, natural exercise, various diseases and medicines, age of menarche, and normal menstrual cycle regulate the acquisition of bone mass in a rather synergic action. Interestingly, De Souza et al. reported that female athletes experiencing both energy and estrogen deficiency present worse bone turnover profile, compared to athletes with only one or none of these disorders [66].

There is a general agreement that physical activity enhances bone formation, thus increasing bone mass density (BMD) [67]. The higher strain levels, associated with growth or extreme physical activity, induce a type of modeling that increases bone mass by accretion on bone surfaces.

Bone mass doubles between the onset of puberty and early adult life [68]. Sex steroids are responsible for the maturation and increase in human skeleton after the onset of puberty. Recent findings in the field of metabolism and endocrinology argue the traditional theory of estrogen-mediated bone resorption in female athletes experiencing menstrual disorders. Thus, it has been suggested that nutritional deprivation and chronic energy deficit cause inadequate bone formation by altering the levels of various hormones affecting bone metabolism, not only estrogens, such as insulin-like growth factor-1 (IGF-1), cortisol, leptin, and ghrelin.

More specifically, IGF-1 is a bone trophic factor important for bone formation [69]. Relevant studies document lower levels of IGF-1 in adolescent athletes with amenorrhea in comparison to sedentary controls [70], while studies of peripubertal elite female RG documented an association of plasma IGF1/IGF-binding protein 3 (IGF1/IGFBP3) ratio with bone mass acquisition [71]. Furthermore, intense physical stress and energy imbalance cause activation of HPA axis and high cortisol levels, suggested to impart detrimental effects on bone [72].

Laboratory research introduced proliferative effects of ghrelin on osteoblasts in cell cultures and studies on animal models indicated that leptin decreases bone mass [73]. Christo et al. studied adolescent athletes and reported higher ghrelin and lower leptin levels in amenorrheic athletes, compared to eumenorrheic athletes and sedentary controls [74]. This study introduced bone age, lean mass, levels of IGF-1, and estradiol, but not ghrelin and leptin, as important positive predictors of bone mass parameters [73]. The involvement of leptin could provide a possible mechanism for an interaction between the nutritional and metabolic bone axes, suggesting a role for leptin as a physiologic regulator of bone mass [75]. Thus, osteopenia characterizing amenorrheic athletes involved in aesthetic sports may represent another adaptive response to chronic undernutrition.

Numerous studies have documented low BMD in athletes with hypoestrogenic amenorrhea, demonstrating lower BMD in amenorrheic athletes compared with regularly cycling athletes [76, 77]. Accordingly, Christo et al. compared bone density in adolescent amenorrheic athletes with eumenorrheic endurance athletes and non-athletic controls and reported lower bone density at the spine, hip and whole body in adolescent amenorrheic athletes compared with the other two groups [70]. In this study, athletes with amenorrhea had significantly lower lumbar BMD z scores, compared with athletes with eumenorrhea and control subjects. Lumbar BMD z scores

<-1 were documented in 38% of athletes with amenorrhea, compared with 16.7% of eumenorrheic athletes and 11% of sedentary controls. Interestingly, in a recent study, Ackerman et al. reported impaired bone microarchitecture, in addition to low BMD, in amenorrheic compared with eumenorrheic and nonathletes [78].

BMD declines as the number of missed menstrual cycles accumulates [79], and the loss of BMD may not be fully reversible [80]. Stress fractures occur more commonly in physically active women with menstrual irregularities and/or low BMD with a relative risk for stress fracture two to four times greater in amenorrheic than eumenorrheic athletes [81]. Studies involving ballet dancers demonstrated higher prevalence of scoliosis and a greater incidence of delayed menarche among the dancers presenting scoliosis [82, 83]. These limited data, though implying a possible connection between idiopathic scoliosis and exercise-induced menstrual disorders, fail to provide convincing evidence of a common pathogenetic mechanism. Furthermore, the prevalence of stress fractures among dancers has been positively correlated with the duration of amenorrhea [84]. Similarly, in runners, the prevalence of stress fractures has been associated with the existence of menstrual disturbances [81].

On the other hand, more recent studies have highlighted that weight-bearing exercise exerts positive impact on bone density. Bembed et al. demonstrated that gymnasts were found to have significantly higher BMD, compared with runners [85]. In addition, Zanker et al. studied retired gymnasts, formerly competing in sports acrobatics during childhood and adolescence, and documented higher BMD, in comparison with women who never participated in structured sport or exercise [86]. These studies support the hypothesis that women involved in sports requiring regular, high-impact and weight-bearing activity on bone mass benefit from an osteogenic advantage.

Moreover, Nichols et al. studied female high school athletes considering both sport-specific type of mechanical loading and menstrual status [87]. This study included eumenorrheic and amenorrheic female adolescents participating in high-/odd-impact sports (soccer, softball, volleyball, tennis, lacrosse, track sprinters, and jumpers) compared to repetitive/nonimpact sports participants (swimmers, cross-country runners, track distance runners participating in events ≥ 800 m). The published data documented higher hip bone density and higher spine bone density in eumenorrheic high-/odd-impact athletes than eumenorrheic repetitive/nonimpact athletes.

In addition, in AG an increase in bone density was observed, which followed the delayed bone age and not the chronological age [88]. Bone acquisition was proportional to the development of puberty according to Tanner stages of breast development, and there was a strong negative influence of early onset of training on bone acquisition, indicating the vulnerability of bone metabolism before the onset of sex steroids production at puberty [88]. Therefore, the early exposure of AG to excess mechanical load exerts its beneficial effect on bone acquisition, leading to a positive net effect. The same appears to be true for RG as well [89]. Elite premenarcheal RG had significantly higher cortical BMD and cortical thickness compared to sedentary controls, indicating that rhythmic gymnastics in premenarcheal girls may induce positive adaptations on the skeleton, especially in cortical bone [89].

Exercise and Reproductive Dysfunction in Males

In contrast to the effect of exercise training on the menstrual cycle in female athletes, the effect of physical activity on the male reproductive system is described far less extensively in the scientific literature. Furthermore, the limited existing data mainly refer to studies of adult athletes. In part this is because males do not have a convenient maturational milestone like menarche [22].

In general, the effects of physical activity on the male reproductive axis vary with the intensity and duration of the activity, the fitness of the individual, and his nutritional–metabolic status. More specifically, early investigations pointed to exercise volume as the variable most affecting reproduction, thus hypothesizing a volume threshold for reproductive disorders [90]. Other studies have suggested that exercise intensity is equally, or even more, deleterious to reproductive function [91].

Studies analyzing hormonal profiles and semen parameters of adult athletes participating in different disciplines (water sports, cycling, and running) report alterations in the reproductive function; however, these changes are rather subclinical and seem to be more pronounced in athletes systematically undergoing high training loads. Specifically, Ayers et al. [92] reported that 10% of a sample of marathon runners exhibited severe oligospermia, while Gebreegziabher et al. [93] reported alterations in sperm morphology in cyclists. Moreover, Vaamonde et al. compared semen parameters of three different disciplines (physically active, water polo, and triathlon) and concluded that the triathletes (undergoing the higher training load) showed a trend towards poorer seminal parameter values than the other two groups [91].

With regard to the effect of intense physical activity on the reproductive potential of young athletes, the data are scarce. Among the few existing data, Gurd et al. reported no significant difference in resting testosterone levels between peripubertal gymnasts and age-matched controls [21], while Daly et al. [94] found no difference in resting serum testosterone between peripubertal gymnasts and controls at any time during a 10-month period. On the other hand, Carli et al. [21] reported that after 43 weeks of swimming training, pubertal athletes had testosterone levels that dropped below pretraining levels. The aforementioned studies provide no conclusive data and highlight the need for further studies emphasizing the effect of physical activity on reproductive function of young males, considering the level of competition, the intensity of exercise, and the energy/metabolic status and evaluating both hormonal profile and semen parameters.

Conclusion

Intensive physical training may lead to detrimental effects on puberty and sexual maturation. However, physical activity does not affect maturation and reproductive health per se but only through its ability to regulate energy balance. Low energy intake combined with increased energy expenditure may compromise normal pubertal progression and result in reproductive dysfunction, leading to serious consequences, mainly involving bone health. Pivotal role in mediating energy balance, pubertal progression, and reproductive function has been attributed to the secretory role of adipose tissue and gut-derived hormones. Thus, further studies are needed, emphasizing on training regimens, dietary patterns, caloric intake, and energy expenditure in sports and exercise in order to establish preventive measures, prompt evaluation, and management of individuals at risk.

References

1. Buck Louis GM, Gray LE Jr, Marcus M, Ojeda SR, Pescovitz OH, Witchel SF, et al. Environmental factors and puberty timing: expert panel research needs. Pediatrics. 2008;121:S192–207.
2. Tanner JM, Whitehouse RH, Marsall WA, Carter BS. Prediction of adult height, bone age, and occurrence of menarche, at age 4 to 16 with allowance for midparental height. Arch Dis Child. 1975;50:14–26.
3. Rogol AD, Clark PA, Roemmich JN. Growth and pubertal development in children and adolescents: effects of diet and physical activity. Ann J Clin Nutr. 2000;72:521–8.
4. Malina RM. Physical growth and biological maturation of young athletes. Exerc Sport Sci Rev. 1994;22:389–433.
5. Claessens A, Lefevre J, Beunen G, Malina RM. The contribution of anthropometric characteristics to performance scores in elite female gymnasts. J Sports Med Phys Fit. 1999;39:355–60.
6. Bonen A. Recreational exercise does not impair menstrual cycles: a prospective study. Int J Sports Med. 1992;13:110–20.
7. Georgopoulos NA, Markou KB, Theodoropoulou A, Benardot D, Leglise M, Vagenakis AG. Growth retardation in artistic compared to rhythmic elite female gymnasts. J Clin Endocrinol Metab. 2002;87(7):3169–73.
8. Georgopoulos NA, Theodoropoulou A, Leglise M, Vagenakis AG, Markou K. Growth and skeletal maturation in male and female artistic gymnasts. J Clin Endocrinol Metab. 2004;89:4377–82.
9. Georgopoulos N, Markou K, Theodoropoulou A, Paraskevopoulou P, Varaki L, Kazantzi Z, et al. Growth and pubertal development in elite female rhythmic gymnasts. J Clin Endocrinol Metab. 1999;84:4525–30.

10. Georgopoulos NA, Markou K, Theodoropoulou A, Vagenakis GA, Benardot D, Leglise M, et al. Height velocity and skeletal maturation in elite female rhythmic gymnasts. J Clin Endocrinol Metab. 2001;86:5159–64.
11. Marshall WA, Tanner JM. Variations in pattern of pubertal changes in girls. Arch Dis Child. 1969;44:291–303.
12. Warren MP. The effects of exercise on pubertal progression and reproductive function in girls. J Clin Endocrinol Metab. 1980;51:1150–57.
13. Zacharias L, Wurtman RJ, Shatzoff M. Sexual maturation in contemporary American girls. Am J Obstet Gynecol. 1970;108:833–46.
14. Erladson MC, Sherar LB, Milwald RL, Miffulli N, Baxter-Jones AD. Growth and maturation of adolescent female gymnasts, swimmers, and tennis players. Med Sci Sports Exerc. 2008;40(1):34–42.
15. Marcus R, Cann C, Madvij P, Minkoff J, Goddard M, Bayer M, et al. Menstrual function and bone mass in elite women distance runners. Ann Intern Med. 1985;102:158–63.
16. Baxter-Jones ADG, Helms P, Baines-Preece J, Preece M. Menarche in intensively trained gymnasts, swimmers and tennis players. Ann Hum Biol. 1994;21:407–15.
17. Peltenburg AL, Erich WBM, Bernink MJE, Zonderland ML, Huisveld IA. Biological maturation, body composition and growth of female gymnasts and control groups of schoolgirls and girls swimmers, aged 8 to 14 years: a cross-sectional survey of 1064 girls. Int J Sports Med. 1984;5:36–42.
18. Schtscherbyna A, Soares EA, de Oliveira FP, Ribeiro BG. Female athlete triad in elite swimmers of the city of Rio de Janeiro, Brazil. Nutrition. 2009;25(6):634–9.
19. Cobb KL, Bachrach LK, Greendale G, Marcus R, Neer RM, Nieves J, et al. Disordered eating, menstrual irregularity, and bone mineral density in female runners. Med Sci Sports Exerc. 2003;35(5):711–9.
20. Castelo-Branco C, Reina F, Montivero AD, Colodrón M, Vanrell JA. Influence of high-intensity training and of dietetic and anthropometric factors on menstrual cycle disorders in ballet dancers. Gynecol Endocrinol. 2006;22(1):31–5.
21. Gurd B, Klentrou P. Physical and pubertal development in young male gymnasts. J Appl Physiol. 2003;95(3):1011–5.
22. Baxter-Jones AD, Helms P, Maffulli N, Baines-Preece JC, Preece M. Growth and development of male gymnasts, swimmers, soccer and tennis players: a longitudinal study. Ann Hum Biol. 1995;22(5):381–94.
23. Frisch RE, Revelle R. Height and weight at menarche and a hypothesis of menarche. Arch Dis Child. 1971;46:695–701.
24. Frisch RE, McArthur JW. Menstrual cycles; Fatness as a determinant of minimum weight for height necessary for their maintenance or onset. Science. 1974;185:949–51.
25. Martos-Moreno GA, Chowen JA, Argente J. Metabolic signals in human puberty: effects of over and undernutrition. Mol Cell Endocrinol. 2010;324(1–2):70–81.
26. Moschos S, Chen JL, Mantzoros CS. Leptin and reproduction; a review. Fertil Steril. 2002;77(3):433–44.
27. Warren MP, Perlroth NE. The effects of intense exercise on the female reproductive system. J Endocrinol. 2001;170:3–11.
28. Torstveit MK, Sundgot-Borgen J. Participation in leanness sports but not training volume is associated with menstrual dysfunction: a national survey of 1276 elite athletes and controls. Br J Sport Med. 2005;39(3):141–7.
29. Loucks AB, Mortola JSF, Girton L, Yen SS. Alterations in the hypothalamic-pituitary-ovarian and the hypothalamic-pituitary-adrenal axis in athletic women. J Clin Endocrinol Metab. 1989;68(2):402–11.
30. Redman LM, Loucks AB. Menstrual disorders in athletes. Sport Med. 2005;35(9):747–55.
31. Trussel J. Statistical flaws in evidence for the Frisch hypothesis that fatness triggers menarche. Hum Biol. 1980;52:711–20.
32. Bronson FH, Manning JM. The energetic regulation of ovulation: a realistic role for body fat. Biol Reprod. 1991;44(6):945–50.
33. Loucks AB. Energy availability, not body fatness, regulates reproductive function in women. Exerc Sport Sci Rev. 2003;31(3):144–8.
34. Williams NI, Helmreichch DL, Parfitt DB, Caston-Balderrama AL, Cameron JL. Evidence for a causal role of low energy availability in the induction of menstrual cycle disturbances during strenuous exercise training. J Clin Endocrinol Metab. 2001;86:5184–93.
35. Loucks AB, Verdun M, Heath EM. Low energy availability, not stress of exercise, alters LH pulsatility in exercising women. J Appl Physiol. 1998;84:37–46.
36. Miller KK, Grinspon S, Gleysteen S, Grieco KA, Ciampa J, Breu J, et al. Preservation of neuroendocrine control of reproductive function, despite severe undernutrition. J Clin Endocrinol Metab. 2004;89(9):4434–8.
37. Kopp W, Blum WF, von Prittwitz S, Ziegler A, Lübbert H, Emons G, et al. Low leptin levels predict amenorrhea in underweight and eating disordered females. Mol Psychiatry. 1997;2:335–40.
38. Launhlin GA, Yen SSC. Hypoleptinemia in women athletes: absence of diurnal rhythm with amenorrhea. J Clin Endocrinol Metab. 1997;82:318–21.
39. Welt CK, Chan JL, Bullen J, Murphy R, Smith P, De Paoli AM, et al. Recombinant human leptin in women with hypothalamic amenorrhea. N Engl J Med. 2004;351:987–97.
40. Rodriguez-Pacheco F, Martinez-Fuentes AJ, Tovar S, Pinilla L, Tena-Sempere M, Dieguez C, et al. Regulation of pituitary cell function by adiponectin. Endocrinology. 2007;148:401–10.

41. LuM, Tang Q, Olefsky JM, Mellon PL, Webster NJ. Adiponectin activates adenosine monophosphate activated protein kinase and decreases luteinizing hormone secretion in L betaT2 gonadotropes. Mol Endocrinol. 2008;22:60–71.
42. Selye H. The effect of adaptation to various damaging agents on the female sex organs in the rats. Endocrinology. 1939;25:615–24.
43. Chen MD, O'Byrne KT, Chiappini SE, Hotchkiss J, Knobil E. Hypoglycemic stress and the gonadotrophin-releasing hormone pulse generator activity in the rhesus monkey: the role of the ovary. Neuroendocrinology. 1992;56:666–73.
44. Chrousos GP, Torpy DJ, Gold PW. Interactions between the hypothalamic-pituitary-adrenal axis and the female reproductive system: clinical implications. Ann Intern Med. 1998;129:229–40.
45. Bullen BA, Skrinar GS, Beitins IZ, von Mering G, Turnbull BA, McArthur JW. Induction of menstrual disorders by strenuous exercise in untrained women. N Engl J Med. 1985;312(21):1349–53.
46. Laughlin GA, Yen SSC. Nutritional and endocrine-metabolic aberrations in amenorrheic athletes. J Clin Endocrinol Metab. 1996;81(12):4301–9.
47. Ding JH, Schecter CB, Drinkwater BL. High serum cortisol levels in exercise associated amenorrhea. Ann Intern Med. 1988;108:530–4.
48. Gindoff PR, Ferin M. Endogenous opioid peptides modulate the effect of corticotrophin-releasing factor on gonadotrophin release in the primate. Endocrinology. 1987;121:837–42.
49. Williams NI, Helmreichch DL, Parfitt DB, Caston-Balderrama AL, Cameron JL. Evidence for a causal role of low energy availability in the induction of menstrual cycle disturbances during strenuous exercise training. J Clin Endocrinol Metab. 2001;86:5184–93.
50. Loucks AB, Verdun M, Heath EM. Low energy availability, not stress of exercise, alters LH pulsatility in exercising women. J Appl Physiol. 1998;84:37–46.
51. Pirke KM, Schweiger V, Laessle R, Dickhaut B, Schweiger M, Waechtler M. Dieting influences the menstrual cycle: vegetarian versus nonvegetarian diet. Fertil Steril. 1986;46:1083–8.
52. Barr SI, Janelle KC, Prior JC. Vegetarian vs nonvegetarian diets, dietary restraint, and subclinical ovulatory disturbances: prospective 6-mo study. Am J Clin Nutr. 1994;60:887–94.
53. De Souza MJ, Metzger DA. Reproductive dysfunction in amenorrheic athletes and anorexic patients: a review. Med Sci Sports Exerc. 1991;23:995–1007.
54. Rogol AD, Weltman JY, Seip RL, Seip RL, Snead DB, Levine S, et al. Durability of the reproductive axis in eumenorrheic women during one year of endurance training. J Appl Physiol. 1992;72:1571–80.
55. Frisch RE, Wyshak G, Vincent L. Delayed menarche and amenorrhea in ballet dancers. N Engl J Med. 1980;303:17–9.
56. Sanborn CF, Martin BJ, Wagner WW. Is athletic amenorrhea specific to runners? Am J Obstet Gynecol. 1982;143:859–61.
57. Bonen A. Recreational exercise does not impair menstrual cycles: a prospective study. Int J Sports Med. 1992;13:110–20.
58. Rosetta L. Female reproductive dysfunction and intense physical training. Oxf Rev Reprod Biol. 1993;15:113–41.
59. Bennell KL, Malcolm SA, Khan KM, Thomas SA, Reid SJ, Brukner PD, et al. Bone mass and bone turnover in power athletes, endurance athletes, and controls. A 12 month longitudinal study. Bone. 1997;20(5):477–84.
60. Sanborn CF, Albrecht BH, Wagner WW Jr. Athletic amenorrhea: lack of association with body fat. Med Sci Sports Exerc. 1987;19:207–12.
61. Shangold MM, Levine HS. The effect of marathon training upon menstrual function. Am J Obstet Gynecol. 1982;143:862–9.
62. De Souza MJ, Miler BE, Loucks AB, Luciano AA, Pescatello LS, Campbell CG, et al. High frequency of luteal phase deficiency and anovulation in recreational women runners: blunted elevation in follicle-stimulating hormone observed during luteal-follicular transition. J Clin Endocrinol Metab. 1998;83:4220–32.
63. Lucas JA, Lucas PR, Vogel S, Gamble GD, Evans MC, Reid IR. Effect of sub-elite competitive running on bone density, body composition and sexual maturity of adolescents females. Osteoporos Int. 2003;14(10):848–56.
64. Constantini NW, Warren MP. Menstrual dysfunction in swimmers: a distinct entity. J Clin Endocrinol Metab. 1995;80(9):2740–4.
65. Theodoropoulou A, Markou K, Vagenakis GA, Benardot D, Leglise M, Kourounis G, et al. Delayed but normally progressed puberty is more pronounced in artistic compared with rhythmic elite gymnasts due to the intensity of training. J Clin Endocrinol Metab. 2005;90(11):6022–7.
66. De Souza MJ, West SL, Jamal SA, Hawker GA, Gundberg CM, Williams NI. The presence of both an energy deficiency and estrogen deficiency exacerbate alterations of bone metabolism in exercising women. Bone. 2008;43:140–8.
67. Marcus R. Mechanisms of exercise effects on bone. In: Bilezikian JP, Raaaaisz LG, Rodan GA, editors Principles of bone biology. San Diego: Academic; 1996. p. 1135–46.
68. Katzman DK, Bachrach LK, Carter DR, Marcus R. Clinical and anthropometric correlates of bone mineral acquisition in healthy adolescent girls. J Clin Endocrinol Metab. 1991;73:1332–9.
69. Fehily AM, Coles RJ, Evans WD, et al. Factors affecting bone density in young adults. Am J Clin Nutr. 1992;56:579–86.
70. Christo K, Prabhakaran R, Lamparello B, Cord J, Miller KK, Goldstein MA, et al. Bone metabolism

in adolescent athletes with amenorrhea, athletes with eumenorrhea, and control subjects. Pediatrics. 2008;121:1127–36.
71. Maïmoun L, Coste O, Galtier F, Mura T, Mariano-Goulart D, Paris F, et al. Bone mineral density acquisition in peripubertal female rhythmic gymnasts is directly associated with plasma IGF1/IGF-binding protein 3 ratio. Eur J Endocrinol. 2010;163(1):157–64.
72. Abad V, Chrousos G, Reynolds J, Nieman LK, Hill SC, Weinstein RS, et al. Glucocorticoid excess during adolescence leads to a major persistent deficit in bone mass and an increase in central body fat. J Bone Miner Res. 2001;16(10):1879–85.
73. Misra M. Bone density in the adolescent athlete. Rev Endocr Metab Disord. 2008;9:139–44.
74. Christo K, Cord J, Mendes N, Miller KK, Goldstein MA, Klibanski A, et al. Acylated ghrelin and leptin in adolescent athletes with amenorrhea, eumenorrheic athletes and controls: a cross sectional study. Clin Endocrinol (Oxf). 2008;69(4):628–33.
75. Miller KK, Parulekar MS, Schoenfeld E, Anderson E, Hubbard J, Klibanski A, et al. Decreased leptin levels in normal weight women with hypothalamic amenorrhea: the effects of body composition and nutritional intake. J Clin Endocrinol Metab. 1998;83:2309–12.
76. Drinkwater BL, Nilson K, Chesnut CH III, Bremner WJ, Shainholtz S, Southworth MB. Bone mineral content of amenorrheic and eumenorrheic athletes. N Engl J Med. 1984;311:277–81.
77. Marcus R, Cann CE, Madvig P, Minkoff J, Goddard M, Bayer M, et al. Menstrual function and bone mass in elite women distance runners. Ann Intern Med. 1985;102:158–63.
78. Ackerman KE, Nazem T, Chapko D, Russell M, Mendes N, Taylor AP, et al. Bone microarchitecture is impaired in adolescent amenorrheic athletes compared with eumenorrheic athletes and nonathletic controls. J Clin Endocrinol Metab. 2011;96(10):3123–33.
79. Drinkwater BL, Bruemner B, Chesnut CH 3rd. Menstrual history as a determinant of current bone density in young athletes. JAMA. 1990;263:545–8.
80. Keen AD, Drinkwater BL. Irreversible bone loss in former amenorrheic athletes. Osteoporos Int. 1997;7:311–5.
81. Warren MP, Brooks-Gunn J, Fox RP, Holderness CC, Hyle EP, Hamilton WG. Osteopenia in exercise associated amenorrhea using ballet dancers as a model: a longitudinal study. J Clin Endocrinol Metab. 2002;87:3162–8.
82. Warren MP, Brooks-Gunn J, Hamilton LH. Scoliosis and fractures in young ballet dancers. Relation to delayed menarche and secondary amenorrhea. N Engl J Med. 1986;314(21):1348–53.
83. Kenanidis E, Potoupnis ME, Papavasiliou KA, Sayegh FE, Kapetanos GA. Adolescent idiopathic scoliosis and exercising: is there truly a liaison? Spine. 2008;33(20):2160–5.
84. Myburgh KH, Hutchins J, Fataar AB, Hough SF, Noakes TD. Low bone density is an etiologic factor for stress fractures in athletes. Ann Intern Med. 1990;113:754–9.
85. Bemben DA, Buchanan TD, Bemben MG, Knehans AW. Influence of type of mechanical loading, menstrual status and training season on bone density in young women athletes. J Strength Cond Res. 2004;18(2):220–6.
86. Zanker CL, Osborne C, Cooke CB, Oldroyd B, Truscott JG. Energy balance, bone turnover and menstrual history of sedentary female former gymnasts, aged 20–32 years. Osteoporos Int. 2004;15(2):145–54.
87. Nichols JF, Rauh MJ, Barrack MT, Barkai HS. Bone mineral density in female high school athletes: interactions of menstrual function and type of mechanical loading. Bone. 2007;41(3):371–7.
88. Markou KB, Mylonas P, Theodoropoulou A, Kontogiannis A, Leglise M, Vagenakis AG, et al. The influence of intensive physical exercise on bone acquisition in adolescent elite female and male artistic gymnasts. J Clin Endocrinol Metab. 2004;89:4383–7.
89. Tournis S, Michopoulou E, Fatouros IG, Paspati I, Michalopoulou M, Raptou P, et al. Effect of rhythmic gymnastics on volumetric bone mineral density and bone geometry in premenarcheal female athletes and controls. J Clin Endocrinol Metab. 2010;95(6):2755–62.
90. De Souza MJ, Miller BE. The effect of endurance training on reproductive function in male runners. A "volume threshold" hypothesis. Sports Med. 1997;23:357–73.
91. Vaamonde D, Silva-Grigoletto ME D, García-Manso JM, Vaamonde-Lemos R, Swanson RJ, Oehninger SC. Response of semen parameters to three training modalities. Fertil Steril. 2009;92(6):1941–6.
92. Ayers JWT, Komesu V, Romani T, Ansbacher R. Anthropomorphic, hormone, and psychologic correlates of semen quality in endurance-trained male athletes. Fertil Steril. 1985;43:917–21.
93. Gebreegziabher Y, Marcos E, McKinon W, Rogers G. Sperm characteristics of endurance trained subjects. Int J Sports Med. 2004;25:247–51.
94. Daly RM, Rich PA, Klein R. Hormonal responses to physical training in high-level peripubertal male gymnasts. Eur J Appl Physiol Occup Physiol. 1998;79:74–81.

Physical Activity and Pregnancy

16

Sarah J. Moss, Andries Fourie van Oort and Yves Schutz

Introduction

Regular physical activity during pregnancy benefits both maternal and infant health [1]. Regardless of the physiological changes women undergo during pregnancy, pregnant women benefit from physical activity just as much as nonpregnant women [2]. The complexity of assessing physical activity during pregnancy hampers the determination of the optimal amount of recreational physical activity for pregnant women [3] and has led to broad physical activity guidelines being proposed for pregnant women. Concurrently, pregnancy is characterised by a reduction in physical activity [4] resulting in discrepancies between physical activity during pregnancy and the guidelines set by various institutional and governmental entities [5–12].

S. J. Moss (✉)
Physical activity, Sport and Recreation Research Focus Area, Faculty of Health Sciences, North-West University, Private bag X6001, Potchefstroom 2531, South Africa
e-mail: Hanlie.moss@nwu.ac.za

A. F. van Oort
Physical activity, Sport and Recreation Research Focus Area, Faculty of Health Sciences, North-West University, Potchefstroom, South Africa

Y. Schutz
Department of Integrative Physiology, University of Fribourg, Fribourg, Switzerland

Physiological Adaptations to Pregnancy

The duration of a pregnancy averages 266 days (38 weeks) after ovulation, or 280 days (40 weeks) after the first day of the last menstrual cycle. This period equals 10 lunar months, or just over 9 calendar months [13]. Physiological changes during pregnancy are divided into a series of stages and sub-stages, and the entire process is then subdivided into three relatively equal trimesters [14].

All maternal physiological systems adapt to the demands of pregnancy; however, the quality, degree and timing of the adaptation varies from one individual to the next and from one organ system to another [15–16]. The adaptations are mostly mediated due to the effects of progesterone and oestrogen that are produced, predominantly by the ovary in the first 12 weeks of pregnancy and thereafter by the placenta [15]. These adaptations enable the foetus and placenta to grow and prepare the mother and baby for parturition [15, 17].

Physiological changes, as a result of pregnancy, represent a serious challenge to all body systems [17]. While these adaptations do not pose major risks for healthy women, the normal physiological changes of pregnancy can place significant strain on already compromised systems, threatening the lives of both the mother and the foetus during parturition [17].

© Springer Science+Business Media New York 2016

D. Vaamonde et al. (eds.), *Exercise and Human Reproduction*, DOI 10.1007/978-1-4939-3402-7_16

Cardiovascular Adaptations During Pregnancy

Profound physiological changes occur in the cardiovascular system during pregnancy [17]. Circulating blood volume increases in order to meet the demands of the developing foetus and placenta. During pregnancy, there are major alterations in blood volume, constituents of cells and coagulation factors [16, 17]. A substantial part of maternal weight gain during pregnancy results from fluid accumulation, specifically plasma volume [16]. This increase in plasma volume supplies the necessary nutrients to the uterus and the placenta and ensures the removal of waste products from the uterus and placenta [14]. The increase in the plasma volume is to counter the decrease in the low pressure circulatory system that resulted due to the increase in vascular dilatation. Overall blood pressure decreases too, more specifically diastolic blood pressure to a greater extent than systolic blood pressure [14]. Blood pressure decreases despite an increase in blood volume and cardiac output, due to a decrease in systemic and pulmonary vascular resistance [18]. In addition to the previously mentioned changes, change to the cardiovascular system includes an increase in cardiac output, the product of heart rate and stroke volume [14, 19]. Initially, the increase in cardiac output is mediated by the increase in stroke volume. As pregnancy progresses, an increase in heart rate becomes the dominant factor to increase the cardiac output [18].

Respiratory Changes During Pregnancy

Numerous changes occur in the maternal respiratory system during pregnancy to ensure sufficient oxygen supply to the placenta for increased foetal energy demands and for foetal physiology [15–17]. The net physiologic change in the respiratory system is a lowering of the maternal PCO_2 to facilitate effective exchange of CO_2 from the foetus to the mother [16, 17]. The oxy-haemoglobin dissociation curves of foetal haemoglobin and adult haemoglobin allow the foetus to extract oxygen effectively from the maternal circulation [16]. The effects are mediated by hormonal factors that influence the respiratory centre, specifically progesterone [20]. An increase in progesterone stimulates the respiratory centre to increase minute volume, lowers the threshold of carbon dioxide concentrations [20] and may also decrease airway resistance, facilitating a greater airflow during maternal respiration [21, 22].

Musculoskeletal Changes During Pregnancy

Hormonal changes, specifically, changes in progesterone and relaxin levels, lead to increased joint laxity and hyper-mobility [23], which could potentially raise the risk of injury during exercise in pregnancy [10]. Increased body weight, as a result of foetal growth, increases the forces imposed on the joints such as the hips and knees [24]. Since the abdomen expands anterior during foetal growth, the centre of gravity shifts during pregnancy, resulting in postural adjustments, specifically an extension of the lumbar spine [14], which realigns the body mass above the base of support [25]. Elongation and decreased tone of the abdominal muscles may ensue because of the prolonged maintenance of the abovementioned position [14]. The combination of weight gain, altered postural alignment and ligamentous laxity causes changes in proprioception and postural balance in pregnant women [26]. The postural changes associated with pregnancy result in pregnant women adapting their stance and gait with a longer double limb support time and changes in the angles of hip, knee and ankles, suggesting an adaptation in locomotion to become more efficient [27] that might also influence energy expenditure of gait during pregnancy.

Endocrine Changes During Pregnancy

Since the development of the foetal origin of disease in later life hypotheses (described later in this chapter), plenty of research focused on the intrauterine environment, specifically with regard to hormonal changes during gestation as summarised by Kuijper et al. [28] in a systematic review that found both endogenous and maternal hormones to influence the foetus. Foetal development and sustained essential physiological functions for both mother and foetus are mediated by an increase in the release of specific hormones [29] such as oestrogen, progesterone, human chorionic gonadotropin, prolactin, adrenocorticotropic hormone, thyroid-stimulating hormone, cortisol and thyroid hormones [30]. The mass of cells that forms on the ovaries, the corpus luteum, is the main source of pregnancy-sustaining hormones during the first 6–8 weeks of gestation [31]. As previously mentioned, the majority of hormonal changes in pregnancy are related to the activity of the placenta [30]. The placenta takes over the role of the corpus luteum later in the pregnancy. The changes to hormones during pregnancy and their effects include:

- Oestrogen, which stimulates glandular tissue and ducts in the breast and increases prostaglandin and oxytocin production [13].
- Progesterone, which mediates vital physiological function during pregnancy, including an increased mobility of the joints [13].
- Relaxin, which functions synergistically with progesterone to decrease uterine activity during pregnancy and to suppress oxytocin release [14]. Relaxin also affects the connective tissue to increase the mobility of the joints, in a similar way to progesterone [26].
- Cortisol secretion, which increases from the second trimester of pregnancy to meet the body's extra metabolic workload [30].
- Human chorionic gonadotropin levels increase, which is linked to changes in appetite, sleep patterns and food tolerance in the first trimester [30].
- Thyroid hormones, both T_3 and T_4, increase, causing the basal metabolic rate to increase during pregnancy [32].

In summary, the changes observed in the physiological systems during pregnancy (Fig. 16.1) simulate the adaptations observed in nonpregnant women who perform regular aerobic exercise to a large degree.

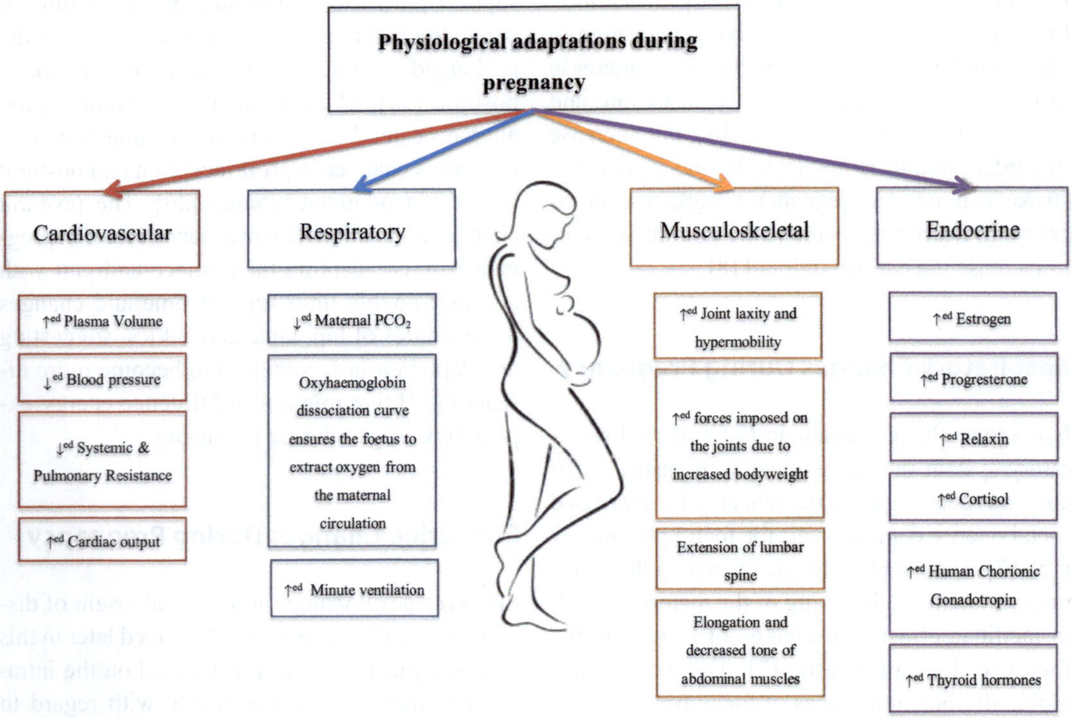

Fig. 16.1 Summary of the physiological adaptations during pregnancy

Metabolic Adaptations to Pregnancy

Energy Intake During Pregnancy

The physiological changes that occur during pregnancy cause an increased demand for dietary energy as a result of increased oxygen consumption, respiration, circulation and renal function of the foetus during development [33]. From conception to birth, all the growth of the foetus is possible because of the nutrients the mother consumes [34]. The nutrient needs during pregnancy and lactation are higher than any other time in a woman's life [34]. This high nutrient demand during pregnancy is met with an increased energy intake, as well as help from the mother's body that maximises absorption and minimises energy expenditure [34].

The energy needs of pregnant women exceed those of nonpregnant women by an additional 340 kilocalories per day during the second trimester and extra 450 kilocalories per day during the third trimester [34]. The additional kilocalories represent 15–20% more food than before pregnancy for an average 2000-kilocalorie daily intake. Ample carbohydrates are essential for fuel to the foetal brain, which ensures that the protein needed for growth is catabolised and used to synthesise glucose [34]. The extra energy demands of pregnancy can be met by an increase in food intake or by the mobilisation of energy fat stores of the mother, particularly those mothers with sufficient energy reserves [35].

The additional energy requirements during pregnancy can be described as the energy needed for maternal tissue and foetal growth, as well as the energy required for the rise in basal metabolic rate and the changes in physical activity [35]. Energy requirements during pregnancy remain controversial because of conflicting data on maternal fat deposition and putative reductions in the mother's physical activity as the pregnancy advances [36].

Energy Expenditure During Pregnancy

Total daily energy expenditure (TDEE) consists of three general factors: resting metabolic rate, thermogenic effect of feeding and physical activity [34, 37]. TDEE for the nonpregnant healthy woman is calculated as the energy expended on resting metabolic rate (60–75%), thermogenic effect of feeding (10%) and physical activity (25–30%). TDEE increases during pregnancy because of tissue growth, an elevated basal metabolic rate and the increased energy costs of moving a heavier body [38].

Resting metabolic rate (RMR) accounts for all the metabolic activities in the human body [34]. Human metabolism involves all the body's chemical reactions of biomolecules that cause anabolism and catabolism. RMR varies dramatically from person to person and for the same individual with a change in circumstances or physical condition (with pregnancy being an extreme physiological condition) [34]. Pregnancy is a dynamic, anabolic state where the human body obtains energy for growth and maintenance [39].

The enhanced work of pregnancy raises the RMR dramatically and demands extra energy [40, 41]. This is calculated by Prentice et al. [42] as 20% in late pregnancy. Forty percent of this variability is explained by the percentage of total body fat before pregnancy and the gain in body weight during pregnancy [35, 41]. Body fat gain accounts for about 55.5±20% of total weight gain during pregnancy [43]. According to Löf et al. [41], factors that are responsible for the variability in RMR response during pregnancy differ in the earlier and later trimesters of pregnancy. Most of the total body fat mass is deposited during the second trimester, with little change taking place in the first and third [44]. Chamberlain and Popkin [33] developed a theoretical model to estimate energy requirements during pregnancy (Fig. 16.2) [45], assuming an average gestational weight gain (GWG) of 12.5 kg (≈0.925 kg protein, ≈3.8 kg fat, and ≈7.8 kg water), which is associated with an increase in RMR [41].

The thermogenic effect of food is attributed to the digestion process and the energy cost of storage of the exogenous macronutrient is proportional to the food energy that is consumed [34]. This diet-induced thermogenesis seems to be unaltered [36, 42, 46–49] or even reduced [44, 50, 51] during pregnancy.

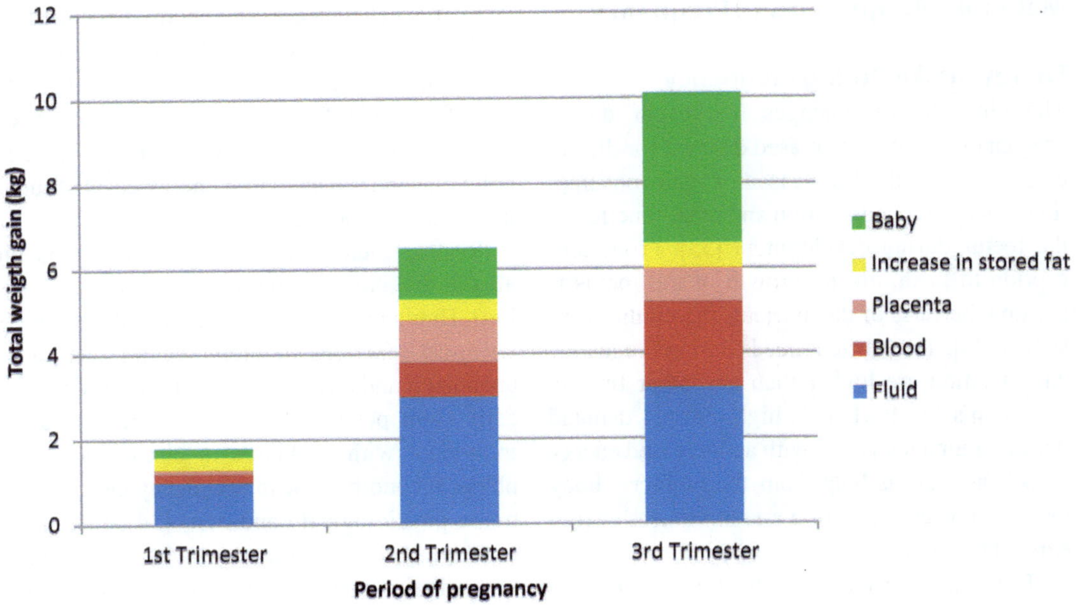

Fig. 16.2 Estimated factors contributing to weight gain during pregnancy. (Based on data from [45])

The most varying factor that determines total energy expenditure is physical activity and is dependent on three factors: muscle mass, body weight and level of activity [34]. The interaction between physical activity and energy metabolism is complex. For example, pregnant women may reduce physical activity energy expenditure by selecting less demanding activities or reducing the pace of activity, although the actual cost might be higher, because of moving a heavier body [38]. However, all pregnant women might not reduce their physical activity because of the knowledge they have of the health benefits of regular physical activity during pregnancy. Over the past 2 years, more studies have focused on the energy expenditure during pregnancy, especially in the wake of the rapid increase in obesity, globally. The measurement of total energy expenditure during pregnancy is controversial, mainly because of conflicting data on the extent of reduction in physical activity as pregnancy advances [35] and the collection of physical activity information with self-report questionnaires.

The energy cost that is attributed to physical activity during pregnancy is generally lower [40, 52–55] and tends to decrease as pregnancy advances [56–60]. Studies show that pregnant Scottish [61] and Dutch [60] women had a slight decrease in absolute energy cost of physical activity, observed in activity diary studies, as their pregnancy advanced. The same results were found in British women by Prentice et al. [42] by means of whole body indirect calorimetry methodology. However, Melzer et al. [35] found this decrease in active energy expenditure insignificant in pregnant women in Sweden and America, but when expressed as per unit of body weight to account for weight differences, this result became significant. Other studies from Sweden and the UK report similar decreases in active energy expenditure per kilogram in the pregnant compared to the nonpregnant state [42, 54]. Preliminary findings of the **H**abitual **A**ctivity **P**atterns during **P**regnanc**Y** (HAPPY)-study in Potchefstroom, South Africa, indicate a 25% reduction in activity energy expenditure from the first to the third trimester of pregnancy. The study included participants from white, black and coloured ethnic groups as well as low-, middle- and high socioeconomic groups [62]. The physical activity levels (PAL) reported can be classified as low activity to sedentary behaviour from the first to the third trimester of pregnancy.

Reasons for this decrease in physical activity are explained in the following section. However, physical activity cannot be observed in isolation when activity energy expenditure is discussed because the energy intake is also important in the energy balance. More details regarding behavioural changes in activity patterns are discussed in the following section.

To better understand the associations between energy intake, energy storage and energy expenditure during pregnancy, studies should be carried out during free-living conditions applying the most objective and reliable methodology [38]. The correct measuring tool is essential to quantify physical activity during pregnancy.

Measurement of Physical Activity During Pregnancy

Critical appraisal of the physical activity during pregnancy and the influence of recreational or habitual physical activity on birth outcomes and maternal health are dependent on valid and reliable objective measurements of physical activity [3]. The relationship between physical activity and birth outcomes is likely to be modest, therefore it is essential to measure recreational physical activity accurately to minimise the possibility that no effect is observed because of a measurement error [3]. The majority of information on physical activity in the pregnant and nonpregnant population is based on subjective physical activity questionnaire-collected data. The current guidelines for physical activity are therefore also based on the research based on the subjective data. Changes in technology have given rise to the development of more objective instruments to determine habitual physical activity, not only in the general population but also in pregnancy.

Subjective Physical Activity Measurements

A great variety of physical activity questionnaires have been developed and validated over the past 20 years. The accuracy of self-reporting questionnaires is influenced by the subjective nature of the term "intensity of physical activity" [63]. Physical activity questionnaires emphasise participation in moderate to vigorous sports while not including household or childcare activity [64]. Indeed, women spend considerable time and energy in moderate intensity activities related to household chores, their job and family care [65]. Interestingly, the accuracy of short- and long-term recollections of physical activity patterns by pregnant women is not known [66]. According to Poudevigne and O'Conner [66] there is a lack of knowledge regarding how accurately women can recall their physical activity patterns during pregnancy.

Direct measurements of the metabolic cost of energy expenditure among pregnant women, as opposed to relying upon values collected among nonpregnant populations, will objectively define the intensity of recreational activity among pregnant women [3]. For this purpose, double-labelled water and indirect calorimetry [67, 68] are used to measure physical activity, but because of the costs, invasiveness and technical sophistication of these methods, their suitability for the general population decreases.

In large samples and population-based studies, questionnaires have been the instrument of choice. Hermann et al. [69] determined the validity of two questionnaires, namely the International Physical Activity Questionnaire (IPAQ) [70, 71] and the Global Physical Activity Questionnaire version 2 (GPAQ) [72]. The GPAQ shows short- and long-term retest reliability and modest validity [69], although it has not been validated in the pregnant population. Specifically during pregnancy, four validated questionnaires are currently being used to determine physical activity [73–76]. A validated, self-administered questionnaire, the Pregnancy Physical Activity Questionnaire (PPAQ) has been used to assess the physical activity levels of pregnant women [74]. Categories in this questionnaire include: household/care-giving, occupational, sport/exercise, transportation and inactivity [77] and asks women to estimate the duration and frequency of time spent per activity during the current trimester of pregnancy. The reliability of the PPAQ for total physical activity was strong ($r=0.78$), with the highest reliability for moderate intensity activity ($r=0.82$). With regards to activity type, the highest reliability was found for occupational activity ($r=0.93$), followed by household/caregiving ($r=0.86$) and sports/exercise ($r=0.83$). The validity of the PPAQ was determined against accelerometry (ActiGraph). The overall correlations between the PPAQ and average counts per minute were within the range of values observed for the published cut points ($r=0.27$ for total activity), while validity coefficients for vigorous activity ($r=0.37$) and sports/exercise ($r=0.48$) were higher using average counts per minute. PPAQ provides an easy method of assessing physical activity patterns in women with uncomplicated pregnancies [77].

Objective Physical Activity Measurements

Both accelerometers [55, 78] and heart rate monitors [79] have been used to measure daily physical activity accurately. However, when these devices are used separately, they have disadvantages [80]. Heart rate is influenced by temperature, humidity, fatigue and emotional stress. [81]. Additional challenges are the loss of data from signal interruptions and delayed heart rate responses [82, 83]. Accelerometers on the other hand are not waterproof and cannot monitor activities in water [80]. Also, static physical activity, such as weight lifting, generates less body movement but requires energy expenditure, which can be problematic when accelerometers are used [84, 85].

To continually measure free-living physical activity, a combination of the abovementioned accelerometers and heart rate monitors are used and could provide more accurate activity profiles by overcoming individual sources of error [84, 86–89]. One such device that combines heart rate and accelerometry is the ActiHeart® (CamNTech, UK) [80], which was first used by Melzer et al. [35] to measure changes in resting and activity-related energy expenditure during pregnancy. The device is currently the only commercially available device that combines acceleration and heart rate, therefore increasing the practical applicability to improve energy estimates compared to traditional acceleration devices [90]. ActiHeart® is a 10 g, waterproof, self-contained logging device that allows activity to be measured synchronously with heart rate at between 15–60 s epochs [91]. The device is worn on the chest and consists of two electrodes that are connected by a short lead and clip onto two standard electrocardiograph (ECG) pads. Free-living data, as assessed by the ActiHeart® and calculated according to branched models, is essential to determine behavioural changes in activity patterns in pregnant women [35]. The ActiHeart® device has shown accurate estimates of energy expenditure versus indirect calorimetry over a wide range of activities (varying from sedentary behaviours to vigorous physical activity) in men and nonpregnant women, although it is not validated specifically for pregnant women [35]. Brage et al. [92] conclude that the ActiHeart® is a reliable and valid tool for the measurement of movement and heart rate in humans at rest and during walking and running. Overall, the ActiHeart® is reliable in measuring and categorising intensities of physical activity [80] in addition to increased monitor-wear compliance in adolescents [93] (Fig. 16.3).

The complexity of assessing physical activity in general, and in particular, during pregnancy, a demanding period characterised by changing physiology, hampers the determination of the optimal dose of recreational physical activity for pregnant women [3]. Because of the well-documented advantages of regular exercise in non-

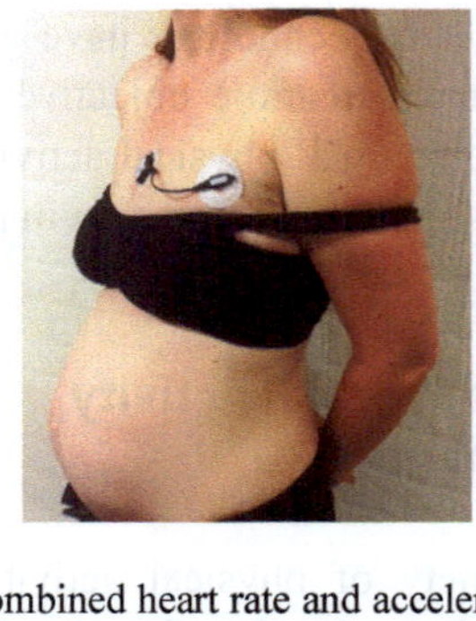

Fig. 16.3 Combined heart rate and accelerometer device (ActiHeart®, CamNtech, UK) placement for the measurement of habitual activity energy expenditure in pregnancy

pregnant women, similar findings are expected during pregnancy. A lack of measuring instruments limits studies on the direct effect of physical activity levels on the growth of the foetus and maternal and foetal birth outcomes. The results are that health professionals have been very conservative in the volume (intensity x duration) and frequency of exercise and physical activity that are recommended to pregnant women. These guidelines have therefore impacted directly on habitual activity patterns during pregnancy.

Physical Activity Patterns During Pregnancy

The physical activity patterns of pregnant women are poorly described [66]. Maternal physical activity tends to decrease during pregnancy because of the minor discomforts that are associated with pregnancy, such as leg cramps, swelling, fatigue, shortness of breath [94], difficulties in movement related to a larger body mass [2] and, sometimes, because of the perception that physical activity may be damaging to the foetus [95, 96].

Physical activity patterns vary across the duration of pregnancy and are generally at a lower level when compared to pre-pregnancy [3, 97]. Prospective studies indicate that recreational, occupational and overall physical activity declines during pregnancy [52, 55]. Physical activity is usually constrained in the first trimester because of nausea, vomiting and profound fatigue [8, 66]. These symptoms usually decrease in the second trimester. Physical limitations—like uterine enlargement and changes in weight distribution [66]— also lead to a decrease in physical activity in the third trimester [8]. Reductions in physical activity, especially in the third trimester, might also be a method to meet the increased energy demands of pregnancy [98]. Physical activity often decreases the most during the third trimester of pregnancy. This decrease in physical activity has sometimes been referred to as the "nesting effect", as pregnant women prepare their home for the arrival of a new baby [66].

Psychological changes, such as a declining body image and depression may make physical activity less attractive during pregnancy [99]. In contrast to this, some of the barriers to physical activity during pregnancy, such as depression and fatigue, can be attenuated by regular exercise [66]. Exercise intensity decreases as many women cease vigorous sport activities when pregnant [100–102]. Evidence indicates that the primary mode of physical activity by pregnant women is low intensity walking [103, 104]. There is a shift in the nature of the activities pregnant women usually perform, to activities that are less vigorous, more comfortable or perceived as safer, like walking and swimming and less bicycling [66, 105, 106]. Work-related physical activity also decreases as pregnancy proceeds [66].

A study done by Löf [38] found that pregnant women, compared with nonpregnant controls, spend less time (1.5 h/24 h) standing and performing moderate activities and more time (1.5 h/24 h) on sedentary activities such as sitting and reclining. Additionally, absolute active energy expenditure decreased by 18 % [38]. The PAL was also significantly lower than the corresponding value for nonpregnant controls per 24-h period [38]. However, as stated by Prentice et al. [42], the use of PAL on pregnant women is not advisable because even if active energy expenditure (total energy expenditure—basal metabolic rate) is unchanged, PAL will still decrease as basal metabolic rate increases during pregnancy. These findings correspond with an American study that confirmed a decrease in active energy expenditure by 13 % as recorded with activity records [40]. However, another study on healthy Swedish women indicated no major effect of pregnancy on activity patterns or on active energy expenditure [54] (Fig. 16.4).

While all of the abovementioned factors contribute to the decreased pattern of physical activity during pregnancy, the strongest predictor of physical activity during pregnancy is the level of physical activity during the year prior to pregnancy [107, 108]. If pregnant women were active as teenagers, they were 13 times more likely to engage in high intensity physical activity during pregnancy as compared to sedentary teens [107]. Highly active women may be more aware of the health benefits of exercise and may have more confidence in their ability to choose an appropriate mode and intensity of exercise [66]. As with

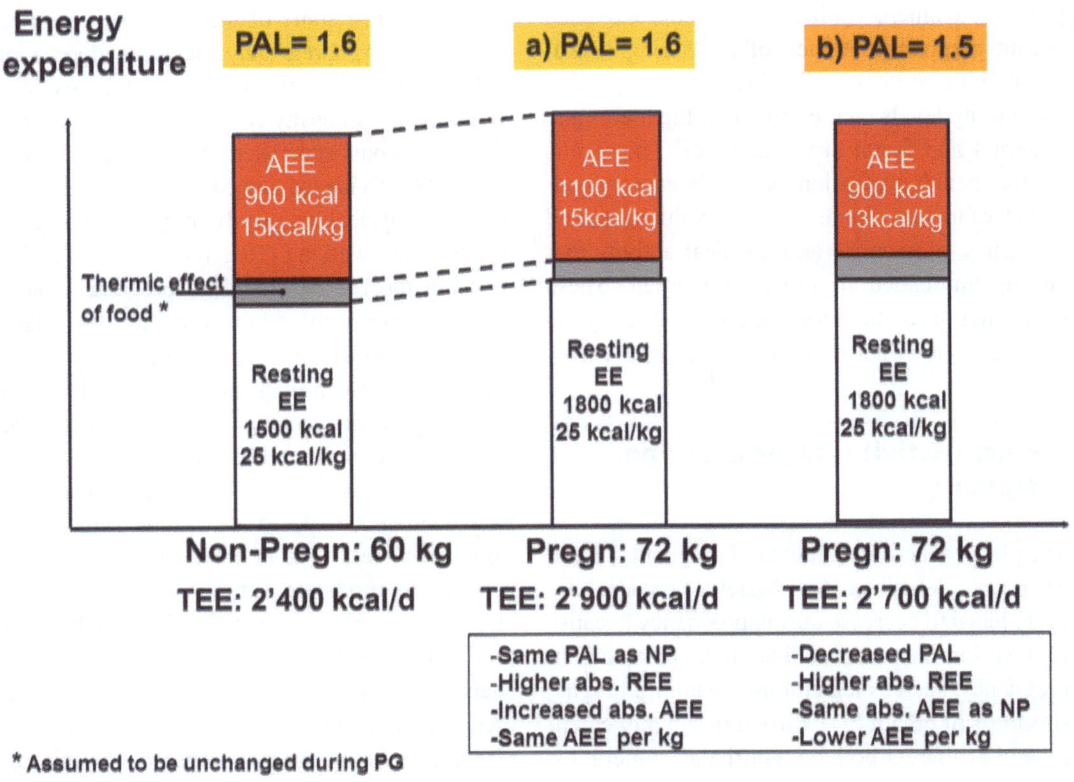

Fig. 16.4 Energy expenditure for nonpregnant versus pregnant women at different physical activity levels. *PAL* physical activity level, *AEE* activity energy expenditure, *EE* energy expenditure, *TEE* total energy expenditure, *NP* nonpregnant; *REE* resting energy expenditure, *kcal* kilocalories, *kcal/d* kilocalories per day, *kg* kilogram

women who were sedentary before pregnancy, some started becoming physically active when they were pregnant, according to a few studies [97, 100, 108, 109]. This indicates that these women consider their pregnancy to be a chance to change their lifestyle [100]. Few studies document longitudinal changes in physical activity during all three trimesters [102, 110, 111]. It is expected that the majority of pregnant women would have low levels of physical activity since PALs of the general nonpregnant population are globally reported to be low.

Very limited research exists pertaining to the physical activity patterns of South African women [112]. Results from a single South African study, determining physical activity subjectively during pregnancy [112], found no change in PALs between the second and third trimester. This contradicts previously mentioned studies that found a decline in physical activity as pregnancy progressed. This contradiction can be explained by the fact that the patients in the study were recruited from a gynaecologist who advocated exercise during pregnancy [112].

Hegaard et al. [100] found that women with a higher body mass index (BMI; more than 25 kg/m^2) decreased their physical activity during pregnancy more than pregnant women with a normal weight (BMI 18.5–24.99 kg/m^2). Changes in physical activity during pregnancy are extremely detrimental because this decrease results in an even higher risk of gestational diabetes, pre-eclampsia or preterm delivery than in women who continued their normal level of physical activity [113–115].

The most extreme type of physical inactivity is bed rest, which is recommended by obstetrics and gynaecology physicians in 20% of all pregnancies [66]. Bed rest is recommended in the hope of preventing or treating a wide variety of conditions, including spontaneous abortion, preterm labour, foetal growth retardation, oedema and pre-eclampsia [116]. Little evidence exists regarding the effectiveness of bed rest on the treatment of these conditions [117]. The adverse effects of bed rest may be even more detrimental than the conditions it is meant to prevent or treat, like decreased sex steroids, insulin resistance, systemic inflammation, mood disturbances and even progressive bone and muscle loss compromising the ability to perform tasks of daily living [118]. Additionally, Poudevigne and O'Conner [66] state that a combination of biological, psychological, social and environmental factors interacts to contribute to changes in physical activity during pregnancy.

Physical activity in the postpartum period is usually decreased, because of the added fatigue of delivery and newborn care [8]. However, less is known about physical activity during the postpartum period and in the change in activity from pregnancy to postpartum [119]. Data from the HAPPY-study that objectively determined physical activity indicate the activity counts in a sample of 70 women decreased by 20 % from the third trimester to 3 months postpartum [62]. According to Pereira et al. [102], walking as a physical activity modality might remain unchanged from pre-pregnancy to postpartum. Usually care-giving physical activity in the postpartum period constitutes the largest proportion of total physical activity [119].

In summary, a reduction in physical activity during pregnancy augments the need to promote regular physical activity of pregnant women as a necessary part of their lifestyle due to the minimal risk and numerous short- and long-term benefits for both the mother and the baby. Education about the benefits of regular physical activity during pregnancy must be included in the planning and implementation of health promotion programmes by medical personnel and physical education staff [120].

Benefits of Regular Physical Activity During Pregnancy

Physical activity is a major determinant of lifelong health [121, 122] and has been associated with reduced morbidity and mortality [123–125] by serving as a primary preventive behaviour for several chronic health conditions including coronary heart disease [126–128], cancer [128], type 2 diabetes [129], [130], stroke [131], metabolic syndrome [132] and osteoporosis [133].

Maternal benefits of physical activity appear to be both physical and psychological in nature [10]. Physical benefits during pregnancy include shorter labour and a lower incidence of operative abdominal and vaginal deliveries and acute foetal distress [2, 128, 134–136]. Benefits for pregnant women also include improved cardiovascular function [2], reduced incidence of muscle cramps and lower limb oedema [137, 138], attenuation of gestational diabetes mellitus [139, 140] and gestational hypertension [24].

Physical activity does not only have physical benefits but also improves psychological health and provides wellbeing benefits [105, 141, 142]. An increased level of physical activity is known to have a protective effect against insomnia, stress, anxiety and depression [143–146], relieve job strain [147] and provide mood stability [66, 148] as well as increased perceived levels of energy during the day [149]. These benefits carry over to the postpartum period [149] and do not compromise infant breast milk acceptance of infant growth [150].

Kalisiak and Spitznagle [151] reviewed clinically controlled trials that demonstrate that there is a moderate amount of evidence proving that exercise during pregnancy in healthy females has positive effects on both the mother and the foetus. While many studies conclude a positive relationship between physical activity and pregnancy outcome, the majority of the studies applied subjective questionnaires to determine the relationships. Therefore, accurate and objective methods to measure levels of physical activity are important when defining an appropriate relationship between physical activity and health outcomes for both the mother and foetus [90].

Recent meta-analyses of randomised control trails determining the effect of structured and supervised exercise during pregnancy report that pregnant women who exercised gained significantly less weight (− 1.13 kg) than women in the control group. The birth weight was however not significantly reduced in the exercise group compared to the control group [152].

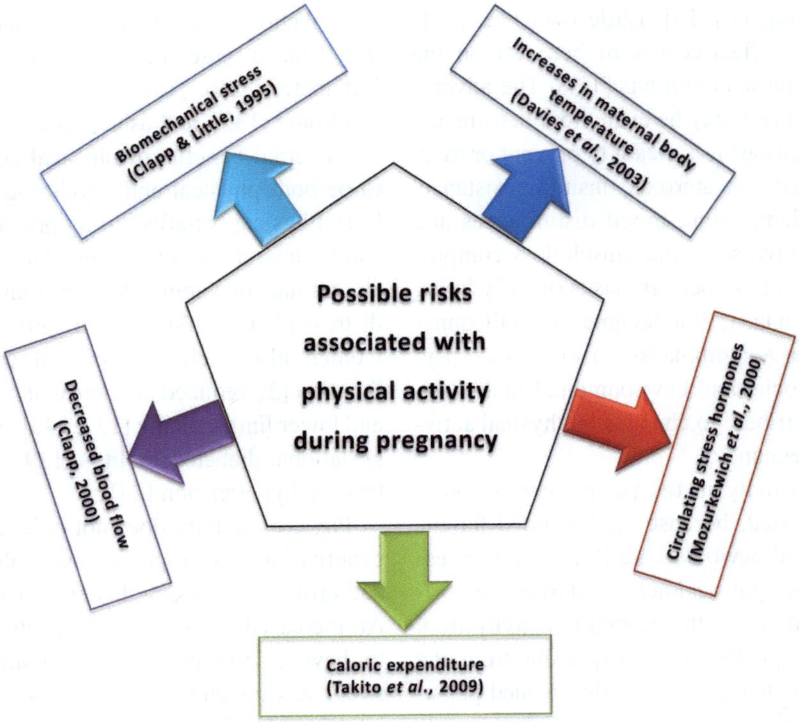

Fig. 16.5 Possible risks associated with physical activity during pregnancy. (Courtesy of Andries Fourie van Oort, M.Sc.)

Risks Associated with Physical Activity During Pregnancy

Physical activity was discouraged until the early twentieth century on the basis of theoretical concerns about exercise-induced injury and adverse foetal and maternal outcomes [31, 144]. These concerns were based on the potentially detrimental effects of exercising on the mother and the foetus, secondary to increases in maternal body temperature, circulating stress hormones, caloric expenditure, decreased blood flow and biomechanical stress [153, 154] as seen in Fig. 16.5 [155].

Biological mechanisms that might contribute to reduced birth weight and length of gestation were theorised by [156]. They suggest that these effects are mediated by the sympathetic nervous system and may also be associated with the release of prostaglandins into the maternal circulation. Physical strain may lead to the release of catecholamines, which may increase maternal blood pressure and uterine contractility and decrease placental function [157].

Another concern of physical training during pregnancy is the subsequent teratogenic effect of hyperthermia in the first trimester [7, 155, 158]. However, this has not been shown to occur in studies of exercising women [8], because an increase in minute ventilation and skin blood flow augment heat dissipation and somewhat inhibit the potential hyperthermic effects of exercise [159]. Even so, exercising while pregnant should preferably take place in a well-ventilated and temperature-controlled environment [7].

The theoretical risk of foetal hypoxia is another concern for the exercising pregnant woman. It was once believed that the demands of exercising muscles divert blood flow from the uteroplacental unit [10]. However, compensatory changes with exercise, such as raised maternal haematocrit and oxygen extraction, appear to prevent the impairment of foetal oxygenation [135, 160]. Takito et al. [161] found that maintaining specific standing postures for a prolonged period could potentially reduce uteroplacental blood flow and lead to decreased foetal growth. Decreased visceral blood flow is suggested to cause potential adverse outcomes, such as congenital malformation, growth retardation, premature labour, brain damage, difficult labour, haemorrhage and maternal musculoskeletal injury [153].

Takito et al. [161] identified high total energy expenditure to potentially be associated with low birth weight, preterm birth and intrauterine growth restriction under the supposition that higher caloric expenditures could withhold energy from the foetus. The risk of maternal musculoskeletal injury due to changes in posture and centre of gravity or fetoplacental injury caused by blunt trauma or stress effects from sudden motions is also a concern [162].

Recommendations of physical activity during pregnancy before the twentieth century were overly conservative [162–171]. Recently, the guidelines have evolved as more reliable research has emerged [14]. The American College of Obstetricians and Gynaecologists (ACOG) found no scientific support that normal pregnant women should limit their exposure to physical activity based on the risks to the foetus and/or mother. However, some studies found that higher daily physical activity is inversely associated with foetal growth [172] and birth weight [173].

Campbell and Mottola [174] found that excessive physical exercise, at a frequency greater than 5 days a week, resulted in a low birth weight. However, their results also showed an equally harmful effect on foetal growth in the group of women who exercised less than two times per week. Magann et al. [175] supported the above-mentioned results and found that less energy expenditure, at work and during leisure time, was associated with an increased risk of preterm birth and low birth weight (< 10th and < 3rd percentile).

The risk–benefit balance of physical activity during pregnancy needs to be assessed. During pregnancy, the risk of a sedentary lifestyle may be more detrimental than an active one [7], since a sedentary lifestyle includes loss of muscular and cardiovascular fitness, excessive weight gain, raised risk of gestational diabetes or pre-eclampsia, development of varicose veins and an increased risk of physical complaints such as dyspnoea, lower back pain and poor psychological adjustment [115, 139, 176]. According to Takito et al. [161], both excessive and insufficient physical activity impact negatively on pregnancy outcomes. Physical activity, done at an appropriate level for the physical condition of the woman, is beneficial to foetal growth, with the extremes being inactivity/sedentarism and a prolonged duration of vigorous intensities, which are potentially harmful to the supply of oxygen for adequate foetal growth [160]. However, women with complicated pregnancies have been discouraged from participating in exercise activities for fear of impacting the underlying disorder or maternal or foetal outcomes [8]. Some publications indicate that high levels of strenuous, high-intensity activity may result in preterm labour in susceptible individuals as well as babies with a low birth weight [177–179].

Absolute contraindications to exercise in pregnancy include haemodynamically significant heart disease, restrictive lung disease, incompetent lung disease, multiple gestation at risk for premature labour (≥ triplets), persistent second- or third-trimester bleeding, placenta praevia after 26 weeks' gestation, ruptured membranes, preterm labour, pre-eclampsia, uncontrolled type-1 diabetes and thyroid disease or other serious systemic disorders like chronic bronchitis and uncontrolled seizures [8]. Relative contraindications to exercise include anaemia (defined by the World Health Organization as < 19 g/dL in pregnant women), unevaluated maternal cardiac arrhythmia, extreme morbid obesity and extreme underweight (BMI 8] (Table 16.1).

However, pregnant women should be advised that adverse pregnancy or neonatal outcomes are not increased for exercising pregnant women [7, 180–186], and maternal and infant health can even be enhanced [144, 180, 187–191]. Table 16.2 provides evidence regarding the effects of physical activity on foetal growth and birth outcomes.

Table 16.1 Absolute and relative contraindicators for exercise during pregnancy. (Reprinted from [5]. With permission from Elsevier)

Relative contraindicators	Absolute contraindicators
Severe anaemia	Haemodynamically significant heart disease
Unevaluated maternal cardiac dysrhythmia	Restrictive lung disease
Chronic bronchitis	Incompetent cervix/cerclage
Poorly controlled type 1 diabetes mellitus	Multiple gestation at risk for premature labour
Extreme morbid obesity	Persistent second- or third-trimester bleeding
Extreme underweight	Placenta praevia after 26 weeks of gestation
History of extremely sedentary lifestyle	Premature labour during current pregnancy
Heavy smoker	Ruptured membranes
Poorly controlled hypertension	Pre-eclampsia/pregnancy-induced hypertension
Orthopaedic limitations	
Poorly controlled seizure disorder	
Poorly controlled hyperthyroidism	
Intrauterine growth restriction in current pregnancy	

Table 16.2 Mapping the evidence: Physical activity and foetal growth. (Randomised controlled trials)

Author	Year	Title	Study design	Method	Foetal growth	Outcome
Alderman et al. [192]	1998	Maternal physical activity in pregnancy and infant size for gestational age	Control: women recruited for an epidemiological investigation of risk factors for craniosynostosis Experimental: mothers were identified by random sampling of Colorado live births records for 1979–1988 matched to birth defect registry cases on month and year of birth	Interviews with the adapted Coronary Artery Risk Development in Young Adult Study (CARDIA) Physical activity history (PAH), which classifies activities into 13 groups based on intensity	Birth weight from birth records. Gestational age was reviewed from medical records of the neonatal exam, interview data from the mother and birth records	Maternal physical activity decreased the risk of large-for-gestational-age infants
Bell et al. [193]	2000	Antenatal exercise and birth weight	Experimental: continued strenuous exercise >=5 times per week from 24 weeks Control: strenuous exercise reduced to <=3 times per week from 24 weeks	Exercise diaries, with details of the baby, labour and delivery	Birth weight and birth rate	Increased mean birth weight
Clapp et al. [194]	2000	Beginning regular exercise in early pregnancy: effect on fetoplacental growth	Experimental: 20 min of aerobic exercise, 3–4 times per week, beginning at 8–9 weeks and continuing until delivery Control: no aerobic exercise	Indirect calorimetry	Gestational weight gain, mid-trimester placental growth rate, placental volume, birth weight, length, ponderal index, head circumference, preterm birth, infant lean mass, fat mass, % fat	Significant, balanced increase in fetoplacental growth in normal pregnancy

Table 16.2 (continued)

Author	Year	Title	Study design	Method	Foetal growth	Outcome
Clapp et al. [195]	2002	Continuing regular exercise during pregnancy: effect of exercise volume on fetoplacental growth	Experimental: 60 min weight-bearing exercise, 5 days per week from 8 to 20 weeks, then reduced to 20 min, 5 times per week from 24 weeks to delivery ('Hi-Lo" group) opposite pattern ('Lo-Hi' group) Control: intermediate intensity, constant pattern (40 min, 5 days per week, from 8 weeks to delivery)	Indirect calorimetry	Placental growth rate, birth weight and placental volume at term	Reduced fetoplacental growth. Proportionally greater increase in fat mass than in lean body mass
Haakstad et al. [196]	2011	Exercise in pregnant women and birth weight: a randomised controlled trial	Experimental group: nulliparous pregnant women (N=52) encouraged to participate in supervised aerobic dance and strength training; 60 min, twice per week; 12 weeks, plus 30 min of self-imposed physical activity on the non-supervised week-days Control group: (N=53)	Questionnaire measured physical activity and sedentary behaviour	Labour and delivery records (infant birth weight, length, head circumference, gestational age at time of delivery and Apgar scores at 1 and 5 min after birth)	Aerobic-dance exercise appeared to be safe and was not associated with any reduction in newborn birth weight, preterm birth rate or neonatal wellbeing
Marquez-Sterling et al. [197]	2000	Physical and psychological changes with vigorous exercise in sedentary primigravidae	Experimental: 1 h aerobic exercise, 3 times per week, for 15 weeks Control: no aerobic exercise during pregnancy	Questionnaires	Physical fitness, gestational weight gain, birth weight, 5-min Apgar score, caesarean section and body image	Low birth weight in experimental group
Prevedel et al. [198]	2003	Maternal and perinatal effects of hydrotherapy in pregnancy	Experimental: aerobic (swimming exercise for 1 h, 3 times per week, for 10 weeks Control: normal activity without aerobic exercise	Maximal oxygen consumption, stroke volume and cardiac output	Physical fitness, foetal heart rate before and after exercise (acute exercise effect) not included in review	Hydrotherapy assisted metabolic and cardiovascular maternal adaptation to pregnancy and did not cause prematurity or weight loss in newborns

Guidelines for Physical Activity During Pregnancy

The ACOG [5] recommends that healthy pregnant women exercise at moderate intensity for at least 30 min, most days of the week [24] while the American College of Sports Medicine [7] encourages an accumulation of 30 min or more of moderate physical activity per day on most, if not all, days of the week. Yet, another recommendation set forth by the US Department of Health and Human Service states in the document "2008 Physical Activity Guidelines for Americans" that pregnant women should engage in a minimum

Table 16.3 A summary of physical activity guidelines during pregnancy as prescribed by various organisations

Body prescribing guidelines	Guideline
ACOG [5]	Healthy pregnant women should exercise at moderate intensity for at least 30 min, most days of the week
ACSM [6]	Encourages pregnant women to accumulate 30 min or more of moderate physical activity per day on most, if not all, days of the week
US Department of Health and Human Services [12]	Pregnant women should engage in a minimum of 150 min of moderate-intensity aerobic activity a week, even if they were not physically active prior to pregnancy
Sports Medicine Australia [11]	Moderate exercise as determined with the Borg scale
Davies et al. [8]	All women without contraindications should be encouraged to participate in aerobic and strength-conditioning exercises as part of a healthy lifestyle during their pregnancy
RCOG [10]	Exercise program should be individualised based on previous physical activity level. Sedentary pregnant women should start with 15 min continuous exercise 3 times per week and increase to 30 min 4–5 times a week
Holan et at. [9]	Sedentary women should be moderately active during pregnancy and gradually increase their activity (up to 30 min per day)
Barsky et al. [7]	In low-risk pregnancies, women should be encouraged to participate in aerobic and strength-conditioning training at a moderate intensity on most or all days of the week

of 150 min of moderate-intensity aerobic activity a week, even if they were not physically active prior to pregnancy [12]. Recommendations in Australia [11], Canada [8], the UK [10] and Norway [9] are similar to the abovementioned American [120]. A recent South African Position Statement [7] supports the guidelines set out by the ACOG [5], the Society of Obstetricians and Gynaecologists of Canada (SOGC) and the Canadian Society of Exercise Physiology [8], but focuses on exercise and does not give guidelines regarding general physical activity during pregnancy (Table 16.3).

The question remains whether pregnant women adhere to these guidelines. Due to the uncertainty regarding the benefits and risks of exercise during pregnancy [199], the adherence of pregnant women to exercise is not reflective of the recommended ACOG guidelines [55, 104, 200]. Additionally, pregnant women often receive mixed messages from friends, family and even their doctors about exercise during pregnancy [199]. While scientific data support the safety of exercise during pregnancy, this knowledge is not always communicated to pregnant women. According to Price et al. [199], exercise must be prescribed to pregnant women in a similar way as the prescription of medicine. In addition, more reliable quantitative-determined data are warranted to provide an evidence-based exercise regimen for pregnant women.

The recommendations for physical activity for pregnant women, as presented in Table 16.3, are similar to the guidelines for nonpregnant women. The only exception is the intensity of the activity. In the guidelines, "moderate activity" is given as the intensity, but the definition for moderate-intensity activity is not defined. When the presented guidelines are compared to the guidelines for maintaining weight after weight loss, which is 60–90 min of activity, it is understandable that women do not comply with the guidelines due to the inherent discrepancies. Finally, the guideline for heart rate should be clarified in consideration with the fitness level of the pregnant women and previous exercise experience and level of fitness prior to pregnancy.

Birth Outcomes

Foetal Growth Parameters and Confounders Thereof

Monitoring the growth of the foetus is a major purpose of antenatal care [201]. The overall term "foetal growth parameters" includes: head and abdominal circumference, femur length, ponderal index (weight in grams x100 divided by length in cubic centimetres), placental weight and expected birth weight [202]. While birth weight is a crude measurement of foetal growth, the measurement of head size and length at birth gives an insight into the timing of growth retardation during intrauterine life [203].

Birth Weight

Although birth weight is not the most objective measurement of foetal growth, it is important with regards to public health [3]. Birth weight is an amalgam of multiple determinants and is a proxy for the many different processes that occur in the months preceding delivery [204]. Birth weight is associated with a broad range of short- and long-term maternal complications (e.g. pre-eclampsia, premature labour), foetal complications (e.g. stillbirth, malformations), neonatal complications (e.g. respiratory distress, infant mortality) and long-term complications (e.g. behavioural disorders, cerebral palsy) [205, 206].

Foetuses delivered with a lower birth weight than expected might become healthy, thriving infants, while others are small because their growth in utero was impaired and have an increased risk for perinatal morbidity and mortality [207, 208]. The cut-off for small-for-gestational-age is a birth weight below the tenth percentile [209]. Low birth weight and foetal growth impairment may be multifactorial in origin, therefore it is vital to have knowledge of possible associations between specific risk factors, pre- and postnatal growth patterns and specific adult health parameters like smoking and physical activity habits [210].

Over the last decade, a new paradigm evolved from the notion that environmental factors in early life and in utero can have profound influences on lifelong health [204]. Reduced foetal growth might also be the origin of cardiovascular disease later in life through programming in foetal life and infancy [203].

Theory of Foetal Origins

Time in the womb can be seen as a critical window during which maturation must be achieved, because failure of maturation is to some extent irrecoverable [203]. The maternal environment influences these critical stages of early life and leads to long-term changes in the body's structure, physiology or metabolism—this is called programming [211, 212]. Relationships between foetal experiences and later risk for adult chronic disease, including cardiovascular disease and its risk factors, cancer, osteoporosis, diabetes, neuropsychiatric outcomes and respiratory diseases, have been demonstrated by a large number of studies [213–216]. The abovementioned relationship, the foetal origins hypothesis, was first proposed by the British epidemiologist David Barker as the "thrifty gene hypothesis" [217]. The foetal origin hypothesis was developed by linking records of births in the early twentieth century with health in later life from the Hertfordshire records [203, 217–225].

The theory of foetal origins suggests that associations with body size at birth underestimate the influence of intrauterine development on later disease. Prevention of coronary heart disease and non-insulin-dependent diabetes may be related to the choices of the mother. Therefore, chronic disorders that manifest later in life may be related to poverty (malnourished mothers give birth to malnourished infants with low birth weight) and prosperity (exposure of an infant with low body weight phenotype to a high caloric diet) [226] In this way, both a low and high birth weight is associated with negative outcomes in later life, showing a U-shaped relationship as observed by Rich-Edwards et al. [227]. Newborns that are small-for-gestational-age tend to preserve body fat at the expense of lean body mass [228], whereas large newborns may also have relatively increased body fat. Hammani et al. [229] suggest that associations between foetal growth and later adiposity are complex. The findings that a low and high birth weight is a strong predictor of diabetes and cardiovascular disease in later life has led to continuing debate about the significance of nature and nurture [230].

Environmental Pollution

Environmental air pollution has been shown to have associations with a low birth weight and its determinants, preterm delivery and intrauterine growth restriction [231–238]. Exposure to an air pollutant like carbon monoxide could lead to decreased oxygen delivery to tissues, including the foetus [239]. Inhaling air pollution particles may lead to increased blood viscosity, which may have an adverse effect on placental function, thereby restricting foetal growth [233]. However, the effect of air pollution on foetal growth is smaller than the effect of high-risk behaviours [239].

Lifestyle

Tobacco smoking, alcohol consumption and illicit drug abuse are increasing among women of childbearing age [240]. Intrauterine growth restriction and low birth weight are the most consistent effect of these high-risk behaviours [240]. Maternal smoking during pregnancy is an extremely important, modifiable risk factor that is associated with adverse perinatal outcomes [241–243], such as intrauterine growth retardation [243, 244], low birth weight [245–248], preterm and very preterm delivery [249], ectopic pregnancy [250], placental pathologies [251] and a significant higher risk of perinatal and infant mortality [252–255]. Specifically, smoking has negative effects on multiple foetal growth parameters including body weight, femur length, limb length, total length, head circumference, chest circumference and abdominal circumference [256–259]. According to Hernandéz-Martínez et al. [261], maternal smoking during pregnancy is also related to cognitive, emotional, temperamental and behavioural problems throughout the child's life.

The effects of smoking could be mediated by the direct toxic effect on the foetus, leading to metabolic alterations, as well as by mechanisms resulting in decreased oxygen delivery [255]. Cigarette smoke contains more than 2500 chemicals and some of these are harmful to the developing foetus and cause adverse pregnancy outcomes [261, 262]. Carbon monoxide readily crosses the placental barrier by passive diffusion, causing a fourfold increase in the level of carboxyhaemoglobin in umbilical cord blood, which inhibits the release of oxygen into foetal tissues [263–266]. This chronic hypoxia alters the physiological development of organs and tissues [261, 267]. Therefore, cigarette smoking during pregnancy is a strong dose-dependent risk factor for small-for-gestational-age [268, 269]. Secondhand smoke showed a similar relationship, according to Horta et al. [248].

Cigarette smoking may confound the relationship between birth weight and later body size [204]. Multiple studies have demonstrated a clear inverse relationship between maternal smoking and childhood weight [270, 271], although [272] suggest an increased risk of obesity later in life among offspring of mothers who smoked during pregnancy. [255] analysed body composition and found that lean body mass was more affected than body fat, and proportional body distribution of subcutaneous fat was not affected in infants from mothers who smoked during pregnancy.

Alcohol consumption during pregnancy has been associated with various pregnancy complications such as miscarriage [273], stillbirth [274] and other multiple birth defects [275–279] such as foetal alcohol syndrome [280, 281] and an increased risk of low birth weight [282, 283].

Drug abuse during pregnancy may lead to complications for the foetus, the newborn and later during childhood [240]. Cannabis, cocaine and heroin specifically have been studied in relation to their effects on foetal growth [240, 284], and findings have proposed that cannabis abuse during pregnancy decreases foetal growth, but this has not been confirmed in follow-up studies [285–287]. Poor pregnancy outcomes, including premature birth and abnormalities of behavioural testing in the offspring, have been associated with cocaine use during pregnancy [240]. Associations with heroin use during pregnancy and an increased incidence of pregnancy complications, including premature delivery, premature rupture of the membranes, intrauterine foetal growth retardation and perinatal mortality have also been confirmed [240].

Another confounder between birth weight and later adiposity may be social and economic factors [204]. Vagero et al. [289] found that babies born to women with a lower social status had lower birth weights. As such, neighbourhood factors that have been associated with an increased risk for a low birth weight include a negative perception of the neighbourhood [290], an average income [291, 292], economic hardship, low housing costs [293] and, interestingly, neighbourhood crime rates [294]. How these factors relate to birth weight remains speculation, but there have been explanations that focus on the stress-related hormonal factors and birth outcomes through biological mechanisms [295–299], whereas others researched the association with maternal health behaviours, such as smoking [300–302]. Although environmental factors play an important role in determining foetal growth, genetics must also be considered.

Genetics

Both genetic and environmental factors are important determinants of foetal growth [230, 303, 304]. As stated by Tower and Baker [305], the growth potential of any foetus is likely to be genetically determined. As an example, Knight et al. [304] found that paternal height is an important, independent determinant of foetal linear growth. Knight et al. [304] concludes that skeletal size is regulated by genetic information, while the adiposity of the newborn is reflected by the maternal intrauterine environment. Another example is that offspring birth weight has a strong association with parental adiposity [306, 307]. Therefore, the associations of maternal and paternal birth weight with offspring birth weight suggest genetic or intergenerational environmental influences [204, 308, 309].

Foetal growth restriction is a complex trait for which no single susceptibility gene can be identified [305]. There are between 100 and 200 imprinted genes and there is increasing evidence that many are involved in pre- and postnatal growth [310]. When the normal imprint is disrupted, malformations in the development of the foetus occur [310]. Vaessen et al. [230] postulate that the Insulin-like Growth Factor-1 (IGF-1) gene imprint disruption may lead to low circulating IGF-1 concentrations, reduced height in adulthood, diminished insulin secreting capacity and a high risk of type-2 diabetes and myocardial infarction. Although genetically established expression of IGF-1 and insulin are important determinants of growth during the foetal period, they do not play a major role in the regulation of body weight in postnatal life [230]. Additionally, the postnatal environment that includes adverse eating and activity habits shared by family members may also lead to a higher birth weight and higher adiposity later in life. Other genetic and environmental factors such as diet and physical activity have more relevant effects on the regulation of weight [230]. A summary of the interactions can be seen in Fig. 16.6 that has been composed from the existing literature.

Labour

Natural birth seems to be the best conclusion of the pregnancy for both the mother and the baby [311] and should therefore be seen as a major goal for all pregnant women [120]. Other methods of childbirth, including a caesarean section, should only be used when justified by the circumstances [120]. From a public health perspective, there is concern regarding the increased rate of caesarean sections during the last decade because this procedure is not risk-free [312]. One possible explanation for this recent rise in caesarean sections includes a rise in maternal obesity [313]. However, this rise cannot be attributed entirely to a worsening of maternal or foetal risk factors [314–316]. Therefore, caesarean sections may be not justified medically, exposing women and babies to surgical risks without proved benefit [317, 318]. Reducing rates of caesarean sections should be a public health priority [312].

In recent years, prenatal physical activity has increasingly been recommended to promote natural birth [99, 120, 134, 165, 319]. Regular physical activity during pregnancy may have other beneficial effects on multiple aspects of the course and outcome of labour and delivery [120] including a shorter delivery [134, 320–323], less frequent need for anaesthesia [134, 324], a lower rate of induction of labour [134, 320], amniotomy [134], episiotomy and perineum lacerations [134, 321, 325] and improved neonatal outcome

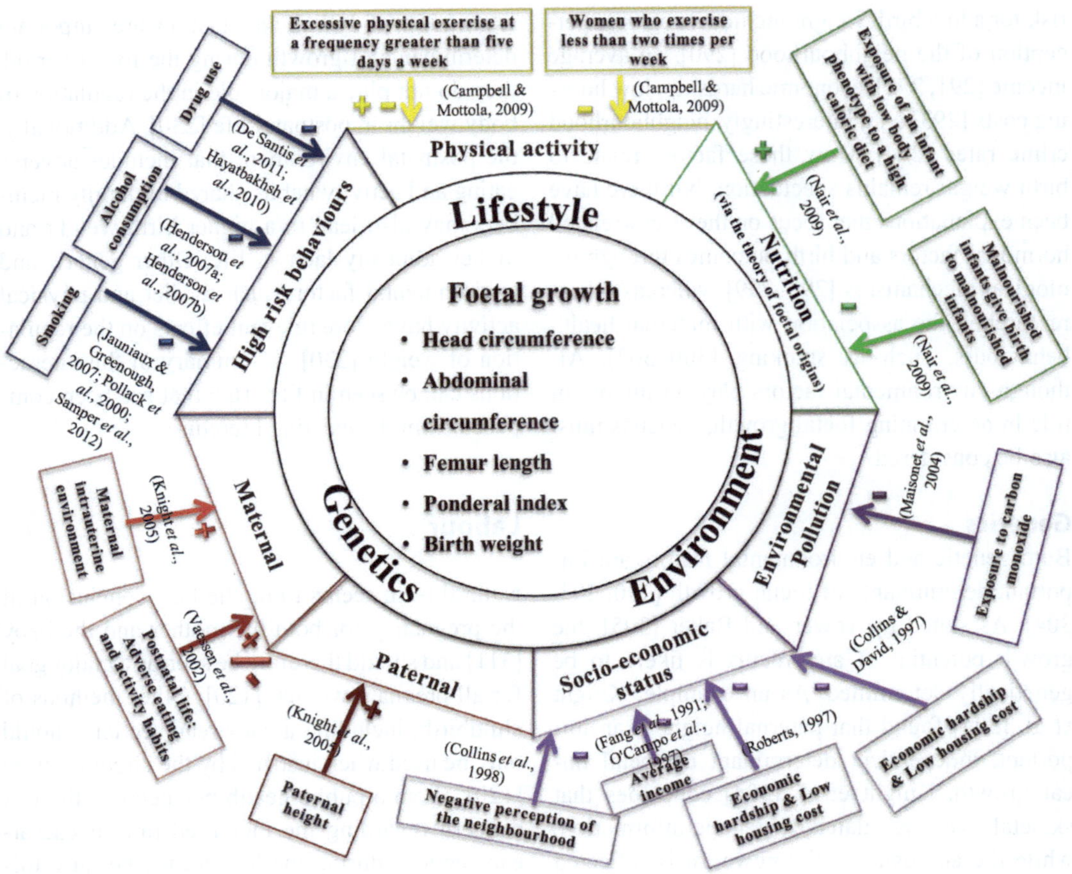

Fig. 16.6 Multifactorial influences on foetal growth. + positive influence/effect, − negative influence/effect

directly after birth [134]. Based on these findings, it is clear that physical activity during pregnancy has physiological benefits on labour. However, as stated by Guskowska [326], pregnant women often experience fear about labour and delivery, which is undoubtedly detrimental. Physical activity might produce anti-anxiety effects that will help to reduce labour anxiety [326].

To conclude, Ghodsi et al. [322] state that physical activity can result in shorter labour, fewer medical interventions, less exhaustion during labour and might also reduce the fear associated with giving birth. Encouraging pregnant women to be physically active could represent a low-cost, low-risk approach to reduce the number of caesarean deliveries [312].

Body Composition at Birth Related to Disease in Later Life

Early environmental influences, as early as in the womb, have long-term effects on body composition and musculoskeletal development as evidenced by the prevalence of obesity, sarcopenia and osteoporosis in later life [327]. This phenomenon is explained by means of foetal programming as previously mentioned, and more specifically, to the body composition of the baby, referred to as developmental plasticity [327]. Developmental plasticity is defined as the ability of a single genotype to produce more than one alternative form of structure, physiological state or behaviour in response to early environmental conditions [327].

During embryonic life, bone and muscle develop from the mesoderm layer, differentiate during the first trimester into dermatomes containing bone and muscle cell precursors [327]. Muscle development starts between 6 and 8 weeks of gestation and progresses until about 18 weeks [328]. Adipose cell formation is determined much later, the critical period varying from 30 weeks of gestation to the first year of postnatal life [329]. These major phases of the developing of muscle and fat are important, because of the high vulnerability of foetal programming occurring during this period of rapid cell division, the so-called critical periods [330].

A low birth weight has implications on fat, muscle and bone distribution in later life [327]. An association between low birth weight and increased adult central distribution of fat exists and has been evident in a couple of studies [327, 331, 332]. Reduced muscle mass and strength have also been implicated due to small size at birth [327]. These abovementioned effects are mediated by mechanisms that include a direct effect on cell number, altered stem cell function and resetting of regulatory hormonal axis [327].

Overall, evidence indicates that a higher birth weight is associated with increased risk of adiposity in childhood and adulthood, as reflected by BMI [204]. According to findings from Silverman et al. [333], increased adiposity was apparent at birth and progressively after the age of 4 years, but not from ages 1 to 3 years. Numerous studies have found direct associations between a higher birth weight and a higher adult BMI [227, 271, 334–339]. Specifically, the magnitude ranges from 0.5 to 0.7 kg/m^2 for each 1-kg increment in birth weight [339, 340].

Maternal Weight Gain During Pregnancy

Women often express concern about weight gain during pregnancy; however, it is important to remember that during pregnancy, all women gain weight due to foetal and maternal health. This weight gain also corresponds directly with foetal birth weight, which is a strong precursor of the health and development of the infant [34]. However, desirable weight gain also depends on BMI before pregnancy. Siega-Riz et al. [341] recommend GWG ranges for women on the basis of BMI as outlined in Table 16.4. The recommended ranges are derived from the observed weight gains of women delivering full-term, healthy infants without complications [40]. The total amount of weight gained in normal-term pregnancies varies considerably between women [41]. Studies show that about one third of mothers in the USA gain more or less the recommended weight; however, there is a lack in current research regarding the effects of physical activity on weight gain during pregnancy in the South African context [112]. One cross-sectional South African study found physically active pregnant women tend to gain less weight than relatively inactive pregnant women [112]. The findings are also supported by a recent meta-analysis from Domenjoz et al. [152] who reported a 1.3 kg less weight gain in women participating in physical activity compared to a non-active control group.

Weight gain during pregnancy is an important factor to consider to determine long-term obesity [342] and predict other health risks such as pre-eclampsia and adverse birth outcomes [343]. Women are usually very self-conscious or concerned about weight gain during pregnancy

Table 16.4 Recomm gestational weight gain ranges for women on the basis of body mass index. (Adapted from [342]. With permission from Elsevier)

Body mass classification	Body mass index (kg/m^2)	Recommended weight gain range (kg)
Low	< 19.8	12.5–18
Normal	19.8–26.0	11.5–16
Overweight	26.0–29.0	7.0–11.5
Obese	≥ 29.0	6

[344]. Brunette et al. [112] conclude that leading a moderately active lifestyle during pregnancy can have definite weight-control benefits, therefore women should be advised to be physically active during their pregnancies to reap the benefits and possibly to prevent the development of postnatal obesity. On the other hand, adopting a sedentary lifestyle, a common trend among pregnant women, results in women gaining weight above the recommended weight gain ranges [345].

Physical Activity in Infertility-Related Conditions

Polycystic Ovarian Syndrome

The most common endocrinopathy affecting women of reproductive age are polycystic ovarian syndrome (PCOS). The condition affects between 4–12 % [346, 347] of women in America. Various diagnostic criteria are used, with the most common being an increase in insulin resistance compared to non-PCOS women independent of obesity [348]. Women suffering from PCOS experience reduced fertility, morphological changes of the ovaries and increased abdominal visceral fat [349]. Although the link between insulin resistance and infertility have not been completely resolved, various studies have indicated in the general population that regular physical activity increases insulin sensitivity, reducing insulin resistance. Researchers were therefore prompted to investigate the effect of physical activity on insulin resistance of women suffering from PCOS. A systematic review including premenopausal women diagnosed with PCOS who were exposed to between 12–24 weeks of exercise reported an improvement of between 23–30 % in fasting insulin [350]. When the effect of diet alone and diet combined with exercise was analysed, an overall improvement in ovulation and/or menstrual cycle was reported in 49 % of the participants. No difference between diet only and diet plus exercise intervention groups were found. The findings from the review suggest that regular physical activity may improve ovulation rates independent of dietary restrictions and changes in body fat. The physical activity interventions seem to enhance the insulin sensitivity which restores the reproductive function.

Amenorrhea

Amenorrhea is considered the most severe form of menstrual abnormality that causes infertility and is reported to be present in 1–44 % of female athletes [351]. The prevalence tends to be higher in athletes of sports where a very low BMI is required or in sports with a large strength component [352]. The mechanism through which exercise disturbs the menstrual cycle is described as a disruption of the hypothalamic–pituitary–ovarian axis. The consequence is that the hypothalamic pulsatile release of gonadotropin-releasing hormone (GnRH) is supressed, which consequently reduces the release of gonadotropins follicle-stimulating hormones (FSH) and luteinizing hormone (LH). An anovulatory and hypoestrogenic state results as a lack of ovarian stimulation [353].

Results from a population-based study in Norway during the mid-1980s with a follow-up one decade later focussing on infertility indicated that an increase in frequency, duration or intensity of physical activity was related to an increase in difficulty conceiving. A 3.2-fold greater chance of being infertile was reported for women exercising most days of the week. Independent of age, smoking and BMI, the risk of infertility increased 2.3 times when exercising to exhaustion [354].

Although regular physical activity and exercise is highly beneficial for most women, adverse effects related to fertility can and do occur. Current evidence indicates that the mechanism appears to be via an energy deficit that is created through a high intensity training program with a concomitant deficit in energy intake [355]. The energy deficit results in a catabolic state, shutting down the reproductive system in order to maintain health.

Summary

Early environmental influences, as early as in the womb, have long-term effects on an individual's health. The maternal environment influences critical stages of early life and leads to long-term changes in the body's structure, physiology and metabolism. A healthy lifestyle during pregnancy, which includes regular physical activity, no smoking and alcohol consumption, is essential. The physical and psychological benefits of regular physical activity during pregnancy are plentiful. Regular physical activity not only provides maternal benefits (decreased GWG, reduced risk of gestational diabetes and pre-eclampsia) but also foetal benefits (decreased risk for small- or large-for-gestational-age) and improved birth outcomes (lower incidence of operative abdominal and vaginal deliveries and a shorter labour period).

Physical activity tends to decrease as pregnancy progresses despite these known benefits. Although scientific data supports the safety of physical activity during pregnancy, this knowledge is not always communicated to pregnant women. The lack of objective and quantitative research regarding physical activity and pregnancy might have led to these uncertainties. Determining physical activity during pregnancy remains problematic due to methodological difficulties. However, the combined heart rate and accelerometer available on the market is a valid and reliable tool for the measurement of physical activity. Free-living data can be assessed and is essential to determine behavioural changes in activity patterns during pregnancy. Accurately determining physical activity will minimise possible inaccuracies of subjectively determined habitual activity patterns by means of questionnaires and could provide better insights into the effect of these patterns on foetal growth.

Determining the influence of habitual physical activity on foetal growth is difficult. Multiple determinants influence foetal growth and these factors have thoroughly been researched. One exception is the influence of habitual physical activity on foetal growth, possibly because of a relatively small relationship. Regular physical activities tend to decrease the risk of small- and large-for-gestational-age. Regular physical activity, in addition, also appears to have advantages for women suffering from infertility due to PCOS, since the restoration of insulin sensitivity improves ovulation rates.

Various institutional and governmental entities have set guidelines specifically for physical activity during pregnancy, but few women follow these guidelines because of uncertainty of the benefits and risks associated with physical activity during pregnancy. These guidelines are not based on longitudinal studies on pregnant women and might be unnecessarily conservative. Future research needs to be aimed at objectively determining the habitual physical activity patterns during pregnancy, as well as guiding governmental organisations to set specific physical activity guidelines and educating women about these guidelines. In addition, the safety of regular physical activity during pregnancy must also be addressed with doctors and health workers.

References

1. Downs DS, Chasan-Taber L, Evenson K, Jenn L, Leo S. Physical activity and pregnancy: past and present evidence and future recommendations. Res Quart Exerc Sport. 2012;83(4):485–502.
2. Melzer K, Schutz Y, Boulvain M, Kayser B. Physical activity and pregnancy: cardiovascular adaptations, recommendations and pregnancy outcomes. Sport Med. 2010;40(6):493–507.
3. Chasan-Taber L, Evenson KR, Sternfeld B, Kengeri S. Assessment of recreational physical activity during pregnancy in epidemiologic studies of birthweight and length of gestation: methodologic aspects. Women Health. 2007;45(4):85–107.
4. Evenson KR, Wen F. Prevalence and correlates of objectively measured physical activity and sedentary behaviour among US pregnant women. Prev Med. 2011;53(1):39–43.
5. ACOG (American College of Obstetricians and Gynecologists). Exercise during pregnancy. and the postpartum period. ACOG Committee Opinion. Int J Gynaecol Obstet. 2002;77(1):79–81.
6. ACSM (American College of Sports Medicine), editor. ACSM's guidelines for exercise testing and prescription. 9th ed. Philadelphia: Lippincott Williams and Wilkins; 2014.

7. Barsky E, Smith T, Patricios J, Collins R, Branfield A, Ramagole M. South African Sports Medicine Association position statement on exercise in pregnancy. S Afr J Sport Med. 2012;24(2):69–71.
8. Davies GA, Wolfe LA, Mottola MF, Mackinnon C. Joint SOGC/CSEP clinical practice guideline: exercise in pregnancy and the postpartum period. J Obstet Gynaecol Can. 2003;28(3):329–41.
9. Holan S, Mathiesen M, Petersen KA. National Clinical Guideline for Antenatal Care. [Internet]. Oslo, Norway: Directorate for Health and Social Affairs; 2005. http://helsedirektoratet.no/publikasjoner/retningslinjer-for-svangerskapsomsorgen-kortversjon/Publikasjoner/a-national-clinical-guideline-for-antenatal-care%E2%80%93short-version.pdf. Accessed 8 July 2013.
10. Royal College of Obstetricians and Gynaecologists [Internet]. RCOG; [updated 2006 Jan 1; cited 2012 Jul 2]. Exercise in Pregnancy (Statement 4); [about 8 screens]. http://www.rcog.org.uk/womens-health/clinical-guidance/exercise-pregnancy.
11. Sports Medicine Australia. Exercise in pregnancy [Internet]. Victoria: Sport and Recreation; 2009. http://sma.org.au/wp-content/uploads/2009/10/WIS-ExPreg.pdf. Accessed 8 July 2013.
12. US Department of Health and Human Services. Physical activity guidelines for americans [Internet]. Office of Disease Prevention and Health Promotion; 2008. http://www.health.gov/paguidelines/pdf/paguide.pdf. Accessed 8 July 2013.
13. Blackburn ST. Maternal, fetal, and neonatal physiology: a clinical perspective. 2nd ed. St. Louis: Mosby; 2003.
14. Kawaguchi JK, Pickering RK. The pregnant athlete, part 1: anatomy and physiology of pregnancy. Athlet Ther Today. 2010;15(2):39–43.
15. Heidemann BH, McClure JH. Changes in maternal physiology during pregnancy. Brit J Anaesth. 2003;3(3):65–8.
16. Norwitz ER, Edusa V, Park JS. Maternal physiology and complications of multiple pregnancy. Semin Perinatol. 2005;29(5):338–48.
17. Carlin A, Alfirevic Z. Physiological changes of pregnancy and monitoring. Best Prac Res Clin Obstet. 2008;22(5):801–23.
18. Capeless EL, Clapp JF. Cardiovascular changes in early phase of pregnancy. Am J Obstet Gynecol. 1989;161(6):1449–53.
19. Holschen JC. The female athlete. Southern Med J. 2004;97(9):852–8.
20. Jensen D, Webb KA, O'Donnell DE. Chemical and mechanical adaptations of the respiratory system at rest and during exercise in human pregnancy. Appl Physiol Nutr Metab. 2007;32(6):1239–50.
21. Garcia-Rio F, Pino JM, Gomez L, Alvarez-Sala R, Villasante C, Villamor J. Regulation of breathing and perception of dyspnoea in healthy pregnant women. Chest. 1996;110(2):446–53.
22. Jensen D, Wolfde LA, Slatkovska L, Webb KA, Davies GAL, O'Donnell DE. Effects of human pregnancy on ventilator chemoreflex response to carbon dioxide. Am J Physiol Regul Integr Comp Physiol. 2005;288(5):1369–75.
23. Calguneri M, Bird HA, Wright V. Changes in joint laxity occurring during pregnancy. Ann Rheum Dis. 1982;41(2):126–8.
24. Artal R, O'Toole M. Guidelines of the American College of Obstetricians and Gynaecologists for exercise during pregnancy and the postpartum period. Brit J Sport Med. 2003;37(1):6–12.
25. Whitcome KK, Shapiro LJ, Lieberman DE. Fetal load and the evolution of lumbar lordosis in bipedal hominins. Nature. 2007;450(7172):1075–8.
26. Wang TW, Apgar BS. Exercise during pregnancy. Am Fam Physician. 1998;57(8):1847–52.
27. Branco M, Santos-Rocha R, Aguiar L, Vieira F, Veloso A. Kinematic analysis of gait in the second and third trimesters of pregnancy. J Preg. 2013;718095. doi:101155/2013/718095.
28. Kuijper EAM, Ket JCF, Caanen MR, Lambalk CB. Reproductive hormone concentrations in pregnancy and neonates: a systematic review. Reprod Biomed Online. 2013;27(1):33–63.
29. Lewis B, Avery M, Jennings E, Sherwood N, Martinson B, Crain AL. The effects of exercise during pregnancy on maternal outcomes: practical implications for practice. Am J Lifestyle Med. 2008;2(5):441–55.
30. Wylie L. Essential anatomy and physiology in maternity care. 2nd ed. United Kingdom: Churchill Livingstone; 2005.
31. Mittlemark RA, Wiswell RA, Drinkwater BL. Exercise in pregnancy. 2nd ed. Baltimore: Lippincott Williams & Wilkins; 1991.
32. Glinoer D. The regulation of thyroid function during normal pregnancy: importance of the iodine nutrition status. Best Prac Res Clin Endocrinol Metab. 2004;18(2):133–52.
33. Chamberlain G, Popkin FB. Clinical physiology in obstetrics. 3rd ed. Nottingham: Blackwell Scientific Publisher; 1998.
34. Whitney E, Rolfes SR. Understanding nutrition. 11th ed. Belmont: Thomson Wadsworth; 2008.
35. Melzer K, Schutz Y, Boulvain M, Kayser B. Pregnancy-related changes in activity energy expenditure and resting metabolic rate in Switzerland. Eur J Clin Nutr. 2009;63(10):1183–91.
36. Poppitt SD, Prentic AM, Jequier E, Schults Y, Whitehead RG. Evidence of energy sparing in Gambian women during pregnancy: a longitudinal study using whole-body calorimetry. Am J Clin Nutr. 1993;57(3):353–64.
37. McArdle WD, Katch FI, Katch VL. Exercise physiology: nutrition, energy, and human performance. 7th ed. Baltimore: Lippincott Williams & Wilkins; 2010.

38. Löf M. Physical activity pattern and activity energy expenditure in healthy pregnant and non-pregnant Swedish women. Eur J Clin Nutr. 2011;65(12):1295–301.
39. Mojtahedi M, De Groot LCP, Boekholt HA, Van Raaij JMA. Nitrogen balance of healthy Dutch women before and during pregnancy. Am J Clin Nutr. 2002;75(6):1078–83.
40. Butte NF, Wong WW, Treuth MS, Ellis KJ, Smith EO. Energy requirements during pregnancy based on total energy expenditure and energy deposition. Am J Clin Nutr. 2004;79(6):1078–87.
41. Löf M, Olausson H, Bostrom K, Janerot-Sjöberg B, Sohlstrom A, Forsum E. Changes in basal metabolic rate during pregnancy in relation to changes in body weight and composition, cardiac output, insulin-like growth factor I, and thyroid hormones in relation to fetal growth. Am J Clin Nutr. 2005;81(3):678–85.
42. Prentice AM, Spaaij CJ, Goldberg GR, Poppitt SD, Van Raaij JM, Totton M, Swann D, Black AE. Energy requirements of pregnant and lactating women. Eur J Clin Nutr. 1996;50(1):82–111.
43. Okereke NC, Huston-Presley L, Saeid BA, Kalhan S, Patrick MC. Longitudinal changes in energy expenditure and body composition in obese women with normal and impaired glucose tolerance. Am J Physiol Endocrinol Metab. 2004;287(3):E472–9.
44. Kopp-Hoolihan LE, Van Loan MD, Wong WW, King JC. Longitudinal assessment of energy balance in well-nourished, pregnant women. Am J Clin Nutr. 1999;69(4):697–704.
45. IOM (Institute of Medicine) and NRC (National Res earch Council) editor. Weight gain during pregnancy: reexamining the guidelines. Rasmussen KM, Yaktine AL. editors. Washington, DC: The National Academic Press; 2009.
46. Bronstein MN, Mak RP, King JC. The thermic effect of food in normal-weight and overweight pregnant women. Brit J Nutr. 1995;74(2):261–75.
47. Nagy LE, King JC. Postprandial energy expenditure and respiratory quotient during early and late pregnancy. Am J Clin Nutr. 1984;40(6):1258–63.
48. Piers LS, Diggavi SN, Thangam S, Van Raaij JM, Shetty PS, Hautvast JG. Changes in energy expenditure, anthropometry, and energy intake during the course of pregnancy and lactation in well-nourished Indian women. Am J Clin Nutr. 1995;61(3):501–13.
49. Spaaij CJ, Van Raaij JN, Van der Heijden LJ, Schouten FJ, Drijvers JJ, De Groot LC, et al. No substantial reduction of the thermic effect of a metal during pregnancy in well-nourished Dutch women. Brit J Nutr. 1994;71(1):335–44.
50. Contaldo F, Scalfi L, Coltorti A, Palo MR D, Martinelli P, Guerritore T. Reduced regulatory thermogenesis in pregnant and ovariectomized women. Int J Vitam Nutr Res. 1987;57(3):299–304.
51. Illingworth PJ, Jung RT, Howie PW, Isles TE. Reduction in postprandial energy expenditure during pregnancy. BMJ (Res C editor). 1987;294(6587):1573–7.
52. Clarke PE, Rousham EK, Gross H, Halligan AW, Bosio P. Activity patterns and time allocation during pregnancy: a longitudinal study of British women. Ann Hum Biol. 2005;32(3):247–59.
53. Lawrence M, Whitehead RG. Physical activity and total energy expenditure of child-bearing Gambian village women. Eur J Clin Nutr. 1988;42(2):145–60.
54. Löf M, Forsum E. Activity patterns and energy expenditure due to physical activity before and during pregnancy in healthy Swedish women. Brit J Nutr. 2006;95(2):296–302.
55. Rousham EK, Clarke PE, Gross H. Significant changes in physical activity among pregnant women in the UK as assessed by accelerometry and self-reported activity. Eur J Clin Nutr. 2006;60(3): 393–400.
56. Forsum E, Kabir N, Sadurkis A, Weterterp K. Total energy expenditure of healthy Swedish women during pregnancy and lactation. Am J Clin Nutr. 1992;56(2):334–42.
57. Heini A, Scuhtz Y, Diaz E, Prentice AM, Whitehead RG, Jequier E. Free-living energy expenditure measured by two independent techniques in pregnant and nonpregnant Gambian women. Am J Physiol. 1994;261(1 Pt 1):E9–17.
58. Lawrence M, Singh J, Lawrence F, Whitehead RG. The energy cost of common daily activities in African women: increased expenditure in pregnancy? Am J Clin Nutr. 1985;42(5):753–63.
59. Singh J, Prentice AM, Diaz E, Coward WA, Ashford J, Sawyer M. Energy expenditure of Gambian women during peak agricultural activity measured by the doubly-labelled water method. Brit J Nutr. 1989;62(2):315–29.
60. Van Raaij JM, Vermaat-Miedema SH, Schonk CM, Peek ME, Hautvast JG. Energy requirements of pregnancy in the Netherlands. Lancet. 1987;2(8565): 953–5.
61. Durnin JV, McKillop FM, Grant S, Fitzgerald G. Energy requirements of pregnancy in Scotland. Lancet. 1987;2(8564):897–900.
62. Moss SJ, Van Oort AF, De Boer MR, Schutz Y. Objectively determined activity energy expenditure during pregnancy and changes in body mass: the HAPPY-study. Oral presentation at the 22nd European College of Sport Science Conference; 2014 Jul 2–5; Amsterdam, The Netherlands.
63. Shephard RJ. Limits to the measurement of habitual physical activity by questionnaires. Brit J Sport Med. 2003;37(3):197–206.
64. Ainsworth BE, Haskell WL, Whitt MC, Irwin ML, Swartz AM, Strath SJ, et al. Compendium of physical activities: an update of activity codes and MET intensities. Med Sci Sport Exerc. 2000;32(9): 498–504.
65. Ainsworth BE, Richardson M, Jacobs DR, Leon AS. Gender differences in physical activity. Women Sport Phys Activ J. 1993;2(1):1–17.
66. Poudevigne MS, O'Conner PJ. A review of physical activity patterns in pregnant women and their relationship to psychological health. Sport Med. 2006;36(1):19–38.
67. Ainslie PN, Reilly T, Westerterp KR. Estimating human energy expenditure; a review of techniques with particular reference to doubly labelled water. Sport Med. 2003;33(9):683–98.

68. Speakman JR. The history and theory of the doubly labelled water technique. Am J Clin Nutr. 1998;68(4):932–8.
69. Herrmann SD, Heumann KJ, Der Ananian CA, Ainsworth BE. Validity and reliability of the global physical activity questionnaire (GPAQ). Meas Phys Educ Exerc Sci. 2013;17(3):221–35.
70. Bauman AE, Sallis JF. Global problems require global studies. Am J Prev Med. 2008;34(6):544–5.
71. Guthold R, Ono T, Strong KL, Chatterji S, Morabia A. Worldwide variability in physical inactivity: a 51-country survey. Am J Prev Med. 2008;34(6): 486–94.
72. Armstrong T, Bull F. Development of the World Health Organization Global Physical Activity Questionnaire (GPAQ). J Public Health. 2006;14(2): 66–70.
73. Aittasalo M, Pasanen M, Fogelholm M, Ojala K. Validity and repeatability of a short pregnancy leisure time physical activity questionnaire. J Phys Activ Health. 2010;7(1):109–18.
74. Chasan-Taber L, Schmidt MD, Roberts DE, Hosmer D, Markenson G, Freedson PS. Development and validation of a pregnancy physical activity questionnaire. Med Sci Sport Exerc. 2004;36(10):1750–60.
75. Evenson KR, Wen F. Measuring physical activity among pregnant women using a structured one-week recall questionnaire: evidence for validity and reliability. Int J Behav Nutr Phys Activ. 2010;7(21): 1–12.
76. Schmidt MD, Freedson PS, Pekow P, Roberts D, Sternfeld B, Chasan-Taber L. Validation of the Kaiser physical activity survey in pregnant women. Med Sci Sport Exerc. 2006;38(1):42–50.
77. Cohen TR, Plourde H, Koski KG. Use of the pregnancy physical activity questionnaire (PPAQ) to identify behaviors associated with appropriate gestational weight gain during pregnancy. J Phys Activ Health. 2013;10(7):1000–7.
78. Stein AD, Rivera JM, Pivarnik JM. Measuring energy expenditure in habitually active and sedentary pregnant women. Med Sci Sport Exerc. 2003;27(5): 634–40.
79. Perkins CC, Pivarnik JM, Paneth N, Stein AD. Physical activity and fetal growth during pregnancy. Obstet Gynecol. 2007;109(1):81–7.
80. Barreira TV, Kang M, Caputo JL, Farley RS, Renfrow MS. Validation of the Actiheart monitor for the measurement of physical activity. Int J Exerc Sci. 2009;2(2):60–71.
81. Eston RG, Rowlands AV, Ingledew DK. Validity of heart rate, pedometry, and accelerometry for predicting the energy cost of children's activities. J App Physiol. 1998;84(1):362–71.
82. Janz KF. Use of heart rate monitors to assess physical activity. In: Welk GJ, editor. Physical activity assessments for health-related research. 1st ed. United States: Human Kinetics; 2002. pp. 143–61.
83. Strath SJ, Swartz AM, Basset DR, O'Brien WL, King GA, Ainsworth BE. Evaluation of heart rate as a method for assessing moderate intensity physical activity. Med Sci Sport Exerc. 2000;32(9):465–70.
84. Freedson PS, Miller K. Objective monitoring of physical activity using motion sensors and heart rate. Res Quart Exerc Sport. 2000;71(2):21–9.
85. Welk GJ. Use of accelerometry-based activity monitors to assess physical activity. In: Welk GJ, editor. Physical activity assessments for health-related research. 1st ed. United States: Human Kinetics; 2002. pp. 125–40.
86. Corder K, Brage C, Mattocks C, Ness A, Riddoch C, Wareham NJ, Ekelund U. Comparison of two methods to assess PAEE during six activities in children. Med Sci Sports Exerc. 2007;39(12):2180–8.
87. Sallis JF, Saelens BE. Assessment of physical activity by self-report: status, limitations, and future directions. Res Quart Exercise Sport. 2000;71(2):1–7.
88. Strath SJ, Bassett DR, Thompson DL, Swarts AM. Validity of the simultaneous heart rate-motion sensor technique for measuring energy expenditure. Med Sci Sport Exerc. 2002;34(5):888–94.
89. Treuth MS. Applying multiple methods to improve the accuracy of activity assessments. In: Welk GJ, editor. Physical activity assessments for health-related research. 1st ed. United States: Human Kinetics; 2002. pp. 213–24.
90. Spierer DK, Hagins M, Rundle A, Pappas E. A comparison of energy expenditure estimates from the Actiheart and Actical physical activity monitors during low intensity activities, walking and jogging. Eur J App Physiol. 2011;111(4):659–68.
91. Brage S, Brage N, Franks PW, Ekelund U, Wareham NJ. Reliability and validity of the combined heart rate and movement sensor Actiheart. Eur J Clin Nutr. 2005;59(4):561–70.
92. Brage S, Brage N, Ekelund U, Franks PW, Wareham NJ. Effect of combined movement and heart rate monitor placement on physical activity estimates during treadmill locomotion and free-living. Euro J Appl Phys. 2006;96(5):517–24.
93. Campbell N, Prapavessis H, Gray C, McGowan E, Rush E, Maddison R. The Actiheart in adolescents: a doubly labelled water validation. Pediatr Exerc Sci. 2012;24(4):589–602.
94. Horns JF, Ratcliffe LP, Leggett JC, Swanson MS. Pregnancy outcomes among active and sedentary primiparous women. J Obstet Gynaecol Neonat Nurs. 1996;25(1):49–54.
95. Cioffi J, Schmied V, Dahlen H, Mills A, Thornton C, Duff M, et al. Physical activity in pregnancy: women's perceptions, practices, and influencing factors. J Midwifery Women Health. 2010;55(5):455–61.
96. Duncombe D, Wertheim EH, Skouteris H, Paxton SJ, Kelly L. Factors related to exercise over the course of pregnancy including women's beliefs about the safety of exercise during pregnancy. Midwifery. 2007;25(4):430–8.
97. Hinton PS, Olson CM. Predictors of pregnancy-associated change in physical activity in a rural white population. Matern Child Health J. 2001;5(1):7–14.
98. Agarwal S, Agarwal A, Agarwal KN, Agarwal DK, Bansal A. Physical activity and pregnancy outcome in rural undernourished women. Indian Pediatr. 2001;38:1017–22.

99. Bungum TJ, Peaslee DL, Jackson AW, Perez MA. Exercise during pregnancy and type of delivery in nulliparae. J Obstet Gynecol Neonat Nurs. 2000;29(3):258–64.
100. Hegaard HK, Damm P, Hedegaard M, Henriksen TB, Ottesen B, Dykes A, et al. Sports and leisure time physical activity during pregnancy in nulliparous women. Matern Child Health J. 2011;15(6):806–13.
101. Mottola MF, Campbell MK. Activity patterns during pregnancy. Can J App Physiol. 2003;28(4): 642–53.
102. Pereira MA, Rifas-Shiman SL, Kleinman KP, Rich-Edwards JW, Peterson KE, Gillman MW. Predictors of change in physical activity during and after pregnancy. Am J Prev Med. 2007;32(4):312–9.
103. Albright C, Maddock JE, Nigg CR. Physical activity before pregnancy and following childbirth in a multiethnic sample of healthy women in Hawaii. Women Health. 2005;42(3):95–110.
104. Evenson KR, Savits DA, Huston SL. Leisure-time physical activity among pregnant women in the U.S. Paediatr Perinat Epidemiol. 2004;18(6):400–7.
105. Costa D D, Rippen N, Dritsa M, Ring A. Self-reported leisure-time physical activity during pregnancy and relationship to psychological well-being. J Psychosom Obstet Gynaecol. 2003;24(2):111–9.
106. Hatch MC, Ji BT, Shu XO, Susser M. Does standing, lifting, climbing or long hours of working during pregnancy have an effect during fetal growth? Epidemiol. 1997;8(5):530–6.
107. Ning Y, Williams MA, Dempsey JC, Sorensen TK, Frederick IO, Luthy DA. Correlates of recreational physical activity in early pregnancy. J Matern Fetal Neonatal Med. 2003;13(6):385–93.
108. Zhang J, Savits DA. Exercise during pregnancy among US women. Ann Epidemiol. 1996;6(1): 53–9.
109. Domingues MR, Barros AJ. Leisure-time physical activity during pregnancy in the 2004 Pelotas Birth Cohort Study. Rev Saude Publ. 2007;41(2):173–80.
110. Barnes DL, Adair LS, Popkin BM. Women's physical activity and pregnancy outcome: a longitudinal analysis from the Philippines. Int J Epidemiol. 1991;20(1):162–72.
111. Lui J, Blair SN, Teng Y, Ness AR, Lawlor DA, Riddoch C. Physical activity during pregnancy in a prospective cohort of British women: results from the Avon longitudinal study of parents and children. Eur J Epidemiol. 2010;26(3):237–47.
112. Brunette EL, Kotze J, Wood PS, Du Toit PJ, Grant CC. An epidemiological study of physical activity patterns and weight gain in physically active and sedentary pregnant women in Tshwane, South Africa. Afr J Phys Health Educ Recr Dance. 2012;18(1):132–43.
113. Dempsey JC, Sorensen TK, Williams MA, Lee IM, Miller RS, Dashow EE, et al. Prospective study of gestational diabetes mellitus risk in relation to maternal recreational physical activity before and during pregnancy. Am J Epidemiol. 2004;159(7):663–70.
114. Juhl M, Anderson PK, Olsen J, Madsen M, Jørgensen T, Nøhr EA, et al. Physical exercise during pregnancy and the risk of preterm birth: a study within the Danish National Birth Cohort. Am J Epidemiol. 2008;167(7):63e1–8.
115. Sørenson TK, Williams MA, Lee IM, Dashow EE, Thompson ML, Luthy DA. Recreational physical activity during pregnancy and risk of preeclampsia. Hypertension. 2003;41(6):1273–80.
116. Goldenberg RL, Cliver SP, Bronstein J, Cutter GR, Andrews WW, Mennemeyer ST. Bed rest in pregnancy. Obstet Gynecol. 1994;84(1):131–6.
117. Crowther CA, Han S. Hospitalisation and bed rest for multiple pregnancy. Cochrane Database Syst Rev. 2010;7:CD000110. doi:10.1002/14651858.CD000110.pub2.
118. Biolo G, Heer M, Nirici M, Strollo F. Microgravity as a model of ageing. Curr Opin Clin Nutr Metab Care. 2003;6(1):31–40.
119. Borodulin K, Evenson KR, Herring AH. Physical activity patterns during pregnancy through postpartum. BMC Women Health. 2009;19(9):32–9.
120. Szumilewicz A, Wojtyla A, Zarębska A, Drobnik-Kozakiewicz I, Sawczyn M, Kwitneiwska A. Influence of prenatal physical activity on the course of labour and delivery according to the new Polish standard for perinatal care. Ann Agric Environ Med. 2013;20(2):380–9.
121. Aaron DL, Jekal YS, LaPorte RE. Epidemiology of physical activity from adolescence to young adulthood. Word Rev Nutr Diet. 2005;94:36–41.
122. Wahlqvist ML. Physical activity for health: an overview. Word Rev Nutr Diet. 2005;95:62–72.
123. Helmrich SP, Ragland DR, Leung RW, Paffenbarger RS. Physical activity and reduced occurrence of non-insulin-dependent diabetes mellitus. N Engl J Med. 1991;325(3):147–52.
124. Kushi L, Fee R, Folsom AR, Mink PJ, Anderson KE, Sellers TA. Physical activity and mortality in postmenopausal women. J Am Med Assoc. 1989;277(16):1287–92.
125. Sandvik L, Erikssen J, Thaulow E, Erikssen G, Mundal R, Rodahl K. Physical fitness as a predictor of mortality among healthy, middle-aged Norwegian men. N Engl J Med. 1993;328(8):533–7.
126. Hu G, Jousilahti P, Barengo NC, Qiao Q, Lakka TA, Tuomilehto J. Physical activity, cardiovascular risk factors, and mortality among Finnish adults with diabetes. Diabetes Care. 2005;28(4):799–805.
127. Lee CD, Blair SN, Jackson AS. Cardiorespiratory fitness, body composition, and all-cause and cardiovascular disease mortality in men. Am J Clin Nutr. 1999;69(3):373–80.
128. Paisley TS, Joy EA, Price RJ. Exercise during pregnancy: a practical approach. Curr Sport Med Rep. 2003;2(6):325–30.
129. Burchfiel CM, Sharp DS, Curb JD, Rodriguez BL, Hwang LJ, Marcus B. Physical activity and incidence of diabetes: the Honolulu heart program. Am J Epidemiol. 1995;141(4):360–8.

130. Sigal JR, Kenny GP, Wasserman DH, Castaneda-Sceppa C, White RD. Physical activity/exercise and type 2 diabetes: a consensus statement from the American Diabetes Association. Diabetes Care. 2006;29(6):1433–8.
131. Ellekjær H, Holmen J, Ellekjaer E, Vatten L. Physical activity and stroke mortality in women: ten-year follow-up of the Nord-Trøndelag health survey, 1984–1986. Stroke. 2000;31(1):14–8.
132. Laaksonen DE, Lakka HM, Lynch J, Lakka TA, Kishanen L, Rauramaa R, et al. Cardiorespiratory fitness and vigorous leisure-time physical activity modify the association of small size at birth with the metabolic syndrome. Diabetes Care. 2003;26(7):2156–64.
133. Warburton DE, Nicol CW, Bredin SS. Health benefits of physical activity: the evidence. Can Med Assoc J. 2006;174(7):801–9.
134. Clapp JF. The course of labor after endurance exercise during pregnancy. Am J Obstet Gynecol. 1990;163(6):1799–805.
135. Sternfeld B. Physical activity and pregnancy outcome: review and recommendations. Sport Med. 1997;23(1):33–47.
136. Wolfe LA, Hall P, Webb KA, Goodman L, Monga M, McGrath MJ. Prescription of aerobic exercise during pregnancy. Sport Med. 1989;8(5):273–301.
137. Arena B, Maffulli N. Exercise in pregnancy: how safe is it? Sport Med Arthroscop Rev. 2002;10(1):15–22.
138. Wallace AM, Boyer DB, Dan A, Hol, Aerobic exercise K. Maternal self-esteem, and physical discomforts during pregnancy. J Nurs-Midwifery. 1986;31(6):255–62.
139. Bung P, Artal R, Khodiguian N, Kjos S. Exercise in gestational diabetes: an optional therapeutic approach? Diabetes. 1991;40(2):182–5.
140. Bung P, Artal R. Gestational diabetes and exercise: a survey. Semin Perinatol. 1996;20(4):328–33.
141. Borg-Stein J, Dugan SA, Gruber J. Musculoskeletal aspects of pregnancy. Am J Phys Med Rehab. 2005;84(3):180–92.
142. Hutchinson SL. Physical activity, recreation, leisure, and sport: essential pieces of the mental health and well-being puzzle [Internet]. Halifax: Recreation Nova Scotia; 2012 [cited 2012 July 6]. http://www.recreationns.ns.ca/wp-content/uploadhere/2012/05/MentalHealthLit.pdf.
143. Adams TB, Moore MT, Dye J. The relationship between physical activity and mental health in a national sample of college females. Women Health. 2007;45(1):69–85.
144. Clapp JF, Rockey R, Treadway JL, Carpenter MW, Artal RM, Warrnes C. Exercise in pregnancy: a short review. Med Sci Sports Exerc. 1992;24(6):294–300.
145. Kritz-Silverstein D, Barrett-Conner E, Corbeau C. Cross-sectional and prospective study of exercise and depressed mood in the elderly. Am J Epidemiol. 2001;153(6):596–603.
146. Strawbridge WJ, Deleger S, Roberts R, Kaplan GA. Physical activity reduces the risk of subsequent depression for older adults. Am J Epidemiol. 2002;156(4):328–34.
147. Yang X, Telama R, Hirvensalo M, Hintsanen M, Heintsa T, Pulkki-Raback, et al. The benefits of sustained leisure-time physical activity on job strain. Occ Med. 2010;60(5):369–75.
148. Poudevigne MS, O'Conner PJ. Physical activity and mood during pregnancy. Med Sci Sport Exerc. 2005;37(8):1374–80.
149. Mottola MF. Exercise in the postpartum period: practical applications. Curr Sport Med Rep. 2002;1(6):362–8.
150. Carey GB, Quinn TJ. Exercise and lactation: are they compatible? Can J App Physiol. 2001;26(1):44–74.
151. Kalisiak B, Spitznagle T. What effect does an exercise program for healthy pregnant women have on the mother, fetus, and child? Am Acad Phys Med Rehab. 2009;1(3):261–7.
152. Domenjoz I, Kayser B, Boulvain M. Effect of physical activity during pregnancy on mode of delivery. Am J Obstet Gynecol. 2014; 21(4):401.e1–11.
153. Clapp JF. Exercise during pregnancy: a clinical update. Clin Sports Med. 2000;19(2):273–86.
154. Shangold MM. Exercise during pregnancy: current state of the art. Can Fam Physician. 1989;35:1675–80.
155. Van Oort AF. The relationship between habitual physical activity patterns of pregnant women and foetal growth parameters: a longitudinal observational study [dissertation]. Potchefstroom: North-West University; 2014.
156. Luke B, Papiernik E. The effects of lifestyle on prematurity. In: Elder MG, Lamont RF, Romero R, editors. Preterm labor. New York: Churchill Livingstone; 1997. pp. 127–52.
157. Mozurkewich EL, Luke B, Avni M, Fredric MW. Working conditions and adverse pregnancy outcome: a meta-analysis. Obstet Gynecol. 2000;95(4):623–35.
158. Edwards MJ. Hyperthermia as a teratogen: a review of experimental studies and their clinical significance. Teratog Carcinog Mutagen. 1986;6(6):563–82.
159. Milunsky A, Ulcickas M, Rothman KJ, Willett W, Jick SS, Jick H. Maternal heat exposure and neural tube defects. J Am Med Assoc. 1992;268(7):882–5.
160. Stevenson L. Exercise in pregnancy: part 2: recommendations for individuals. Can Fam Physician. 1997;(43):107–111.
161. Takito MY, Benício MH, Neri LC. Physical activity by pregnant women and outcomes for newborns: a systematic review. Revis Saúd Públic. 2009;43(6):1059–69.
162. Clapp JF, Little KD. The interaction between regular exercise and selected aspects of women's health. Am J Obstet Gynecol. 1995;173(1):2–9.
163. Clapp JF. The effects of maternal exercise on early pregnancy outcome. Am J Obstet Gynecol. 1989;161(6):1453–7.

164. Clapp JF, Lopez B, Harcar-Swvcik R. Neonatal behavioural profile of the offspring of women who continued to exercise regularly throughout pregnancy. Am J Obstet Gynecol. 1999;180(1):91–4.
165. Clapp JF, Simonian S, Lopez B, Appleby-Wineberg S, Harcar-Sevcik R. The one-year morphometric and neurodevelopmental outcome of the offspring of women who continued to exercise regularly throughout pregnancy. Am J Obstet Gynecol. 1998;178(3):594–9.
166. Hall DC, Kaufmann DA. Effects of aerobic and strength conditioning on pregnancy outcomes. Am J Obstet Gynecol. 1987;157(5):1199–203.
167. Hatch MC, Shu XO, Mclean DE, Levin B, Begg M, Reuss L, et al. Maternal exercise during pregnancy, physical fitness, and fetal growth. Am J Epidemiol. 1993;137(10):1105–14.
168. Kardel KR, Kase T. Training in pregnant women: effects on fetal development and birth. Am J Obstet Gynecol. 1998;178(2):280–6.
169. Klebanoff MA, Shiono PH, Carey JC. The effect of physical activity during pregnancy on preterm delivery and birth weight. Am J Obstet Gynecol. 1990;163(5 Pt 1):1450–6.
170. Kulpa PJ, White BM, Visscher R. Aerobic exercise in pregnancy. Am J Obstet Gynecol. 1987;156(6):1395–403.
171. O'Neill ME. Maternal rectal temperature and fetal heart rate responses to upright cycling in late pregnancy. Brit J Sport Med. 1996;30(1):32–5.
172. Sternfeld B, Quesenberry CP, Eskenazi B, Newman LA. Exercise during pregnancy and pregnancy outcome. Med Sci Sport Exerc. 1995;27(5):634–40.
173. Magann EF, Evans SF, Weitz B, Newnham J. Antepartum, intrapartum, and neonatal significance of exercise on healthy low-risk pregnant working women. Obstet Gynecol. 2002;99(3):466–72.
174. Rao S, Kanade A, Margetts BM, Yajnik CS, Lubree H, Rege S, et al. Maternal activity in relation to birth size in rural India: the Pune Maternal Nutrition Study. Eur J Clin Nutr. 2003;57(4):531–42.
175. Campbell MK, Mottola MF. Recreational exercise and occupational activity during pregnancy and birth weight: a case-control study. Am J Obstet Gynecol. 2001;184(3):403–8.
176. Magann EF, Evans SF, Newnham JP. Employment, exertion, and pregnancy outcome: assessment by kilocalories expended each day. Am J Obstet Gynecol. 1996;175(1):182–7.
177. Wolfe LA, Mottola MF. Validation of guidelines for aerobic exercise in pregnancy. In: Kumbhare DA, Basmajian JV, editors. Decision making and outcomes in sport rehabilitation. New York: Churchill Livingstone; 2000. pp. 205–22.
178. Bell RJ. The effect of vigorous exercise during pregnancy on birth weight. J Sci Med Sport. 2002;5(1):32–6.
179. Derbyshire E, Davies GJ, Costarelli V, Dettmar PW. Habitual patterns of physical activity during pregnancy and postnatally. Matern Health. 2008;16(1):20–4.
180. Riemann MK, Kanstrup Hansen IL. Effects on the foetus of exercise in pregnancy. Scand J Med Sci Sport. 2000;10(1):12–9.
181. Artal R. Exercise and pregnancy. Clin Sport Med. 1992;11(2):363–77.
182. Bell RJ, O'Neill M. Exercise and pregnancy: a review. Birth. 1994;21(2):85–9.
183. Dewey KG, McCrory MA. Effects of dieting and physical activity on pregnancy and lactation. Am J Clin Nutr. 1994;59(2S):446-53.
184. Jarski RW, Tripett DL. The risks and benefits of exercise during pregnancy. J Fam Prac. 1990;30(2):185–9.
185. Lokey EA, Tran ZV, Wells CL, Meyers BC, Tran AC. Effects of physical exercise on pregnancy outcomes: a meta-analytic review. Med Sci Sport Exerc. 1991;23(11):1234–9.
186. Schick-Boschetto B, Rose NC. Exercise in pregnancy. Obstet Gynecol Sur. 1991;47(1):10–3.
187. Snyder JL. Aerobic exercise during pregnancy. J Am Board Fam Prac. 1990;3(1):50–3.
188. Clapp JF. Exercise and fetal health. J Develop Physiol. 1991;15(1):9–14.
189. Hutch R, Erkkola R. Pregnancy and exercise-exercise and pregnancy. A short review. Brit J Obstet Gynaecol. 1990;97(3):208–14.
190. McMurray RG, Mottola MF, Wolfe LA, Artal R, Millar L, Pivarnik JM. Recent advances in understanding maternal and fetal responses to exercise. Med Sci Sport Exerc. 1993;25(12):1305–21.
191. Revelli A, Durandom A, Massobrio M. Exercise and pregnancy: a review of maternal and fetal effects. Obstet Gynecol Sur. 1992;47(6):355–67.
192. Warren MP. Exercise in women: effects on reproductive system and pregnancy. Clin Sport Med. 1991;10(1):131–9.
193. Alderman BW, Zhao H, Holt VL, Watts DH, Beresford AA. Maternal physical activity in pregnancy and infant size for gestational age. Ann Epidemiol. 1998;8(8):513–9.
194. Bell RJ, Palma S. Antenatal exercise and birth weight. Aus N Z J Obstet Gynaecol. 2000;40(1):70–3.
195. Clapp JF, Kim H, Burciu B, Lopez B. Beginning regular exercise in early pregnancy: effect on fetoplacental growth. Am J Obstet Gynecol. 2000;183(6):1484–8.
196. Clapp JF, Kim H, Burciu B, Schmidt S, Petry K, Lopez B. Continuing regular exercise during pregnancy: effect of exercise volume on fetoplacental growth. Am J Obstet Gynecol. 2002;186(1):142–7.
197. Haakstad LAH, Bø K. Exercise in pregnant women and birth weight: a randomized controlled trial. BMC Pregnancy Childbirth. 2011;(11):66–73.
198. Marquez-Sterling S, Perry AC, Kaplan TA, Halberstein RA, Signorile JF. Physical and psychological changes with vigorous exercise in sedentary primigravidae. Med Sci Sport Exerc. 2000;32(1):58–62.
199. Prevedel T, Calderon I, Abadde J, Borges V, Rudge M. Maternal and perinatal effects of hydrotherapy in pregnancy. Rev Brasil Ginecol Obstet. 2003;25(1):53–9.

200. Price BB, Amini SB, Kappeler K. Exercise in pregnancy: effect on fitness and obstetric outcomes—a randomized trial. Med Sci Sport Exerc. 2012;44(12):2263–70.
201. Macera CA, Ham SA, Yore MM, Jones DA, Ainsworth BE, Kimsey CD, et al. Prevalence of physical activity in the United States: behavioral risk factor surveillance system. Prev Chron Dis. 2001;2(2):A17.
202. Hall MH, Chng PK, MacGillivray I. Is routine antenatal care worthwhile? Lancet. 1980;2(8185):78–80.
203. Juhl M, Olsen J, Anderson PK, Nøhr EA, Anderson AN. physical exercise during pregnancy and fetal growth measures: a study within the Danish National Birth Cohort. Am J Obstet Gynecol. 2010;202(1):1e1–8.
204. Barker DJP, Osmond C, Simmonds SJ, Wield GA. The relation of small head circumference and thinness at birth to death from cardiovascular diseases in adult life. BMJ. 1993;306(6875):422–6.
205. Oken E, Gillman MW. Fetal origins of obesity. Obes Res. 2003;11(4):496–506.
206. Martin JA, Hamilton BE, Sutton PD, Ventura SJ, Menacker F, Munson ML. Births: final data for 2003. Nat Vital Stat Rep. 2005;54(2):1–116.
207. Massett HA, Greenup M, Ryan CE, Staples DA, Green NS, Maibach EW. Public perceptions about prematurity: a national survey. Am J Prev Med. 2003;24(2):120–7.
208. Gardosi J, Mul T, Mongelli M, Fagan D. Analysis of birthweight and gestational age in antepartum stillbirths. Brit J Obstet Gynaecol. 1998;105(5):524–30.
209. Lobos H, Rennie JM, Lees C. The natural history of fetal growth restriction in women with abnormal uterine artery Doppler. Prenat Diag. 2005;25(4):331–2.
210. Breeze ACG, Lees CC. Prediction and perinatal outcomes of fetal growth restriction. Semin Fetal Neonat Med. 2007;12(5):383–97.
211. Vielwerth SE, Jensen RB, Larsen T, Greisen G. The impact of maternal smoking on fetal and infant growth. Early Hum Dev. 2007;83(8):491–5.
212. Lucas A. Programming by early nutrition in man. In: Bock GR, Whelan J, editors. The childhood environment and adult disease. Chichester: Wiley; 1991. pp. 38–50.
213. Lucas A. Role of nutritional programming in determining adult morbidity. Arch Dis Child. 1994;71(4):288–90.
214. Ekbom A, Hsieh CC, Lipworth L, Wolk A, Pontén J, Adami HO, et al. Perinatal characteristics in relation to incidence of and mortality from prostate cancer. BMJ (Res C editor). 1996;313(7053):337–41.
215. Innes K, Byers T, Schymura M. Birth characteristics and subsequent risk for breast cancer in very young women. Am J Epidemiol. 2000;152(12):1121–8.
216. Karter AJ, Rowell SE, Ackerman LM, Mitchell BD, Ferrara A, Selby JV, et al. Excess maternal transmission of type 2 diabetes. Diabetes Care. 1999;22(6):938–43.
217. Shaheen SO, Sterne JA, Montgomery SM, Azima H. Birth weight, body mass index and asthma in young adults. Thorax. 1999;54(5):396–402.
218. Barker DJP. Fetal origins of coronary heart disease. BMJ. 1995;311(6998):171–4.
219. Barker DJP, Osmond C, Golding J, Kuh D, Wadsworth MEJ. Growth in utero, blood pressure in childhood and adult life, and mortality from cardiovascular disease. BMJ. 1989;298(6673):564–7.
220. Barker DJP, Winter PD, Osmond C, Margetts B. Weight in infancy and death from ischemic heart disease. Lancet. 1989;2(8663):577–80.
221. Gupta R, Gupta VP. Meta-analysis of coronary heart disease in India. Indian Heart J. 1996;48(3):241–5.
222. Hales CN, Barker DJP, Clark PMS, Cox LJ, Fall CHD, Osmond C, et al. Fetal and infant growth and impaired glucose tolerance at age 64. BMJ. 1991;303(6809):1019–22.
223. Law CM, Shiell AW. Is blood pressure inversely related to birth-weight? The strength of evidence from a systematic review of the literature. J Hypertension. 1996;14(8):935–41.
224. Mckeigue PM, Shah B, Marmot MG. Relation of central obesity and insulin resistance with high diabetes prevalence and cardiovascular risk in South Asia. Lancet. 1991;377(8738):330–6.
225. Stien CE, Fall CHD, Kumaran K, Osmond C, Cox V, Barker DJP. Fetal growth and coronary heart disease in South India. Lancet. 1996;348(9037):1269–73.
226. Yajnik CS, Fall CHD, Vaidya U, Pandit AN, Bavdekar A, Bhat DS, et al. Fetal growth and glucose and insulin metabolism in four year old Indian children. Diabetic Med J Brit Diabetic Assoc. 1995;306(4):422–6.
227. Nair L, Nair MKC, Chacko DS. Markers of fetal onset adult diseases. Indian Pediatr. 2009;46:S48–54.
228. Rich-Edwards JW, Colditz GA, Stampfer MJ, Manson JE, Rosner B, Hankinson SE, et al. Birth-weight and the risk for type 2 diabetes mellitus in adult women. Ann Int Med. 1999;130(4 Pt 1):278–84.
229. Hediger ML, Overpeck MD, Kuczmarski RJ, McGlynn A, Maurer KR, Davis WW. Muscularity and fatness of infants and young children born small- or large-for-gestational-age. Pediatrics. 1998;102(5):E60–7.
230. Hammami M, Walters JC, Hockman EM, Koo WW. Disproportionate alterations in body composition of large for gestational age neonates. J Pediatr. 2001;138(6):817–21.
231. Vaessen N, Janssen JA, Heutink P, Hofman A, Lamberts SWJ, Oostra BA, et al. Association between genetic variation in the gene for insulin-like growth factor-I and low birthweight. Lancet. 2002;359(9311):1036–7.
232. Bobak M. Outdoor air pollution, low birth weight, and prematurity. Environ Health Perspect. 2000;108(2):173–6.
233. Dejmek J, Selevan SG, Benes I, Solansky I, Sram RJ. Fetal growth and maternal exposure to particulate matter during pregnancy. Environ Health Perspect. 1999;107(6):475–80.

234. Ha EH, Hong YC, Lee BE, Woo BH, Schwartz J, Christiani DC. Is air pollution a risk factor for low birth weight in Seoul? Epidemiology. 2001;12(6):643–8.
235. Maisonet M, Bush TJ, Correa A, Jaakkola JK. Relation between ambient air pollution and low birth weight in the northeastern United States. Environ Health Perspect. 2001;109(3):351–6.
236. Ritz B, Yu F. The effect of ambient carbon monoxide on low birth weight among children born in Southern California between 1989 and 1993. Environ Health Perspect. 1999;107(1):17–25.
237. Ritz B, Yu F, Chapa G, Fruin S. Effect of air pollution on preterm birth among children born in Southern California between 1989 and 1993. Epidemiol. 2000;11(5):502–11.
238. Wang X, Ding H, Ryan L, Xu X. Association between air pollution and low birth weight: a community-based study. Environ Health Persp. 1997;105(5):514–20.
239. Xu X, Ding H, Wang X. Acute effects of total suspended articles and sulphur dioxides on preterm delivery: a community-based cohort study. Arch Environ Health. 1995;50(6):407–15.
240. Maisonet M, Correa A, Misra D, Jaakkola JJK. A review of the literature on the effects of ambient air pollution on fetal growth. Environ Res. 2004;95(1):106–15.
241. De Santis M, De Luca C, Mappa I, Quattrocchi T, Angelo L, Cesari E. Smoking, alcohol consumption and illicit drug use in an Italian population of pregnant women. Eur J Obstet Gynecol Reprod Biol. 2011;159(1):106–10.
242. Jauniaux E, Greenough A. Short and long term outcomes of smoking during pregnancy. Early Hum Dev. 2007;83(11):697–8.
243. Pollack H, Lantz PM, Frohna JG. Maternal smoking and adverse birth outcomes among singletons and twins. Am J Pub Health. 2000;90(3):395–341.
244. Samper MP, Jiménez-Muro A, Nerín I, Marqueta A, Ventura P, et al. Maternal active smoking and newborn body composition. Early Hum Dev. 2012;88(3):141–5.
245. Figueras F, Meler E, Eixarch E, Francis A, Coll O, Gratacos E, et al. Association of smoking during pregnancy and fetal growth restriction: subgroups of higher susceptibility. Eur J Obstet Gynecol Reprod Biol. 2008;138(2):171–5.
246. Barker DJP, Gluckman PD, Robinson JS. Conference report: fetal origins of adult disease-report of the first international study group. Placenta. 1995;16(3):317–20.
247. Bernstein IM, Mongeon JA, Badger GJ, Solomon L, Heil SH, Higgins ST. Maternal smoking and its association with birth weight. Obstet Gynecol. 2005;106(5):986–91.
248. Källen K. The impact of maternal smoking during pregnancy on delivery outcome. Eur J Pub Health. 2001;11(3):329–33.
249. Horta BL, Victora CG, Menezes AM, Halpern R, Barros FC. Low birth weight, preterm births and intrauterine growth retardation in relation to maternal smoking. Paediatr Perinat Epidemiol. 1997;11(2):140–51.
250. Fantuzzi G, Aggazzotti G, Righi E, Faccinetti F, Bertucci E, Kanitz S. Preterm delivery and exposure to active and passive smoking during pregnancy: a case-control study from Italy. Paediatr Perinat Epidemiol. 2007;21(3):194–200.
251. Dekeyser-Boccara J, Milliez J. Smoking and ectopic pregnancy: is there a causal relationship? J Gynecol. 2005;34(1):119–23.
252. Jauniaux E, Burton GJ. Morphological and biological effects of maternal exposure to tobacco smoke on the feto-placental unit. Early Hum Dev. 2007;83(11):699–706.
253. Cnattingius S, Lambe M. Trends in smoking and overweight during pregnancy: prevalence, risk of pregnancy complications and adverse pregnancy outcomes. Semin Perinatol. 2002;26(4):286–95.
254. Kyrklund-Blomberg NB, Genuser G, Cnattingius S. Placental abruption and perinatal death. Paediatr Perinat Epidemiol. 2001;15(3):290–7.
255. Mitchell EA, Milerad J. Smoking and the sudden infant death syndrome. Rev Environ Health. 2006;21(2):81–104.
256. Wisborg K, Kesmodel U, Henriksen TB, Olsen SF, Secher NJ. Exposure to tobacco smoke in utero and the risk of stillbirth and death in the first year of life. Am J Epidemiol. 2001;154(4):322–7.
257. Andersson K, Arner P. Systemic nicotine stimulates human adipose tissue lipolysis through local cholinergic and catecholaminergic receptors. Int J Obes Metab Dis. 2001;25(8):1225–33.
258. Bernstein IM, Horbar JD, Badger GJ, Ohlsson A, Golan B. Morbidity and mortality among very-low-birth-weight neonates with intrauterine growth restriction: the Vermont Oxford Network. Am J Obstet Gynecol. 2000;182(1):198–206.
259. Cliver SP, Goldenberg MD, Cutter GR, Hoffman HJ, Davis RO, Nelson KG. The effect of cigarette smoking on neonatal anthropometric measurements. Obstet Gynecol. 1995;85(4):625–30.
260. Reeves S, Bernstein I. Effects of maternal tobacco-smoke exposure on fetal growth and neonatal size. Expert Rev Obstet Gynecol. 2008;3(6):719–39.
261. Hernández-Martínez C, Val VA, Subías JE, Sans JC. A longitudinal study on the effects of maternal smoking and secondhand smoke exposure during pregnancy on neonatal neurobehavior. Early Hum Dev. 2012;88(6):403–8.
262. Bruchova H, Vasikova A, Merkerova M, Milcova A, Topinka J, Balascak I, et al. Effect of maternal tobacco smoke exposure on the pacental transcriptome. Placenta. 2010;31(3):186–91.
263. Zhang J, Ratcliffe JM. Paternal smoking and birthweight in Shanghai. Am J Pub Health. 1993;83(2):207–10.

264. Eskenazi B, Prehn AW, Christianson RE. Passive and active maternal smoking as measured by serum cotinine: the effect on birthweight. Am J Pub Health. 1995;85(3):395–8.
265. Hansen C, Sorensen LD, Asmussen I, Autrup H. Transplacental exposure to tobacco smoke in human-adduct formation in placenta and umbilical cord vessels. Teratog Carcinog Mutagen. 1992;12(2):51–60.
266. Jauniaux E, Gulbis B, Acharya G, Thiry P, Rodeck C. Maternal tobacco exposure and cotinine levels in fetal fluids in the first half of pregnancy. Obstet Gynecol. 1999;93(1):25–9.
267. Luck W, Nau H, Hansen R, Stelding R. Extent of nicotine and cotinine transfer to the human fetus, placenta and amniotic fluid of smoking mothers. Dev Pharmacol Therap. 1985;8(6):384–95.
268. Lichtensteiger W, Ribary U, Schiumpf M, Odermatt B, Widemer HR. Prenatal adverse effects of nicotine on the developing brain. Prog Brain Res. 1988;73:137–57.
269. Rasmussen S, Irgens LM. The effects of smoking and hypertensive disorders on fetal growth. BMC Pregnancy Childbirth. 2006;6:16–23.
270. Windham GC, Hopkins B, Fenster L, Swan SH. Prenatal active or passive tobacco smoke exposure and the risk of preterm delivery or low birth weight. Epidemiol. 2000;11(4):427–33.
271. Morley R, Leeson PC, Lister G, Lucas A. Maternal smoking and blood pressure in 7.5 to 8 year old offspring. Arch Dis Child. 1995;72(2):120–4.
272. Williams S, Poulton R. Twins and maternal smoking: ordeals for the fetal origins hypothesis: a cohort study. BMJ. 1999;318(7188):897–900.
273. Power C, Jefferis BJ. Fetal environment and subsequent obesity: a study of maternal smoking. Int J Epidemiol. 2002;31(2):413–9.
274. Maconochie N, Doyle P, Prior S, Simmons R. Risk factors for the first trimester miscarriage—results from a UK-population-based case-control study. Int J Obstet Gynaecol. 2007;1114(2):170–86.
275. Burd L, Roberts D, Olson M, Odendaal H. Ethanol and the placenta: a review. J Matern-Fetal Neonat Med. 2007;20(5):361–75.
276. Barr HM, Bookstein FL, O'Malley KD, Connor PD, Huggins JE, Streissguth AP. Binge drinking during pregnancy as a predictor of psychiatric disorders on the structured clinical interview for DSM-IV in young adult offspring. Am J Psyc. 2006;163(6):1061–5.
277. Lazzaroni F, Bonassi S, Magnani M, Calvi A, Repetto E, Serra F, et al. Moderate maternal drinking and outcome of pregnancy. Eur J Epidemiol. 1993;9(6):599–606.
278. Little RE, Wendt JK. The effects of maternal drinking in the reproductive period: an epidemiologic review. J Subst Abuse. 1991;3(2):187–204.
279. O'Leary CM, Nassar N, Kurinczuk JJ, Bower C. The effect of maternal alcohol consumption on fetal growth and preterm birth. Int J Obstet Gynaecol. 2009;116(3):390–400.
280. Warren KR, Foudin LL. Alcohol-related birth defects—the past, present, and future. Alcohol Res Health. 2001;25(3):153–8.
281. Chiriboga CA. Fetal alcohol and drug effects. Neurologist. 2003;9(6):267–79.
282. Sokol RJ, Delaney-Black V, Nordstrom B. Fetal alcohol spectrum disorder. J Am Med Assoc. 2003;290(22):2996–9.
283. Henderson J, Gray R, Brocklehurst P. Systematic review of effects of low-moderate prenatal alcohol exposure on pregnancy outcome. Int J Obstet Gynaecol. 2007;114(3):243–52.
284. Henderson J, Kesmodel U, Nordstrom B. Systematic review of the fetal effects of prenatal binge-drinking. J Epidemiol Community Health. 2007;61(12):1069–73.
285. Hayatbakhsh MR, Kingsbury AM, Flenady V, Gilshenan KS, Hutchinson DM, Najman JM. Illicit drug use before and during pregnancy at a tertiary maternity. Drug Alcohol Rev. 2010;30(2):181–7.
286. Hatch EE, Bracken MB. Effect of marihuana use in pregnancy on fetal growth. J Ethnopharmacol. 1986;20(3):986–93.
287. Fried PA, Watkinson B, Willan A. Marijuana use during pregnancy and decreased length of gestation. Am J Obstet Gynecol. 1984;150(1):23–7.
288. Hingson R, Alpert JJ, Day N, Dooling E, Kayne H, Morelock S, et al. Effects of maternal drinking and marijuana. Pediatr. 1982;70(4):539–45.
289. Zuckerman R, Frank DA, Hingson R, Amaro H, Levenson SM, Kayne H, et al. Effects of maternal marijuana and cocaine use on fetal growth. Int J Gynecol Obstet. 1989;30(3):289–90.
290. Vagero D, Koupilova I, Leon DA, Lithell UB. Social determinants of birthweight, ponderal index and gestational age in Sweden in the 1920s and the 1980s. Acta Paediatr. 1999;88(4):445–53.
291. Collins J, David R, Symons R, Handler A, Wall S, Andes S. African-American mothers' perception of their residential environment, stressful life events, and very low birthweight. Epidemiol. 1998;9(3):286–9.
292. Fang J, Madhavan S, Alderman M. Low birth weight: race and maternal nativity—impact of community income. Pediatr. 1999;103(1):1–6.
293. O'Campo P, Xu X, Wang M-C, Caughy M. Neighborhood risk factors for low birthweight in Baltimore: a multilevel analysis. Am J Pub Health. 1997;87(7):1113–8.
294. Roberts EM. Neighborhood social environments and the distribution of low birthweight in Chicago. Am J Pub Health. 1997;87(4):597–603.
295. Collins J, David R. Urban violence and African-American pregnancy outcome: an ecologic study. Ethnic Dis. 1997;7(3):184–90.
296. Copper R, Goldenberg R, Das A, Elder N, Swain M, Norman G, et al. The Preterm Prediction Study: maternal stress is associated with spontaneous preterm birth at less than thirty five weeks' gestation. Am J Obstet Gynecol. 1996;175(5):1286–92.

297. Hickey CA, Cliver SP, Mulvihill FX, McNeal SF, Hoffman HJ, Goldenberg RL. Employment-related stress and preterm delivery: a contextual examination. Pub Health Rep. 1995;110(4):410–8.
298. Hoffman S, Hatch M. Stress, social support and pregnancy outcome: a reassessment based on recent research. Paediatr Perinat Epidemiol. 1996;10(4):380–405.
299. Sandman CA, Wadhwa PD, Chicz-DeMet A, Dunkel-Schetter C, Porto M. Maternal stress, HPA activity, and fetal/infant outcome. Ann NY Acad Sci. 1997;814(1):266–75.
300. Wadhwa P, Dunkel-Schetter C, Shicz-DeMet A, Porto M, Sandman C. Prenatal psychosocial factors and the neuroendocrine axis in human pregnancy. Psychosom Med. 1996;58(5):432–46.
301. LeClere FB, Wilson JB. Smoking behaviour of recent mothers, 18–44 years of age, before and after pregnancy: United States, 1990. Adv Data. 1997;288:1–11.
302. Wakefield M, Gillies P, Graham H, Madeley R, Symonds M. Characteristics associated with smoking cessation during pregnancy among working class women. Addiction. 1993;88(10):1423–30.
303. Walsh RA. Effects of maternal smoking on adverse pregnancy outcomes: examination of the criteria of causation. Hum Biol. 1994;66(6):1059–92.
304. Hattersley AT, Tooke JE. The fetal insulin hypothesis: an alternative explanation of the association of low birthweight with diabetes and vascular disease. Lancet. 1999;353(9166):1789–92.
305. Knight B, Shields BM, Turner M, Powell RJ, Yajnik CS, Hattersley AT. Evidence of genetic regulation of fetal longitudinal growth. Early Hum Dev. 2005;81(10):823–31.
306. Tower C, Baker P. The genetics of fetal growth restriction: implications for management. Rev Gynaecol Prac. 2006;6(1–2):99–105.
307. Guillaume M, Lapidus L, Beckers F, Lambert A, Björntorp P. Familial trends of obesity through three generations. Int J Obes Relat Metab Disord. 1995;19(3):5–9.
308. Okun N, Verma A, Mitchell BF, Flowerdew G. Relative importance of maternal constitutional factors and glucose intolerance of pregnancy in the development of newborn macrosomia. J Matern-Fetal Med. 1997;6(5):285–90.
309. Magnus P, Gjessing HK, Skrondal A, Skjaerven R. Paternal contribution to birth weight. J Epidemiol Community Health. 2001;55(12):873–7.
310. Skjaerven R, Wilcox AJ, Oyen N, Magnus P. Mothers' birth weight and survival of their offspring. BMJ (Res C editor). 1997;314(7091):1376–80.
311. Preece MA, Moore GE. Genomic imprinting, uniparental disomy and foetal growth. Trends Endocrinol Metab. 2000;11(7):270–5.
312. Odent M. New reasons and new ways to study birth physiology. Int J Gynecol Obstet. 2001;75(1):39–45.
313. Bovbjerg ML, Siega-Riz AM. Exercise during pregnancy and cesarean delivery: north Carolina PRAMS, 2004–2005. Birth. 2009;36(3):200–7.
314. Chu SY, Bachman DJ, Callaghan WM, Whitlock EP, Dietz PM, Berg CJ, et al. Association between obesity during pregnancy and increased use of health care. N Engl J Med. 2008;3358(14):1444–53.
315. Bailit JL, Love TE, Mercer B. Rising caesarean rates: are patients sicker? Am J Obstet Gynecol. 2004;191(3):800–3.
316. Declercq E, Meacker F, Macdorman M. Maternal risk profiles and the primary cesarean rate in the United States, 1991–2002. Am J Pub Health. 2006;96(5):867–72.
317. Kabir AA, Steinmann WC, Myers L, Khan MM, Herrera EA, Yu S, et al. Unnecessary delivery in Louisiana: an analysis of birth certificate data. Am J Obstet Gynaecol. 2004;190(1):10–9.
318. Baicker K, Buckles KS, Chandra A. Geographic variation in the appropriate use of caesarean delivery. Health Aff. 2006;25(5):w355–67.
319. Shearer EL. Cesarean section: medical benefits and costs. Soc Sci Med. 1993;37(10):1223–31.
320. Melzer K, Schutz Y, Soehnchen N, Othenin-Girard V, Martinez de Tejada B, Irion O, et al. Effects of recommended levels of physical activity on pregnancy outcomes. Am J Obstet Gynecol. 2010;202(3):226.e1–6.
321. Beckmann CR, Beckman CA. Effect of a structured antepartum exercise program on pregnancy and labor outcome in primiparas. J Reprod Med. 1990;35(7):704–9.
322. Valgesoo T, Linkberg R. Effect of different physical exercises on pregnancy outcome. Acta Med Baltic. 1997;4(1):101–6.
323. Ghodsi Z, Asltoghiri M, Hajiloomohajerani M. Exercise and pregnancy: duration of labor stages and perineal tear rates. Proc Soc Behav Sci. 2012;(31):441–5.
324. Wong SC, Mkenzie DC. Cardiorespiratory fitness during pregnancy and its effect on outcome. Int J Sport Med. 1987;8(2):79–83.
325. Baciuk EP, Pereira RI, Cecatti JG, Braga AF, Cavalcante SR. Water aerobics in pregnancy: cardiovascular response, labor and neonatal outcomes. Reprod Health. 2008;21(5):10–21.
326. Salvesen KL, Mørkved S. Randomised controlled trial of pelvic floor muscle training during pregnancy. BMJ (Res C editor). 2004;329(7462):378–80.
327. Guszkowska M. Physical activity in relation to affetive states and labor anxiety in pregnant women. Med Sport. 2011;15(3):114–9.
328. Sayer AA, Cooper C. Fetal programming of body composition and musculoskeletal development. Early Hum Dev. 2005;81(9):735–44.
329. Barbet JP, Thornell LE, Butler-Browne GS. Immunocytochemical characterisation of two generations of fibres during the development of the human quadriceps muscle. Mech Dev. 1991;35(1):3–11.
330. Brook CG. Evidence for a sensitive period in adipose-cell replication in man. Lancet. 1972;2(7778):624–7.
331. McCance RA, Widdowson EM. The determinants of growth and form. P Roy Soc Lond. 1974;185(1078):1–17.

332. Law CM, Barker DJP, Osmond C, Fall CHD, Simmonds SJ. Early growth and abdominal fatness in adult life. J Epidemiol Community Health. 1992;46(3):184–6.
333. Rogers I. The influence of birthweight and intrauterine environment on adiposity and fat distribution in later life. Int J Obes Rel Metab Dis. 2003;27(7):755–77.
334. Silverman BL, Rizzo T, Green OC, Cho NH, Winter RJ, Ogata ES, et al. Long-term prospective evaluation of offspring of diabetic mothers. Diabetes. 1991;40(Suppl 2):121–5.
335. Fall CHD, Osmond C, Barker DJP, Clark PM, Hales CN, Stirling Y, et al. Fetal and infant growth and cardiovascular risk factors in women. BMJ. 1995;310(6977):428–32.
336. Gale CR, Martyn CN, Kellingray S, Eastell R, Cooper C. Intrauterine programming of adult body composition. J Clin Endocrinol Metab. 2001;86(1):267–72.
337. Parsons TJ, Power C, Logan S, Summerbell CD. Childhood predictors of adult obesity: a systematic review. Int J Obes Relat Metabc Dis. 1999;23(8):1–107.
338. Parsons TJ, Power C, Manor O. Fetal and early life growth and body mass index from birth to early adulthood in 1958. British cohort: longitudinal study. BMJ. 2001;323(7325):1331–5.
339. Rich-Edwards JW, Stampfer MJ, Manson JE, Rosner B, HanKinon SE, Colditz GA, et al. Birth weight and risk of cardiovascular disease in a cohort of women followed up since 1976. BMJ. 1997;315(7105):396–400.
340. Sørenson HT, Sabroe S, Rothman KJ, Gillman M, Fischer P, Sørensen TIA. Relation between weight and length at birth and body mass index in young adulthood. BMJ (Res C editor). 1997;315(7116):1137.
341. Loos RJ, Beunen G, Fagard R, Derom C, Vlietinck R. Birth weight and body composition in young adult men—a prospective twin study. Int J Obes Relat Metab Disord. 2001;25(10):1537–45.
342. Siega-Riz AM, Viswanathan M, Moos MK, Deierlein A, Mumford S, Knaack J, et al. A systematic review of outcomes of maternal weight gain according to the Institute of Medicine recommendations: birthweight, fetal growth, and postpartum weight retention. Am J Obstet Gynecol. 2009;201(4):339.e1–14.
343. Rooney BL, Schauberger CW. Excess pregnancy weight gain and long-term obesity: one decade later. Obstet Gynecol. 2002;100(2):245–52.
344. Cedergren M. Effects of gestational weight gain and body mass index on obstetric outcome in Sweden. Int J Gynecol Obstet. 2006;93(3):269–74.
345. Devine CM, Bove CF, Olson CM. Continuity and change in women's weight orientations and lifestyle patterns and the postpartum period: the influence of life course trajectories and transitional events. Soc Sci Med. 2000;50(4):567–82.
346. American Pregnancy Association [Internet]. Eating for two when over/or under weight. At what rate should I gain weight during my pregnancy? [updated 2014 Jun; cited 2013 Jan 22]. 2008. Promoting Pregnancy Wellness; [about 8 screens]. http://americanpregnancy.org/pregnancyhealth/eatingfortwo.html.
347. Azziz R, Woods KS, Reyna R, Key TJ, Knochenhauer ES, Yildiz BO. The prevalence and features of the polycystic ovary syndrome in an unselected population. J Clin Endocrinol Metab. 2004;89(6):2745–49.
348. March WA, Moore VM, Willson KJ, Phillips DI, Norman RJ, Davies MJ. The prevalence of polycystic ovary syndrome in a community sample assessed under contrasting diagnostic criteria. Hum Reprod. 2010;25(2):544–51.
349. Teede HJ, Hutchison SK, Zoungas S. The management of insulin resistance in polycystic ovary syndrome. Trends Endocrinol Metab. 2007;18(7):273–9.
350. Lord J, Thomas R, Fox B, Acharya U, Wilkin T. The central issue? Visceral fat mass is a good marker of insulin resistance and metabolic disturbance in women with polycystic ovary syndrome. Brit J Obstet Gynaecol. 2006;113(10):1203–9.
351. Harrison CL, Lombard CB, Moron LJ, Teede HJ. Exercise therapy in polycystic ovary syndrome: systemic review. Hum Reprod Update. 2011;17(2):171–83.
352. De Souza MJ, Toombs RJ, Scheid JL, O'Donnell E, West SL, Williams NI. High prevalence of subtle and severe menstrual disturbances in exercising women: confirmation using daily hormone measures. Hum Reprod. 2010;25(2):491–503.
353. Christo K, Prabhakaran R, Lamparello B, Cord J, Miller KK, Goldstein MA, Gupta N, Herzog DB, Klibanski A, Misra M. Bone metabolism in adolescent athletes with amenorrhea, athletes with eumenorrhea, and control subjects. Pediatrics. 2008;121(6):1127–36.
354. De Souza MJ, Williams NI. Physiological aspects and clinical sequelae of energy deficiency and hypoestrogenism in exercising women. Hum Reprod Update. 2004;10:433–48.
355. Gudmundsdottir SL, Flanders WD, Augestad LB. Physical activity and fertility in women: the North-Trøndelag health study. Hum Reprod. 2009;24(12):3196–204.
356. Olive DL. Exercise and fertility: an update. Curr Opin Obstet Gynecol. 2010;22(4):259–63.

Impact of Combined Oral Contraceptive Use on Exercise and Health in Female Athletes

17

Heather C. M. Allaway, Rebecca J. Mallinson and Mary Jane De Souza

Introduction

In a recent report from the Centers for Disease Control and Prevention, 44 % of women between the ages of 15 and 24 years use hormonal contraceptives [1]. Of these women, 49 % use oral contraceptive (OC) preparations and approximately another 14 % use other forms of hormonal contraceptives [1]. The prevalence of OC use among athletic women is increasing and is now estimated to match the prevalence of use in the general population [2, 3]. The increased use of combined hormonal contraceptives (containing both estrogen and progestin) in the athletic community is likely due to the reduction in cycle-length variability and the consistent 28-day "cycle" that is achieved with administration of exogenous sex steroids and subsequent systematic control of endogenous sex hormone concentrations [3]. The effect of OC preparations on athletic performance and health has not been conclusively answered as early investigators utilized a diverse number of OC preparations, range of participant fitness levels, and timing of experiments within the OC pill cycle. Most research studies have been cross sectional and were not carried out using the most commonly prescribed contraceptives today (low and ultra-low OC preparations and the vaginal ring).

Modern combined hormonal contraceptives can be provided in a variety of types and formulations. These include, but are not limited to, OC pills (monophasic, biphasic, and triphasic), the contraceptive transdermal patch, and the contraceptive vaginal ring. Current combined hormonal contraceptives typically contain one of the two types of synthetic estrogen, ethinyl estradiol (EE) or manestrol, while the progestin component is typically one of eight different forms. The biological properties of the progestogen derivatives used in contraceptives relate to the potency and the relative binding affinity [4]. Progestins with a higher relative binding affinity for the progesterone receptor exert their progestational effects with smaller doses. Progestins with high relative binding affinity for the androgen receptor cause undesirable side effects that counteract the positive effects produced by the synthetic estrogen [4].

Since the introduction of the OC pill, the dose of the estrogen component has been decreased. The high-dose OC preparations contain 50 µg/d or more of the estrogen component, low-dose OC preparations contain less than 50 µg/d (generally 20–35 µg/d of the estrogen component), and ultra-low-dose OC preparations contain 15 µg/d of the estrogen component [5, 6]. Low and ultra-low OC pills are the most commonly prescribed pills today [6].

M. J. De Souza (✉) · R. J. Mallinson
Department of Kinesiology, Pennsylvania State University, 104 Noll Laboratory, University Park, PA 16802, USA
e-mail: mjd34@psu.edu

H. C. M. Allaway
Department of Kinesiology, Pennsylvania State University, University Park, PA 16802, USA

© Springer Science+Business Media New York 2016

D. Vaamonde et al. (eds.), *Exercise and Human Reproduction*, DOI 10.1007/978-1-4939-3402-7_17

The progestin component has undergone four developmental generations since the introduction of the OC pill. The first generation was the first to demonstrate the desired activity on the reproductive axis and include norethindrone and medroxyprogesterone acetate [7–9]. The successive generations were designed to minimize the side effects and increase the safety profile (i.e., to decrease the risk of blood clots). The second generation includes levonorgestrel and norgestrel, the third generation includes norgestimate and etonogestrel, and the fourth generation includes drospirenone and nomegestrol acetate [7–9]. All conventional 28-day hormonal contraceptive regimens provide exogenous steroids for 21 days (active pill phase) followed by a 7-day hormone-free phase. The hormone-free phase, which allows for breakthrough bleeding, can consist of either inactive/placebo pills or the cessation of taking any pills for 7 days. Monophasic OC formulations contain the same dose of estrogen and progestin in all active pills, whereas biphasic OC formulations contain a constant estrogen dose, but the progestin dose increases in the second half of the active pill phase [10]. Triphasic OC formulations have two doses of estrogen (higher in the second week of the active pill phase than the first or third week) and the progestin increases in three steps during the active pill phase [10]. The contraceptive transdermal patch delivers 20 µg of EE daily with a third-generation progestin, norelgestromin [11], and the contraceptive vaginal ring delivers 15 µg EE daily with a third-generation progestin, etonogestrel [12].

The purpose of this brief review is to elucidate the current understanding of the effects of OC preparations on factors that influence exercise performance and the health of athletes. Information regarding the impact of the contraceptive transdermal patch and vaginal ring on exercise performance is not currently available. This review will focus on the effects of OC preparations on the factors that affect exercise performance, including substrate utilization, aerobic and anaerobic capacity, ventilatory capacity, and anaerobic strength, and factors that affect the health of female athletes, including body composition, bone health, and menstrual function.

Factors That Affect Exercise Performance

Substrate Utilization

The new low- and ultra-low-dose and third-generation progestin OC preparations minimize the side effects of early preparations on insulin resistance, decreased glucose tolerance, and high plasma cholesterol and triglyceride levels [3]. However, current formulations of ultra-low-dose OC preparations have not been extensively evaluated to determine the differences in substrate utilization throughout the active pill phase or hormone-free phase and during exercise. It has been hypothesized that during the active pill phase, with high EE, there would be a glycogen sparing effect and increased lipid use during exercise [13–16]. However, progestins are hypothesized to oppose the lipolytic effects induced by EE [13–16]. These hypotheses were based on observations of increased lipolysis and reduced carbohydrate oxidation during exercise with high estrogen in the follicular phase of the natural menstrual cycle and an opposition to lipolysis in the luteal phase with high progesterone and estrogen [17–19]. However, in rats and humans, the use of exogenous sex steroids has been shown to interfere with substrate utilization [13, 20]. A few researchers have utilized various modes (e.g., cycle ergometer and treadmill) and intensities of exercise to investigate changes of fuel utilization during exercise when combined with OC use.

Inconsistent results have been reported with regard to substrate availability following endurance exercise between *monophasic* OC users and nonusers. For example, Bonen et al. [14] investigated substrate utilization during exercise in monophasic OC users compared to non-OC users. During 30 min of exercise at 40% of maximal oxygen consumption (VO_{2max}), a shift to high plasma free fatty acids and decreased plasma glucose concentrations was observed in monophasic OC users compared to non-OC users; however, no differences between the active pill and hormone-free phases were observed [14]. Similarly, Bemben et al. [13] reported a decrease in carbohydrate utilization and lower plasma glucose in the 40th and 50th minutes of a 90 min treadmill test at 50 % VO_{2max} in monophasic (35 μg EE) and multiphasic (35 μg EE) OC users during the active pill phase compared to the luteal phase in non-OC users. However, no difference in fat oxidation was observed between OC users and non-OC users [13]. In contrast, a cross-sectional analysis by Sunderland et al. [21] investigated the impact of long-term (12 months) monophasic (20–30 μg EE) OC use on substrate utilization in regularly active women and failed to observe any changes in blood glucose concentrations between the active pill and hormone-free phases, and between OC users and non-OC users following a 30-s sprint treadmill exercise [21].

In support of the proposed hypothesis that high EE would spare glycogen and encourage lipid utilization but high progestin concentrations would oppose lipolysis, Redman et al. [22] investigated the impact of the third week of the active pill phase and the hormone-free phase of *triphasic* OC use on metabolism in five elite female rowers. During three consecutive triphasic OC cycles increased glucose (37 and 8 %) and reduced plasma triglyceride (8 and 31 %) concentrations were reported at rest and post-anaerobic exercise in the hormone-free phase compared to the active pill phase [22]. Similarly, in the menstrual cycle before and following 4 months of triphasic OC use, Casazza et al. [15] evaluated lipid utilization during exercise in eight active, eumenorrheic women and reported greater triglyceride mobilization during 60 min of leg ergometer exercise at 45 % of VO_{2max} in the third week of the active pill phase (21.6 %) and at 65 % of VO_{2max} during the active pill (20.4 %) and hormone-free phase (21.6 %) compared to pre-OC use [15]. However, no differences were observed in free fatty acid oxidation, but re-esterification of free fatty acids was not investigated [15]. In addition, Jacobs et al. [23] observed increased free fatty acid appearance, disappearance, and oxidation during exercise at 45 and 65 % of peak oxygen uptake (VO_{2peak}) compared to during rest in eight active women during the natural menstrual cycle prior to OC initiation and following 4 months of triphasic OC use. They also observed an increase in free fatty acid re-esterification and a decrease in the proportion of plasma free fatty acid rate of disappearance at rest and during exercise with triphasic OC use compared to pre-OC use. Suh et al. [24] investigated the effects of 4 months of triphasic OC use on substrate metabolism in eight active women; no difference in the rate of glucose appearance was observed between the third week of the active pill phase and the hormone-free phase at rest or during exercise at 45 and 65 % VO_{2peak}. Further, Suh et al. [24] did not observe any differences in glucose or lipid oxidation rates between the natural menstrual cycle and triphasic OC use or between the third week of the active pill phase and the hormone-free phase of the OC cycle. A decrease in the rate of glucose appearance was observed at rest and during exercise at 45 and 65 % VO_{2peak} during triphasic OC use compared to the menstrual cycle prior to OC use [24]. The investigations of the effect of *triphasic* OC use on substrate metabolism to date used differing modes and durations of exercise [15, 22–24], and there appears to be a shift toward increased free fatty acid mobilization, while substrate oxidation does not show a clear difference between phases of the OC cycle (active pill and hormone-free phases) or cross-sectionally between triphasic OC users and non-OC users.

Limited research has been conducted to evaluate differences in substrate utilization with OC use in various prandial states. Tremblay et al. [25] investigated measures of substrate oxidation during 120 min of cycle ergometer exercise at 57 % of VO_{2max} following ingestion of 2 g/kg of glucose between triphasic OC users and non-OC users and reported no differences in exogenous and endogenous carbohydrate oxidation rates. However, Issaco et al. [26] reported a greater reliance on lipids during 45 min of exercise at 65 % of VO_{2max} in the fasting state compared to the post-prandial state in 21 active women using a monophasic (20–30 μg EE) OC preparation. However, a greater reliance on lipids during exercise in the fasted state compared to the post-prandial state was also observed in non-OC users, and there were no differences in lipid reliance between OC users and non-OC users [26].

In summary, current research findings do not indicate consistent changes in substrate utilization during exercise in women using monophasic and triphasic OC preparations. It is possible that during shorter exercise tests, where there is less reliance on glycogen and lipid utilization, less opportunity is available for the exogenous steroids to exert an influence over substrate flux [10, 27]. An insufficient number of studies have been conducted at various durations and intensities of exercise and durations of OC use to definitively determine whether OCs have an impact on substrate utilization during aerobic and anaerobic exercise. Further research is also needed to determine the effects of transdermal and vaginal hormonal contraceptives on substrate utilization during exercise in athletic women.

Exercise Capacity

The availability and use of glucose and lipids as a fuel source during exercise are known to impact aerobic and anaerobic capacity [28]. With the use of OC pills, early reports indicate an alteration of (1) fat and carbohydrate metabolism, as previously described, (2) movement of glucose into muscle (glucose flux), and (3) insulin sensitivity [13–16, 20]. These early observations of alterations in the proportion of fuel availability, glucose flux, and insulin sensitivity led to theories of the impact of OC use and phase of OC cycle on both aerobic and anaerobic capacity.

During the active pill phase, EE may exert a glycogen sparing effect, which is proposed to enhance sustained aerobic capacity [29]. During the hormone-free phase, when sex steroid hormone concentrations are lowest, the carbohydrate metabolism is upregulated and may enhance anaerobic capacity [29, 30]. It is noteworthy that this review will focus on the effects of OC use on factors influencing exercise capacity, which are commonly assumed to correlate with athletic performance [31, 32], and will *not* focus on athletic performance per se, which is defined as the complex interaction between physiological, tactical, technical, and psychological factors [32].

Aerobic Capacity

The large majority of investigators have evaluated the effects of monophasic OC preparations on aerobic capacity in both trained [33–37] and untrained [36, 38, 39] women. Few investigators have evaluated the influence of biphasic or triphasic OC preparations on aerobic capacity [23, 24, 40, 41]. Differences in aerobic capacity have been evaluated in both cross-sectional [33, 35–37] and longitudinal studies [23, 24, 40, 41]. Researchers have also focused on evaluating the variation in aerobic capacity between the active pill phase and the hormone-free phase [33, 38].

In *untrained* women using *monophasic* OC pills, study results have been inconsistent [36, 38, 39]. Early work indicated a significant increase in VO_{2peak} for a standardized workload in untrained women following two cycles of high-dose (50 µg EE) monophasic OC use when compared with baseline measures (assessed during the menstrual cycle prior to OC initiation) [39]. However, more recently, investigators have suggested that low-dose (20–35 µg EE) monophasic OC use for 12 months had no effect on oxygen consumption (VO_2) in untrained women during the hormone-free phase or the final week of the active pill phase [38]. Similarly, Rebelo et al. [36] reported no difference in VO_{2peak} in sedentary women who had been using a low-dose (20 µg EE) monophasic OC for 18 months compared to non-OC users.

Varying results have also been reported in studies evaluating the impact of *monophasic* OC pill use in *trained* women, both in recreational and in elite athletes [33, 34, 36, 37, 42]. In recreationally active women who had been using a low-dose (20–30 µg EE) monophasic OC for a minimum of 18 months, submaximal VO_2 was reduced by 3–6% during the active pill phase compared to the hormone-free phase [33]. Other reports in recreationally active women using OCs for a minimum of 12 months demonstrate a reduced VO_{2peak} and a lower VO_2 at the anaerobic threshold, with no differences reported in time to exhaustion during a submaximal aerobic test compared to non-OC users [35]. Likewise, Notelovitz et al. [43] described a 7–8% decrease in VO_{2peak} following 6 months of low-dose

(35 µg EE) OC use in trained women, while the non-OC user control group had a 7.5% increase in VO_{2peak} during the same timeframe. However, in 2010, Rebelo et al. [36] did not observe a significant difference in VO_{2peak} nor VO_2 at the anaerobic threshold of trained women who had been using a low-dose (20 µg EE) monophasic OC for a minimum of 18 months compared to non-OC users. Similarly, in trained rowers, who had been on a low-dose (20 µg EE) OC preparation for a minimum of 3 months, no significant differences in measurements of VO_{2max} and VO_2 at the aerobic-anaerobic transition were observed between day 8 or day 20 of a monophasic OC pill cycle [37]. Studies of monophasic OC use in highly trained women also indicate that there is no significant effect of OC preparations on aerobic capacity [34].

Due to the relatively equal proportion of studies that have shown a decrease or no significant change in VO_2 with OC use in *untrained* and *trained* women, the impact of *monophasic* OC use on aerobic capacity remains unclear. In summary, the conflicting results in VO_2 among *untrained and trained* women using a *monophasic* OC have been reported to be secondary to a wide variety of causes, that include (1) differences in progestational and androgenic activity of the progestins within the contraceptives in the studies, (2) duration of OC use (no use, 3, 6, 12 or 18 months of use prior to study initiation), (3) varying training status of the study participants, (4) small sample sizes that may not power studies adequately for primary study outcomes, and (5) variation in the exercise protocols utilized in each research study [10, 29]. Further research will be necessary to resolve this issue.

Very few investigators have evaluated the impact of *triphasic* OC preparations on aerobic capacity in *trained* women [23, 24, 40, 41]. In a study of trained athletes over two triphasic OC pill cycles, a 4.7% decrease in VO_{2peak} but no change in endurance performance, as measured by time to exhaustion, was observed [41]. Similarly, a study of triphasic OC pills over four [24] and six [23] cycles demonstrated a decrease in VO_{2peak} of 11–15% in active women, agreeing with results from a study conducted by Casazza et al. [40] which demonstrated an 11% decrease in VO_{2peak} among recreationally active women using a triphasic OC for 4 months. In summary, triphasic OC preparations appear to decrease VO_2 in trained athletes during use of up to 6 months. No studies to date have investigated the impact of triphasic OC use (1) of long duration (>6 months) or (2) in untrained women.

Ventilatory Capacity

Early research on the menstrual cycle has shown that the natural rise in progesterone during the luteal phase increases chemosensitivity of the lungs to hypoxia and hypercapnia [44]; thus, monophasic OC preparations with high doses of progestin and the third phase of the triphasic OC may also increase the chemosensitivity of the lungs and increase ventilatory capacity. In agreement with this hypothesis, a few studies conducted in trained women using monophasic OC preparations demonstrated an increase in ventilation (VE) [37, 45]; however, these results have not been consistent, particularly when considering the ventilation response to OC preparations in untrained women or with a different OC formulation, i.e. triphasic OC preparations.

For example, during a 1-h endurance test performed by *trained* cyclists taking *monophasic* OC preparation mean VE and mean ventilation per oxygen consumption (VE/VO_2) were 7 and 5% higher, respectively, during the active pill phase compared to measures taken early and late in the hormone-free phase [45]. However, in trained rowers administered a monophasic OC, there was a tendency toward an increased ventilatory response during the hormone-free phase demonstrated by increased VE and VE/VO_2 at VO_{2max} (1.6 and 6.3%, respectively) compared to the active pill phase [37].

On the other hand, no significant differences in VE were observed in *untrained* women, who had been using a *monophasic* OC preparation (20–30 µg EE) for a minimum of 18 months and performed submaximal treadmill exercise during any phase (active pill and hormone-free) of a monophasic OC pill cycle [33]. Further, Redman et al. [46] evaluated ventilatory measures in untrained women who had been using contraceptives for a minimum of 6 months. Participants changed their OC use in a cross-over design to a 35 μg EE monophasic OC with high (1000 μg norethisterone) or low (500 μg norethisterone) progesterone concentration. VE and VE/VO_2 measured at VO_{2peak} were not different between progesterone concentrations; however, VE and VE/VO_2 were 10.5 and 8.5 % higher, respectively, at rest during use of the high progesterone OC compared to the low progesterone OC [46]. Rebelo et al. [36] evaluated VE in active and sedentary OC users (20 μg EE; minimum use 18 months) and non-OC users and did not observe any differences among the four groups. Further, Joyce et al. [35, 42] did not observe any differences in VE between *untrained or trained* OC users (minimum use 12 months) and non-users.

Contrary to the hypothesis that the third week of the *triphasic* OC preparation may increase ventilatory capacity due to the high progestational content, the majority of studies have demonstrated no effect of triphasic OC preparation use on VE in both *untrained and trained* women. For example, in *untrained* women who utilized a triphasic OC for 4 months, VE measured in the active pill and hormone-free phases were not significantly different compared to measurements taken during the follicular or luteal phase of the menstrual cycle prior to OC initiation [40]. Similarly, in *trained* women, VE did not differ between measurements taken following 4 months of triphasic OC use during the active pill and hormone-free phases nor compared to the follicular and luteal phases in the menstrual cycle prior to OC initiation [24]. Further, VE did not change with a single cycle of a triphasic OC in trained women compared to the menstrual cycle prior to OC initiation [41].

Overall, OC use (monophasic or triphasic formulations) does not appear to have an effect on ventilatory capacity. The conflicting results observed with monophasic OC use can be attributed to the initial fitness level of the participants, the intensity and duration of the exercise, and/or the androgenic activity of the progestin in the OC preparations used. Further research is necessary to confirm the results from studies evaluating triphasic OC use.

Anaerobic Exercise

Few studies have been conducted on the influence of OC preparations on anaerobic performance, including capacity and strength. Variation in anaerobic performance during an OC cycle could be caused by the impact of EE and progestins on substrate utilization, buffering capacity, and neuromuscular function [47].

Anaerobic Capacity

During short-duration maximal exercise, the maximal amount of ATP resynthesized via anaerobic metabolism (phosphocreatine and glycolysis) is considered anaerobic capacity [29]. During a menstrual cycle, a low estrogen environment and increased circulating aldosterone following a drop in progesterone (as observed at the end of the luteal phase) upregulate carbohydrate metabolism, which is necessary for the anaerobic production of ATP [29]. Further, increases in circulating aldosterone may increase body fluid and electrolyte retention, thus increasing buffering and anaerobic capacity [48]. As such, in accordance with the influence of endogenous steroid hormones on substrate utilization and buffering capacity, it is plausible that anaerobic capacity would be greatest during the hormone-free phase of the OC cycle [29]. Currently, available literature does not provide hypotheses surrounding the impact of OC use on anaerobic capacity when compared to non-OC users. Production of lactate, a by-product of anaerobic metabolism, has been evaluated in women using monophasic and triphasic OC preparations, thus serving as an indicator of the impact of OC use on anaerobic capacity.

The majority of studies, however, do not support the proposed hypothesis that anaerobic capacity is enhanced during the hormone-free phase. For example, Bonen et al. [14] evaluated lactate concentrations following a walk to elicit 85 % VO_{2max} in *monophasic* OC users (30–50 μg EE) and observed no differences between phases of the OC cycle [14]. Similarly, Bernardes et al. [18] investigated anaerobic capacity in a mixed group of women using *monophasic* and *triphasic* OC preparations of a similar EE dose (30–40 μg EE) and found no variation in blood lactate between the active pill phase and the hormone-free phase following intermittent exercise (80% VO_{2max}) tests. Likewise, Lynch et al. [49] investigated the impact of low-dose (30–35 μg EE) *monophasic* OC administration on intermittent exercise (five by 20-s treadmill runs at increasing speed on a 10.5% incline) in *recreationally active* women and observed no significant difference in peak blood lactate between OC users and non-OC users; however, peak blood lactate was significantly higher during week 1 compared to week 2 (11.2 vs. 9.6 mmol/L) of the active pill phase of OC users. Notably, in contrast to their previous report, Lynch et al. [38] observed no difference in blood lactate concentrations between week 1 and week 3 of the active pill phase after repeating the intermittent exercise test on *untrained* women who had been using a low-dose OC preparation (20–35 μg EE) for at least 12 months. Interestingly, neither of the studies by Lynch et al. [38, 49] evaluated differences between the active pill and hormone-free phases. Following high intensity, intermittent exercise in the heat, no differences in blood lactate concentrations were observed between OC cycle phases in *trained* women using *monophasic* (20–35 μg EE) OC preparations [50]. In a study by Redman et al. [22], conducted among 6 highly *trained* rowers who had been taking a *triphasic* OC for a minimum of 12 months, a significant increase in glucose and decrease in plasma triglyceride with no difference in lactate concentrations were observed in the hormone-free phase compared to the third week of the active pill phase following a 1000 m simulated row test. The participants were tested in three consecutive OC cycles and the results were consistent between the active pill phase and hormone-free phase [22]. In 2011, Sunderland et al. [21] also evaluated the impact of *monophasic* OC use (20-30ug EE) on blood lactate concentration following an all-out 30-s sprint. Blood lactate concentrations were not different between the active pill phase and hormone-free phase in OC users [21]. These results indicate that there is no difference in carbohydrate metabolism between OC cycle phases during tests of short, intense activity when compared with studies of aerobic and submaximal endurance exercise [27].

Recently, however, findings by Rechichi et al. [27] do support the hypothesis that anaerobic capacity is greater during the hormone-free phase of the OC cycle. For example, Rechichi et al. [27] measured a 23% decrease in peak blood lactate following a 200 m time trial in the hormone-free phase compared to late in the active pill phase in competitive swimmers using a monophasic OC (30 μg EE) preparation, indicating an increase in buffering capacity.

In addition to comparing differences between phases of the OC cycle, three teams of investigators also reported comparisons between OC users and non-OC users. In 1991, Bonen et al. [14] evaluated lactate concentrations following a walk to elicit 85% VO_{2max} in monophasic OC users (30–50 μg EE) and non-OC users. No differences in blood lactate concentrations were observed between OC users and non-OC users [14]. Sunderland et al. [50] investigated high-intensity intermittent exercise in the heat in trained women on monophasic (20–35 μg EE) OC preparations and non-OC users and found no differences in blood lactate concentrations. However, in 2011, Sunderland et al. [21] found significantly higher blood lactate concentrations following an all-out 30-s sprint in OC users compared to non-OC users. Of three available reports comparing OC users and non-OC users, this was the first report demonstrating a difference in blood lactate concentrations between OC users and non-OC users. The differences in the available data are due to the large variability in EE concentrations as well as the variation in the exercise evaluated and the conditions of the test.

The majority of available data to date do not support the hypothesis that anaerobic capacity would be greater during the hormone-free phase compared to the active pill phase in OC users. The limited comparisons of anaerobic capacity between OC users and non-OC users indicate the exogenous hormones in OC preparations have a diminished capacity to alter aldosterone and lactate buffering capacity; however, further research is needed to conclude if there is a general impact of OC use (compared to non-OC users) on anaerobic capacity. Data regarding blood lactate accumulation following anaerobic exercise during use of monophasic or triphasic OC preparations suggest the impact of aldosterone on buffering capacity is not consistent with changes observed in the natural menstrual cycle. Thus, future studies should investigate the alterations in the progesterone/aldosterone ratio at more than one time point during the active pill and hormone-free phases. It is also possible that duration of activity is a significant factor in the ability of exogenous hormones from OC preparations to impact anaerobic capacity. With shorter duration tests the influence of sex steroids on lipid and glycogen utilization is limited; thus there may be less opportunity for the exogenous steroids to exert their influence [10, 29].

Anaerobic Strength

It has been proposed that endogenous estrogens, when highest, may have a positive impact on muscle strength, while progesterone inhibits the effects of estrogen [51]. However, EE may not influence the estrogen receptors within the skeletal muscle in the same way as endogenous estrogen or the progestin consumed with OC use may influence the interaction of EE with the neuromuscular pathway [47]. Rechichi et al. [47] evaluated reactive strength with a 45 cm drop height test in team sport *athletes* taking a *monophasic* OC preparation and found reactive strength was approximately 11 % lower during the hormone-free phase (early or late) compared to the active pill phase. In contrast, Sarwar et al. [52] observed no differences with handgrip strength or isometric quadriceps strength between active pill and hormone-free phases of a monophasic OC cycle. Similarly, Elliot et al. [53] found no differences in dynamic or isometric leg strength between the active pill and hormone-free phases in 14 women using a monophasic OC (30–35 μg EE) preparation. In addition, Elliot et al. [53] did not observe differences in dynamic or isometric leg strength between the 14 monophasic OC users and 7 eumenorrheic women. A study by Peters et al. [54] on trained athletes using monophasic OC (30 μg EE) preparation showed no difference in maximal leg isokinetic strength through extension or flexion between the active pill and hormone-free phases of the OC cycle. Similarly, Ekenros et al. [55] did not observe any differences in isokinetic knee extensor strength or isometric handgrip strength between monophasic (20–35 μg EE) OC users and non-OC users nor between phases of an OC cycle. Further testing is required to determine if there is an effect of OC use on reactive strength; however, the available data indicates that isometric strength is not influenced by *monophasic* OC use or phase of the monophasic OC cycle. Further research is needed to determine the impact of *triphasic* OC use on all aspects of muscular strength.

Competitive Exercise Performance

As previously discussed, factors that influence performance may be altered by use of OC preparations; however, what is the cumulative effect on competitive performance? There are currently few studies that have evaluated field measures of performance, such as a time trial or competitive event [27]. As such, limited information is known about how OC use will ultimately affect the outcome of an individual athlete's competitive performance. Overall, of the studies that have assessed more generally applicable measures of performance, it is found that OC use does not appear to benefit athletic performance. For example, in five female rowers who had been using a triphasic OC preparation for 12 months, Redman et al. [22] found 1000 m simulated rowing times were 3-s faster during the hormone-free phase compared to the third week of the active pill phase in three consecutively tested OC cycles. Rechichi et al. [27] also demonstrated this apparent lack of beneficial influence of OC use on athletic performance among six competitive swimmers and water polo players using a monophasic OC (30 μg EE) preparation; they observed no significant difference in 200-m swim time between the active pill phase and the hormone-free phase. Likewise, a few investigators have evaluated time to exhaustion as a proxy measure of endurance performance and have shown no difference in time to exhaustion between OC users and non-OC users [35, 41, 56], nor between phases of the OC cycle [56].

Conflicting results have been reported by investigators during tests of peak power output. Casazza et al. [40] reported that 4 months of OC use in six moderately active women revealed a significant 8 % decrease in peak power output as evaluated on a cycle ergometer, indicating that OC use may impair peak exercise capacity. On the other hand, Redman et al. [46] reported improved peak power output (1.5 %) as evaluated on a cycle ergometer in 26 sedentary women using a monophasic OC preparation with a high progesterone content (1000 µg norethisterone) compared with a low progesterone preparation (500 µg norethisterone), indicating that OC preparations with higher progesterone content may enhance peak exercise capacity. However, the lack of large studies that assess field measures of performance highlights the need for more research in this area and limits the knowledge about how OC use may ultimately impact competitive performance in female athletes.

Factors That Affect the Health of Athletes

Body Composition and Bone Health

Body Composition

In athletic girls and women, changes in body composition, particularly in the fat mass compartment, caused by OC use would be important in determining changes in athletic performance. Available research has focused on a broad population of women, while there is limited information available specifically regarding changes in body composition in female athletes using OC preparations. In general, investigators have demonstrated an increase in body mass, in particular fat mass, with OC use among female athletes. For example, Coney et al. [57] observed a nonsignificant increase of $\geq$ 1 kg in body mass over 6 months of *monophasic* OC use in 40 % of participants in a pooled analysis of two phase III randomized, placebo-controlled trials. Furthermore, the use of monophasic OC for 6 months by active women showed a 2 kg increase in body mass compared to active controls [43]. However, following a month without use of OC pills, the participants returned to their baseline weight [43]. Rickenlund et al. [58] observed an increase in body weight and fat mass following 10 months of monophasic OC use in female, endurance athletes who had oligomenorrhea/amenorrhea prior to OC use. Likewise, a 3 and 9 % increase in body weight and fat mass, respectively, was observed following 4 months of *triphasic* OC use in active women, while no change in fat-free mass was observed [40]. Similarly, Jacobs et al. [23] and Suh et al. [24] demonstrated significant increases in body mass (1.7–2.5 %) and percent body fat (5.6–10 %) over 4–6 months of triphasic OC use in active women. Lebrun et al. [41] observed a significant increase in body mass and percent body fat with the use of a triphasic OC in trained women over two pill cycles.

In contrast, results from a few studies reveal a decrease or no change in body mass or fat mass. In adolescent girls administered OC preparations for the first time, a significant decrease in body fat percentage (0.1 %) and a nonsignificant increase (0.6 %) in lean body mass after 6 months of use were observed [59]. Thai women using two different *monophasic* OC pill types (35 µg/d or 30 µg/d EE) showed a trend of loss in body mass of 1.5 and 1.1 kg, respectively, over 6 months [60]. On the other hand, in collegiate cross-country runners randomized to the use of a monophasic OC, there was little difference in weight or fat mass gain compared to no treatment following a minimum of 6 months of OC use [61]. Women who had regular menses prior to initiation of OC use showed a significant increase in lean body mass compared to no treatment; however, there was no association of OC use and lean body mass change among women with oligomenorrhea prior to OC initiation [61]. The differences observed between studies on the general population and specific athletic populations are most adequately explained by the difference in training status of the participants; however, differences in progestational or androgenic activity of the progestin and EE concentrations in the monophasic and triphasic OC pills used in each study may also explain some of the variations in results.

In a review by Gallo et al. [62], no large effect of OC preparations on weight gain was evident; however, there was insufficient evidence to rule out an association. The changes observed over long-duration monophasic and triphasic OC use, though small, are meaningful differences in an athletic performance context. An increase in body fat, even small, could be viewed as detrimental to performance in many sports, most notably aesthetic sports where body shape is imperative (i.e., gymnastics, distance running, and dance) and in weight-classification events where a pre-event weigh-in determines the competition category (i.e., rowing and weightlifting). Overall, the aforementioned studies suggest that athletic women may experience an increase in body mass and percent body fat during long-term use of any type and formulation of OC. The weight gain observed in studies has been hypothesized to be due to fluid retention, increased subcutaneous fat, anabolic effects on appetite, and androgenic effects on muscle mass; however, no dose–response relationship with weight gain has been observed between the EE concentrations of the various OC formulations that have been examined [62].

Bone Health

Published data on the influence of OC preparations on bone mass, another component of body composition, among physically active girls and women are limited and inconclusive. However, results from a few published studies suggest that OC preparations may have detrimental effects on bone health, especially when combined with exercise, thereby initiating concern about the use of OC preparations in female athletes.

In the only prospective study to date that assessed bone mineral density (BMD) and bone mineral content (BMC) among women taking OC preparations and participating in a 24-month exercise training program, Weaver et al. [63] reported a significant decrease in BMD and BMC at the lumbar spine after 6 months of OC use and exercise training. Interestingly, this change was significantly different when compared with the women participating in the exercise training program but not taking an OC preparation and the women taking an OC preparation but not exercising who both demonstrated a significant gain in lumbar spine BMD after 6 months [63]. After 24 months of training, lumbar spine BMD of the women who were taking an OC preparation and exercising had returned to baseline, but the women who were taking an OC preparation and not exercising demonstrated a continued gain in lumbar spine BMD [63]. Although not statistically significant, women who were taking OC preparations and participating in the exercise program had smaller gains in femoral neck cross-sectional moment of inertia and cross-sectional area, two important indicators of bone strength, when compared with women who were neither taking OC preparations nor exercising [64]. Further, in a cross-sectional study, Hartard et al. [65] explored the history of OC use and regular physical activity on BMD among young women; those who had a long history of both OC use and physical activity had lower BMD than those with a short history of OC use and a long history of physical activity. In agreement with these findings, a retrospective analysis of female endurance athletes aged 18–35 years revealed that BMD at both the hip and the lumbar spine was significantly lower in the athletes who reported OC use for more than 3 years or greater than 50 % of the time since menarche compared with control athletes [66]. Furthermore, age at initiation of OC use was a strong positive predictor of BMD at the lumbar spine, indicating the potentially negative effects that OC use may have on BMD during key years of bone mineral accrual [66].

It appears that OC use may compromise the skeletal benefits of regular physical activity; however, the underlying reason why OC use in combination with exercise may be particularly detrimental to bone health is unclear. It must be noted that even within the general population of women, the influence of OC preparations on bone health lacks clarity, with studies demonstrating an increase [67], decrease [68, 69], and no change [6, 68, 70–74] in BMD during OC use lasting 12–36 months.

The skeletal consequences that may be associated with OC use are proposed to stem from the hepatic first-pass effect of EE. When administered orally, doses of estrogen greater than what is naturally in the circulation must be given due to the reduced bioavailability of the hormone after active metabolism by the liver [75]. The synthesis of hormones, clotting factors, growth factors, and binding proteins by the liver can be affected by this first-pass effect through the liver [75]. Thus, it is speculated that the first-pass effect of exogenous estrogen through the liver suppresses hepatic production of insulin-like growth factor-1 (IGF-1) and upregulates the synthesis of certain binding proteins, such as IGF binding protein-1 (IGFBP-1), which bind to IGF-1 further reducing its bioavailability [75]. IGF-1 is a protein known to have strong anabolic effects on bone tissue and may stimulate bone formation, as evidenced by the positive association between circulating IGF-1 concentrations and a marker of bone formation during childhood and adolescence [76]. In support of the proposed negative effect of OC administration on hepatic production of IGF-1, Hansen et al. [77] reported significantly lower serum concentrations of IGF-1 and P1NP (amino terminal propeptide of type I collagen), a marker of bone formation, 24 h after an exercise bout in women who were taking OC preparations compared to women who were not using an OC.

Current studies indicate that long-term use of OC preparations may increase body weight and percent body fat, while causing a decrease in BMD and BMC in athletic women. Changes in both bone and fat composition are likely to have a negative impact on aerobic and anaerobic performance. Further research is necessary to confirm available results, determine mechanisms of action on changes in body composition, and evaluate the effects of all forms of hormonal contraceptives on body composition and bone health.

Menstrual Function and Contraceptive Use in Female Athletes

Up to 60% of female athletes present with the most severe menstrual disturbance, amenorrhea [78]. The underlying cause of exercise-associated amenorrhea is low energy availability, or insufficient energy to perform the daily physiological and locomotive functions of life [79]. The energy deficit contributes to a cascade of physiological adaptations to conserve fuel, including metabolic adaptations that suppress the reproductive axis. (For a detailed explanation of the characteristics and consequences of an energy deficiency in female athletes, refer to Chaps. 11 and 12.) The metabolic and reproductive suppression that occurs in an energy-deficient environment contributes to low bone mass. The combination of low energy availability, amenorrhea, and low bone mass is referred to as the female athlete triad [80]. Correcting the low energy availability that leads to the menstrual dysfunction and poor bone health, via an increase in energy intake or a decrease in energy expenditure, should be the mainstay of clinical practice [81, 82]. However, the increase in energy intake and/or decrease in energy expenditure that often leads to weight gain can be a challenging treatment strategy for many clinicians and female athletes. As such, clinicians may prescribe OC preparations to female athletes who present with amenorrhea in order to "regulate" the menstrual cycle [83].

As described in the 2014 Female Athlete Triad Consensus Statement [81, 82], pharmacological treatment, such as OC preparations, should only be considered for a female athlete with the Triad if there is no positive response to 1 year of non-pharmacological treatment (increasing energy intake and/or decreasing energy expenditure) and if the athlete experiences a new fracture. More specifically, pharmacological treatment may be considered in athletes who have undergone non-pharmacological treatment but continue to experience health consequences of amenorrhea such as infertility, vaginal dryness, and dyspareunia, or impaired bone health [81, 82].

However, the efficacy of OC preparations in improving bone health in female athletes with the Triad is unclear [81, 82, 84]. Furthermore, spontaneous menses is not restored with the use of OC preparations; rather, the induced withdrawal bleeding that occurs with OC preparations instigates a false sense of security to the athlete [81, 82]. The root cause of the menstrual disturbances and poor bone health, that is, the low energy availability, is not addressed, but masked, with administration of OC preparations. For this reason, OC preparations alone are not effective for treating menstrual disturbances that occur as a result of an energy deficit and, if used, should be administered in combination with nonpharmacological treatment [81, 82]. It must be emphasized that the cornerstone of treatment of the female athlete triad is reversal of the low energy availability that leads to the menstrual dysfunction and poor bone health. The engagement of a multidisciplinary team that includes a physician, sports dietician, and mental health professional is necessary to guide the athlete through recovery to restoration of a healthy energy state and menstrual status, which are important to the overall and long-term health and well-being.

Conclusions and Future Research

The purpose of this brief review was to elucidate the current understanding of the effects of combined OCs on factors that influence exercise performance and the health of athletes. The scope of the review was limited to OC preparations as there is currently no data available regarding the impact of the transdermal patch or vaginal ring contraceptive use on physiologic factors associated with exercise performance. The effects of OC preparations on physiologic factors related to performance are complicated due to the large variation in OC formulations available. Older formulations used in the earliest studies available will have had a greater physiologic impact on athletic performance compared to the newer, low-dose formulations.

Available data examining physiology and performance within a single OC cycle and across multiple OC cycles, regardless of duration of prior OC use, indicate the potential for variation in (1) aerobic performance due to an altered ventilatory response [37, 45], (2) anaerobic performance due to alterations in substrate utilization and buffering capacity [21, 27], and (3) reactive strength [29, 47]. Most data that are available on the effects of OC preparations on factors influencing performance include data on substrate utilization [3, 13–26], aerobic capacity [23, 24, 33–41], and body composition [23, 24, 41, 43, 57, 59–62], while less is understood regarding the effects of OC use on other factors that influence exercise performance including core body temperature, cardiovascular responses, anaerobic capacity, muscle strength or power, and postexercise recovery [10]. There is little evidence to suggest that the acute exogenous hormonal fluctuations observed across a single OC cycle have a significant effect on variables that impact aerobic performance. The variations in types of OC preparations used and the dosage of progesterone within the available studies relate to the observed variability in ventilation, VO_2, and substrate metabolism [29].

Results in the small number of studies to date are conflicting and disagreements abound between investigators regarding the effects and mechanisms involved in the variation in physiology and performance at different phases (active pill and hormone-free phases) within a single OC cycle. The current cross-sectional studies with small sample sizes should be viewed with caution due to the absence of randomization and variation in formulations used by participants [10]. Further studies on monophasic, triphasic, transdermal, and vaginal contraceptives are needed to evaluate the impact of exogenous steroids on all aspects of athletic performance. Future trials should be appropriately randomized and controlled [10]. There will likely be high inter-individual variability in response to the exogenous hormones contained in each hormonal contraceptive evaluated.

Variations between the experimental findings in available studies are likely caused by (1) the use of different types of OC agents (monophasic vs. triphasic preparations), (2) differences in exogenous hormone concentrations of the different OC formulations (as well as the androgenicity and potency of the progestin), (3) variation in defining the phases of an OC cycle and determination of testing days within an OC cycle, (4) small sample sizes in individual studies, (5) variation in the training status of participants, (6) variation in the exercise protocols used to test aerobic and anaerobic performance between investigations, and (7) variation in OC exposure prior to study initiation [10, 29]. The day of testing during a hormonal contraceptive cycle is important especially due to variation in dosing of exogenous steroids across a cycle [10]. In monophasic OC preparations, as well as transdermal and vaginal contraceptives, the same dose of EE and progestin is delivered across the entire active hormone phase followed by 7 days free from hormones. However, in triphasic OC preparations, there is a need to evaluate the impact of all three portions of the active pill phase and during the hormone-free phase to ensure that observed effects do not vary across the OC cycle [10]. There is also a need to account for the duration of hormonal contraceptive use when comparing the effects of a single OC cycle or multiple cycles observed in studies. The effects of OC usage on physiologic variables impacting exercise performance may change with the duration of OC use [10]. It is quite possible that the effects are more strongly observed within the first two hormonal contraceptive cycles, and, thereafter, the impact of OC use on exercise performance is negligible.

More research is necessary to determine the effects of the most commonly prescribed contraceptives (i.e., monophasic and triphasic OCs and the vaginal ring) on endurance performance. The current findings are unclear as to whether variation in oxygen uptake, ventilation, and exercise economy are influenced by changes in exogenous steroids used in monophasic and triphasic OCs. The influence of training status (sedentary, recreationally active, or elite), dose of exogenous steroids, and the duration of OC use on endurance performance still requires research.

Future studies should address the aforementioned issues in comparability, as well as examine the differences in effects of short-term and long-term consumption on athletic performance, off-label extension of cycles, and the effects of transdermal and vaginal contraceptives on performance. Expanding research to examine the differences in duration of use, off-label extension of cycles, as well as transdermal and vaginal contraceptives will assist in determining the mechanisms behind the impact of exogenous steroids on physiologic variables of performance. Strong consideration of the training status of participants, sample size, type of hormonal contraceptive, and days of testing during the hormonal contraceptive cycle should be made in all future studies. A wide variety of training statuses (e.g., sedentary, recreationally active, trained, and elite) have been evaluated to various degrees; however, the effects of OCs on athletic performance may be more important to elite athletes. Therefore, interpretation of results based on statistics and meaningful differences that are not statistically significant should also be considered. To allow determination of meaningful and statistical differences, future studies should ensure appropriate randomization for the design while maintaining adequate power when assessing the effects of hormonal contraception on performance. Evaluation of a single formulation within each study is important to assess the impact of specific EE and progestin potencies and androgenicities on exercise performance and will be necessary in the development of guidelines of OC use for athletes.

It is prudent that any female athlete considering hormonal contraception should talk with the general practitioner and consider not only the hormonal contraceptive formulation but also its potential impact on overall health and performance variables. The type of hormonal contraceptive (e.g., OC, transdermal contraceptive, or vaginal contraceptive) and the potency and androgenicity of the progestin determine the potential effects on performance and should be considered when deciding which hormonal contraceptive, if any, should be taken and when during the training period a hormonal contraceptive regimen should be initiated. The correct hormonal contraceptive choice for each athlete may be different; therefore, trying various formulations available on the market in an individualized manner for each athlete in conjunction with a general practitioner may be necessary. Further, it must be emphasized that OC use may not promote optimal health in athletes with the female athlete triad. As such, allowing a wide range of information to be available to athletes and support staff is important in allowing guidelines for OC use in athletes to be developed and based on sound scientific evidence.

References

1. Jones J, Mosher W, Daniels K. Current contraceptive use in the United States, 2006–2010, and changes in patterns of use since 1995. Natl Health Stat Report. 2012(60):1–25.
2. Brynhildsen J, Lennartsson H, Klemetz M, Dahlquist P, Hedin B, Hammar M. Oral contraceptive use among female elite athletes and age-matched controls and its relation to low back pain. Acta Obstet Gynecol Scand. 1997;76(9):873–8.
3. Bennell K, White S, Crossley K. The oral contraceptive pill: a revolution for sportswomen? Br J Sports Med. 1999;33(4):231–8.
4. Carr BR. Uniqueness of oral contraceptive progestins. Contraception. 1998; 58(3 Suppl):23 (S-27 S; quiz 67 S).
5. Burkman R, Bell C, Serfaty D. The evolution of combined oral contraception: improving the risk-to-benefit ratio. Contraception. 2011;84(1):19–34.
6. Nappi C, Di Spiezio Sardo A, Acunzo G, Bifulco G, Tommaselli GA, Guida M, Di Carlo C. Effects of a low-dose and ultra-low-dose combined oral contraceptive use on bone turnover and bone mineral density in young fertile women: a prospective controlled randomized study. Contraception. 2003;67(5):355–9.
7. Lawrie TA, Helmerhorst FM, Maitra NK, Kulier R, Bloemenkamp K, Gulmezoglu AM. Types of progestogens in combined oral contraception: effectiveness and side-effects. Cochrane Database Syst Rev. 2011(5):CD004861.
8. Oslakovic S, Zadro R. Comparison of the impact of four generations of progestins on hemostatic variables. Clin Appl Thromb Hemost. 2014;20(4):448–55.
9. Szarewski A, Mansour D, Shulman LP. 50 years of "The Pill": celebrating a golden anniversary. J Fam Plann Reprod Health Care. 2010;36(4):231–8.
10. Burrows M, Peters CE. The influence of oral contraceptives on athletic performance in female athletes. Sports Med. 2007;37(7):557–74.
11. Rubinstein ML, Halpern-Felsher BL, Irwin CE Jr. An evaluation of the use of the transdermal contraceptive patch in adolescents. J Adolesc Health. 2004;34(5):395–401.
12. Roumen FJ, D.R. Mishell J. The contraceptive vaginal ring, NuvaRing((R)), a decade after its introduction. Eur J Contracept Reprod Health Care. 2012;17(6):415–27.
13. Bemben DA, Boileau RA, Bahr JM, Nelson RA, Misner JE. Effects of oral contraceptives on hormonal and metabolic responses during exercise. Med Sci Sports Exerc. 1992;24(4):434–41.
14. Bonen A, Haynes FW, Graham TE. Substrate and hormonal responses to exercise in women using oral contraceptives. J Appl Physiol (1985). 1991;70(5):1917–27.
15. Casazza GA, Jacobs KA, Suh SH, Miller BF, Horning MA, Brooks GA. Menstrual cycle phase and oral contraceptive effects on triglyceride mobilization during exercise. J Appl Physiol (1985). 2004;97(1):302–9.
16. Spellacy WN. Carbohydrate metabolism during treatment with estrogen, progestogen, and low-dose oral contraceptives. Am J Obstet Gynecol. 1982;142(6 Pt 2):732–4.
17. Ashley CD, Kramer ML, Bishop P. Estrogen and substrate metabolism: a review of contradictory research. Sports Med. 2000;29(4):221–7.
18. Bernardes RP, Radomski MW. Growth hormone responses to continuous and intermittent exercise in females under oral contraceptive therapy. Eur J Appl Physiol Occup Physiol. 1998;79(1):24–9.
19. D'Eon TM, Sharoff C, Chipkin SR, Grow D, Ruby BC, Braun B. Regulation of exercise carbohydrate metabolism by estrogen and progesterone in women. Am J Physiol Endocrinol Metab. 2002;283(5):E1046–55.
20. Campbell SE, Febbraio MA. Effect of ovarian hormones on mitochondrial enzyme activity in the fat oxidation pathway of skeletal muscle. Am J Physiol Endocrinol Metab. 2001;281(4):E803–8.
21. Sunderland C, Tunaley V, Horner F, Harmer D, Stokes KA. Menstrual cycle and oral contraceptives' effects on growth hormone response to sprinting. Appl Physiol Nutr Metab. 2011;36(4):495–502.
22. Redman LM, Weatherby RP. Measuring performance during the menstrual cycle: a model using oral contraceptives. Med Sci Sports Exerc. 2004;36(1):130–6.
23. Jacobs KA, Casazza GA, Suh SH, Horning MA, Brooks GA. Fatty acid reesterification but not oxidation is increased by oral contraceptive use in women. J Appl Physiol (1985). 2005;98(5):1720–31.
24. Suh SH, Casazza GA, Horning MA, Miller BF, Brooks GA. Effects of oral contraceptives on glucose flux and substrate oxidation rates during rest and exercise. J Appl Physiol (1985). 2003;94(1):285–94.
25. Tremblay J, Peronnet F, Massicotte D, Lavoie C. Carbohydrate supplementation and sex differences in fuel selection during exercise. Med Sci Sports Exerc. 2010;42(7):1314–23.
26. Isacco L, Thivel D, Pelle AM, Zouhal H, Duclos M, Duche P, Boisseau N. Oral contraception and energy intake in women: impact on substrate oxidation during exercise. Appl Physiol Nutr Metab. 2012;37(4):646–56.
27. Rechichi C, Dawson B. Oral contraceptive cycle phase does not affect 200-m swim time trial performance. J Strength Cond Res. 2012;26(4):961–7.
28. Powers SK, Howley ET. Exercise metabolism. In: Powers SK, Howley ET, editors. Exercise physiology: theory and application to fitness and performance. McGraw Hill: New York; 2012 p. 68–90.
29. Rechichi C, Dawson B, Goodman C. Athletic performance and the oral contraceptive. Int J Sports Physiol Perform. 2009;4(2):151–62.
30. Akin JW. Contraception. In: Ireland ML, Nattiv A, editors. The female athlete. Saunders: Philadelphia; 2002 p. 157–64.
31. Saris WH, Antoine JM, Brouns F, Fogelholm M, Gleeson M, Hespel P, Jeukendrup AE, Maughan RJ, Pannemans D, Stich V. PASSCLAIM—physical performance and fitness. Eur J Nutr.

2003;42(Suppl 1):I50–95.
32. Bangsbo J, Mohr M, Poulsen A, Perez-Gomez J, Krustrup P. Training and testing the elite athlete. J Exerc Sci Fit. 2006;4(1):1–13.
33. Giacomoni M, Falgairette G. Decreased submaximal oxygen uptake during short duration oral contraceptive use: a randomized cross-over trial in premenopausal women. Ergonomics. 2000;43(10):1559–70.
34. Huisveld IA, Hospers JE, Bernink MJ, Erich WB, Bouma BN. The effect of oral contraceptives and exercise on hemostatic and fibrinolytic mechanisms in trained women. Int J Sports Med. 1983;4(2):97–103.
35. Joyce S, Sabapathy S, Bulmer A, Minahan C. Effect of long-term oral contraceptive use on determinants of endurance performance. J Strength Cond Res. 2013;27(7):1891–6.
36. Rebelo AC, Zuttin RS, Verlengia R, Cesar Mde C, de Sa MF, da Silva E. Effect of low-dose combined oral contraceptive on aerobic capacity and anaerobic threshold level in active and sedentary young women. Contraception. 2010;81(4):309–15.
37. Vaiksaar S, Jurimae J, Maestu J, Purge P, Kalytka S, Shakhlina L, Jurimae T. No effect of menstrual cycle phase and oral contraceptive use on endurance performance in rowers. J Strength Cond Res. 2011;25(6):1571–8.
38. Lynch NJ, De Vito G, Nimmo MA. Low dosage monophasic oral contraceptive use and intermittent exercise performance and metabolism in humans. Eur J Appl Physiol. 2001;84(4):296–301.
39. McNeill AW, Mozingo E. Changes in the metabolic cost of standardized work associated with the use of an oral contraceptive. J Sports Med Phys Fitness. 1981;21(3):238–44.
40. Casazza GA, Suh SH, Miller BF, Navazio FM, Brooks GA. Effects of oral contraceptives on peak exercise capacity. J Appl Physiol (1985). 2002;93(5):1698–702.
41. Lebrun CM, Petit MA, McKenzie DC, Taunton JE, Prior JC. Decreased maximal aerobic capacity with use of a triphasic oral contraceptive in highly active women: a randomised controlled trial. Br J Sports Med. 2003;37(4):315–20.
42. Joyce S, Sabapathy S, Bulmer AC, Minahan C. The effect of prior eccentric exercise on heavy-intensity cycling: the role of gender and oral contraceptives. Eur J Appl Physiol. 2014;114(5):995–1003.
43. Notelovitz M, Zauner C, McKenzie L, Suggs Y, Fields C, Kitchens C. The effect of low-dose oral contraceptives on cardiorespiratory function, coagulation, and lipids in exercising young women: a preliminary report. Am J Obstet Gynecol. 1987;156(3):591–8.
44. England SJ, Farhi LE. Fluctuations in alveolar CO2 and in base excess during the menstrual cycle. Respir Physiol. 1976;26(2):157–61.
45. Rechichi C, Dawson B, Goodman C. Oral contraceptive phase has no effect on endurance test. Int J Sports Med. 2008;29(4):277–81.
46. Redman LM, Scroop GC, Westlander G, Norman RJ. Effect of a synthetic progestin on the exercise status of sedentary young women. J Clin Endocrinol Metab. 2005;90(7):3830–7.
47. Rechichi C, Dawson B. Effect of oral contraceptive cycle phase on performance in team sport players. J Sci Med Sport. 2009;12(1):190–5.
48. Gaebelein CJ, L.C. Senay J. Vascular volume changes during cycling and stepping in women at two hydration levels. Eur J Appl Physiol Occup Physiol. 1982;48(1):1–10.
49. Lynch NJ, Nimmo MA. Effects of menstrual cycle phase and oral contraceptive use on intermittent exercise. Eur J Appl Physiol Occup Physiol. 1998;78(6):565–72.
50. Sunderland C, Nevill M. Effect of the menstrual cycle on performance of intermittent, high-intensity shuttle running in a hot environment. Eur J Appl Physiol. 2003;88(4–5):345–52.
51. Phillips SK, Sanderson AG, Birch K, Bruce SA, Woledge RC. Changes in maximal voluntary force of human adductor pollicis muscle during the menstrual cycle. J Physiol. 1996;496(Pt 2):551–7.
52. Sarwar R, Niclos BB, Rutherford OM. Changes in muscle strength, relaxation rate and fatiguability during the human menstrual cycle. J Physiol. 1996;493(Pt 1):267–72.
53. Elliott KJ, Cable NT, Reilly T. Does oral contraceptive use affect maximum force production in women? Br J Sports Med. 2005;39(1):15–9.
54. Peters C, Burrows M. Androgenicity of the progestin in oral contraceptives does not affect maximal leg strength. Contraception. 2006;74(6):487–91.
55. Ekenros L, Hirschberg AL, Heijne A, Friden C. Oral contraceptives do not affect muscle strength and hop performance in active women. Clin J Sport Med. 2013;23(3):202–7.
56. Bryner RW, Toffle RC, Ullrich IH, Yeater RA. Effect of low dose oral contraceptives on exercise performance. Br J Sports Med. 1996;30(1):36–40.
57. Coney P, Washenik K, Langley RG, DiGiovanna JJ, Harrison DD. Weight change and adverse event incidence with a low-dose oral contraceptive: two randomized, placebo-controlled trials. Contraception. 2001;63(6):297–302.
58. Rickenlund A, Carlstrom K, Ekblom B, Brismar TB, Von Schoultz B, Hirschberg AL. Effects of oral contraceptives on body composition and physical performance in female athletes. J Clin Endocrinol Metab. 2004;89(9):4364–70.
59. Bonny AE, Secic M, Cromer BA. A longitudinal comparison of body composition changes in adolescent girls receiving hormonal contraception. J Adolesc Health. 2009;45(4):423–5.
60. Tantbirojn P, Taneepanichskul S. Clinical comparative study of oral contraceptives containing 30 microg ethinylestradiol/150 microg levonorgestrel, and 35 microg ethinylestradiol/250 microg norgestimate in Thai women. Contraception. 2002;66(6):401–5.
61. Procter-Gray E, Cobb KL, Crawford SL, Bachrach LK, Chirra A, Sowers M, Greendale GA, Nieves JW, Kent K, Kelsey JL. Effect of oral contraceptives on weight and body composition in young female runners. Med Sci Sports Exerc. 2008;40(7):1205–12.

62. Gallo MF, Lopez LM, Grimes DA, Schulz KF, Helmerhorst FM. Combination contraceptives: effects on weight. Cochrane Database Syst Rev. 2006(1):CD003987.
63. Weaver CM, Teegarden D, Lyle RM, McCabe GP, McCabe LD, Proulx W, Kern M, Sedlock D, Anderson DD, Hillberry BM, Peacock M, Johnston CC. Impact of exercise on bone health and contraindication of oral contraceptive use in young women. Med Sci Sports Exerc. 2001;33(6):873–80.
64. Burr DB, Yoshikawa T, Teegarden D, Lyle R, McCabe G, McCabe LD, Weaver CM. Exercise and oral contraceptive use suppress the normal age-related increase in bone mass and strength of the femoral neck in women 18–31 years of age. Bone. 2000;27(6):855–63.
65. Hartard M, Bottermann P, Bartenstein P, Jeschke D, Schwaiger M. Effects on bone mineral density of low-dosed oral contraceptives compared to and combined with physical activity. Contraception. 1997;55(2):87–90.
66. Hartard M, Kleinmond C, Kirchbichler A, Jeschke D, Wiseman M, Weissenbacher ER, Felsenberg D, Erben RG. Age at first oral contraceptive use as a major determinant of vertebral bone mass in female endurance athletes. Bone. 2004;35(4):836–41.
67. Berenson AB, Radecki CM, Grady JJ, Rickert VI, Thomas A. A prospective, controlled study of the effects of hormonal contraception on bone mineral density. Obstet Gynecol. 2001;98(4):576–82.
68. Berenson AB, Breitkopf CR, Grady JJ, Rickert VI, Thomas A. Effects of hormonal contraception on bone mineral density after 24 months of use. Obstet Gynecol. 2004;103(5 Pt 1):899–906.
69. Hartard M, Kleinmond C, Luppa P, Zelger O, Egger K, Wiseman M, Weissenbacher ER, Felsenberg D, Erben RG. Comparison of the skeletal effects of the progestogens desogestrel and levonorgestrel in oral contraceptive preparations in young women: controlled, open, partly randomized investigation over 13 cycles. Contraception. 2006;74(5):367–75.
70. Endrikat J, Mih E, Dusterberg B, Land K, Gerlinger C, Schmidt W, Felsenberg D. A 3-year double-blind, randomized, controlled study on the influence of two oral contraceptives containing either 20 microg or 30 microg ethinylestradiol in combination with levonorgestrel on bone mineral density. Contraception. 2004;69(3):179–87.
71. Gai L, Jia Y, Zhang M, Gai P, Wang S, Shi H, Yu X, Liu Y. Effect of two kinds of different combined oral contraceptives use on bone mineral density in adolescent women. Contraception. 2012;86(4):332–6.
72. Gargano V, Massaro M, Morra I, Formisano C, Carlo CD, Nappi C. Effects of two low-dose combined oral contraceptives containing drospirenone on bone turnover and bone mineral density in young fertile women: a prospective controlled randomized study. Contraception. 2008;78(1):10–5.
73. Nappi C, Di Spiezio Sardo A, Greco E, Tommaselli GA, Giordano E, Guida M. Effects of an oral contraceptive containing drospirenone on bone turnover and bone mineral density. Obstet Gynecol. 2005;105(1):53–60.
74. Sordal T, Grob P, Verhoeven C. Effects on bone mineral density of a monophasic combined oral contraceptive containing nomegestrol acetate/17beta-estradiol in comparison to levonorgestrel/ethinylestradiol. Acta Obstet Gynecol Scand. 2012;91(11):1279–85.
75. Leung KC, Johannsson G, Leong GM, Ho KK. Estrogen regulation of growth hormone action. Endocr Rev. 2004;25(5):693–721.
76. Leger J, Mercat I, Alberti C, Chevenne D, Armoogum P, Tichet J, Czernichow P. The relationship between the GH/IGF-I axis and serum markers of bone turnover metabolism in healthy children. Eur J Endocrinol. 2007;157(5):685–92.
77. Hansen M, Miller BF, Holm L, Doessing S, Petersen SG, Skovgaard D, Frystyk J, Flyvbjerg A, Koskinen S, Pingel J, Kjaer M, Langberg H. Effect of administration of oral contraceptives in vivo on collagen synthesis in tendon and muscle connective tissue in young women. J Appl Physiol (1985). 2009;106(4):1435–43.
78. Gibbs JC, Williams NI, De Souza MJ. Prevalence of individual and combined components of the female athlete triad. Med Sci Sports Exerc. 2013;45(5):985–96.
79. Loucks AB, Verdun M, Heath EM. Low energy availability, not stress of exercise, alters LH pulsatility in exercising women. J Appl Physiol (1985). 1998;84(1):37–46.
80. Nattiv A, Loucks AB, Manore MM, Sanborn CF, Sundgot-Borgen J, Warren MP. American College of Sports Medicine position stand. The female athlete triad. Med Sci Sports Exerc. 2007;39(10):1867–82.
81. De Souza MJ, Nattiv A, Joy E, Misra M, Williams NI, Mallinson RJ, Gibbs JC, Olmsted M, Goolsby M, Matheson G. 2014 female athlete triad coalition consensus statement on treatment and return to play of the female athlete triad: 1st International Conference held in San Francisco, California, May 2012 and 2nd International Conference held in Indianapolis, Indiana, May 2013. Br J Sports Med. 2014;48(4):289.
82. De Souza MJ, Nattiv A, Joy E, Misra M, Williams NI, Mallinson RJ, Gibbs JC, Olmsted M, Goolsby M, Matheson G. 2014 female athlete triad coalition consensus statement on treatment and return to play of the female athlete triad: 1st International Conference held in San Francisco, CA, May 2012, and 2nd International Conference held in Indianapolis, IN, May 2013. Clin J Sport Med. 2014;24(2):96–119.
83. Carlson JL, Curtis M, Halpern-Felsher B. Clinician practices for the management of amenorrhea in the adolescent and young adult athlete. J Adolesc Health. 2007;40(4):362–5.
84. Mallinson RJ, De Souza MJ. Current perspectives on the etiology and manifestation of the "silent" component of the female athlete triad. Int J Womens Health. 2014;6:451–67.

18 Oxidative Stress and Infertility: A Possible Link to Exercise

Pieter Johann Maartens, Jason Peng, Ashok Agarwal, Diana Vaamonde and Stefan S. du Plessis

List of Abbreviations

ATP	Adenosine triphosphate
ART	Assisted reproductive technologies
CRH	Corticotropin-releasing hormone
ERK	Extracellular-signal-regulated kinases
FSH	Follicle-stimulating hormone
GnRH	Gonadotropin-releasing hormone
HPT	Hypothalamus–pituitary–testis
JNK	C-Jun N-Terminal Kinases
LH	Luteinizing hormone
MAPK	Mitogen-activated protein Kinases
MDA	Malondialdehyde
OS	Oxidative stress
PUFA	Polyunsaturated fatty acids
RNS	Reactive nitrogen species
ROS	Reactive oxygen species
SHBG	Sex-hormone-binding globulin

S. S. du Plessis (✉)
Division of Medical Physiology, Department of Biomedical Sciences, Stellenbosch University, P.O. Box 19063, Tygerberg 7505, Cape Town, South Africa
e-mail: ssdp@sun.ac.za

P. J. Maartens
Division of Medical Physiology, Faculty of Medicine and Health Sciences, Stellenbosh University, Cape Town, Tygerberg, South Africa

J. Peng
Center for Reproductive Medicine, Cleveland Clinic Foundation, Cleveland, OH, USA

A. Agarwal
American Center for Reproductive Medicine, Cleveland Clinic Foundation, Cleveland, OH, USA

D. Vaamonde
Department of Morphological Sciences, School of Medicine, Gynemed and Reproductive Care Center, University of Cordoba, International Network on Physical Exercise and Fertility (INPEF), Cordoba, Spain
e-mail: fivresearch@yahoo.com

Introduction

Infertility can be defined as the reduction in or absence of the capacity of a man and/or a woman to reproduce [1]. The term is generally used to reference the reproductive state of a couple who are sexually active without the use of contraceptives and yet are unable to achieve spontaneous natural pregnancy after a year of attempt. Both male and female reproductive impediments can contribute to infertility, and approximately 15% of the population in high-income countries and between 9 and 30% in low-income countries are affected [2–4]. One of the biggest issues remains that of the idiopathic component of infertility and the extent to which various lifestyle factors, such as exercise, possibly affect this phenomenon [5].

Oxidative stress (OS) is defined as an imbalance of reactive oxygen species (ROS) production and the detoxification of these molecules by antioxidative processes in the body. Antioxidants have a protective effect acting as scavengers of surplus ROS, and thus any external influence that can disturb this delicately balanced homeostasis is regarded a threat to the health of individuals [6–9]. ROS are free radicals that are natural by-products of energy production and cellular metabolism. Interestingly enough, they are required in physiological amounts as second messengers

© Springer Science+Business Media New York 2016

D. Vaamonde et al. (eds.), *Exercise and Human Reproduction*, DOI 10.1007/978-1-4939-3402-7_18

in signaling cascades as well as for immunological function. Furthermore, they are vital for the maturation and capacitation of spermatozoa and play a key role in fertilization. There is, however, a high association between pathological levels of ROS, the consequent onset of OS, and infertility. It is now generally accepted that OS accounts for approximately 30–80 % of these idiopathic infertility cases [10–14]. Despite this plausible link, couples are rarely screened or treated for elevated ROS levels [15].

Exercise has long been propagated by healthcare professionals as a natural remedy to ailing psychological, emotional, spiritual, and physical health. Sporting activities have vastly increased during recent decades due to both the evidence for improved health and the growing market for sport as a profession. Simultaneously, awareness of noncommunicable diseases and their risk factors has grown, and great emphasis is placed on the attributing effect of an unhealthy and sedentary lifestyle to the development of obesity and other health afflictions. Numerous studies have reported the beneficial outcome of exercise in combating and reversing such adverse effects [16, 17]. Positive associations between exercise and general indicators of fertility, such as semen parameters and hormone levels, have also been reported in several studies [18, 19]. The international increase in interest and participation in sports, both recreational and professional, has led to concern among researchers that ignorant and insufficient knowledge of training regimes could lead to excessive exercise that could cause homeostatic disturbances and elicit harmful side effects [20, 21]. Several studies have linked exercise to both OS and subfertility [22–26]. However, more conclusive research is necessary to question the intensities at which exercise is beneficial and detrimental to bodily functions. Bearing in mind that exercise and OS may constitute just some of the underlying contributing factors to infertility, this chapter aims to address OS as one of the main factors influencing infertility as well as highlighting a possible link among exercise and the aforementioned.

Table 18.1 Different types of reactive oxygen species (ROS)

Radicals		Non-radicals	
Hydroxyl	OH^-	Hypochloric acid	HOCl
Superoxide	$O_2^{-\bullet}$	Hydrogen peroxide	H_2O_2
Thyl	$RS^{-\bullet}$	Lipid peroxide	LOOH
Peroxyl	$RO_2^{\bullet}$	Ozone	O_3
Lipid peroxyl	$LOO^{\bullet}$	Singlet oxygen	$^{-1}O_2$

ROS and OS

Free radicals are molecules (oxygen or nitrogen) that have one or more unpaired electrons, making them highly reactive and susceptible to radical formation. There are three general forms of free radicals. The primary form of ROS is the superoxide anion radical, and the secondary subforms are all derived directly or indirectly from this radical [9, 15]. These secondary ROS are hydrogen peroxide, peroxyl radicals, and hydroxyl radicals (Table 18.1). The third group, known as the reactive nitrogen species (RNS), consists of nitrogen compound free radicals such as peroxynitrite, peroxy-nitrous acid, nitroxyl anions, and nitrous oxide [9]. ROS production results, as part of normal bodily functions, as a product of adenosine triphosphate (ATP) production via oxidative phosphorylation in the mitochondria [15, 27]. ROS is primarily produced by leukocytes but also by spermatozoa in the male reproductive system as part of natural metabolism. Studies have shown that the rate of ROS production in leukocytes is 1000 times greater than that of spermatozoa [28]. The body does, however, have natural defenses that are capable of inactivating ROS. These are known as the antioxidant enzymes, and their function is explained in Fig. 18.1. External influences can cause the production of excessive levels of ROS that overwhelm the natural defense mechanisms and result in damage to biomolecules. This process is termed OS [29, 30].

All cellular components including nucleic acids, lipids, and proteins are potentially OS targets as ROS are present in almost all tissues [31]. Free radicals predominantly attack the closest stable molecule altering that molecule and its

Superoxide Dismutase:

- Neutralizes superoxide anions by forming hydrogen peroxide and oxygen as products.

$$2O_2^- + 2H^+ \longrightarrow H_2O_2 + O_2$$

Catalase and Glutathione:

- Neutralize hydrogen peroxide anions by forming water and oxygen as products.

$$H_2O_2 + H_2O_2 \longrightarrow H_2O + O_2$$

Fig. 18.1 The primary antioxidant enzymes and their function

characteristics. ROS can be involved in a cascade of reactions which can damage a wide variety of biomolecules [32, 33]. OS can lead to oxidation of membrane lipids, DNA-related carbohydrates and amino acids, thereby affecting cell function and endangering cell survival [9, 29, 34]. The reproductive system is specifically vulnerable to oxidative damage as the plasma membranes of spermatozoa and testicular tissue are particularly rich in polyunsaturated fatty acids (PUFA) [35, 36]. Damaged sperm plasma membranes result in reduced sperm motility and ability to fertilize the oocyte. DNA damage has also been observed to be a common effect of OS. Damage, such as single and double strand breaks to the spermatozoon's DNA affects the embryo's paternal genetic contribution, and thus OS can have a telling influence on fertilization and development of the embryo [15]. Infertile patients presenting with normozoospermia, who are categorized as idiopathic infertile patients, generally present with higher levels of ROS and lower levels of antioxidants. This observation emphasizes the link between idiopathic infertility and OS and the need for more knowledge with regard to this subject [37, 38]. However, it is important to take note that a delicate balance exists between ROS and antioxidants, especially within the reproductive system. This is considered necessary for processes such as spermatogenesis to occur routinely, and it is only when this homeostasis is disturbed that malfunction occurs. An ideal example of this concept is hydrogen peroxide, which plays an integral role in tyrosine phosphorylation and the acrosome reaction. Hydrogen peroxide is therefore essential for proper binding of the spermatozoa to the zona pellucida [9, 29, 34]. Catalase, the antioxidant reducing hydrogen peroxide into water and oxygen, has also been indicated to be of importance for the preservation of sperm motility. Thus, the maintenance of a proper oxidative status in the reproductive system is essential to fertility and disturbing this harmony promotes subfertility [15].

Sources of ROS

While noted in the previous section that ROS are produced as a natural by-product of ATP generation, certain lifestyle choices and environmental exposures can also elicit excess ROS production and lead to OS. It is therefore important to identify possible sources of OS to improve oxidative infertility treatment/management. The following exposures have been linked to OS (as shown in Fig. 18.2):

- Tobacco usage has been linked to increased ROS production and OS. Studies have shown a 48% increase in seminal leukocyte concentration and a 107% increase in seminal ROS levels in smokers [39]. Decreased levels of antioxidants (specifically vitamins C and E) have likewise been observed in the seminal plasma of smokers [40, 41]. Smokers are also at a greater risk for DNA fragmentation than nonsmokers [39, 42, 43].

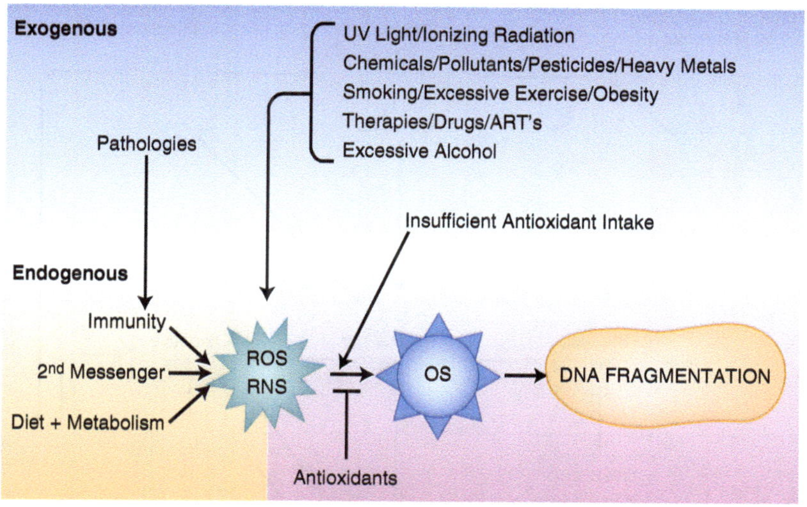

Fig. 18.2 Endogenous and exogenous sources of reactive oxygen species *(ROS)* and reactive nitrogen species *(RNS)* that can lead to oxidative stress *(OS)* if the balance with antioxidants is disturbed

- Diet and alcohol consumption affect ROS production. It is well established that the accumulation of adipose tissue in obesity leads to the release of pro-inflammatory cytokines, increased testicular temperature, and increased ROS generation by leukocytes [44–47]. Unhealthy diets, such as the antioxidant-deficient diet associated with excessive alcohol consumption, have also been linked to OS. Ethanol consumption has been shown to increase ROS production as well [15, 48–50].
- Environmental influences such as chemicals, ionizing radiation, and UV light exposure have all been linked to OS. Phthalates (plasticizers found in commonplace items such as food packaging and medical devices), pesticides, and heavy metals lead to cellular and DNA damage via OS [51–56]. Drugs, such as aspirin, increase enzymatic activity which can promote OS. Even in widely used methods, such as assisted reproductive technologies (ART), an increase in the likelihood of OS is observed as spermatozoa are exposed to centrifugation techniques, among others, while seminal antioxidants are removed during washing and cryopreservation [11–13, 57].
- Natural immune response that results from pathological infection, for example inflammation via leukocytes and macrophages, promotes OS [58, 59]. This can be observed in genital tract infections or current and past *Chlamydial* infections [60–62]. Prolonged periods of ischemia followed by spontaneous or surgical restoration of blood flow can furthermore lead to increased activation of leukocytes in the testicles thereby resulting in OS, germinal cell necrosis, and ultimately subfertility or infertility [15, 63, 64].
- Exercise is a source of stress that requires the body to produce large amounts of energy. With the resulting increase in metabolism, the increase in ROS production and decrease in antioxidant levels is inevitable [27–30]. This theory will subsequently be explored in further detail during the latter parts of this chapter.

The Effects of ROS and OS on Fertility

Mechanism of Cell Injury Due to OS

Cellular dysfunction can be caused by OS through any or a combination of the following mechanisms (as shown in Fig. 18.3): lipid peroxidation, DNA damage, redox-dependent signaling pathways, and apoptosis.

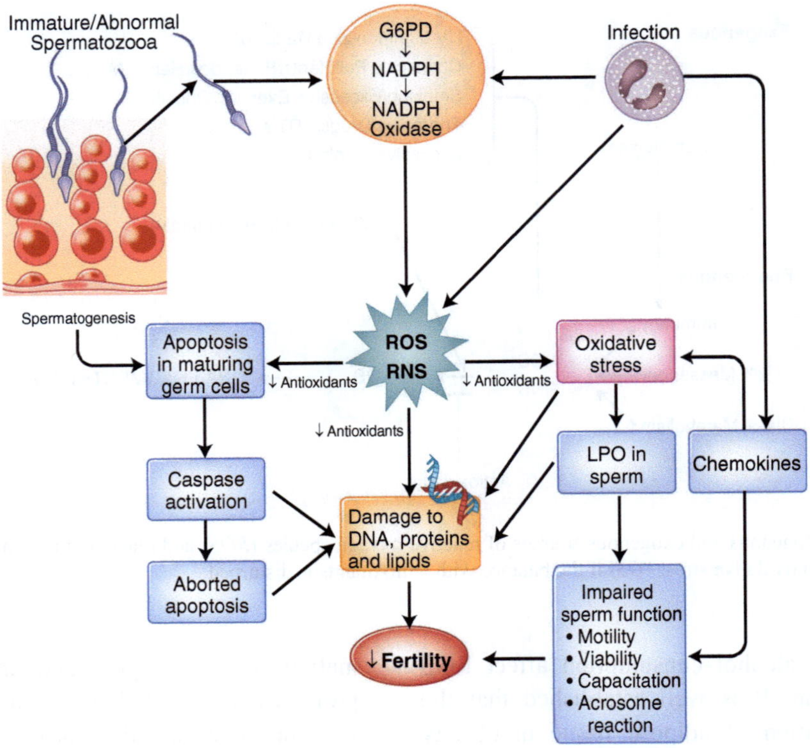

Fig. 18.3 Possible mechanisms of ROS/OS induced decrease in sperm function, DNA damage, and fertility. *ROS* reactive oxygen species, *RNS* reactive nitrogen species, *LPO* lipid peroxidation, *G6PD* glucose-6-phosphate dehydrogenase, *NADPH* nicotinamide adenine dinucleotide phosphate

As mentioned previously, PUFA present in cell membranes are especially susceptible to oxidative insult resulting in lipid peroxidation. Break down or peroxidation of these fatty acids leads to loss of membrane fluidity as well as the formation of various oxidatively modified products which are toxic to cells [7, 65]. Phosphodiester backbones and DNA bases are some of the other sites that are primarily susceptible to OS. In this instance, ROS-mediated peroxidative damage results in DNA fragmentation and cellular damage.

Increases in ROS have been observed to induce redox-dependent signaling, thereby modifying the activity of various intracellular signaling molecules and pathways. Such pathways can activate tyrosine kinases, which inhibit tyrosine phosphatase activity, while modifying the activity of the mitogen-activated protein kinases (MAPK). Some of these kinases such as p38 MAPK, c-Jun N-terminal kinase (JNK), and extracellular-signal-regulated kinases (ERK) [66] may initiate a chain of reactions that ultimately lead to apoptosis [67]. Studies have also linked the acceleration of the process of apoptosis to ROS-induced DNA damage [68].

Effects of OS on Female Fertility

Female infertility is most commonly observed to be of somatic cell origin and has an endocrine involvement, often amenable to pharmacological treatment [69, 70].

Various reviews have associated reproductive oxidative toxicity to electron transfer–ROS–OS associations [71]. The excess of free radicals in the female reproductive system can lead to reproductive pathologies of the genital tract [72]. Studies have found definite links midst the onset of

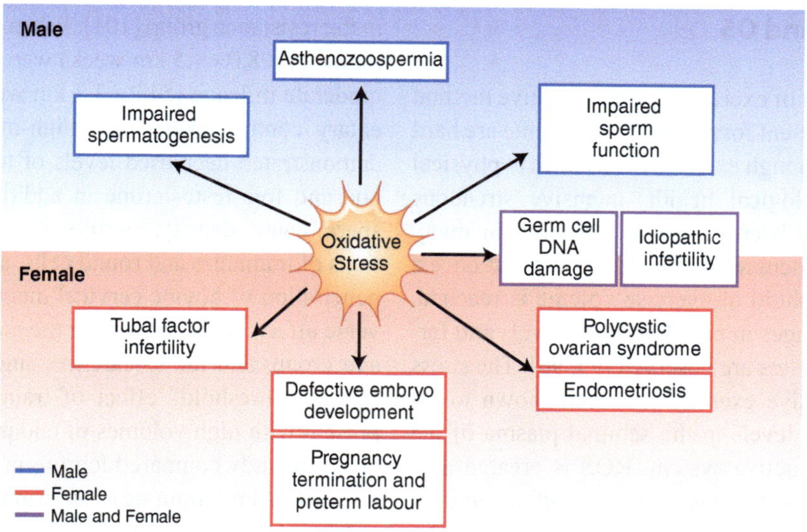

Fig. 18.4 The effect of oxidative stress on fertility

OS and the development of endometriosis, tubal factor infertility, polycystic ovarian disease, unexplained infertility, adverse embryonic development, preterm labor, and recurrent pregnancy loss (see Fig. 18.4) [72–76]. OS in the female reproductive tract can also severely affect oogenesis and embryo development. These aforementioned pathologies are attributed to various mechanisms including lipid peroxidation, DNA damage, inhibition of protein synthesis, mitochondrial alterations, and depletion of ATP [77–79].

Effects of OS on Male Fertility

The presence of free radicals in semen samples was reported as early as 1943 when a loss of sperm motility was observed in an oxygenated medium [80, 81]. This effect could be alleviated by the addition of catalase, an antioxidant enzyme, responsible for the reduction of hydrogen peroxide. OS was thus identified as the causative factor for the adverse effects displayed by spermatozoa [80].

The most commonly observed cause of male infertility is defective sperm function. With regard to idiopathic infertility, most men who are categorized as infertile present with sufficient amounts of spermatozoa and have normal levels of endocrine function, but the gametes that are produced are often morphologically flawed [80]. Spermatozoa and gametes seem to suffer multiple defects that researchers attribute to the influence of OS (shown in Fig. 18.4) [82]. Inept characteristics of spermatozoa include impaired motility, impaired ability to penetrate the cervical mucus as well as the inability to timeously acrosome react, bind to the zona pellucida, and fuse with the oocyte's membrane [83–85]. The lipid peroxidation and axonemal protein phosphorylation associated with OS have been suggested as possible mechanisms for decreased sperm motility [86].

Another major contributing factor is the lack of naturally occurring antioxidant enzymes in the cytoplasm of spermatozoa [87]. Mitochondria are located in the spermatozoa midpiece and are generally responsible for oxidative phosphorylation that energizes the spermatozoon and generates ROS as a by-product. Mitochondrial DNA, when compared to nuclear DNA, is 10–17 times faster in accumulating mutations and polymorphisms. Such mutations may also result in ultrastructural defects and abnormal sperm morphology [88–91]. Free radicals are able to attack DNA at multiple points, that is, the pyrimidine and purine bases as well as the deoxyribose backbone. If DNA damage accumulates, it eventually leads to poor blastocyst formation in vitro and higher rates of miscarriage [9, 92–94].

Exercise and OS

The benefits of exercise as a preventative method and/or treatment for metabolic syndrome are hard to ignore. Though exercise contributes to physical and psychological health, intensive strenuous exercise has been linked to infertility in many studies as discussed below. It appears that once a certain threshold of exercise volume is reached, clinical changes in both hormonal levels and fertility parameters are observed [95, 96]. The stress from excessive exercise has been shown to increase ROS levels in the seminal plasma of the male reproductive system. ROS is created as a by-product of aerobic exercise and respiration and oxygen consumption increases 20-fold from rest to high activity. It is thus postulated that ROS can leak from the mitochondria due to elevated oxygen flow through the mitochondrial electron-transport pathway as muscle-based aerobic metabolism produces large amounts of ROS [97]. Raised temperatures, heat stress, and dehydration may lead to amplified rates of oxidative DNA damage in germ cells and hence more mutations in the resulting spermatozoa [98]. Exercise has also been correlated with leukocyte activation and the promotion of OS [24]. The observed link of excessive exercise and infertility may thus be directly attributable to OS. A related mechanism of action is believed to adversely affect the female reproductive system. There is, however, some debate as to exactly how and to what extent this takes place and as to how the difference in the hormonal profiles of the different genders affects the oxidative profile of the body [99].

Studies conducted on males have demonstrated that high levels of endurance cycling (40 min/day at least 3 days/week) negatively affect sperm morphology [100]. A cross-sectional study evaluated the difference between the hormonal profiles of endurance-trained athletes (runners) and resistance-trained athletes (weight lifting) and found that plasma levels of total testosterone and serum levels of free testosterone were significantly lower in both these types of exercise as compared to the controls. Sperm density, motility, and morphology were significantly lowered in the endurance group, while sperm penetration of the cervical mucus was significantly lowered in the resistance group [101]. When high-mileage runners (108.0 ± 4.5 km/week) were compared to moderate mileage (54.2 ± 3.7 km/week) and sedentary control groups, the high-mileage group demonstrated decreased levels of total testosterone and free testosterone in addition to altered sperm count, density, motility, increased populations of immature and round cells, and decreased penetration of bovine cervical mucus. These adverse effects were not seen in the moderate-mileage group, and the researchers suggested that a "volume-threshold" effect of training could be present with high volumes of endurance running [102]. A study compared long-term moderate-intensity treadmill running (~60 % maximal oxygen uptake- VO_2max) and high-intensity treadmill running (~80 % VO_2max) over a 60-week period integrating five sessions per week of exercise, each session lasting 120 min. The study evaluated the hypothalamus–pituitary–testis (HPT) axis by monitoring levels of sex-hormone-binding globulin (SHBG), luteinizing hormone (LH), and follicle-stimulating hormone (FSH) responses to gonadotropin-releasing hormone (GnRH). Long-term high-intensity training was associated with declined sperm parameters after 24 weeks of exercise and both high- and low-intensity groups showed decreased serum- and free testosterone levels and decreased levels of LH and FSH after 12 weeks of exercise. SHBG increased in both groups after 12 weeks of exercise, while blunted LH and FSH responses to GnRH were observed in both groups. These disturbances were rectified after a 36-week recovery period. The group concluded that long-term strenuous treadmill exercises have a deleterious effect on reproduction. They proposed a mechanism of increased cortisol secretion during training mobilizing fuel stores and subsequently inhibiting GnRH secretion in addition to directly inhibiting the HPT axis function at the hypothalamic–pituitary level as well as inhibiting Leydig cell function via corticotropin-releasing hormone (CRH) receptors, the effect being an altered HPT axis and manifesting as a decrease in LH, FSH, and testosterone levels [103]. Therefore, when examining exercise in relation to male fertility, the intensity, type, and amount of exercise are important.

Acute exhaustive training in humans (pedaling >60 rev/min, VO_2max until exhaustion) was linked to a 26% increase in plasma lipid peroxides as markers of OS, while moderate- to low-intensity training (<70% VO_2max) decreased lipid peroxides by 10.3% [25]. In an attempt to explain this phenomenon, some studies have suggested that mitochondria may play less of a role than initially thought and that heme proteins might play more of a determining role in the onset of OS [26]. Other factors, such as the decreased testosterone and antioxidant (e.g., glutathione) levels may result in increased levels of immature spermatozoa which may stimulate ROS production due to incomplete cytoplasm extrusion [104, 105].

In vivo animal studies investigating the link between infertility, exercise, and OS reported some interesting results. Acute exhaustive running (running 17 m/min until exhaustion) was tested in rats and correlated with increased erythrocyte lipid peroxidation and leukocyte activity within a 24 h-follow-up period [24]. A study using Wistar rats investigated the link between intensive chronic exercise and OS in the male reproductive system. When the experimental group, subjected to intensive swimming exercises, was compared to the control group, a decrease in both plasma testosterone and LH was observed. Furthermore, a detrimental effect on spermatogenesis was noted, elevated levels of lipid peroxidation were found, and the antioxidant activities of superoxide dismutase, catalase, and glutathione were decreased [106]. The authors believed these observations to be responsible for decreased reproductive activities such as steroidogenesis and spermatogenesis. Similar results were found in a study done by the same group examining the effects of different gradients of exercise on subjects. The study reported that the most pronounced results were found in the group subjected to the highest level of exercise [107]. Another study compared sedentary mice to mice exposed to a lifelong regular running plan (1.75 km/day). The study found that running protected against age-related histological changes as well as age-related OS. Running was also associated with fewer biomarkers for lipid peroxidation and protein oxidation, while sedentary mice had elevated levels of antioxidants. The study suggested that this was a mechanism to counteract the oxidative damage that comes with age. The results from these studies therefore clearly suggest that while intensive/exhaustive exercise is detrimental to reproductive health properly sustained amounts of exercise can help reduce the risk of OS [108].

Comparable results were found in human studies. When comparing OS biomarkers and antioxidant levels in elite athletes to recreationally active men, recreationally active men presented with elevated levels of antioxidants. These results pointed to them developing better antioxidant defenses compared to elite athletes. This observation was also accompanied by reduced biomarkers of OS and decreased rates of sperm DNA fragmentation [109]. Another study compared elite athletes (regular 2 h sessions of high-intensity endurance training for 4–5 days per week, 180–190 beats/min, and a maximum oxygen consumption of 58–67 mL/min/kg), recreationally active men (low-to-moderate intensity recreational physical activities, 127–132 beats/min, and a maximum oxygen consumption of 47–53 mL/min/kg), and sedentary men (maximum oxygen consumption of less than 37 mL/min/kg). The study found elite athletes to have a higher number of seminal OS biomarkers (seminal 8-Isoprostane, ROS, and malondialdehyde (MDA), and lower levels of antioxidants (super oxide dismutase, catalase, and total antioxidant capacity) than both of the other groups. The recreationally active men had higher levels of antioxidants and lower amounts of OS biomarkers compared to both elite athletes and sedentary, non-active males [110].

The effects of OS, as well as the adverse effects of excess exercise, on the female reproductive system have been well documented. Excess exercise has been associated with delayed menarche, primary and secondary amenorrhea, oligomenorrhea, and decreased fertility even prevalent when using in vitro fertilization as treatment. Such occurrences are especially prevalent among athletes, vary with athletic discipline and level of competition, and are primarily attributed to hypothalamic dysfunction and disturbances in GnRH pulsatility but also to increased levels of stress and energy imbalances [22, 111–114].Studies conducted on the oxidative profile of females that exercise, however, seem to be in much lesser quantity and far less conclusive about which OS associated mechanism is responsible for these adverse effects [99]. This observation could be explained by the reluctance of researchers to work with female subjects due to the increased variability (as observed during the menstrual cycle) associated with the hormonal differences between men and women. Studies have found that females have lesser levels of OS and higher levels of antioxidant enzyme activity at rest compared to men [115–117]. Studies have also associated acute exercise with differences in vitamin C, E, and glutathione levels amid males and females [118]. Estrogen has also been linked to several antioxidant properties in both in vitro and in vivo studies and some researchers have postulated that this proves females to be less prone to OS and thus explains their longer life expectancy [119–122]. In response to these claims, many research groups have investigated the significance in exercise-associated OS between men and women and found no such difference [113, 114, 118, 123, 124]. Though the evidence of female reproductive irregularities due to exercise induced OS seems to be less pronounced and rather inconclusive, researchers still maintain that the most probable mechanism of action is induced via OS [99].

Conclusion

While a great amount of literature is available on exercise, OS, and reproductive dysfunction, the link between all three is still important to explore. This may reveal major mechanisms and biomarkers in infertility that might aid with diagnosing and treating patients in the future. It has been well established that OS is detrimental to reproduction. With regard to exercise, most studies report that moderate exercise is good for reproductive parameters, while intensive chronic exercise is detrimental to reproduction. The literature clearly attributes these observations to oxidative mechanisms, while the effect of the differences in the hormonal profile of different genders is not well understood and should be further investigated. Thus, the general belief that health benefits result from repeated exercise can be endorsed by health-care professionals as long as the exercise remains in moderation. The threshold with regard to intensive exercise and reproductive health, applicable especially to professional athletes, is less clear and more research and careful clinical discretion is required.

References

1. Brink A, Lochner J. Infertility, Obesity, Cigarette Smoke. In: Brink A, Lochner J, editors. Pharos dictionary for the health sciences. Cape Town: Pharos Dictionaries; 2011. p. 359, 725, 869.
2. Healy D, Trounson A, Andersen A. Female infertility: causes and treatment. Lancet. 1994;343:1539–44.
3. World Health Organization Task force on the diagnosis and treatment of infertility. Workshop on the investigation of subfertile couple. In: Ratnam S, Eng-Soon T, Anandakumar C, editors. Releasing hormones: and genetics and immunology in human reproduction. Advances in fertility and sterility. Carnforth: Parthenon Publishing; 1987. p. 5–56.
4. Ombelet W, Cooke I, Dyer S, Serour G, Devroey P. Infertility and the provision of infertility medical services in developing countries. Hum Reprod Upd. 2008;14(6):605–21.
5. Arce J, De Souza M. Exercise and male factor infertility. Sport Med. 1993;15(3):146–69.
6. Sikka SC, Rajasekaran M, Hellstrom WJ. Role of oxidative stress and antioxidants in male infertility. J Androl. 1995;16(6):464–8.
7. Sharma RK, Agarwal A. Role of reactive oxygen species in male infertility. Urology. 1996;48(6):835–50.
8. Sikka SC. Relative impact of oxidative stress on male reproductive function. Curr Med Chem. 2001;8(7):851–62.
9. Hwang K, Lamb D. Molecular mechanisms of antioxidants in male infertility. In: Parekattil SJ, Agarwal A, editors. Male infertility. New York: Springer Verlag; 2012. p. 45–54.
10. Zini A, de Lamirande E, Gagnon C. Reactive oxygen species in semen of infertile patients: levels of superoxide dismutase- and catalase-like activities in seminal plasma and spermatozoa. Int J Androl. 1993;16(3):183–8.
11. Iwasaki A, Gagnon C. Formation of reactive oxygen species in spermatozoa of infertile patients. Fertil Steril. 1992;57(2):409–16.

12. Ochsendorf FR, Thiele J, Fuchs J, Schuttau H, Freisleben HJ, Buslau M, et al. Chemiluminescence in semen of infertile men. Andrologia. 1994;26(5):289–93.
13. Shekarriz M, DeWire DM, Thomas AJ Jr, Agarwal A. A method of human semen centrifugation to minimize the iatrogenic sperm injuries caused by reactive oxygen species. Europ Urol. 1995;28(1):31–5.
14. Shekarriz M, Thomas AJ Jr, Agarwal A. Incidence and level of seminal reactive oxygen species in normal men. Urology. 1995;45(1):103–7.
15. Tremellen K. Oxidative stress and male infertility-a clinical perspective. Hum Reprod Update. 2008;14(3):243–58.
16. Palmer N, Bakos H, Owens J, Setchell B, Lane M. Diet and exercise in an obese mouse fed a high-fat diet improve metabolic health and reverse perturbed sperm function. Am J Phys Endocrinol Metab. 2012;302(7):E768–80.
17. Khullar K, Agarwal A, Du Plessis SS. A hormonal, physical, and proteomic view of obesity-induced effects on male infertility and possible lifestyle modifications. Asian Pac J Reprod. 2012;1(2):161–8.
18. Vaamonde D, Da Silva-Grigoletto M, Garcia-Manso J. Sperm and hormonal differences between physically active and sedentary subjects: European congress of sport sciences. Proceedings of the 14th Annual Congress of the European College of Sport Sciences; Olso, Norway; June 2009; Editors: Loland S, Bø K, Fasting K, Hallèn J, Ommundsen Y, Roberts G, Tsolakidis E; Gamlebyen Grafiske A, Oslo, Greenland; 2009.
19. Vaamonde D, Da Silva-Grigoletto M, Garcia-Manso J, Vaamonde-Lemos R. Improved values of gonadotropins in physically active subjects: European congress of sport sciences. Proceedings of the 15th Annual Congress of the European Congress of Sport Sciences; June 2010; Middle East Technical University, Antalya, Turkey; 2010.
20. Vaamonde D, Da Silva-Grigoletto M, Garcia-Manso J, Vaamonde-Lemos R, Swanson RJ, Oehninger SC. Response of semen parameters to three training modalities. Fertil Steril. 2009;92(6):1941–6.
21. Mastorakos G, Pavlatou M, Diamanti-Kandarakis E, Chrousos G. Exercise and the stress system. Hormones. 2005;4(2):73–89.
22. Olive DL. Exercise and fertility: an update. Curr Opin Obstet Gyne. 2010;22(4):259–63.
23. Ihara H, Shino Y, Morita Y, Kawaguchi E, Hashizume N, Yoshida M. Is skeletal muscle damaged by the oxidative stress following anaerobic exercise? J Clin Lab Anal. 2001;15(5):239–43.
24. Temiz A, Baskurt OK, Pekcetin C, Kandemir F, Gure A. Leukocyte activation, oxidant stress and red blood cell properties after acute, exhausting exercise in rats. Clin Hemor Microcirc. 2000;22(4):253–9.
25. Lovlin R, Cottle W, Pyke I, Kavanagh M, Belcastro AN. Are indices of free radical damage related to exercise intensity. Europ J App Phys Occup Phys. 1987;56(3):313–6.
26. Cooper CE, Vollaard NB, Choueiri T, Wilson MT. Exercise, free radicals and oxidative stress. Biochem Soc Transac. 2002;30(2):280–5.
27. Valko M, Leibfritz D, Moncol J, Cronin MT, Mazur M, Telser J. Free radicals and antioxidants in normal physiological functions and human disease. Int J Biochem Cell Biol. 2007;39(1):44–84.
28. Plante M, de Lamirande E, Gagnon C. Reactive oxygen species released by activated neutrophils, but not by deficient spermatozoa, are sufficient to affect normal sperm motility. Fertil Steril. 1994;62(2):387–93.
29. Ochsendorf FR. Infections in the male genital tract and reactive oxygen species. Hum Reprod Update. 1999;5(5):399–420.
30. Cocuzza M, Sikka SC, Athayde KS, Agarwal A. Clinical relevance of oxidative stress and sperm chromatin damage in male infertility: an evidence based analysis. Int Braz J Urol. 2007;33(5):603–21.
31. Maneesh M, Jayalekshmi H. Role of reactive oxygen species and antioxidants on pathophysiology of male reproduction. Indian J Clinical Biochem. 2006;21(2):80–9.
32. Makker K, Agarwal A, Sharma R. Oxidative stress & male infertility. Indian J Med Res. 2009;129(4):357–67.
33. Gorczyca W, Gong J, Darzynkiewicz Z. Detection of DNA strand breaks in individual apoptotic cells by the in situ terminal deoxynucleotidyl transferase and nick translation assays. Cancer Res. 1993;53(8):1945–51.
34. de Lamirande E, Cagnon C. Human sperm hyperactivation and capacitation as parts of an oxidative process. Free Rad Biol Med. 1993;14(2):157–66.
35. Radak Z, Sasvari M, Nyakas C, Pucsok J, Nakamoto H, Goto S. Exercise preconditioning against hydrogen peroxide-induced oxidative damage in proteins of rat myocardium. Arch Biochem Biophys. 2000;376(2):248–51.
36. Ghosh D, Das UB, Ghosh S, Mallick M, Debnath J. Testicular gametogenic and steroidogenic activities in cyclophosphamide treated rat: a correlative study with testicular oxidative stress. Drug Chem Toxicol. 2002;25(3):281–92.
37. Pasqualotto FF, Sharma RK, Kobayashi H, Nelson DR, Thomas AJ Jr, Agarwal A. Oxidative stress in normospermic men undergoing infertility evaluation. J Androl. 2001;22(2):316–22.
38. Agarwal A, Sharma RK, Nallella KP, Thomas AJ Jr, Alvarez JG, Sikka SC. Reactive oxygen species as an independent marker of male factor infertility. Fertil Steril. 2006;86(4):878–85.
39. Saleh RA, Agarwal A, Sharma RK, Nelson DR, Thomas AJ Jr. Effect of cigarette smoking on levels of seminal oxidative stress in infertile men: a prospective study. Fertil Steril. 2002;78(3):491–9.
40. Fraga CG, Motchnik PA, Wyrobek AJ, Rempel DM, Ames BN. Smoking and low antioxidant levels increase oxidative damage to sperm DNA. Mutat Res. 1996;351(2):199–203.

41. Mostafa T, Tawadrous G, Roaia MM, Amer MK, Kader RA, Aziz A. Effect of smoking on seminal plasma ascorbic acid in infertile and fertile males. Andrologia. 2006;38(6):221–4.
42. Sepaniak S, Forges T, Fontaine B, Gerard H, Foliguet B, Guillet-May F, et al. Negative impact of cigarette smoking on male fertility: from spermatozoa to the offspring. J Gyne Obstet Biol Reprod. 2004;33(5):384–90.
43. Trummer H, Habermann H, Haas J, Pummer K. The impact of cigarette smoking on human semen parameters and hormones. Hum Reprod. 2002;17(6): 1554–9.
44. Banks S, King SA, Irvine DS, Saunders PT. Impact of a mild scrotal heat stress on DNA integrity in murine spermatozoa. Reproduction. 2005;129(4):505–14.
45. Ishii T, Matsuki S, Iuchi Y, Okada F, Toyosaki S, Tomita Y, et al. Accelerated impairment of spermatogenic cells in SOD1-knockout mice under heat stress. Free Radical Res. 2005;39(7):697–705.
46. Perez-Crespo M, Pintado B, Gutierrez-Adan A. Scrotal heat stress effects on sperm viability, sperm DNA integrity, and the offspring sex ratio in mice. Molec Reprod Develop. 2008;75(1):40–7.
47. Singer G, Granger DN. Inflammatory responses underlying the microvascular dysfunction associated with obesity and insulin resistance. Microcirculation. 2007;14(4–5):375–87.
48. Koch OR, Pani G, Borrello S, Colavitti R, Cravero A, Farre S, et al. Oxidative stress and antioxidant defenses in ethanol-induced cell injury. Molec Aspect Med. 2004;25(1–2):191–8.
49. Villalta J, Ballesca JL, Nicolas JM, Martinez de Osaba MJ, Antunez E, Pimentel C. Testicular function in asymptomatic chronic alcoholics: relation to ethanol intake. Alcohol Clin Exp Res. 1997;21(1):128–33.
50. Wu D, Cederbaum AI. Alcohol, oxidative stress, and free radical damage. Alcoh Res Health. 2003;27(4):277–84.
51. Agarwal DK, Maronpot RR, Lamb JCt, Kluwe WM. Adverse effects of butyl benzyl phthalate on the reproductive and hematopoietic systems of male rats. Toxicology. 1985;35(3):189–206.
52. Kasahara E, Sato EF, Miyoshi M, Konaka R, Hiramoto K, Sasaki J, et al. Role of oxidative stress in germ cell apoptosis induced by di(2-ethylhexyl) phthalate. Biochem J. 2002;365(Pt 3):849–56.
53. Hauser R, Meeker JD, Singh NP, Silva MJ, Ryan L, Duty S, et al. DNA damage in human sperm is related to urinary levels of phthalate monoester and oxidative metabolites. Hum Reprod. 2007;22(3):688–95.
54. Chitra KC, Sujatha R, Latchoumycandane C, Mathur PP. Effect of lindane on antioxidant enzymes in epididymis and epididymal sperm of adult rats. Asian J Androl. 2001;3(3):205–8.
55. Latchoumycandane C, Chitra KC, Mathur PP. 2,3,7,8-tetrachlorodibenzo- p-dioxin (TCDD) induces oxidative stress in the epididymis and epididymal sperm of adult rats. Arch Toxicol. 2003;77(5):280–4.
56. Xu DX, Shen HM, Zhu QX, Chua L, Wang QN, Chia SE, et al. The associations among semen quality, oxidative DNA damage in human spermatozoa and concentrations of cadmium, lead and selenium in seminal plasma. Mutat Res. 2003;534(1–2):155–63.
57. Agarwal A, Said TM. Oxidative stress, DNA damage and apoptosis in male infertility: a clinical approach. BJU Int. 2005;95(4):503–7.
58. Roos D. The involvement of oxygen radicals in microbicidal mechanisms of leukocytes and macrophages. Klin Wochens. 1991;69(21–23):975–80.
59. Mazzilli F, Rossi T, Marchesini M, Ronconi C, Dondero F. Superoxide anion in human semen related to seminal parameters and clinical aspects. Fertil Steril. 1994;62(4):862–8.
60. Padron OF, Brackett NL, Sharma RK, Lynne CM, Thomas AJ Jr, Agarwal A. Seminal reactive oxygen species and sperm motility and morphology in men with spinal cord injury. Fertil Steril. 1997;67(6):1115–20.
61. Brackett NL, Ibrahim E, Grotas JA, Aballa TC, Lynne CM. Higher sperm DNA damage in semen from men with spinal cord injuries compared with controls. J Androl. 2008;29(1):93–9. (discussion 100-1).
62. Segnini A, Camejo MI, Proverbio F. Chlamydia trachomatis and sperm lipid peroxidation in infertile men. Asian J Androl. 2003;5(1):47–9.
63. Turner TT, Bang HJ, Lysiak JL. The molecular pathology of experimental testicular torsion suggests adjunct therapy to surgical repair. J Urol. 2004;172(6–2):2574–8.
64. Filho DW, Torres MA, Bordin AL, Crezcynski-Pasa TB, Boveris A. Spermatic cord torsion, reactive oxygen and nitrogen species and ischemia-reperfusion injury. Molec Aspect Med. 2004;25(1–2):199–210.
65. Jones R, Mann T, Sherins R. Peroxidative breakdown of phospholipids in human spermatozoa, spermicidal properties of fatty acid peroxides, and protective action of seminal plasma. Fertil Steril. 1979;31(5), 531–7.
66. Bahorun T, Soobratte MA, Luximon-Ramma V, Aruoma OI. Free radicals and antioxidants in cardiovascular health and disease. Internet J Med Update. 2006;1(2):25–41.
67. Agarwal A, Allamaneni SS. Oxidants and antioxidants in human fertility. Midd East Fertil Soc J. 2004;9(3):187–97.
68. Sikka SC. Role of oxidative stress and antioxidants in andrology and assisted reproductive technology. J Androl. 2004;25(1):5–18.
69. Duckitt K. Infertility and subfertility. Clin Evid. 2003;9:2044–73.
70. Eskandari N. Infertility. In: Cherney A, editors. Current obstetrics and gynecologi diagnosis and treatment. 9th edn. New York: McGraw-Hill; 2003. p. 979–1000.
71. Kovacic P, Jacintho J. Reproductive toxins: pervasive theme of oxidative stress and electron transfer. Curr Med Chem. 2001;8(7):863–92.

72. Agarwal A, Gupta S, Sharma R. Role of oxidative stress in female reproduction. Reprod Biol Endocrinol. 2005;3:28.
73. Agarwal A, Gupta S, Sharma R. Oxidative stress and its implications in female infertility—a clinician's perspective. Reprod Biomed Online. 2005;11(5):641–50.
74. Bedaiwy M, Falcone T, Sharma R, Goldberg J, Attaran M, Nelson D, et al. Prediction of endometriosis with serum and peritoneal fluid markers: a prospective controlled trial. Hum Reprod. 2002;17(2):426–31.
75. Pressman E, Cavanaugh J, Mingione M, Norkus E, Woods J. Effects of maternal antioxidant supplementation on maternal and fetal antioxidant levels: a randomized, double-blind study. Am J Obstet Gynecol. 2003;189(6):1720–5.
76. Wall P, Pressman E, Woods J. Preterm premature rupture of the membranes and antioxidants: the free radical connection. J Perinat Med. 2002;30(6):447–57.
77. Cooke M, Evans M, Dizdaroglu M, Lunec J. Oxidative DNA damage: mechanisms, mutation, and disease. Faseb J. 2003;17(10):1195–214.
78. Halliwell B, Gutteridge J. Free radicals and antioxidant protection: mechanisms and significance in toxicology and disease. Hum Toxicol. 1988;7(1):7–13.
79. Ray S, Lam T, Rotollo J, Phadke S, Patel C, Dontabhaktuni A, et al. Oxidative stress is the master operator of drug and chemically-induced programmed and unprogrammed cell death: Implications of natural antioxidants in vivo. Biofactors. 2004;21(1–4):223–32.
80. Aitken R, Baker M. Oxidative stress and male reproductive biology. Reprod Fertil Dev. 2004;16(5):581–8.
81. MacLeod J. The role of oxygen in the metabolism and motility of human spermatozoa. Am J Physiol. 1943;138: 512–8.
82. Cummins J, Jequier A, Kan R. Molecular biology of human male infertility: links with aging, mitochondrial genetics, and oxidative stress? Mol Reprod Dev. 1994;37(3):345–62.
83. Aitken J, Buckingham D, Harkiss D. Analysis of the extent to which sperm movement can predict the results of ionophore-enhanced functional assays of the acrosome reaction and sperm-oocyte fusion. Hum Reprod. 1994;9(10)1867–74.
84. Liu D, Baker H. A new test for the assessment of sperm-zona pellucida penetration: relationship with results of other sperm tests and fertilization in vitro. Hum Reprod. 1994;9(3):489–96.
85. Zouari R, De Almeida M, Rodrigues D, Jouannet P. Localization of antibodies on spermatozoa and sperm movement characteristics are good predictors of in vitro fertilization success in cases of male autoimmune infertility. Fertil Steril. 1993;59(3):606–12.
86. Agarwal A, Makker K, Sharma R. Clinical relevance of oxidative stress in male factor infertility: an update. Am J Reprod Immunol. 2008;59(1):2–11.
87. Saleh R, Agarwal A. Oxidative stress and male infertility: from research bench to clinical practice. J Androl. 2002;23(6):737–52.
88. Bogenhagen D. Repair of mtDNA in vertebrates. Am J Hum Gen. 1999;64(5):1276–81.
89. Liu CY, Lee CF, Hong CH, Wei YH. Mitochondrial DNA mutation and depletion increase the susceptibility of human cells to apoptosis. Ann N Y Acad Sci. 2004;1011:133–45.
90. Taylor RW, Turnbull DM. Mitochondrial DNA mutations in human disease. Nat Rev Gene. 2005;6(5):389–402.
91. Wang X, Sharma RK, Gupta A, George V, Thomas AJ, Falcone T, et al. Alterations in mitochondria membrane potential and oxidative stress in infertile men: a prospective observational study. Fertil Steril. 2003;80(Suppl 2):844–50.
92. Zorn B, Vidmar G, Meden-Vrtovec H. Seminal reactive oxygen species as predictors of fertilization, embryo quality and pregnancy rates after conventional in vitro fertilization and intracytoplasmic sperm injection. Int J Androl. 2003;26(5):279–85.
93. Meseguer M, de los Santos MJ, Simon C, Pellicer A, Remohi J, Garrido N. Effect of sperm glutathione peroxidases 1 and 4 on embryo asymmetry and blastocyst quality in oocyte donation cycles. Fertil Steril. 2006;86(5):1376–85.
94. Meseguer M, Martinez-Conejero JA, O'Connor JE, Pellicer A, Remohi J, Garrido N. The significance of sperm DNA oxidation in embryo development and reproductive outcome in an oocyte donation program: a new model to study a male infertility prognostic factor. Fertil Steril. 2008;89(5):1191–9.
95. Hall HL, Flynn MG, Carroll KK, Brolinson PG, Shapiro S, Bushman BA. Effects of intensified training and detraining on testicular function. Clin J Sport Med. 1999;9(4):203–8.
96. Vaamonde D, Da Silva-Grigoletto ME, García-Manso JM, Cunha-Filho JS, Vaamonde-Lemos R. Sperm morphology normalcy is inversely correlated to cycling kilometers in elite triathletes. Revista Andaluza de Medicina del Deporte. 2009;2(2):43–6.
97. Peake J, Suzuki K, Coombes J. The influence of antioxidant supplementation on markers of inflammation and the relationship to oxidative stress after exercise. J Nutr Biochem. 2007;18(6):357–71.
98. Ivell R. Lifestyle impact and the biology of the human scrotum. Reprod Biol Endocrinol. 2007;5:15.
99. Fisher-Wellman K, Bloomer R. Acute exercise and oxidative stress: a 30 year history. Dyn Med. 2009;8(1):1.
100. Gebreegziabher Y, Marcos E, McKinon W, Rogers G. Serm characteristics of endurance trained cyclists. Int J Sport Med. 2004;25(04):247–51.
101. Arce JC, De Souza MJ, Pescatello LS, Luciano AA. Subclinical alterations in hormone and semen profile in athletes. Fert Steril. 1993;59(2):398–404.
102. De Souza MJ, Arce JC, Pescatello LS, Scherzer HS, Luciano AA. Gonadal hormones and semen quality in male runners. A volume threshold effect of endurance training. Int J Sport Med. 1994;15(7):383–91.

103. Safarinejad MR, Azma K, Kolahi AA. The effects of intensive, long-term treadmill running on reproductive hormones, hypothalamus-pituitary-testis axis, and semen quality: a randomized controlled study. J Endocrinol. 2009;200(3):259–71.
104. du Plessis SS, Kashou A, Vaamonde D, Agarwal A. Is there a link between exercise and male factor infertility? Open Reprod Sci J. 2011;3:105–13.
105. Gomez-Cabrera MC, Domenech E, Vina J. Moderate exercise is an antioxidant: upregulation of antioxidant genes by training. Free Rad Biol Med. 2008;44(2):126–31.
106. Manna I, Jana K, Samanta PK. Effect of intensive exercise-induced testicular gametogenic and steroidogenic disorders in mature male Wistar strain rats: a correlative approach to oxidative stress. Acta Phys Scan. 2003;178(1):33–40.
107. Manna I, Jana K, Samanta PK. Effect of different intensities of swimming exercise on testicular oxidative stress and reproductive dysfunction in mature male albino Wistar rats. Indian J Exp Biol. 2004;42(8):816–22.
108. Chigurupati S, Son TG, Hyun DH, Lathia JD, Mughal MR, Savell J, et al. Lifelong running reduces oxidative stress and degenerative changes in the testes of mice. J Endocrinol. 2008;199(2):333–41.
109. Tartibian B, Maleki BH. Correlation between seminal oxidative stress biomarkers and antioxidants with sperm DNA damage in elite athletes and recreationally active men. Clin J Sport Med. 2012;22(2):132–9.
110. Hajizadeh Maleki B, Tartibian B, Eghbali M, Asri-Rezaei S. Comparison of seminal oxidants and antioxidants in subjects with different levels of physical fitness. Andrology. 2013;1(4):607–14.
111. Warren M, Perlroth N. The effects of intense exercise on the female reproductive system. J Endocrinol. 2001;170(1), 3–11.
112. Sanborn C, Albrecht B, Wagner W. Athletic amenorrhea: lack of association with body fat. Med Sci Sport Exerc. 1987;19:207–12.
113. Singh K. Menstrual disorders in college students. Am J Obs Gyn. 1981;1210:299–302.
114. Glass A, Deuster P, Kyle S, Yahiro J, Vigersky R, Schoomaker E. Amenorrhea in Olympic marathon runners. Fertil Steril. 1987;48:740–5.
115. Goldfarb A, McKenzie M, Bloomer R. Gender comparisons of exercise-induced oxidative stress: influence of antioxidant supplementation. Appl Physiol Nutr Metab. 2007;32(6):1124–31.
116. Rush J, Sandiford S. Plasma glutathione peroxidase in healthy young adults: influence of gender and physical activity. Clin Biochem. 2003;36(5):345–51.
117. Bloomer R, Fisher-Wellman K. Blood oxidative stress biomarkers: Influence of sex, exercise training status, and dietary intake. Gen Med. 2007;5(3):218–28.
118. Tiidus P, Bombardier E, Hidiroglou N, Madere R. Gender and exercise influence on tissue antioxidant vitamin status in rats. J Nutr Sci Vitaminol (Tokyo). 1999;45(6):701–10.
119. Ruiz-Larrea M, Garrido M, Lacort M. Estradiol-induced effects on glutathione metabolism in rat hepatocytes. J Biochem. 1993;113(5):563–7.
120. Kaikkonen J, Porkkala-Sarataho E, Tuomainen TP, Nyyssonen K, Kosonen L, Ristonmaa U, Lakka H, Salonen R, Korpela H, Salonen J. Exhaustive exercise increases plasma/serum total oxidation resistance in moderately trained men and women, whereas their VLDL + LDL lipoprotein fraction is more susceptible to oxidation. Scand J Clin Lab Invest. 2002;62(8):599–607.
121. Ginsburg G, O'Toole M, Rimm E, Douglas P, Rifai N. Gender differences in exercise-induced changes in sex hormone levels and lipid peroxidation in athletes participating in the Hawaii Ironman triathlon. Ginsburg-gender and exercise-induced lipid peroxidation. Clin Chim Acta. 2001;305(1–2):131–9.
122. Sastre J, Borras C, Garcia-Sala D, Lloret A, Pallardo F, Vina J. Mitochondrial damage in aging and apoptosis. Ann N Y Acad Sci. 2002;959:448–51.
123. Matuszczak Y, Farid M, Jones J, Lansdowne S, Smith M, Taylor A, Reid M. Effects of N-acetylcysteine on glutathione oxidation and fatigue during handgrip exercise. Musc Nerve. 2005;32(5):633–8.
124. Bloomer R, Davis P, Consitt L, Wideman L. Plasma protein carbonyl response to increasing exercise duration in aerobically trained men and women. Int J Sports Med. 2007;28(1):21–5.

Nutritional Deficiencies and Impairment of Fertility in Athletes

19

Juan Marcelo Fernández

Abbreviations

FFQ	Food frequency questionnaire
FSH	Follicle-stimulating hormone
GnRH	Gonadotropin-releasing hormone
HPG	Hypothalamic–pituitary–gonadal
LEA	Low energy availability
LH	Luteinizing hormone
NPY	Neuropeptide Y
KISS	Kisspeptin
RAA	Reduced antioxidant availability
ROS	Reactive oxygen species

Low Energy Availability (LEA) and Fertility Control

The reproductive function has been shown to be costly in terms of energy and thus less of a priority than the conservation of essential metabolic fuels and basic physiological functions in humans [1] (Fig. 19.1). At the same time, the neuroendocrine mechanisms which support the reproductive function act as true sensors of environmental characteristics (food, water, psychological well-being, etc.) and indicate the right time and place for the successful reproduction of individuals [2]. In fact, in an environment of LEA, individuals suffer from metabolic stress, which is capable of blocking the hypothalamic–pituitary–gonadal (HPG) axis. Fertility depends on the complex intercommunication of the important set of neural and endocrine tissues which make up the HPG axis.

Under normal conditions, activation of the HPG axis begins with the pulsatile secretion of the main intermediary between the tissues of the axis, that is, the gonadotropin-releasing hormone (GnRH), released from the hypothalamus [3].

This decapeptide hormone has an affinity for specific receptors on the gonadotropic cells of the anterior pituitary, which induce the synthesis and release of the gonadotropins, follicle-stimulating hormone (FSH) and luteinizing hormone (LH). In men, LH stimulates testicular production of testosterone by the Leydig cells and androgen-binding protein by the Sertoli cells, while in women, it stimulates ovarian androgen production by thecal cells.

In conditions of LEA, a disruption in the pulsatile secretion of GnRH is produced, with either a reduction in the frequency or increased pulsatile amplitude of LH. This results in disturbances of gonadal function with decreasing steroid levels. In humans, this occurs in both men and women, but especially in the latter, for whom the energy cost of maintaining the reproductive system is significantly higher [4]. In men, the result is expressed in terms of a progressive reduction in plasma testosterone levels and reduced spermatogenesis. Meanwhile, in women, it produces either

J. M. Fernández (✉)
Sport and Clinical Nutrition, Nutrition Group, Nutrir Medical Nutrition and Exercise Clinic, Andalusian Society of Sports Medicine (S.A.M.E.D.E.), Avenida Aeropuerto 28 Local, 14004 Cordoba, Spain
e-mail: j.marfer.lopez@gmail.com

© Springer Science+Business Media New York 2016

D. Vaamonde et al. (eds.), *Exercise and Human Reproduction*, DOI 10.1007/978-1-4939-3402-7_19

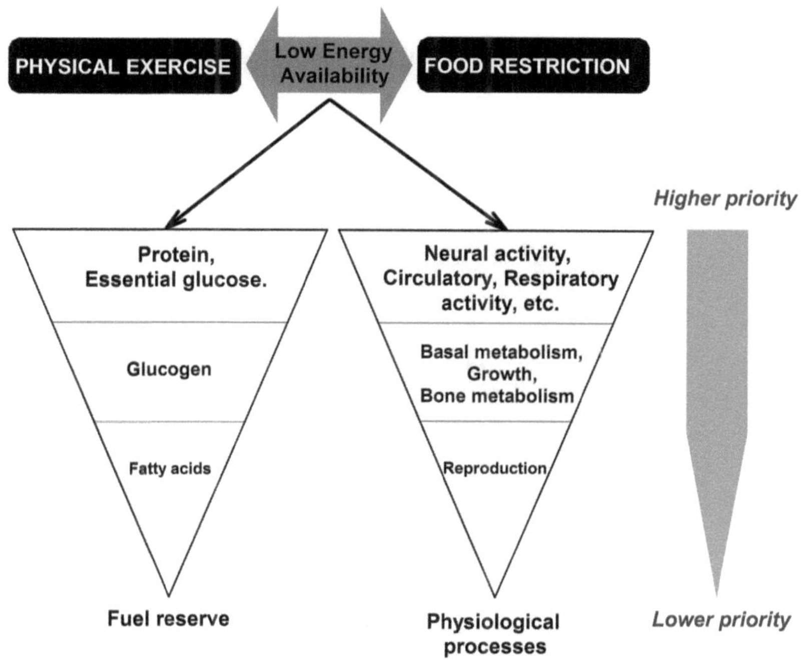

Fig. 19.1 Conservation of metabolic fuels and basic physiological functions in low energy availability conditions

a delay in the onset of menarche (primary amenorrhea), irregular menstrual cycles (oligomenorrhea), or the total loss of menstrual cycles (secondary amenorrhea). In adult women, the main causes of these disturbances are the shortening of the luteal phase of the menstrual cycle and/or a lengthening of the follicular phase, or alternatively, a fault in the secretory function of the corpus luteum in not releasing enough progesterone [5].

Signs of LEA and Blockage of HPG

Mechanistically, the hypothesis that "critical body fat" is the sole initiator of disturbances in fertility in LEA conditions has become obsolete [6]. Deregulation of the reproductive axis seems to be initiated earlier by a complex interaction of a number of neuropeptides (Fig. 19.2) capable of modulating both hypothalamic appetite control and the individual's reproductive endocrinology [7, 8]. Among these, leptin and ghrelin are two important metabolic messengers responsible for signaling the state of the individual's intake, energy reserves, and nutritional status to the hypothalamus (Table 19.1).

Particularly, leptin could act as an "on-switch" for neuroendocrine changes which can lead to a state of infertility in LEA [9–11]. In the hypothalamus and largely on the anterior pituitary (gonadotropes), the abundant expression of the leptin receptor indicates a direct stimulatory effect on the HPG axis, resulting in a dose-related release of LH, FSH, and prolactin [12–14]. Therefore, in animals and humans in an LEA situation, the levels of this hormone correlate directly with the secretion of the gonadotropins LH and FSH. In those areas where the action of leptin is not direct, as in the case of neurons in the preoptic area, this action is mediated by other neuropeptides (related to leptin) such as neuropeptide Y, kisspeptin, and pro-opiomelanocortin [15, 16]. Furthermore, the secretion of leptin and leptin receptor expression in different reproductive tissues (e.g., placenta, ovary, and endometrium) indicate that leptin may have autocrine and paracrine activity with endocrine and immunomodulatory effects. Not only would this allow for controlled ovarian function but also allow key processes such as embryo implantation and placentation [17].

However, the multifaceted influence of the neuropeptides and hormones on the neuroendo-

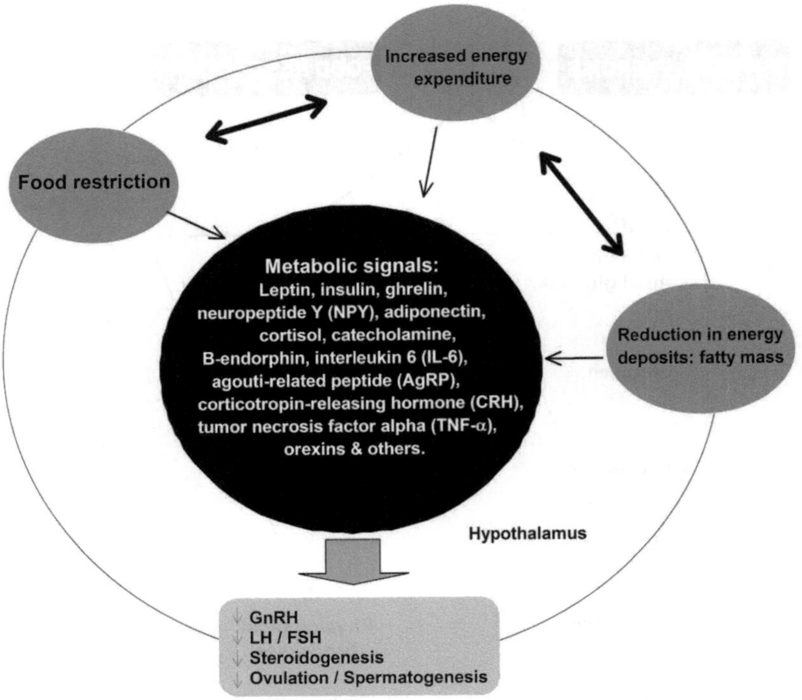

Fig. 19.2 Main metabolic modulators of reproductive function sensitive to low energy availability

Table 19.1 Synthesis, main functions, and regulators of leptin and ghrelin in energy metabolism

Molecule	Location of main synthesis	Function	Regulators of circulating levels	Effects
Leptin	Adipose tissue	Suppresses appetite	Energy stores	Decreases with decrease in percent total body fat
		Signals the hypothalamus on the amount of stored energy	Gender	Higher in females compared to males
		Affects energy expenditure	Food intake	Increases in postprandial condition and with glucose uptake
			Exercise	Decreases
Ghrelin	Stomach	Stimulates appetite; enhances acid secretion and gastric motility	Energy stores	Increases with decrease in total body fat
		Indicates the status of stored energy to the hypothalamus	Gender	Higher in females compared to males
		Increases carbohydrate use and reduces lipolysis	Food intake	Decreases in postprandial condition, with glucose uptake and insulin release

crine metabolism, along with the observation in animal models that reproductive failure still continues even when there are normal levels of one or more of them (e.g., sufficient levels of leptin), proves that there is no single type of hypothalamic sensor which activates changes in the HPG axis. Therefore, the current focus of study for different research groups around the world is the possible hypothalamic pathways which are activated (e.g., GnRH neurons, first-order neurons like NPY- or KISS-1-expressing neurons, and gamma-aminobutyric acid (GABA)-nergic neurons) and their complex interaction with the signals of peripheral metabolic changes. These

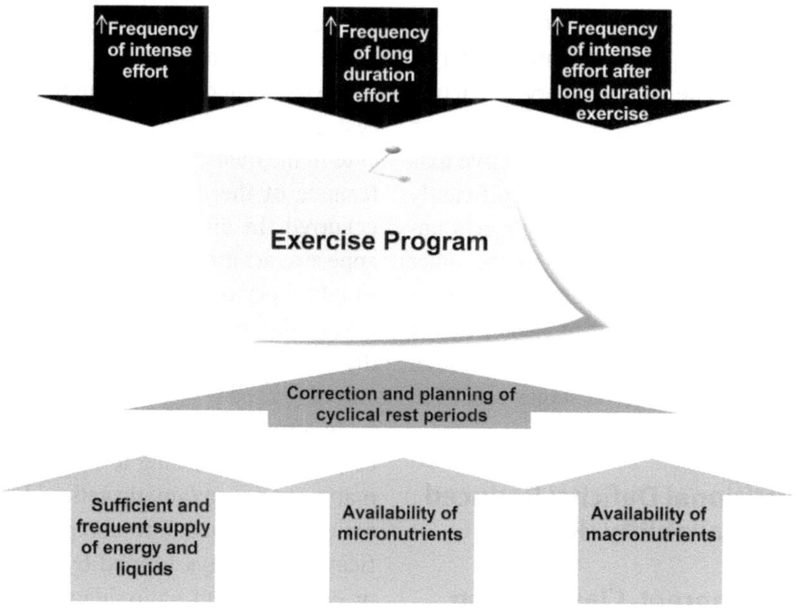

Fig. 19.3 Characteristics of a training program which can lead to low energy availability and general measures to prevent it

lines of work are producing new knowledge and study hypotheses about how energy balance exerts a critical influence on fertility [18, 19].

LEA, Exercise, and Fertility

Leaving aside the population who suffer from crises of subnutrition, athletes seem to be an important risk group for experiencing states of subfertility or infertility associated with LEA. In their case, LEA could result from two general situations: (a) a reduction in energy intake, secondary to nutritional restriction (while maintaining a constant energy expenditure increased by exercise), and (b) a sharp increase in energy expenditure dependent on exercise, in combination with food restriction or noncompensatory energy intake [20] (Fig. 19.3).

The origin and magnitude of the energy crisis created under these circumstances seem to be important in explaining the intensity of disturbances in the individuals' fertility. Different studies in both animal models and humans have shown that it is dietary restriction, rather than the increase in energy expenditure, that is the main factor in the equation responsible for neuroendocrine dysregulation. Along these lines, a study carried out to compare the independent effect of dietary restriction and exercise as metabolic stressors showed that dietary restriction generates significantly greater fluctuations in daily leptin secretion in young women [21].

This would explain the reversal of the reproductive alterations that occurs after an adequate nutritional intake is restored in both humans and trained animals [22, 23]. It could also be related to the fact that many of the different messengers involved in the physiology of the hypothalamic–pituitary–gonadal axis are, as stated previously, particularly sensitive to alimentary, postprandial, and metabolic signals.

Moreover, in practice, the combination of both factors (energy restriction and an exponential increase in energy expenditure) may well be the most common situation, and this is potentially capable of causing clinically relevant LEA. Therefore, mild to moderate exercise, accompanied by dietary restriction, is capable of causing only a small negative energy balance and weight loss, and even a slight exposure to steroids, but it will not cause real changes in the subject's fertility [24, 25]. Meanwhile, when dietary restriction is added to a short-term increase in training, the possibility of disruption of the reproductive axis associated with LH pulsatility is significantly increased, as has been observed in subjects undergoing moderate training [26]. On the other hand, the combination of both factors at greater intensity can cause severe states of energy deficit and reduce LH concentrations to levels similar to those observed in prepubertal stages [26, 27].

Specific Nutritional Deficits: Reduced Antioxidant Availability (RAA)

Antioxidants: Concept, Classification and Their Relation to Human Fertility

In general, an antioxidant compound can be defined as an atom or a molecule that avoids or blocks reactive oxygen species (ROS), thus preventing oxidative damage of other molecules. Its mechanism of action is based on direct interaction with ROS, forming a less active radical, or blocking oxidative chain reactions that lead to damage of substrates, such as lipids, proteins, carbohydrates, and DNA. A broader definition would also include those molecules responsible for repairing oxidative damage caused by ROS.

In reproductive function, antioxidant compounds have been shown to play an important role in countering the action of ROS and preventing oxidative stress, which is characterized by damage to sensitive lipid structures and the cell DNA aimed at fertilization [28]. In human males, an impaired or depleted antioxidant defense and an oxidative environment surrounding the sperm can alter their development and maturation, and can cause oxidative damage to their plasma membranes and cell apoptosis. These phenomena produce morphological and functional changes expressed in terms of deficient sperm count, morphology, and motility [29–31], which are the predictors most commonly used nowadays to define a man's reproductive capacity.

Meanwhile, in women, there is a complex balance (which is not yet fully understood) between antioxidants and ROS throughout the whole process, from the growth and development of the oocyte in the ovary to follicle growth and the maintenance of the corpus luteum if pregnancy has occurred. In all these phenomena, antioxidants appear to act mainly as promoters, while ROS act as inhibitory or apoptotic agents, from the selection of the dominant oocyte to the regression of the corpus luteum when pregnancy has not occurred [32, 33].

In terms of classification, all antioxidants can be grouped, according to their nature, into enzymatic and nonenzymatic antioxidants. Enzymatic antioxidants constitute complex cellular detoxification pathways formed by numerous families of enzymes with antioxidant capacity. Whereas non-enzymatic antioxidants exert their antioxidant action directly, whether by chelating transition metals and stopping them from catalyzing ROS production or allowing the activity of some antioxidant enzymes.

Nonenzymatic antioxidants are of particular interest because of their relation to dietary intake, and of these, there are a variety of compounds that can act on an intracellular or extracellular level, or in both compartments (Table 19.2). In this regard, it has been demonstrated in animal

Table 19.2 Classification of nonenzymatic antioxidants by location

Location	Compound	General characteristics
Preferably extracellular	Transferrin Lactoferrin Ceruloplasmin Haptoglobin Albumin	Provided by the diet or modulated by diet and the individual's nutritional status
Intra- and/or extracellular	Glutathione (intracellular) Methionine Urate (extracellular) Ascorbate Tocopherols Cysteine Taurine Selenium Zinc Others	Supplied by the diet or synthesized endogenously from nutrients and can react directly, not catalytically, so that they can be consumed in the process

models that the antioxidants naturally present in foods, once ingested, have sufficient bioavailability to significantly improve the damage to the reproductive organs caused by experimentally induced oxidative stress [34].

Intake of Antioxidant Nutrients and Reproductive Capacity

Regular physical exercise and a healthy diet provide obvious benefits in the prevention and treatment of chronic diseases such as diabetes, metabolic syndrome, and some cancers [35–37]. A healthy diet is one that, in addition to providing the energy required for all physiological processes, contributes the different nutrients which are functionally essential for good health. Among these substances, the antioxidants usually ingested in food have constituted an important line of research and have furthered our understanding of the pathophysiology and therapy used for different health disorders, including infertility.

The relationship between antioxidant intake and fertility in women is still largely unknown. A recent study including a large sample size assessed the relationship between time to pregnancy and antioxidant intake in women undergoing treatment for unexplained infertility (n=437; age =21–39 years) [38]. The detailed analysis of the mean intake of total, dietary, and dietary supplement sources of beta-carotene and vitamins C and E showed that increased intake of these antioxidant vitamins was associated with shorter time to pregnancy, depending on age and body mass index (BMI). However, more studies are needed to evaluate the effect of different antioxidants and their sources on female fertility, as well as the influence of other cofactors that may affect the oxidative balance, such as exercise.

On the other hand, several studies have linked a low habitual intake of dietary antioxidants with problems in fertility, associated with phenomena of oxidative damage in men (Table 19.3). In particular, the level of vitamin C intake seems to have a positive relationship with semen volume and sperm motility in healthy young adults [39–41]. Its antioxidant potential, its activity in an aqueous medium, and its presence in high concentrations in seminal plasma are arguments that have been used to explain the importance of this nutrient. Similarly, higher intake levels of beta-carotene and lycopene have been associated with increased sperm concentration and higher sperm quality and motility [40, 41]. Other antioxidants such as vitamin E and selenium have also been reported to improve sperm motility in healthy individuals [41] .

However, the available evidence is not particularly robust since many of the associations established between the different antioxidant nutrients and the fertility parameters analyzed have not produced uniform results within the different studies. A possible cause of this controversy could be found in the methods used to measure dietary intake in fertility studies. It is certain that the food frequency questionnaire (FFQ) is the dietary assessment instrument of choice for large-scale nutritional epidemiological studies. However, these same studies have also shown that the use of FFQ presents important limitations of validity and accuracy, overestimating or underestimating the real intakes, and altering the associations between diet and health outcomes. The sample size in fertility studies is obviously one of the main limitations for the interpretation of associations between antioxidant intake parameters of fertility. In addition, the FFQ assessments in studies that include populations with heterogeneity of age, body size, and socioeconomic status may lack validity and accuracy when dietary information obtained has not been statistically adjusted [46, 47]. Interestingly, none of the studies shown in Table 19.3 have considered the level of physical activity or exercise daily as co-variables in their research design.

Regarding the quality of dietary information, not all studies investigating the association between antioxidant intake and fertility published to date (Table 19.3) have made an analysis using energy-adjusted nutrient intake. In this sense, there is a consensus between nutritional epidemiologists, proposing that energy-adjusted nutrient intake is essential to improve the accuracy of the specific dietary composition measured by FFQ, allowing detection of moderate statistical asso-

Table 19.3 Intake of antioxidants and fertility biomarkers in men

Subject/sample size (n)	Antioxidants analyzed	Method of analyzing intake	Effect on fertility
20–40-year-old, oligo- and/or astheno- and/or teratozoospermic nonsmoking men (n=32) vs. age-matched normal healthy donors (n=32) [42]	Dietary intake of vitamin C, vitamin E, beta-carotene, folate, selenium, and zinc	Food frequency questionnaire (FFQ), semiquantitative with 116 food items	Poor sperm concentration, Motility, and morphology are associated with low intake of zinc, folate, and vitamin E
22–80-year-old nonsmoking men without fertility problems (n=80) [43]	Daily dietary and supplement intake of vitamin C, vitamin E, beta-carotene, zinc, and folate	100-item modified block FFQ	Sperm with less oxidative DNA damage in men (especially older men) with higher intake of vitamins C and E, zinc, and folate
18–23-year-old healthy young men (n=215) [39]	Dietary intakes of cryptoxanthin, vitamin C, lycopene, alpha-carotene and beta-carotene, lutein + zeaxanthin, folate, vitamin D, and vitamin B complex	Semiquantitative FFQ of 101 items	Positive association between cryptoxanthin, vitamin C, lycopene, and beta-carotene and the total motile sperm count. Semen volume increased with higher intakes of vitamin C, lycopene, and beta-carotene
20–70-year-old healthy nonsmoking men (n=89) [44]	Dietary intake plus supplement intake for vitamin C, vitamin E, beta-carotene, folate, and zinc	Self-administered 100-item modified block FFQ. Nutrient intakes were not calorie-adjusted	Inverse relationship between folate intake (diet + supplements) and the frequency of sperm aneuploidy. No evidence for zinc, vitamin C, vitamin E, or beta-carotene
Normozoospermic and oligoasthenoteratozoospermic men (n=30 and 31, respectively) [40]	Dietary intake for vitamin C, vitamin E, beta-carotene, selenium, folate, and lycopene	Semiquantitative FFQ of 93 food items	A low intake of vitamin C, folate, and lycopene is associated with poor semen quality (volume, concentration, motility, and morphology)
20–80-year-old healthy nonsmoking men (n=87) [45]	Dietary and supplementary intake of vitamin C, vitamin E, and beta-carotene	Self-administered 100-item modified block FFQ. Nutrient intakes were not calorie-adjusted	No association between increased intake of vitamin C, vitamin E, beta-carotene, or their composite and improved sperm chromatin integrity as measured by the DNA fragmentation index
20–80-year-old healthy nonsmoking men (n=97) [41]	Dietary and supplementary intake of zinc, folate, vitamins C and E, and beta-carotene	100-item self-administered modified block FFQ. Nutrient intakes were not calorie-adjusted	Positive associations between vitamin C and sperm count, between vitamin E and progressive motility, and between beta-carotene and sperm concentration and progressive motility. No associations for folate and zinc

ciations in large health cohort studies [47, 48]. However, neither the energy-adjusted nutrient intake nor the use of 24-h or multiple-day food records chosen as instruments for calibration/validation of FFQ ensures the absence of *bias,* the magnitude of which is unknown. This is because 24-h or multiple-day food records not only imperfect the measurements they perform but also share with FFQ the origin of that imperfection; therefore, they are not independent and there is doubt about their usefulness as a reference method [49] .

Furthermore, to date, there are no dietary biomarkers capable of serving as instruments of valid reference. An example is the case of vitamin C and beta-carotene for which different confounders (physical activity, smoking, comorbidities, etc.) have made it impossible to detect a valid relationship between the measured plasma levels or its metabolites and referred dietary intake [50]. In this regard, recent data have shown that even when using a 7-day food diary and an antioxidant intake questionnaire to determine the total antioxidant intake, only a small correlation (correlation 0.29, 90 % confidence limits ±0.27) with blood antioxidant biomarkers can be observed [51].

Finally, enough is known to ensure that FFQ is technically overdependent on the respondents' memory: They have to try to remember their food intake over long periods of time, usually 12 months. Furthermore, over these periods, the sensitivity to reflect seasonal changes in the consumption of antioxidant-rich foods such as different varieties of fruit and vegetables is low.

All these problems can significantly limit the possibility of analyzing and interpreting the causality between the intake of dietary antioxidants and declining fertility parameters. The minimum criterion for studies investing the effect of diet on fertility is to utilize the FFQ and subsequent calculation of energy-adjusted nutrient intake in order to obtain a more accurate dietary composition. Measurement of relevant antioxidants in seminal plasma should also be considered to give greater support to the associations between intake and fertility parameters.

Epidemiology of Dietary Intake of Antioxidants in Athletes

The content of antioxidant nutrients in an athlete's diet, as in the general population, is not necessarily linked to the energy it supplies. In dietary restriction conditions, antioxidant intake is usually a linear function of the energy input, while in states of overnutrition, a high energy input combined with low content in antioxidant nutrients can occur [52]. This is what happens in the globalized Western dietary patterns and trends, which are high-energy and low-nutrient density diets featuring a low intake of fruit, vegetables, and seeds but a high intake of carbohydrates and/or fats. Moreover, dietary patterns and the quality of an athlete's diet seem to depend on multiple factors including personal characteristics (e.g., sex), sociocultural conditions, and even the type of sport they do [53].

Conversely, the competitive level does not seem to be directly related to lower availability of dietary antioxidants. In this regard, different studies have shown that elite athletes have an adequate dietary intake of antioxidant vitamins (especially vitamins C and E), and in some cases higher than their recommended daily intake (RDI) [54].

A normal intake of fruits and vegetables in these athletes is usually sufficient to ensure an adequate supply of fat and water-soluble vitamins and also precursors of glutathione synthesis, such as lipoic acid [55]. The latter is found in the form of lipoyl-lysine in different plant foods such as spinach, broccoli, tomatoes and green peas, and in foods derived from animals, especially offal and its derivatives.

Restrictive Dietary Patterns and RAA

Some athletes choose to apply restrictions to their energy intake or exclude one or more food groups from their diet. These strategies comprise almost completely excluding dietary oils and fats rich in fat-soluble vitamins or limiting the dietary intake of fruit, vegetables, and whole grains. As a result, they may have a deficit intake of antioxidant nutrients [53]. This occurs most often in sports in which the athletes are weight conscious because body weight is a decisive factor in the competitive category, the esthetics of performing certain movements or the overall performance of a test (e.g., dance and gymnastics).

In addition, these behaviors tend to be more prevalent among female athletes than among men involved in the same sport [56]. Another increasingly common condition among athletes at all levels is the realization of fad diets to achieve rapid weight loss. The very-low-carbohydrate ketogenic diets are an example of this, where

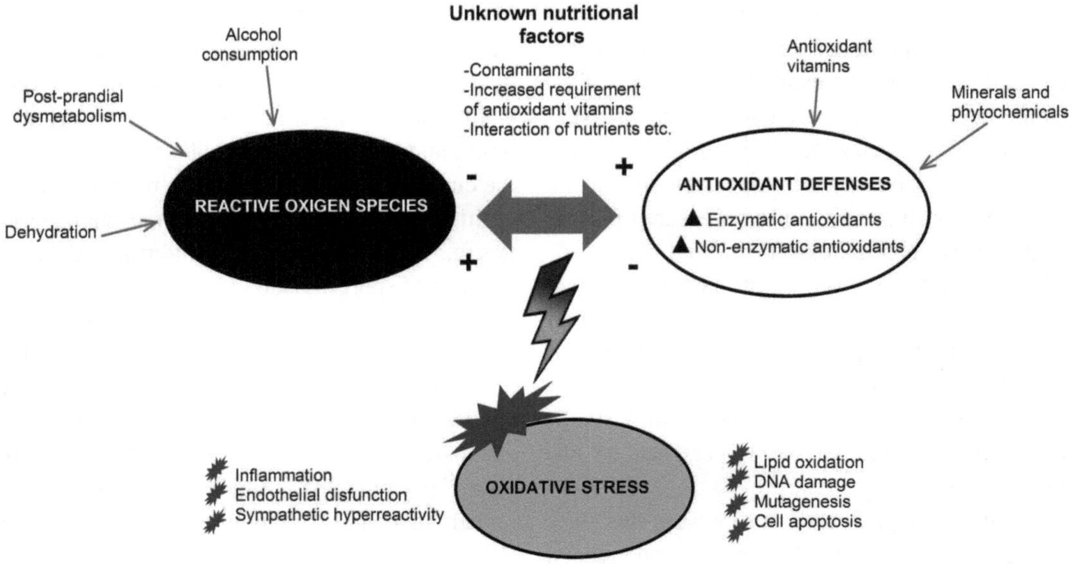

Fig. 19.4 Oxidative stress of nutritional origin. Multiple factors related to food upregulate reactive oxygen species production and downregulate the antioxidant defense system, leading to oxidative stress and cellular damage

the consumption of fruit and certain vegetables is often eliminated or drastically reduced. In this regard, some evidence has shown that a 4-week diet low in carbohydrates and high in protein causes a slight reduction in plasma retinol, vitamin E (α-tocopherol), and β-cryptoxanthin, which implies the need for vitamin supplementation while following such diets [57]. However, to date, the effect of ketogenesis on oxidative status and fertility parameters in athletes has not been studied; therefore, future studies are necessary to shed light on this area.

Nonrestrictive Dietary Patterns and RAA

Several studies have shown that diets high in fat, especially saturated fat, and sugars are positively associated with the prevalence of altered sperm count and motility in humans [58–61]. At the same time, these dietary patterns inherently involve a low variety and/or quantity of ingested fruit, berries, nuts and legumes, tomatoes, red wine, and vegetable oil—in other words, RAA. In this regard, increased fruit and vegetable consumption (especially tomatoes, dark green vegetables, and oranges) has been linked to a lower risk of asthenozoospermia and higher sperm motility in both fertile and infertile men [40, 62, 63].

From a mechanistic point of view, accumulated data from multiple lines of clinical evidence have shown that high-calorie meals rich in processed, easily digestible, quickly absorbable foods cause pro-oxidative phenomena, such as supraphysiological postprandial spikes in blood glucose and lipids [64]. Conversely, fruits and vegetables are rich in antioxidants such as vitamin C, beta-carotene, and vitamin E, which are essential for maintaining antioxidant defense against the ROS produced by spermatozoa, in physiological (under normal conditions) or supraphysiological quantities (in metabolic stress conditions). Thus, these kinds of dietary patterns, on the one hand, may favor an increased formation of ROS and, on the other hand, may lead to the deterioration of antioxidant defenses leading to oxidative stress and damage [65] (Fig. 19.4).

Athletes at different competitive levels are not exempt from this westernization of their diet, which tends toward overnutrition and/or impaired antioxidant capacity. There are different reasons why athletes maintain an excessive intake of refined carbohydrates, protein, and/or fat at the expense of a diet rich in antioxidant nutrients. This is the case of athletes who do not follow healthy behavior patterns in their diet or whose diet is not properly regulated due to lack of knowledge and/or advice on healthy sports nutrition. An attempt to increase performance (e.g., in endurance-based sports) or to avoid gastrointestinal distress during periods of intense training may also be factors which lead to an excessive intake of carbohydrates and/or proteins and a low consumption of fruit and vegetables.

So, Can It Be Said That RAA in an Athlete's Diet Can Affect His/Her Reproductive Capacity?

There is still very little information on athletes about the direct relationship between the content of dietary antioxidant nutrients and oxidative status in their reproductive tissues. However, there is evidence that metabolic stress caused by the level of physical training can break the oxidative balance in the sensitive tissues related to reproduction (e.g., sperm). In this regard, two cross-sectional studies on healthy young subjects have shown higher levels of seminal ROS and lipid peroxidation, and significant reductions in antioxidant defenses, in elite athletes compared with recreationally active men [66, 67].

On the one hand, these findings are consistent with other studies that have shown the importance of the exercise load (intensity × duration) on increased production of ROS and the occurrence of oxidative stress in athletes [68]. On the other hand, they lend credit to the hypothesis of an increased need for antioxidants in an athlete's diet to prevent oxidative stress during periods of intensive effort or training.

However, another interesting aspect yet to be confirmed is the clinical relevance of oxidative damage on fertility in individuals subjected to conditions of exhaustive exercise. In this regard, previous studies on animal models have shown that medium-term intensive training induces oxidative stress-dependent reproductive dysfunction, and also that this situation can be avoided when alpha-tocopherol succinate is injected subcutaneously [69, 70]. More recently, research carried out on humans has also shown that long-term intensive training causes oxidative damage and a fall in seminal antioxidant capacity in healthy male amateur road cyclists [71]. No less interesting is the evidence showing that supplementation with 70 g of natural honey before each session of intense exercise causes an attenuation of seminal plasma levels of cytokines and oxidative stress biomarkers, and an improvement in seminal antioxidants [72].

Based on the information currently available, we can consider reduced fertility in some athletes to be "fairly likely" as a result of the low availability of antioxidants, especially in times of exhaustive effort. First, the load of exercise may act as a metabolic stressor, a multifaceted physiological source of ROS which increases the need for antioxidants. Second, the low availability of antioxidant nutrients could weaken or deplete the defenses, leading to oxidative damage in sensitive tissues for fertility (Fig. 19.5).

Finally, not only further studies are needed on the antioxidant–fertility relationship, but a more sensitive research design is required to isolate the effect of multiple confounding factors. In this regard, recent evidence has shown that other characteristics of food, different from the antioxidant content but able to co-exist in a dietary pattern with RAA, can worsen the reproductive capacity of humans. One example of this is the report in a recent study showing that animal fats present in full-fat dairy food could, due to the content in environmental estrogens, affect sperm quality in healthy young individuals [73].

Similarly, the intake of trans fatty acid, determined using an FFQ, was related to poorer quality sperm (sperm concentration, motility, morphology, and total count) in healthy young men [74]. The latter nutrient has already been studied in animal models for its detrimental effect on various fertility parameters [75, 76].

Conclusions

Complex neuroendocrine changes occurring in conditions of LEA can affect the fertility of men and especially women in varying degrees. This situation is the result of the activity of a complex circuit of fuel regulators, where the hypothalamus is the primary sensor that processes information and reacts to the fall of peripheral energy re-

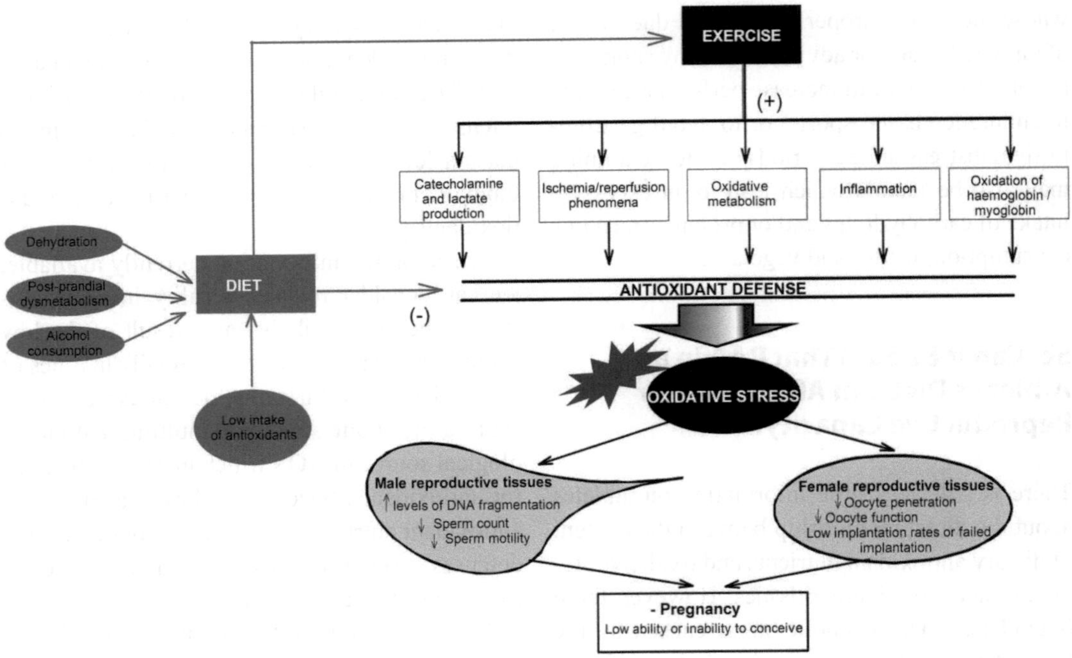

Fig. 19.5 Diet–exercise interaction, oxidative stress, and fertility. A pro-oxidant diet, that is one with a low supply of antioxidant nutrients and the presence of other stress factors, may have a cumulative effect on the sources of reactive oxygen species (ROS) in physical exercise. When ROS production exceeds the physiological quantities due to exercise or strenuous training and the antioxidant defenses are not capable of recycling due to reduced antioxidant availability in the diet, the occurrence of oxidative stress may possibly affect the functionality and structure of reproductive tissues

serves. An important role in this system is played by the messengers whose job is to communicate, at different levels, the occurrence of an energy crisis. Leptin and ghrelin, two known regulators of appetite and satiety, act centrally on anteroventebral periventricular neurons and on those of the arcuate nucleus to communicate the decrease in peripheral fat and energy reserves. Therefore, although the intensity and/or duration of physical exercise can cause LEA, dietary restriction in athletes appears to be especially influential in the disruption of the hypothalamic hypophysial gonadal axis and the occurrence of aberrations in fertility.

In addition, regardless of energy intake, the availability of antioxidant compounds, which counter the occurrence of oxidative stress and damage, is essential for the maintenance of proper reproductive capacity. In athletes worried about their body weight, the exclusion of one or more food groups related to the contribution of antioxidant nutrients could be a risk behavior which endangers their oxidative balance. Similarly, a dietary pattern which is energy-dense and nutritionally weak could convert the diet into a cofactor of oxidative risk. The reduced availability of antioxidants does not favor the body's antioxidant defense system, while different postprandial and metabolic phenomena have an accumulated effect on the very sources of ROS produced by exercise and may favor the occurrence of oxidative stress. Further studies are needed to evaluate the effect of different fad diets, such as high-protein diets, on the oxidative status and fertility of athletes.

References

1. Wade GN, Schneider JE. Metabolic fuels and reproduction in female mammals. Neurosci Biobehav Rev. 1992;16(2):235–72.
2. Evans JJ, Anderson GM. Balancing ovulation and anovulation: integration of the reproductive and energy balance axes by neuropeptides. Hum Reprod Update. 2012;18:313–32.

3. Bliss SP, Navratil AM, Xie J, Roberson MS. GnRH signaling, the gonadotrope and endocrine control of fertility. Front Neuroendocrinol. 2010;31(3):322–40.
4. Wade GN, Jones JE. Neuroendocrinology of nutritional infertility. Am J Physiol Regul Integr Comp Physiol. 2004;287(6):R1277–96.
5. Beitins IZ, McArthur JW, Turnbull BA, Skrinar GS, Bullen BA. Exercise induces two types of human luteal dysfunction: confirmation by urinary free progesterone. J Clin Endocrinol Metab. 1991;72(6):1350–8.
6. Bronson FH, Manning JM. The energetic regulation of ovulation: a realistic role for body fat. Biol Reprod. 1991;44(6):945–50.
7. Budak E, Fernández Sánchez M, Bellver J, Cerveró A, Simón C, Pellicer A. Interactions of the hormones leptin, ghrelin, adiponectin, resistin, and PYY3-36 with the reproductive system. Fertil Steril. 2006;85(6):1563–81.
8. Fernandez-Fernandez R, Martini AC, Navarro VM, Castellano JM, Dieguez C, Aguilar E, Pinilla L, Tena-Sempere M. Novel signals for the integration of energy balance and reproduction. Mol Cell Endocrinol. 2006;25;254–255:127–32.
9. Chan JL, Mantzoros CS. Role of leptin in energy-deprivation states: normal human physiology and clinical implications for hypothalamic amenorrhoea and anorexia nervosa. Lancet. 2005;366(9479): 74–85
10. Hausman GJ, Barb CR, Lents CA. Leptin and reproductive function. Biochimie. 2012;94(10):2075–81.
11. Gamba M, Pralong FP. Control of GnRH neuronal activity by metabolic factors: the role of leptin and insulin. Mol Cell Endocrinol. 2006;254–255:133–9.
12. Fei H, Okano HJ, Li C, Lee GH, Zhao C, Darnell R, Friedman JM. Anatomic localization of alternatively spliced leptin receptors (Ob-R) in mouse brain and other tissues. Proc Natl Acad Sci USA. 1997;94(13):7001–5.
13. Zamorano PL, Mahesh VB, De Sevilla LM, Chorich LP, Bhat GK, Brann DW. Expression and localization of the leptin receptor in endocrine and neuroendocrine tissues of the rat. Neuroendocrinology. 1997;65(3):223–8.
14. Jin L, Burguera BG, Couce ME, Scheithauer BW, Lamsan J, Eberhardt NL, Kulig E, Lloyd RV. Leptin and leptin receptor expression in normal and neoplastic human pituitary: evidence of a regulatory role for leptin on pituitary cell proliferation. J Clin Endocrinol Metab. 1999;84(8):2903–11.
15. Czaja K, Łakomy M, Sienkiewicz W, Kaleczyc J, Pidsudko Z, Barb CR, Rampacek GB, Kraeling RR. Distribution of neurons containing leptin receptors in the hypothalamus of the pig. Biochem Biophys Res Commun. 2002;298(3):333–7.
16. Quennell JH, Mulligan AC, Tups A, Liu X, Phipps SJ, Kemp CJ, Herbison AE, Grattan DR, Anderson GM. Leptin indirectly regulates gonadotropin-releasing hormone neuronal function. Endocrinology. 2009;150(6):2805–12.
17. Pérez-Pérez A, Sánchez-Jiménez F, Maymó J, Dueñas JL, Varone C, Sánchez-Margalet V. Role of leptin in female reproduction. Clin Chem Lab Med. 2014. doi:10.1515/cclm-2014-0387.
18. Pralong FP. Insulin and NPY pathways and the control of GnRH function and puberty onset. Mol Cell Endocrinol. 2010;324(1–2):82–6.
19. Roa J. Role of GnRH neurons and their neuronal afferents as key integrators between food intake regulatory signals and the control of reproduction. Int J Endocrinol. 2013;2013:518046.
20. Orio F, Muscogiuri G, Ascione A, Marciano F, Volpe A, Sala G L, Savastano S, Colao A, Palomba S. Effects of physical exercise on the female reproductive system. Minerva Endocrinol. 2013;38(3):305–19.
21. Hilton LK, Loucks AB. Low energy availability, not exercise stress, suppresses the diurnal rhythm of leptin in healthy young women. Am J Physiol Endocrinol Metab. 2000;278(1):E43–9.
22. Loucks AB, Verdun M, Heath EM. Low energy availability, not stress of exercise, alters LH pulsatility in exercising women. J Appl Physiol. 1998;84(1):37–46.
23. Williams NI, Helmreich DL, Parfitt DB, Caston-Balderrama A, Cameron JL. Evidence for a causal role of low energy availability in the induction of menstrual cycle disturbances during strenuous exercise training. J Clin Endocrinol Metab. 2001;86(11):5184–93.
24. Loucks AB, Thuma JR. Luteinizing hormone pulsatility is disrupted at a threshold of energy availability in regularly menstruating women. J Clin Endocrinol Metab. 2003;88(1):297–311.
25. Williams NI, Reed JL, Leidy HJ, Legro RS, De Souza MJ. Estrogen and progesterone exposure is reduced in response to energy deficiency in women aged 25–40 years. Hum Reprod. 2010;25(9):2328–39.
26. Williams NI, Young JC, McArthur JW, Bullen B, Skrinar GS, Turnbull B. Strenuous exercise with caloric restriction: effect on luteinizing hormone secretion. Med Sci Sports Exerc. 1995;27(10):1390–8.
27. De Souza MJ, West SL, Jamal SA, Hawker GA, Gundberg CM, Williams NI. The presence of both an energy deficiency and estrogen deficiency exacerbate alterations of bone metabolism in exercising women. Bone. 2008;43:140–8.
28. Agarwal A, Gupta S, Sikka S. The role of free radicals and antioxidants in reproduction. Curr Opin Obstet Gynecol. 2006;18(3):325–32.
29. Saalu LC. The incriminating role of reactive oxygen species in idiopathic male infertility: an evidence based evaluation. Pak J Biol Sci. 2010;13(9):413–22.
30. Benedetti S, Tagliamonte MC, Catalani S, Primiterra M, Canestrari F, De Stefani S, Palini S, Bulletti C. Differences in blood and semen oxidative status in fertile and infertile men, and their relationship with sperm quality. Reprod Biomed Online. 2012;25(3):300–6.

31. Hosseinzadeh Colagar A, Karimi F, Jorsaraei SG. Correlation of sperm parameters with semen lipid peroxidation and total antioxidants levels in astheno- and oligoasheno- teratospermic men. Iran Red Crescent Med J. 2013;15(9):780–5.
32. Al-Gubory KH, Garrel C, Faure P, Sugino N. Roles of antioxidant enzymes in corpus luteum rescue from reactive oxygen species-induced oxidative stress. Reprod Biomed Online. 2012;25(6):551–60.
33. Agarwal A, Aponte-Mellado A, Premkumar BJ, Shaman A, Gupta S. The effects of oxidative stress on female reproduction: a review. Reprod Biol Endocrinol. 2012;10:49.
34. Türk G, Ceribasi S, Sönmez M, Ciftçi M, Yüce A, Güvenç M, Ozer Kaya S, Cay M, Aksakal M. Ameliorating effect of pomegranate juice consumption on carbon tetrachloride-induced sperm damages, lipid peroxidation, and testicular apoptosis. Toxicol Ind Health. doi: 10.1177/0748233713499600. Accessed 30 Sept 2013.
35. Booth FW, Roberts CK, Laye MJ. Lack of exercise is a major cause of chronic diseases. Compr Physiol. 2012;2(2):1143–211.
36. Huang CJ, Webb HE, Zourdos MC, Acevedo EO. Cardiovascular reactivity, stress, and physical activity. Front Physiol. 2013;4:314.
37. Willett WC, Stampfer MJ. Current evidence on healthy eating. Annu Rev Public Health. 2013;34:77–95.
38. Ruder EH, Hartman TJ, Reindollar RH, Goldman MB. Female dietary antioxidant intake and time to pregnancy among couples treated for unexplained infertility. Fertil Steril. 2014;101(3):759–66.
39. Mínguez-Alarcón L, Mendiola J, López-Espín JJ, Sarabia-Cos L, Vivero-Salmerón G, Vioque J, Navarrete-Muñoz EM, Torres-Cantero AM. Dietary intake of antioxidant nutrients is associated with semen quality in young university students. Hum Reprod. 2012;27(9):2807–14.
40. Mendiola J, Torres-Cantero AM, Vioque J, Moreno-Grau JM, Ten J, Roca M, Moreno-Grau S, Bernabeu R. A low intake of antioxidant nutrients is associated with poor semen quality in patients attending fertility clinics. Fertil Steril. 2010;93(4):1128–33.
41. Eskenazi B, Kidd SA, Marks AR, Sloter E, Block G, Wyrobek AJ. Antioxidant intake is associated with semen quality in healthy men. Hum Reprod. 2005;20(4):1006–12.
42. Nadjarzadeh A, Mehrsai A, Mostafavi E, Gohari MR, Shidfar F. The association between dietary antioxidant intake and semen quality in infertile men. Med J Islam Repub Iran. 2013;27(4):204–9.
43. Schmid TE, Eskenazi B, Marchetti F, Young S, Weldon RH, Baumgartner A, Anderson D, Wyrobek AJ. Micronutrients intake is associated with improved sperm DNA quality in older men. Fertil Steril. 2012;98(5):1130–7.e1.
44. Young SS, Eskenazi B, Marchetti FM, Block G, Wyrobek AJ. The association of folate, zinc and antioxidant intake with sperm aneuploidy in healthy nonsmoking men. Hum Reprod. 2008;23(5):1014–22.
45. Silver EW, Eskenazi B, Evenson DP, Block G, Young S, Wyrobek AJ. Effect of antioxidant intake on sperm chromatin stability in healthy nonsmoking men. J Androl. 2005;26(4):550–6.
46. Willett W. Dietary diaries versus food frequency questionnaires-a case of undigestible data. Commentary. Int J Epidemiol. 2001;30(2):317–9.
47. Kipnis V, Subar AF, Midthune D, Freedman LS, Ballard-Barbash R, Troiano RP, Bingham S, Schoeller DA, Schatzkin A, Carroll RJ. Structure of dietary measurement error: results of the OPEN biomarker study. Am J Epidemiol. 2003;158(1):14–21.
48. LS1 F, Schatzkin A, Midthune D, Kipnis V. Dealing with dietary measurement error in nutritional cohort studies. J Natl Cancer Inst. 2011;103(14):1086–92.
49. Kipnis V, Midthune D, Freedman L, Bingham S, Day NE, Riboli E, Ferrari P, Carroll RJ. Bias in dietary-report instruments and its implications for nutritional epidemiology. Public Health Nutr. 2002;5(6 A):915–23.
50. Kaaks RJ. Biochemical markers as additional measurements in studies of the accuracy of dietary questionnaire measurements: conceptual issues. Am J Clin Nutr. 1997;65(4 Suppl):1232S–9S.
51. Braakhuis AJ, Hopkins WG, Lowe TE. Effect of dietary antioxidants, training, and performance correlates on antioxidant status in competitive rowers. Int J Sports Physiol Perform. 2013;8(5):565–72.
52. Cetin I, Berti C, Calabrese S. Role of micronutrients in the periconceptional period. Hum Reprod Update. 2010;16(1):80–95.
53. American Dietetic Association; Dietitians of Canada; American College of Sports Medicine, Rodriguez NR, Di Marco NM, Langley S. American college of sports medicine position stand. nutrition and athletic performance. Med Sci Sports Exerc. 2009;41(3):709–31.
54. Slattery KM, Coutts AJ, Wallace LK. Nutritional practices of elite swimmers during an intensified training camp: with particular reference to antioxidants. J Sports Med Phys Fitness. 2012;52(5):501–5.
55. Packer L, Cadenas E. Lipoic acid: energy metabolism and redox regulation of transcription and cell signaling. J Clin Biochem Nutr. 2011;48(1):26–32.
56. Burke LM, Slater G, Broad EM, Haukka J, Modulon S, Hopkins WG. Eating patterns and meal frequency of elite Australian athletes. Int J Sport Nutr Exerc Metab. 2003;13(4):521–38.
57. Johnstone AM, Lobley GE, Horgan GW, Bremner DM, Fyfe CL, Morrice PC, Duthie GG. Effects of a high-protein, low-carbohydrate v. high-protein, moderate-carbohydrate weight-loss diet on antioxidant status, endothelial markers and plasma indices of the cardiometabolic profile. Br J Nutr. 2011;106(2):282–91.
58. Gaskins AJ, Colaci DS, Mendiola J, Swan SH, Chavarro JE. Dietary patterns and semen quality in young men. Hum Reprod. 2012;27(10):2899–907.
59. Attaman JA, Toth TL, Furtado J, Campos H, Hauser R, Chavarro JE. Dietary fat and semen quality

among men attending a fertility clinic. Hum Reprod. 2012;27(5):1466–74.
60. Chiu YH, Afeiche MC, Gaskins AJ, Williams PL, Mendiola J, Jørgensen N, Swan SH, Chavarro JE. Sugar-sweetened beverage intake in relation to semen quality and reproductive hormone levels in young men. Hum Reprod. 2014;29(7):1575–84.
61. Afeiche MC, Gaskins AJ, Williams PL, Toth TL, Wright DL, Tanrikut C, Hauser R, Chavarro JE. Processed meat intake is unfavorably and fish intake favorably associated with semen quality indicators among men attending a fertility clinic. J Nutr. 2014;144(7):1091–8.
62. Eslamian G, Amirjannati N, Rashidkhani B, Sadeghi MR, Hekmatdoost A. Intake of food groups and idiopathic asthenozoospermia: a case-control study. Hum Reprod. 2012;27(11):3328–36.
63. Braga DP, Halpern G, Figueira Rde C, Setti AS, Iaconelli A Jr, Borges E Jr. Food intake and social habits in male patients and its relationship to intracytoplasmic sperm injection outcomes. Fertil Steril. 2012;97(1):53–9.
64. O'Keefe JH, Gheewala NM, O'Keefe JO. Dietary strategies for improving post-prandial glucose, lipids, inflammation, and cardiovascular health. J Am Coll Cardiol. 2008;51(3):249–55.
65. Wahlqvist ML. Antioxidant relevance to human health. Asia Pac J Clin Nutr. 2013;22(2):171–6.
66. Maleki BH, Tartibian B, Eghbali M, Asri-Rezaei S. Comparison of seminal oxidants and antioxidants in subjects with different levels of physical fitness. Andrology. 2013;1(4):607–14.
67. Tartibian B, Maleki BH. Correlation between seminal oxidative stress biomarkers and antioxidants with sperm DNA damage in elite athletes and recreationally active men. Clin J Sport Med. 2012;22(2):132–9.
68. Gomes EC, Silva AN, de Oliveira MR. Oxidants, antioxidants, and the beneficial roles of exercise-induced production of reactive species. Oxid Med Cell Longev. 2012;2012:756132.
69. Manna I, Jana K, Samanta PK. Effect of intensive exercise-induced testicular gametogenic and steroidogenic disorders in mature male Wistar strain rats: a correlative approach to oxidative stress. Acta Physiol Scand. 2003;178(1):33–40.
70. Manna I, Jana K, Samanta PK. Intensive swimming exercise-induced oxidative stress and reproductive dysfunction in male wistar rats: protective role of alpha-tocopherol succinate. Can J Appl Physiol. 2004;29(2):172–85.
71. Maleki BH, Tartibian B, Vaamonde D. The effects of 16 weeks of intensive cycling training on seminal oxidants and antioxidants in male road cyclists. Clin J Sport Med. 2014;24(4):302–7.
72. Tartibian B, Maleki BH. The effects of honey supplementation on seminal plasma cytokines, oxidative stress biomarkers, and antioxidants during 8 weeks of intensive cycling training. J Androl. 2012;33(3):449–61.
73. Afeiche M, Williams PL, Mendiola J, Gaskins AJ, Jørgensen N, Swan SH, Chavarro JE. Dairy food intake in relation to semen quality and reproductive hormone levels among physically active young men. Hum Reprod. 2013;28(8):2265–75.
74. Chavarro JE, Mínguez-Alarcón L, Mendiola J, Cutillas-Tolín A, López-Espín JJ, Torres-Cantero AM. Trans fatty acid intake is inversely related to total sperm count in young healthy men. Hum Reprod. 2014;29(3):429–40.
75. Cerri RL, Juchem SO, Chebel RC, Rutigliano HM, Bruno RG, Galvão KN, Thatcher WW, Santos JE. Effect of fat source differing in fatty acid profile on metabolic parameters, fertilization, and embryo quality in high-producing dairy cows. J Dairy Sci. 2009;92(4):1520–31.
76. Demeter RM, Schopen GC, Lansink AG, Meuwissen MP, van Arendonk JA. Effects of milk fat composition, DGAT1, and SCD1 on fertility traits in Dutch Holstein cattle. J Dairy Sci. 2009;92(11):5720–9.

20 Nutritional Strategies to Reduce Potential Fertility Problems Induced by Exercise. Nutritional and Exercise Strategies to Improve Fertility Disorders

Diana Vaamonde, Juan Marcelo Fernández, Carolina Algar-Santacruz and Juan Manuel García-Manso

It is a fact that many athletes undergoing high training loads show alterations in reproductive potential. These alterations are frequently associated with the training and nutritional intake of these athletes. However, a problem is raised since the paradox of appropriate performance is associated to quantity and quality of training and to a predetermined nutritional plan in which caloric intake and the type of nutrient are key to reach elevated sports performance. Yet, if both aspects are not adequately balanced, they may become a risk factor for athletes who want to keep an intact reproductive potential.

D. Vaamonde (✉)
Department of Morphological Sciences, School of Medicine, University of Cordoba, International Network on Physical Exercise and Fertility (INPEF), Cordoba, Spain
e-mail: fivresearch@yahoo.com

J. M. Fernández
Sport and Clinical Nutrition, Nutrition Group, Nutrir Medical Nutrition and Exercise Clinic, Andalusian Society of Sports Medicine, (S.A.M.E.D.E.), Avenida Aeropuerto 28 Local, 14004 Cordoba, Spain
e-mail: j.marfer.lopez@gmail.com

C. Algar-Santacruz
Scientific Sport Association, Nutrir, Nutrición Médica y Ejercicio, Córdoba, Spain

J. M. García-Manso
Department of Physical Education, Universidad de Las Palmas de GranCanaria, C/ Consuela la Maestra 29, C Santa María de Guía, Islas Canarias 35017, Spain
e-mail: jgarciamanso@gmail.com

Energy Intake

In practical terms, besides the stability of the weight of an athlete, other factors could be indicative of an energy deficit as a possible cause of dysregulation of fertility in the athlete. Table 20.1 shows the main targets (signs, symptoms, behaviors, or characteristics) that the coach or health professional should consider with regard to the athlete's training and nutrition plan in order to look for evidence of a negative energy balance.

Determination of Referred Energy Intake

When clinical or behavioral evidence predicts an energy deficit as a possible dysregulator of fertility, the intervention of a nutrition professional could be important [1]. If this happens, the first step is to verify that the athlete's energy intake is not sufficient by itself or in relation to the needs caused by training. Establishing this relationship is not a simple task. The use of reported energy intake (REI) as a predictor of caloric deficit requires a valid and accurate measure. A valid REI accurately reflects the energy that the athlete might have ingested over a period of time. A precise REI is a measure close to reality that is obtained from repeated determinations (e.g., a re-

© Springer Science+Business Media New York 2016

D. Vaamonde et al. (eds.), *Exercise and Human Reproduction*, DOI 10.1007/978-1-4939-3402-7_20

Table 20.1 Main targets to look for evidence of a negative energy balance in athletes

Focus	Signs, symptoms, behaviors, and/or characteristics
Athlete	Physical signs of nutritional deficiency (capillary fragility, dry skin, gingival bleeding, etc.)
	Immune system depression with increase in infectious diseases
	Drastic changes in body weight
	Body fat deposits below the healthy level
	Antisocial or atypical behavior in circumstances relating to food (meetings, meals, etc.)
Sports	Sports of high energy demand especially in long-duration exercise
	Periods of increased load training (volume and/or intensity)
	Ideal image requirements and defined body weight
	Excessive stress and psychosocial stress associated with athletic performance
Food	Low level of knowledge about healthy nutrition and sports nutrition
	Restrictive eating behavior
	Excessive protein intake and aversion to eating carbohydrates and fats
	Background of dieting and/or unbalanced diets

ported mean energy intake of 3500 kcal observed in an athlete using three 24-h recordings of food and drink intake is considered as valid and precise, when a 7-day-diet questionnaire with weight method for food and drink shows a mean intake of 3554 kcal/day for the same athlete).

In addition, it is recommended to evaluate the number of meals that the athlete ingests throughout the day. The portion size of the main foods with highly energetic nutrients (e.g., carbohydrates and fats) should also be determined with the help of visual materials such as photographs and scale models.

Strategies to Increase Energy Intake of Athletes with Possible Fertility Problems as a Result of Negative Energy Balance

Subjects with a large volume and/or intensity of training could be subjected to energy demands that are difficult to satisfy in terms of food and meals. Furthermore, unlike exercise performed for a short duration at high intensity, appetite suppression often occurs at the end of a long-duration exercise at low or moderate intensity. For these reasons, the following dietary/behavioral strategies should be especially taken into account:

1. Carbohydrates and fats are the main fuels to burn and their use as energy substrates varies proportionally according to the intensity and duration of effort. Nevertheless, it is carbohydrates which, when ingested in adequate amounts, would determine energy intake sufficient for physical performance and the health of athletes [2].
2. Between 4 and 11 servings of bread, cereal, rice, and pasta should be consumed according to the calculation of the energy and carbohydrate needs for each athlete depending on the type of exercise.
3. Vegetable fats and oils should be sufficiently consumed and not restricted to below 20 % of daily energy intake [3, 4].
4. The intake of fluids containing carbohydrates is a useful recommendation for athletes with appetite suppression induced by exercise [5, 6].

5. Educating female athletes to maintain a healthy weight and adopt a practice of sufficient food intake taken at appropriate time intervals in relation to exercise is a good way to increase energy intake and nutrients in these athletes. Moreover, this practice could make a key difference to competitiveness against other athletes.
6. Educating the athlete about the global importance of specific nutrients in the athlete's diet, and avoiding mistakes and prejudices which may cause difficulty in achieving a sufficient energy intake.
7. Changing erroneous beliefs with regard to intake of specific supplements such as minerals, vitamins, or proteins before a competition, as this can correct a long-term unbalanced and insufficient diet.
8. Educating the female athlete on the fact that cessation of menstruation not only affects fertility, but it is also associated with reduced bone mineral density and potentially increases the risk of stress fractures. In this regard, food intake is clearly one of the modifiable factors and is an important strategy.

Reduced Availability of Antioxidant Compounds

As stated earlier, the first step in correcting specific nutritional deficiencies that can affect fertility of an athlete is to ensure adequate global energy intake. Moreover, adequate intake of antioxidants and minerals is needed because of the importance of these nutrients.

It is also interesting to note that different dietary patterns have proven to be effective in improving oxidative and inflammatory status in healthy subjects or subjects with different chronic diseases such as obesity, diabetes, metabolic syndrome (MetS), etc. [7–9]. Although most of the previously published studies have examined the effect of an increase in the availability of antioxidants on cellular phenomena associated with metabolic and cardiovascular risk, there is now sufficient evidence to show improved fertility through antioxidant nutritional therapy [10, 11].

Specifically, the Mediterranean diet has emerged as a dietary pattern with significant effect on the oxidative status in healthy individuals of different age groups [12, 13]. It is a dietary pattern characterized by abundant intake of minor components with antioxidants derived from varied and moderate consumption of fruits, vegetables, extra-virgin olive oil, and red wine.

From other cultural, or recent nutritional habits, dietary patterns and other foods have been proposed as they include high-antioxidant-potential compounds. Nutrients, such as honey, curcumin, omega-3 acids, or trans-resveratrol, could be included as examples among this type of substances.

It has been reported that honey has a protective role against oxidative stress produced during intensive training cycle, reducing markers of inflammation and oxidative stress and increasing levels of endogenous antioxidant systems [14, 15].

Meanwhile, curcumin present in curry, either alone or as an adjuvant with vitamin E, protects seminal glands, as well as sperm and testicular tissue, against toxic damage [16–18]. However, more research is needed about the effect of curcumin, as some studies have reported that, at least in animal models, curcumin could alter the onset of puberty in female mice as well as sperm quality and rate of live births in mice because of estrogenic/antiandrogenic activity and disruption of pregnancy [19].

Polyphenolic antioxidant compounds derived from grapes (especially proanthocyanidins), as in the case of resveratrol, are also common in Mediterranean diet (wine, grapes, peanuts, etc). In recent years, due to reported beneficial effects, it has drawn much interest among scientists having assessed its anti-inflammatory, antiviral [20], and antitumoral [21] properties and its potential effect on cardiopathies [22].

Although, strictly speaking, omega-3 fatty acids are not antioxidants, they are important components in many diets and seem to exert antioxidant-like properties, increasing total antioxidant capacity and decreasing inflammation and oxidative stress in tissues. Diets rich in fish are high in omega-3, which has been reported to increase both the male and female reproductive potential [23–25]. In females, omega-3 seems to improve folliculogenesis and oocyte quality as well as the prognosis in assisted reproductive technique (ART) procedures [24]. Moreover, there is evidence that these compounds help improve placental function by decreasing oxidative stress and inflammation [25]. In males, some studies have reported improved morphology and even a positive effect on oligoasthenoteratozoospermia [26].

In more western-style diets, walnuts can provide the benefits observed when consuming fish as they are also omega-3-rich fruits [27]. However, it seems that there is an altered relationship between omega-3 and omega-6 acids, similar to that of elevated linoleic acid (LA) omega-6/alpha linoleic acid (ALA) omega-3 ratio, which may affect female reproductive physiology, due to alterations in progesterone production, ovulation rate, and/or oocyte quality [28]. Moreover, the same authors have observed an identical effect in rat sperm, where an altered LA omega-6/ALA omega-3 ratio affects sperm density and motility. Mouse plasma progesterone levels are affected by different dietary omega-6/omega-3 ratios [28].

We could also highlight the Okinawan diet, which is a traditional Japanese dietary pattern that could be comparable to the Mediterranean diet and is characterized by a low calorie intake but rich in vegetables and fruits with reduced intake of meat, refined grains, saturated fat, sugar, salt, and full-fat dairy products [29]. Because of these characteristics, this is a phytonutrient and antioxidant-rich diet.

Strategies to Increase Antioxidant Food Intake

Obviously, an athlete with his/her own cultural characteristics and high energy demands as a result of his/her own sports practice (e.g., mainly carbohydrates in long-distance runners and proteins in the case of bodybuilders) may not meet all his/her dietary characteristics that define these dietary patterns and its healthy antioxidants. However, it would be desirable to adopt common strategies and habits to those dietary patterns that have proven to have increased daily intake of vitamins C and E, selenium, beta-carotene, and flavonols, including quercetin. These compounds have recently been associated with a significant improvement in fertility, especially leading to increased sperm count and mobility. The main dietary measures to enhance oxidative status according to current scientific evidence are:

a. Increasing consumption of fruits, to three to five servings a day, with particular emphasis on selecting brightly colored fruits, citrus, and others that are known to be antioxidant rich, such as pomegranate.
b. Reducing consumption of animal and refined esterified fats and increasing consumption of vegetable oils. The daily consumption of extra-virgin olive oil is particularly interesting.
c. Consuming at least two servings of vegetables a day, at least one of them raw.
d. Performing a moderate daily intake of nuts, such as walnuts.
e. Using green or white tea as a liquid pre-exercise hydration or rehydration of the athlete, and adding carbohydrates when its input is needed.
f. Daily consumption of one glass of red wine is recommended, provided this is not a strange habit for the athlete.

Exercise and Nutrition Strategies As Therapeutic Treatment of Pathologies Associated with Fertility Disorders

MetS and obesity and polycystic ovary syndrome (PCOS) are pathologies that frequently involve fertility problems. Although many metabolic abnormalities, with possible implications on fertility (e.g., hypertension, insulin resistance, inflammation, and oxidative stress), may be present in obese or MetS or PCOS subjects, there are two common components that worsen these alterations: excess weight and physical inactivity.

Metabolic Syndrome and Obesity

Obesity and MetS have been linked, both in men and women, to lower fertility rates and worsen the prognosis in ARTs [30–33]. Recognizing and treating patients with obesity, and especially those with associated MetS, can help improve not only fertility but also sexual and overall health [34].

Obesity has been associated with poorer sperm quality, oocyte quality, and embryo development. In men, poor sperm quality has been revealed by reduced sperm binding to hyaluronan-coated slides in men with high body mass index (BMI) and other unhealthy lifestyles such as smoking [35]. Moreover, in patients with MetS, it was observed that varicocelectomy improved semen quality, yet this improvement was not as effective as in patients without MetS. This seems to indicate that MetS can be a factor for male infertility [36]. The importance of obesity and MetS seems evident from a number of interventional studies showing that treatment with diet either alone or in conjunction with an exercise regime improves fertility [37]. However, with regard to surgical approaches to reduce obesity (bariatric surgery), there is no clear consensus as to whether this intervention helps in improving the fertility potential as evidenced by contradictory results from different studies [38–41]. These conflicting results may arise from confounding factors that were not taken into account in these studies. Therefore, it must be noted that careful patient selection and accurate clarification of their infertility cause and other health issues that may be present along with their obesity state are needed for obtaining proper knowledge.

In women, obesity has been found to affect mitochondrial metabolic function and increase mitochondrial reactive oxygen species (ROS) production, altering the initial stages of embryonic development [31]. Mitochondria are critical components in oocyte quality and embryo development as evidenced by studies revealing that defective mitochondrial biogenesis along with insufficient mitochondrial mass leads to failed oocyte maturation and hampered embryo development [42, 43]. Therefore, mitochondrial quality and quantity are required for successful fertilization and embryo development [31, 44].

Overweight and obesity were related to lower live birth rates in women undergoing ART treatment. In these cases, short-term weight loss intervention was related to higher metaphase II (MII) oocyte (mature) yield but not to clinical outcomes [45]. Other studies have also proven the efficacy of short-term nutritional and exercise intervention in increasing pregnancy rates [46, 47].

Polycystic Ovary Syndrome

PCOS is a common complex, heterogeneous disorder that affects 5–10 % of women, normally appears in adolescence, and is one of main causes of female subfertility/infertility. In this condition, the ovaries contain many cystic follicles that are associated with chronic anovulation and overproduction of androgens. Symptoms may include anovulation, irregular menstrual periods, obesity, excessive growth of central body hair (hirsutism), and infertility. It can be associated with other systemic disorders, being commonly linked to MetS and obesity (obesity in up to 60 % of PCOS subjects depending on country), thus having a severe impact on quality of life [48].

Palliative Recommendations for Subjects with Obesity, Metabolic Syndrome, and Polycystic Ovary Syndrome

Although PCOS is commonly treated with pharmacologic agents such as clomiphene citrate, due to the fact that this disorder is frequently associated with obesity and/or MetS, the recommendations that can be given with regard to nutrition and exercise are common. The changing of lifestyles is a key pillar in the treatment to improve the reproductive capacity of these individuals, requiring even the intervention on the psychological status of these patients to promote adherence to lifestyle changes. Thus, the two main lines of treatment are modifications leading to the acquisition of healthy nutritional habits and a more active lifestyle.

Healthy Nutritional Habits

In order to improve the fertility potential of subjects with the above-mentioned pathologies, reducing body weight could allow for attenuating the negative effects associated with these pathologies [49]. It has been shown that weight reduction leads to increased fertility in women with obesity, MetS, and PCOS. Controlling obesity with dietary intervention is one of the main strategies used to promote weight loss.

Different nutritional strategies with caloric restriction have been proposed for long-term sustained weight loss and improvement of these conditions: short-term hypocaloric diet in women with PCOS led to a significant weight loss and a significant improvement in reproductive and metabolic abnormalities [50]; a low-carbohydrate, high-protein diet in in vitro fertilization (IVF) patients led to increased blastocyst formation rate and clinical pregnancy rate [51]. Although nutritional strategies alone seem to favor reproductive outcomes [52], it is suggested that diet and lifestyle interventions be implemented as a combined approach for subfertility in overweight and obese men.

However, one must be careful as extreme rapid dieting and acute very-low-calorie diets have been associated with poor natural reproductive and ART outcomes. Therefore, this type of patients should be offered the necessary advice and support for the needed weight loss and compliance to the dietary strategies (Table 20.2). When dealing with these patients, one should have a well-structured, realistic approach to a weight loss of approximately 5–10% of initial weight. Moreover, structuring phases favors adherence to the program and prevents loss of motivation. In PCOS, weight loss of 5% or greater will help in correcting ovulatory dysfunction or in reducing the dose needed for ovulation-inducing drugs [57].

Moreover, new theories, based on increasing dietary protein at the expense of carbohydrates, are gaining popularity for the treatment of obesity and PCOS [10, 51, 58]. Increased protein

Table 20.2 Main strategies used to promote weight loss through diet

Dietary strategy	Proposed protocol	Potential systemic benefits
Caloric restriction	Progressive reduction of calorie intake in the diet	Phasing out calories in a diet of negative energy balance and fat mass loss
		Reeducation of food intake habits
Overall reduction of dietary fat	Restricting dietary fat to between 25 and 35% of total energy intake [53]	Reduced caloric intake
		Improved postprandial status
Reduction of saturated fat	Less than or equal to 10% of total energy intake	Favors blood lipid control
		Improves oxidative status
		Improves endothelial dysfunction (ATP III)
Increase viscous (soluble) fibers (mainly in oat products, psyllium, and pectin) intake	10–25 gr/day	Reduces glycemic and insulinemic response of other foods [54]
		Increases gastric emptying time and satiety [55]
Reduction of glycemic load of diet	Selection of low-glycemic-index food	Increased availability of fats for oxidative metabolism
	Reduction of high-glycemic-index food	Improved triglyceride levels and higher levels of high-density lipoprotein cholesterol
		Reduced C-reactive protein (CRP) concentrations [56]

ATP III Adult Treatment Panel III

intake seems to facilitate short-term weight reduction (e.g., Zone diet), moderately reducing triglycerides levels and improving insulin sensitivity [59]. However, future studies are needed to determine the long-term maintenance of results achieved with these diets and their effect on the embryos at the different stages.

Most likely, the most adequate strategy would be to combine adequate nutrition with a carefully planned exercise intervention. Supplementation of antioxidant such as trans-resveratrol may help decrease BMI and improve reproductive potential in these patients [60, 61]. However, other authors have observed that resveratrol is unable to improve insulin sensitivity in rats with PCOS fed with normal chow [62]. Therefore, resveratrol may not be the most adequate candidate in this regard and should be taken cautiously.

Continuous Level of Physical Activity

An adequate exercise program is the first-line treatment with dietary changes to achieve weight reduction in obese patients with MetS or PCOS. Alterations in reproductive function due to physical activity and physical training have already been investigated, although with inconsistent conclusions due to a number of factors, such as training status, gender, and the different exercise protocols used [14, 15, 63, 64].

Nevertheless, intensive, strenuous training for competition seems to lead to altered hormonal profiles [65–67], testicular atrophy [68, 69], genitourinary problems [70, 71], altered semen parameters [72], altered oxidative status [14, 15], and menstrual abnormalities [73]. However, few negative effects have been described when performing regular moderate exercise; and in this regard, active subjects show better hormone and semen profiles [63].

Increased adherence is achieved when physical exercise is integrated into a comprehensive program that includes group therapy and patient-specific nutrition. In the case of patients with PCOS, adherence to these changes not only achieves better range of objectives in weight and general well-being of the patient but also allows a better response to the drugs used to correct infertility.

The *Clinical Guidelines on the Identification, Evaluation, and Treatment of Overweight and Obesity in Adults* suggest performing physical exercise for 30–45 min, three to five times per week. All adults should set a long-term goal to accumulate at least 30 min or more of moderate-intensity physical activity on most, but preferably all, days of the week. We understand by moderate-intensity physical activity (60–70 % VO_{2max}; equivalent to 75–80 % HR_{max}) as any type of activity (cycling, running, swimming, or strength training) performed at least three times per week during a minimum duration of approximately 12 weeks [74].

Most of the studies published refer to training involving at least three 30-min aerobic sessions per week (e.g., 90 min/week) without dietary restriction or resistance exercise [75–77], although two studies reporting improvement included these components [78, 79].

Nevertheless, we would like to note that the activity adopted does not necessarily have to be of continuous low-intensity aerobic exercise. Using intense intervallic works (short-term, high-intensity interval training) may also provide beneficial effects on an elevated number of metabolic and vascular risk factors in overweight/obese, sedentary men [80, 81]. In these protocols, duration of each repetition must be short enough (≈5 s for supramaximal exercises and ≈30 s for submaximal exercises) and done at ample duration (≈twice the effort duration) in order to get an elevated work volume during the session without getting to fatigue level.

Also, the inclusion of resistance training (RT) as an integral part of an exercise therapy program has been endorsed on *Appropriate Intervention Strategies for Weight Loss and Prevention of Weight Regain in Adults* by the *American College of Sports Medicine* [82], the *Dietary Guidelines for Americans 2005* (USDHHS and USDA), and other of the *American Heart Association* [83] and the *American Diabetes Association* [84].

The *American College of Sports Medicine* [82] proposes to perform, at least, 150 min of moderate exercise per week to improve the health status in overweight and obese individuals. They also include a recommended goal of 200–300 min of leisure time activity per week for long-term weight maintenance. In the *Dietary Guidelines for Americans,* it is proposed to undertake at least 30 min of exercise on most days to improve health and 60 min of exercise on most days for weight loss and weight control.

In line with this, several studies show how exercise at least three times per week allows for reduction of fat percentage and risk factors associated with normal-weight and overweight sedentary subjects [85–87].

Endometriosis

Endometriosis is a pathological condition commonly observed in women with infertility (6–10% of women during their reproductive years; [88]). Endometriosis is characterized by the presence and growth of endometrial cells outside the uterine cavity, most commonly in the peritoneum [89]. These cells are influenced by hormonal changes and respond in a way that is similar to the cells found inside the uterus [90]. Endometriosis is characterized by a range of symptoms and severity, including chronic pelvic pain and infertility, with common presence of inflammation, scarring, and adhesions. As a result of these, many women may also suffer from infertility [91, 92]. Moreover, it has been suggested that endometriotic lesions release factors which are detrimental to gametes or embryos [93].

The role of modifiable exogenous factors such as nutrition and exercise in the development and/or prevention of this disease is not well understood. Nevertheless, recent evidence suggests there may be nutritional and exercise strategies to help ease the condition or even prevent it [94]. In an animal model study [95], it was found that fish oil could induce regression of surgically induced endometriosis. In humans [96], it was observed that the degree of endometriotic lesions was positively related to red meat consumption and inversely related to fruits and green vegetables consumption.

It has also been observed that N-acetyl-L-cysteine, besides having a beneficial effect on sports performance [97], also exerts a complex action on endometrial cells, involving regulation of gene expression and protein activity and location, with all of it converging into decreased proliferation and a switch towards a differentiating, less invasive, and less inflammatory phenotype [98].

It has been observed that markers of inflammation and interleukin-6 (IL-6) in women with endometriosis are modulated with fatty acid intake [99]. Although controversies exist [100], it has been observed that omega-3 fatty acids exert a protective effect on endometriosis risk; conversely, other foods such as red meat, trans fats, and coffee have affected this risk in a negative manner. Other authors have reported similar findings, encouraging increased omega-3 fatty acid and decreased trans fats intake in order to modify endometriosis risk [94].

Imbalance between ROS and antioxidant in the peritoneal fluid of some women has been shown to lead to oxidative stress and endometriosis [101–102]. In the presence of oxidative stress, ROS might increase the growth and adhesion of endometrial cells in the peritoneal cavity, leading to endometriosis and infertility [102].

Nutritional Proposal

Among the different nutrients in a diet, some seem to be especially interesting for the prevention and treatment of this pathology [103].

- Increased long-chain omega-3 fatty acid consumption was associated with a decreased risk of endometriosis, while trans fat intake was associated with an increased risk of endometriosis [94]. Omega-3 diets decrease the levels of inflammatory markers as well as the extension of endometriotic lesions. As mentioned earlier in other parts of the chapter, the omega-3/omega-6 ratio seems to be of great importance for the improvement of the pathology; as such, an altered ratio is related to endometriosis development [104].

- Diets with foods containing moderate amount of beta-carotenes could be adequate, even recommendable for people with endometriosis. However, elevated intake of beta-carotenes (e.g., spinach, asparagus, red peppers, carrots, pumpkins, peas, etc.), in spite of their antioxidant capacity, could be detrimental for people with this pathology. Causes are unknown, but [103] it is reported that the negative effects are seen when patients consume a high dose of these products, especially of green vegetables, along with elevated amounts of fruits (especially melon, apricot, watermelon, strawberry, papaya, etc.). The effect noticed in these patients could be due to the pesticides contained in these foods.
- Intake of vitamins B, C, and E has been related to decreased endometriotic lesions, but this effect could be related not to these vitamins per se but to the intake of foods that are rich in these micronutrients [105]. The volume of cysts is also diminished by vitamin C intake [106]. Much amount of these vitamins is ingested in diet as fruits; however, it must be taken into account that higher servings of fruit per day in diet could also be linked to a greater risk of suffering from endometriosis due to the pesticides that these foods could contain [103].
- Moderate amounts of fresh fruit, especially of ecological origin, are associated with decreased risk [96]. This seems to be in line with that reported by Trabert as pesticides being the potential reason behind elevated endometrioses risk in people with high vegetable and fruit consumption.
- Though still a controversial aspect, dietary vitamin D intake and plasma 25-hydroxyvitamin D (25(OH)D) concentration could be linked to decreased endometriosis risk [74]. A biological plausibility for the role of vitamin D, as an immunomodulator and anti-inflammatory agent, in the pathogenesis and treatment of endometriosis is suggested by Sayegh et al. [107].
- Some observational studies have shown that plant-based diets and diets high in fiber increase estrogen excretion and decrease concentrations of bioavailable estrogen, and thus may lower endometriosis risk [103, 108].
- A 12-month treatment with gluten-free diets has been observed to improve chronic pelvic pain related to endometriosis in 75 % of the analyzed patients. In any case, there was no observed worsening of pain in any of the treated patients and there was an increased perception of overall well-being and quality of life [109].

Proposed Physical Activity

Despite the possibility of a certain degree of free radical being generated as a result of physical activity, and the effect this could exert on the development of inflammatory processes associated with endometrial tissue, there is evidence that regular physical activity has a protective effect on endometriosis, which possibly is favored by a hormetic mechanism [110].

The beneficial effects of exercise could be related to increase in cytokines and their anti-inflammatory potential [111]. The cytokine response to exercise is characterized by a constant increase in plasma IL-6 concentration [112, 113], in parallel with an enhanced expression of IL-6 mRNA in contracting muscles [114].

In addition, regular exercise is associated with changes in levels of circulating estrogens, with a reduction that could have a beneficial effect on the endometrium [115]. This effect can provide a protective effect since endometriosis is an estrogen-dependent disease and physical activity may increase levels of sex hormone-binding globulin (SHBG), which would reduce estrogen bioavailability [116, 117]. Physical activity also reduces insulin resistance and hyperinsulinemia [116], cell invasion, and proliferation and increases apoptosis on endometriosis lesions [117].

Endometriosis risk has been observed to be low in women who regularly exercise compared to those who do not [118, 119]. This observation, however, could be biased as women experiencing symptoms before being diagnosed may not engage in physical activity as much as healthy women do [119]. Total physical activity levels were weakly associated with confirmed endometriosis. Endometriosis risk was reduced by 11% in the most active group when compared to the least active (≥42 metabolic equivalent (MET)-h/week vs. <3 MET-h/week). Similar trend was observed in patients with no infertility but not in patients with infertility. When analyzing physical activity profile of the women 4 years prior to diagnosis, the observation was a 9% reduction in risk for the more physically active women compared to less active women [119]. This observation is similar to the observation obtained from the most recent reported data [118] that women who reported frequent and regular high-intensity activity (>30 min/session; >three times per week) for several years (2 years prior to the reference date) had a reduced endometrioma risk (76%). Also, a nonsignificant reduction in risk was observed for women who reported such activity at ages 12–21 years. Moreover [120], it was observed that implementing a physical and psychological intervention protocol (one time per week; 2.5 h/session) in women with endometriosis was effective in reducing perceived stress, normalizing cortisol levels, increasing vitality, and improving physical functioning.

Moderate and regular physical exercise, independent of the characteristics of activity (e.g., running, swimming, cycling, aerobic, or training with loads), will have a beneficial effect on endometriosis. For healthy women that are not involved in a specific sports training modality, it is recommended to engage in recreational or leisure activities that imply movement (e.g., walking, jogging, or cycling), games, sports, or exercises fulfilling the following characteristics:

- Minimum of 180 min/week of moderate-intensity aerobic physical activity, or 90 min/week of vigorous aerobic physical activity, or an equivalent combination of moderate and vigorous activities [121, 122]. Intense aerobic physical activity shall be practiced in sessions in which the cumulative work is greater than 15 min. Using pedometers may be useful in controlling the activity performed by the subjects, recommending that even subjects with low-level physical activity reach 10,000 daily steps.
- These activities may be done through practice of cyclic modalities (e.g., running, rowing, cycling, etc.) or with group activities of similar intensity (e.g., aerobic classes, CrossFit, etc.). Group activities add socializing and psychological elements to the activity and therefore may be especially interesting for some population subtypes [123].
- To obtain greater health benefits, or in women with greater physical status, moderate aerobic physical activity can be increased up to 300 min/week, or up to 150 min/week in the case of intense physical activity, preferably aerobic, or an equivalent combination of moderate and vigorous activities.
- It would be recommendable, at least twice a week, to perform activities aimed at strengthening the big muscle groups.

Inappropriate Lifestyles Leading to Infertility

Nowadays, there are many unhealthy lifestyle factors that have been linked to decreased semen quality; among these, we should highlight unhealthy nutritional habits, sedentarism, and substance abuse such as tobacco, alcohol, and different drugs [124, 125].

Alimentary Habits and Inadequate Nutritional Status

Alimentary habits of humans (food origin, caloric intake, number of meals, meal schedules, etc.) clearly reflect a person's cultural, economic, and geographic environment. As a result of these circumstances, the habits adopted by many are far from those considered as adequate and healthy.

An inadequate diet may lead to many health problems; among these, fertility problems should be highlighted. It has been reported in men that high BMI and alcohol negatively affect important sperm parameters such as concentration, velocity, and morphology [126]. Conversely, cereal consumption and the number of meals done throughout the day positively influence the same parameters [126].

Needless to say, the IVF setting is a unique one, in which female and male parameters cannot be easily separated or linked to the ART procedure outcome. Nonetheless, alcohol and coffee intake in the male partner and smoking in the female partner have been linked to negative effects on intracytoplasmic sperm injection (ICSI) fertilization rate. Implantation rate has been observed to be negatively affected by frequent consumption of red meat and by the female BMI, and also by uncontrolled weight loss dieting [126]. Also, in this regard, poor semen quality has been related to higher intake of products that could incorporate xenobiotics, mainly xenoestrogens or certain anabolic steroids [127–130]. The xenoestrogens (highly lipophilic substances) that may accumulate in fat-rich foods, such as meat, are believed to negatively influence semen quality [128]. Similarly, subjects with higher skim milk and lower dairy products intake exhibit better semen parameters [128, 129]. We must be aware that these compounds are virtually everywhere and may exert negative effects on gametes, embryos, and, therefore, reproductive potential. On the other hand, higher antioxidant and micronutrients intake has been reported to positively influence sperm quality [126].

Sedentarism

In men, higher prevalence of sedentarism has been associated with low-normal sperm concentration [131]. An important component of this relationship is linked to obesity problems and pathologies associated with MetS; however, some work positions with none or low physical demand may result in increased scrotal temperature that could negatively affect male fertility [132]. Other studies detect a decrease in sperm concentration, which, although not statistically significant, suggests that sedentary work is a risk factor for abnormal semen characteristics [133].

Tobacco, Alcohol, and Drug Use

There is evidence linking tobacco use to alterations in female fertility [134–138], which argues that cigarette smoking in women is associated with an increase in both time to conception and risk of primary infertility. Also, smoking, or simply cigarette smoke exposure, is related to decreased ovarian weight and follicle numbers, and increased oxidative stress with greater number of autophagosomes in granulosa cells of ovarian follicles. In men, smoke-induced toxins primarily hamper sperm motility and seminal fluid quality [139].

The use of recreational drugs may be a risk factor for both male and female fertility [140, 141]. In females, marijuana may alter ovulatory function [140], suppress plasma prolactin [141] and luteinizing hormones [142, 143], and can also affect pregnancy. In males, the use of this drug exerts negative effects on the hypothalamic–pituitary–testicular axis [141] and reduces testosterone released from Leydig cells, modulates apoptosis of Sertoli cells, decreases spermatogenesis, sperm motility, sperm capacitation, and acrosome reaction [144]. Cocaine and other drugs exert similar effects [141]. In males, the maintained and elevated use of cocaine negatively affects the sexual act (erection and ejaculation; [145]) and spermatogenesis as a consequence of the incidence on hormonal balance (increment of prolactin and decrease of free testosterone; [146]). Opiates (e.g., methadone and heroin) are also commonly used drugs in certain social sectors. Their frequent use also affects the sexual act [147], sperm quality [148], and, probably, female fertility [149].

An elevated alcohol intake may be associated with lower fertility potential and chance of conception and with higher miscarriage rate. Thus, couples with fertility problems should greatly, or even completely, limit alcohol intake [150]. Alcohol intake is associated with decreased fecundability in women, even when weekly intake amounts to five or less drinks [151]. The level of consumption did not affect the average time to conception and risk of primary infertiliy [134]. In men and male animals, alcohol abuse can result in impotency, infertility, hypogonadism, and sperm morphology and production problems [152]. However, dose-dependent effects of alcohol on human spermatogenesis are not well established [139, 153, 154].

Final Remarks

In order to keep a healthy reproductive potential, both athletes and nonathletes should engage in good habits regarding nutrition and exercise. Yet, it is understood that competitive sports practice requires training levels that could be considered as not healthy, and nutritional strategies can be implemented aimed at counteracting the possible negative effects on the reproductive system. In this regard, maintaining or achieving an ideal weight, if allowed by the demands of the sports practice, is of paramount importance for reproductive processes, although we acknowledge that this may be against the requirements imposed on the athletes, especially for competition purposes. Therefore, we understand some of these strategies may not be implemented at least until the athlete stops competing and intends to have an offspring. With regard to nonathletes, several exercise strategies can be implemented in trying to cure or alleviate reproductive disorders or health-related issues that can have a toll on reproduction.

References

1. Delimaris I, Piperakis SM. The importance of nutritional factors on human male fertility: a toxicological approach. J Transl Toxicol. 2014;1(1):52–9.
2. Burke LM, Hawley JA, Wong SH, Jeukendrup AE. Carbohydrates for training and competition. J Sports Sci. 2011;29(Suppl 1):S17–27.
3. Rodriguez NR, Di Marco NM, Langley S, American College of Sports Medicine, American Dietetic Association Dietitians of Canada, American College of Sports Medicine. American College of Sports Medicine position stand. Nutrition and athletic performance. Med Sci Sports Exerc. 2009;41(3):709–31.
4. Hausswith C, Le Meur Y. Physiological and nutritional aspects of post-exercise recovery: specific recommendations for female athletes. Sports Med. 2011;41(10):861–82.
5. Burke LM, Kiens B, Ivy JL. Carbohydrates and fat for training and recovery. J Sports Sci. 2004;22(1):15–30.
6. Maughan RJ, Burke LM. Practical nutritional recommendations for the athlete. Nestle Nutr Inst Workshop Ser. 2011;69:131–49.
7. Lopez-Garcia E, Schulze MB, Fung TT, Meigs JB, Rifai N, Manson JE, Hu FB. Major dietary patterns are related to plasma concentrations of markers of inflammation and endothelial dysfunction. Am J Clin Nutr. 2004;80(4):1029–35.
8. Salas-Salvadó J, Garcia-Arellano A, Estruch R, Marquez-Sandoval F, Corella D, Fiol M, Ros E. Components of the Mediterranean-type food pattern and serum inflammatory markers among patients at high risk for cardiovascular disease. Eur J Clin Nutr. 2007;62(5):651–9.
9. Stancliffe RA, Thorpe T, Zemel MB. Dairy attentuates oxidative and inflammatory stress in metabolic syndrome. Am J Clin Nutr. 2011;94(2):422–30.
10. Mora- Esteves C, Shin D. Nutrient supplementation: improving male fertility fourfold. Semin Reprod Med. 2013;31(4):293–300.
11. Showell MG, Brown J, Clarke J, Hart RJ. Antioxidants for female subfertility. Cochrane Database Syst Rev. 2013;8:CD007807.
12. Dai J, Jones DP, Goldberg J, Ziegler TR, Bostick RM, Wilson PW, Vaccarino V. Association between adherence to the Mediterranean diet and oxidative stress. Am J Clin Nutr. 2008;88(5):1364–70.
13. Sari I, Baltaci Y, Bagci C, Davutoglu V, Erel O, Celik H, Aksoy M. Effect of pistachio diet on lipid parameters, endothelial function, inflammation, and oxidative status: a prospective study. Nutrition. 2010;26(4):399–404.
14. Tartibian B, Maleki B. Correlation between seminal oxidative stress biomarkers and antioxidants with sperm DNA damage in elite athletes and recreationally active men. Clin J Sport Med. 2012;22:132–9.
15. Tartibian B, Maleki B. The effects of honey supplementation on seminal plasma cytokines, oxidative stress biomarkers, and antioxidants during 8 weeks of intensive cycling training. J Androl. 2012;33:449–61.
16. Sahoo DK, Roy A, Chainy GB. Protective effects of vitamin E and curcumin on L-thyroxine-induced rat testicular oxidative stress. Chem Biol Interact. 2008;176(2):121–8.
17. Oguzturk H, Ciftci O, Aydin M, Timurkaan N, Beytur A, Yilmaz F. Ameliorative effects of curcumin against acute cadmium toxicity on male reproductive system in rats. Andrologia. 2012;44(4):243–9.
18. Karbalay-Doust S, Noorafshan A. Ameliorative effects of curcumin on the spermatozoon tail length, count, motility and testosterone serum level in metronidazoletreated mice. Prague Med Rep. 2011;112(4):288–97.
19. Murphy CJ, Tang H, Van Kirk EA, Shen Y, Murdoch WJ. Reproductive effects of a pegylated curcumin. Reprod Toxicol. 2012;34(1):120–4.

20. Frémont L. Biological effects of resveratrol. Life Sci. 2000;66(8):663–73.
21. Sauer H, Wartenberg M, y Hescheler J. Reactive oxygen species as intracellular messengers during cell growth and differentiation. Cell Physiol Biochem: Int J Exp Cell Physiol Biochem Pharmacol. 2001;11:173–86.
22. Bhat KPL, Kosmeder JW, Pezzuto JM. Biological effects of resveratrol. Antioxid Redox Signal. 2001;3:1041–64.
23. Safarinejad MR, Safarinejad S. The roles of omega-3 and omega-6 fatty acids in idiopathic male infertility. Asian J Androl. 2012;14(4):514–5.
24. Moallem U, Shafran A, Zachut M, Dekel I, Portnick Y, Arieli A. Dietary α-linolenic acid from flaxseed oil improved folliculogenesis and IVF performance in dairy cows, similar to eicosapentaenoic and docosahexaenoic acids from fish oil. Reproduction. 2013;146(6):603–14. doi:10.1530/REP-13-0244.
25. Jones ML, Mark PJ, Waddell BJ. Maternal dietary omega-3 fatty acids and placental function. Reproduction. 2014;147(5):R143–52.
26. Attaman JA, Toth TL, Furtado J, Campos H, Hauser R, Chavarro JE. Dietary fat and semen quality among men attending a fertility clinic. Hum Reprod. 2012;27(5):1466–74.
27. Robbins WA, Xun L, FitzGerald LZ, Esguerra S, Henning SM, Carpenter CL. Walnuts improve semen quality in men consuming a Western-style diet: randomized control dietary intervention trial. Biol Reprod. 2012;87(4):101.
28. Oliva LL, Santillán ME, Ryan LC, Bianconi S, Vincenti LM, Martini AC, Ponzio MF, Stutz G. Mouse plasma progesterone levels are affected by different dietary ω6/ω3 ratios. Horm Metab Res. 2014;46(2):120–5.
29. Willcox DC, Willcox BJ, Todoriki H, Suzuki M. The Okinawan diet: health implications of a low-calorie, nutrient-dense, antioxidant-rich dietary pattern low in glycemic load. J Am Coll Nutr. 2009;28(sup4):500 S–16.
30. Du Plessis SS, Cabler S, McAlister DA, Sabanegh E, Agarwal A. The effect of obesity on sperm disorders and male infertility. Nat Rev Urol. 2010;7(3):153–61.
31. Igosheva N, Abramov AY, Poston L, Eckert JJ, Fleming TP, Duchen MR, McConnell J. Maternal diet-induced obesity alters mitochondrial activity and redox status in mouse oocytes and zygotes. PLoS ONE. 2010;5(4):e10074. doi:10.1371/journal.pone.0010074.
32. Bakos HW, Henshaw RC, Mitchell M, Lane M. Paternal body mass index is associated with decreased blastocyst development and reduced live birth rates following assisted reproductive technology. Fertil Steril. 2011;95(5):1700–4.
33. Kuzbari O, Hammoud AO. Obesity and male infertility: is there an effect on embryogenesis? In: Carrell DT, editor. Paternal influences on human reproductive success. Cambridge: Cambridge University Press; 2013. pp. 141–7.
34. Lotti F, Corona G, Vignozzi L, Rossi M, Maseroli E, Gacci M, Forti G, Maggi M. Metabolic syndrome correlates with prostate volume and biochemical and ultrasound signs of prostate inflammation in male members of infertile couples. Endocr Abstr. 2013;32:P653. doi:10.1530/endoabs.32.P65.
35. Wegner CC, Clifford AL, Jilbert PM, Henry MA, Gentry WL. Abnormally high body mass index and tobacco use are associated with poor sperm quality as revealed by reduced sperm binding to hyaluronan-coated slides. Fertil Steril. 2010;93(1):332–4.
36. Ozturk U, Sener NC, Nalbant I, Karabacak OR, Ulusoy MG, Imamoglu MA. The effect of metabolic syndrome upon the success of varicocelectomy. Sci World J. 2012;2012:985201.
37. Panidis D, Tziomalos K, Papadakis E, Vosnakis C, Chatzis P, Katsikis I. Lifestyle intervention and anti-obesity therapies in the polycystic ovary syndrome: impact on metabolism and fertility. Endocrine. 2013;44(3):583–90.
38. Reis LO, Zani EL, Saad RD, Chaim EA, de Oliveira LC, Fregonesi A. Bariatric surgery does not interfere with sperm quality–a preliminary long-term study. Reprod Sci. 2012;19(10):1057–62.
39. Sermondade N, Massin N, Boitrelle F, Pfeffer J, Eustache F, Sifer C, Czernichow S, Lévy R. Sperm parameters and male fertility after bariatric surgery: three case series. Reprod Biomed Online. 2012;24(2):206–10.
40. Lazaros L, Hatzi E, Markoula S, Takenaka A, Sofikitis N, Zikopoulos K, Georgiou I. Dramatic reduction in sperm parameters following bariatric surgery: report of two cases. Andrologia. 2012;44(6):428–32.
41. Facchiano E, Scaringi S, Veltri M, Samavat J, Maggi M, Forti G, Luconi M, Lucchese M. Age as a predictive factor of testosterone improvement in male patients after bariatric surgery: preliminary results of a monocentric prospective study. Obes Surg. 2013;23(2):167–72.
42. Jansen RP, Burton GJ. Mitochondrial dysfunction in reproduction. Mitochondrion. 2004;4:577–600.
43. Van Blerkom J. Mitochondria as regulatory forces in oocytes, preimplantation embryos and stem cells. Reprod Biomed Online. 2008;16:553–69.
44. Tachibana M, Sparman M, Sritanaudomchai H, Ma H, Clepper Woodward J, Li Y, Ramsey C, Kolotushkina O, Mitalipov S. Mitochondrial gene replacement in primate offspring and embryonic stem cells. Nature. 2009;461:367–72.
45. Chavarro JE, Ehrlich S, Colaci DS, Wright DL, Toth TL, Petrozza JC, Hauser R. Body mass index and short-term weight change in relation to treatment outcomes in women undergoing assisted reproduction. Fertil Steril. 2012;98(1):109–16.
46. Moran LJ, Norman RJ. The obese patient with infertility: a practical approach to diagnosis and treatment. Nutr Clin Care. 2002;5(6):290–7.

47. Brewer CJ, Balen AH. The adverse effects of obesity on conception and implantation. Reproduction. 2010;140(3):347–64.
48. Fauser BCJM, Tarlatzis BC, Rebar RW, Legro RS, Balen AH, Lobo R, et al. Consensus on women's health aspects of polycystic ovary syndrome (PCOS): the Amsterdam ESHRE/ASRM-Sponsored 3rd PCOS Consensus Workshop Group. Fertil Steril. 2012;97(1):28–38.
49. Westphal LM, Polan ML, Trant AS, Mooney SB. A nutritional supplement for improving fertility in women. J Reprod Med. 2004;49(4):289–93.
50. Stamets K, Taylor DS, Kunselman A, Demers LM, Pelkman CL, Legro RS. A randomized trial of the effects of two types of short-term hypocaloric diets on weight loss in women with polycystic ovary syndrome. Fertil Steril. 2004;81(3):630–7.
51. Russell JB, Abboud C, Williams A, Gibbs M, Pritchard S, Chalfant D. Does changing a patient's dietary consumption of proteins and carbohydrates impact blastocyst development and clinical pregnancy rates from one cycle to the next? Fertil Steril. 2012;98(3):S47.
52. Håkonsen LB, Thulstrup AM, Aggerholm AS, Olsen J, Bonde JP, Andersen CY, Bungum M, Emst EH, Hansen ML, Ernst EH, Ramlau-Hansen CH. Does weight loss improve semen quality and reproductive hormones? Results from a cohort of severely obese men. Reprod Health. 2011;8(24):3–8.
53. Kaur JA. Comprehensive review on metabolic syndrome. Cardiol Res Pract. 2014;2014:943162.
54. American Diabetes Association (ADA). Evidence based nutrition principles and recommendations for the treatment and prevention of diabetes and related complications. Diabetes Care. 2002;25(1):202–12.
55. Wanders AJ, van den Borne JJ, de Graaf C, Hulshof T, Jonathan MC, Kristensen M, Mars M, Schols HA, Feskens EJ. Effects of dietary fibre on subjective appetite, energy intake and body weight: a systematic review of randomized controlled trials. Obes Rev. 2011;12(9):724–39.
56. Esfahani A, Wong JM, Mirrahimi A, Srichaikul K, Jenkins DJ, Kendall CW. The glycemic index: physiological significance. J Am Coll Nutr. 2009;28(Suppl):439 S–5.
57. Holzer H, Casper R, Tulandi T. A new era in ovulation induction. Fertil Steril. 2006;85(2):277–84.
58. Norman RJ, Noakes M, Wu R, Davies MJ, Moran L, Wang JX. Improving reproductive performance in overweight/obese women with effective weight management. Hum Reprod Update. 2004;10:267–80.
59. Moran L, Norman RJ. Understanding and managing disturbances in insulin metabolism and body weight in women with polycystic ovary syndrome. Best Pract Res Clin Obstet Gynaecol. 2004;18(5):719–36.
60. Liu M, Yin Y, Ye X, Zeng M, Zhao Q, Keefe DL, Liu L. Resveratrol protects against age-associated infertility in mice. Hum Reprod. 2013;28(3):707–17.
61. Cabello E. Respuesta a la hiperestimulación ovárica en un modelo murino de obesidad. Potencial terapéutico del resveratrol. Trabajo Fin de Master. Máster en Biología y Tecnología de la Reproducción. Universidad de Oviedo; 2013.
62. Benrick A, Maliqueo M, Miao S, Villanueva JA, Feng Y, Ohlsson C, Duleba AJ, Stener-Victorin E. Resveratrol is not as effective as physical exercise for improving reproductive and metabolic functions in rats with dihydrotestosterone-induced polycystic ovary syndrome. Evid Based Complement Alternat Med. 2013;2013:964070.
63. Vaamonde D, Da Silva-Grigoletto ME, García-Manso JM, Barrera N, Vaamonde-Lemos R. Physically active men show better semen parameters and hormone values than sedentary men. Eur J Appl Physiol. 2012;112:3267–73.
64. Maleki BH, Tartibian B, Vaamonde D. The effects of 16 weeks of intensive cycling training on seminal oxidants and antioxidants in male road cyclists. Clin J Sport Med. 2014;24(4):302–7.
65. Hackney AC. Effects of endurance exercise on the reproductive system of men: the exercise-hypogonadal male condition. J Endocrinol Invest. 2008;31:932–8.
66. Safarinejad MR, Azma K, Kolahi AA. The effects of intensive, long-term treadmill running on reproductive hormones, hypothalamus-pituitary-testis axis, and semen quality: a randomized controlled study. J Endocrinol. 2009;200:259–71.
67. Vaamonde D, Da Silva-Grigoletto ME, Garcia-Manso JM, Vaamonde-Lemos, Swanson R, Oehninger SC. Response of semen parameters to three training modalities. Fertil Steril. 2009;92:1941–6.
68. Lucia A, Chicharro JL, Perez M, Serratosa L, Bandres F, Legido JC. Reproductive function in male endurance athletes: sperm analysis and hormonal profile. J Appl Physiol. 1996;81:2627–36.
69. Munkelwitz R, Gilbert BR. Are boxer shorts really better? A critical analysis of the role of underwear type in male subfertility. J Urol. 1998;160:1329–33.
70. Leibovitch I, Mor Y. The vicious cycling: bicycling related urogenital disorders. Eur Urol. 2005;47(3):277–86.
71. Asplund C, Barkdull T, Weiss BD. Genitourinary problems in bicyclists. Curr Sports Med Rep. 2007;6:333–9.
72. Gebreegziabher Y, Marcos E, McKinonW, Rogers G. Sperm characteristics of endurance trained cyclists. Int J Sports Med. 2004;25:247–51.
73. Torstveit MK, Sundgot-Borgen J. Participation in leanness sports but not training volume is associated with menstrual dysfunction: a national survey of 1276 elite athletes and controls. Br J Sports Med. 2005;39(3):141–7.
74. Harrison CL, Lombard CB, Moran LJ, Teede HJ. Exercise therapy in polycystic ovary syndrome: a systematic review. Hum Reprod Update. 2011;17(2):171–83.
75. Vigorito C, Giallauria F, Palomba S, Cascella T, Manguso F, Lucci R, de Lorenzo A, Tafuri D, Lombardi C, Colao A, Orio F. Beneficial effects of a three-month structured exercise training program on car-

diopulmonary functional capacity in young women with polycystic ovary syndrome. J Clin Endocrinol Metab. 2007;92(4):1379–84.
76. Giallauria F, Palomba S, Maresca L, Vuolo L, Tafuri D, Lombardi G, Colao A, Vigorito C, Orio F. Exercise training improves autonomic function and inflammatory pattern in women with polycystic ovary syndrome (PCOS). Clin Endocrinol (Oxf). 2008;69(5):792–8.
77. Palomba S, Giallauria F, Falbo A, Russo T, Oppedisano R, Tolino A, Colao A, Vigorito C, Zullo F, Orio F. Structured exercise training programme versus hypocaloric hyperproteic diet in obese polycystic ovary syndrome patients with anovulatory infertility: a 24-week pilot study. Hum Reprod. 2008;23(3):642–50.
78. Bruner B, Chad K, Chizen D. Effects of exercise and nutritional counseling in women with polycystic ovary syndrome. Appl Physiol Nutr Metab. 2006;31(4):384–91.
79. Thomson RL, Buckley JD, Noakes M, Clifton PM, Norman RJ, Brinkworth GD. The effect of a hypocaloric diet with and without exercise training on body composition, cardiometabolic risk profile, and reproductive function in overweight and obese women with polycystic ovary syndrome. J Clin Endocrinol Metab. 2008;93(9):3373–80.
80. Trapp EG, Chisholm DJ, Freund J, Boutcher SH. The effects of high-intensity intermittent exercise training on fat loss and fasting insulin levels of young women. Int J Obes. 2008;32(4):684–91.
81. Whyte LJ, Gill JM, Cathcart AJ. Effect of 2 weeks of sprint interval training on health-related outcomes in sedentary overweight/obese men. Metabolism. 2010;59(10):1421–8.
82. Pescatello LS, Franklin BA, Fagard R, Farquhar WB, Kelley GA, Ray CA. American College of Sports Medicine position stand. Exercise and hypertension. Med Sci Sports Exerc. 2004;36(3):533–53.
83. Pollock ML, Franklin BA, Balady GJ, et al. Resistance exercise in individuals with and without cardiovascular disease: benefits, rationale, safety, and prescription: an advisory from the American Heart Association. Circulation. 2001;101:828–33.
84. Sigal RJ, Kenny GP, Wasserman DH, Castaneda-Sceppa C. Physical activity/exercise and type 2 diabetes. Diabetes Care. 2004;27(10):2518–39.
85. Cauza E, Hanusch-Enserer U, Strasser B, Ludvik B, Metz-Schimmerl S, Pacini G, Wagner O, Georg P, Prager R, Kostner K, Dunky A, Haber P. The relative benefits of endurance and strength training on the metabolic factors and muscle function of people with type 2 diabetes mellitus. Arch Phys Med Rehabil. 2005;86(8):1527–33.
86. Shaw I, Shaw BS. Consequence of resistance training on body composition and coronary artery disease risk. Cardiovasc J S Afr. 2005;17(3):111–6.
87. Sarsan A, Ardiç F, Özgen M, Topuz O, Sermez Y. The effects of aerobic and resistance exercises in obese women. Clin Rehabil. 2006;20(9):773–82.
88. Mcleod BS, Retzloff MG. Epidemiology of endometriosis: an assessment of risk factors. Clin Obstet Gynecol. 2010;53(2):389–96.
89. Bianconi L, Hummelshoj ME, Coccia P, Vigano G, Vittori J, Veit R, Music A, Tomassini T, D'Hooghe T. Recognizing endometriosis as a social disease: the European Union-encouraged Italian Senate approach. Fertil Steril. 2007;88:1285–7.
90. Guo SW. An overview of the current status of clinical trials on endometriosis: issues and concerns. Fertil Steril. 2014;101(1):183–90.
91. Viganò P, Parazzini F, Somigliana E, Vercellini P. Endometriosis: epidemiology and aetiological factors. Best Pract Res Clin Obstet Gynaecol. 2004;18(2):177–200.
92. Viganò P, Somigliana E, Panina P, Rabellotti E, Vercellini P, Candiani M. Principles of phenomics in endometriosis. Hum Reprod Update. 2012;18(3):248–59.
93. Akhter N, Jebunnaher S. Evaluation of female infertility. J Med. 2012;13(2):200–9.
94. Missmer SA, Chavarro JE, Malspeis S, Bertone-Johnson ER, Hornstein MD, Spiegelman D, Barbieri RL, Willet WC, Hankinson SE. A prospective study of dietary fat consumption and endometriosis risk. Hum Reprod. 2010;25(6):1528–35.
95. Covens AL, Christopher P, Casper RF. The effect of dietary supplementation with fish oil fatty acids on surgically induced endometriosis in the rabbit. Fertil Steril. 1988;49:698–703.
96. Parazzini F, Chiaffarino F, Surace M, Chatenoud L, Cipriani S, Chiantera V, Benzi G, Fedele L. Selected food intake and risk of endometriosis. Hum Reprod. 2004;19:1755–9.
97. Trewin AJ, Petersen AC, Billaut F, McQuade LR, McInerney BV, Stepto NK. N-acetylcysteine alters substrate metabolism during high-intensity cycle exercise in well-trained humans. Appl Physiol Nutr Metab. 2013;38(12):1217–27.
98. Pittaluga E, Costa G, Krasnowska E, Brunelli R, Lundeberg T, Porpora MG, Santucci D, Parasassi T. More than antioxidant: n-acetyl-L-cysteine in a murine model of endometriosis. Fertil Steril. 2010;94(7):2905–8.
99. Baer DJ, Judd JT, Clevidence BA, Tracy RP. Dietary fatty acids affect plasma markers of inflammation in healthy men fed controlled diets: a randomized crossover study. Am J Clin Nutr. 2004;79:969–73.
100. Parazzini F, Viganò P, Candiani M, Fedele L. Diet and endometriosis risk: a literature review. Reprod Biomed Online. 2013;26(4):323–36.
101. Donnez J, Van Langendonckt A, Casanas-Roux F, Van Gossum JP, Pirard C, Jadoul P, Squifflet J, Smets M. Current thinking on the pathogenesis of endometriosis. Gynecol Obstet Invest. 2002;54(Suppl 1):52–8.
102. Jackson LW, Schisterman EF, Dey-Rao R, Browne R, Armstrong D. Oxidative stress and endometriosis. Hum Reprod. 2005;20(7):2014–20.

103. Trabert B, Peters U, De Roos AJ, Scholes D, Holt VL. Diet and risk of endometriosis in a population-based case–control study. Br J Nutr. 2011;105(03):459–67.
104. Netsu S, Konno R, Odagiri K, Soma M, Fujiwara H, Suzuki M. Oral eicosapentaenoic acid supplementation as possible therapy for endometriosis. Fertil Steril. 2008;90(4 Suppl):1496–502.
105. Darling AM, Chavarro JE, Malspeis S, Harris HR, Missmer SA. A prospective cohort study of Vitamins B, C, E, and multivitamin intake and endometriosis. J Endometr. 2013;5(1):17–26.
106. Durak Y, Kokcu A, Kefeli M, Bildircin D, Çelik H, Alper T. Effect of vitamin C on the growth of experimentally induced endometriotic cysts. J Obstet Gynaecol Res. 2013;39(7):1253–8. doi:10.1111/jog.12050. (Epub 2013 May 30).
107. Sayegh L, Fuleihan GEH, Nassar AH. Vitamin D in endometriosis: a causative or confounding factor? Metabolism. 2014;63(1):32–41.
108. Kaneda N, Nagata C, Kabuto M, et al. Fat and fiber intakes in relation to serum estrogen concentration in premenopausal Japanese women. Nutr Cancer. 1997;27:279–83.
109. Marziali M, Venza M, Lazzaro S, Lazzaro A, Micossi C, Stolfi VM. Gluten-free diet: a new strategy for management of painful endometriosis related symptoms? Minerva Chir. 2012;67(6):499–504.
110. Radak Z, Chung HY, Koltai E, Taylor AW, Goto S. Exercise, oxidative stress and hormesis. Ageing Res Rev. 2008;7(1):34–42.
111. Bonocher CM, Montenegro ML, Rosa E, Silva JC, Ferriani RA, Meola J. Endometriosis and physical exercises: a systematic review. Reprod Biol Endocrinol. 2014;12:4.
112. Ostrowski K, Rohde T, Zacho M, Asp S, Pedersen BK. Evidence that interleukin-6 is produced in human skeletal muscle during prolonged running. J Physiol. 1998;508:949–53.
113. Pedersen AM, Pedersen BK. The anti-inflammatory effect of exercise. J Appl Physiol. 2005;98:1154–62.
114. Steensberg AC, Keller RL, Starkie T, Osada MA, Febbraio BK, Pedersen. IL-6 and TNF-a expression in, and release from, contracting skeletal muscle. Am J Physiol Endocrinol Metab. 2002;283:E1272–8.
115. Warren MP, Perlroth NE. The effects of intense exercise on the female reproductive system. J Endocrinol. 2001;170:3–11.
116. Stoll BA. Adiposity as a risk determinant for postmenopausal breast cancer. Int J Obes Relat Metab Disord. 2000;24:527–33.
117. Montenegro M, Bonocher C, Rosa e Silva JC, Meola J, Ferriani RA. Influence of aerobic exercise on endometriosis induced in rat. Fertil Steril. 2013;100(3):S372.
118. Dhillon PK, Holt VL. Recreational physical activity and endometrioma risk. Am J Epidemiol. 2003;158(2):156–64.
119. Vitonis AF, Hankinson SE, Hornstein MD, Missmer SA. Adult physical activity and endometriosis risk. Epidemiology. 2010;21(1):16. (Cambridge, Mass.).
120. Friggi-Sebe-Petrelluzzi K, Garcia MC, Petta CA, Ribeiro DA, de Oliveira Monteiro NR, Céspedes IC, Spadari RC. Physical therapy and psychological intervention normalize cortisol levels and improve vitality in women with endometriosis. J Psychosom Obstet Gynecol. 2012;33(4):191–8.
121. Boutcher SH. High-intensity intermittent exercise and fat loss. J Obes. 2011;2011:868305.
122. De Araujo ACC, Roschel H, Picanço AR, do Prado DML, Villares SMF, de Sa Pinto AL, Gualano B. Similar health benefits of endurance and high-intensity interval training in obese children. PloS ONE. 2012;7(8):e42747.
123. Carratalá V, García A. Diferencias en las motivaciones y actividades de ocio y tiempo libre entre adolescentes deportistas y no deportistas. Eur J Hum Mov. 2010;5:111–31. (Motricidad).
124. Chavarro JE, Rich-Edwards JW, Rosner BA, Willett WC. Caffeinated and alcoholic beverage intake in relation to ovulatory disorder infertility. Epidemiology. 2009;20(3):374 (Cambridge, Mass.).
125. Sharpe RM. Environmental/lifestyle effects on spermatogenesis. Philos Trans R Soc B: Biol Sci. 2010;365(1546):1697–712.
126. Braga DPAF, Halpern G, Figueira RDCS, Setti AS, Iaconelli A Jr, Borges E Jr. Food intake and social habits in male patients and its relationship to intracytoplasmic sperm injection outcomes. Fertil Steril. 2012;97(1):53–9.
127. Santti R, Mäkelä S, Strauss L, Korkman J, Kostian ML. Phytoestrogens: potential endocrine disruptors in males. Toxicol Ind Health. 1998;14(1–2):223–37.
128. Rozati R, Reddy PP, Reddanna PA, Mujtaba R. Role of environmental estrogens in the deterioration of male factor fertility. Fertil Steril. 2002;78(6):1187–94.
129. Mendiola J, Torres-Cantero AM, Moreno-Grau JM, Ten J, Roca M, Moreno-Grau S, Bernabeu R. Food intake and its relationship with semen quality: a case-control study. Fertil Steril. 2009;91(3):812–8.
130. Mendiola J, Torres-Cantero AM, Vioque J, Moreno-Grau JM, Ten J, Roca M, Bernabeu R. A low intake of antioxidant nutrients is associated with poor semen quality in patients attending fertility clinics. Fertil Steril. 2010;93(4):1128–33.
131. Magnusdottir EV, Thorsteinsson T, Thorsteinsdottir S, Heimisdottir M, Olafsdottir K. Persistent organochlorines, sedentary occupation, obesity and human male subfertility. Hum Reprod. 2005;20(1):208–15.
132. Thonneau P, Bujan L, Multigner L, Mieusset R. Occupational heat exposure and male fertility: a review. Hum Reprod. 1998;13(8):2122–5.
133. Støy J, Hjøllund NHI, Mortensen JT, Burr H, Bonde JP. Semen quality and sedentary work position. Int J Androl. 2004;27(1):5–11.

134. Joesoef MR, Beral V, Aral SO, Rolfs RT, Cramer DW. Fertility and use of cigarettes, alcohol, marijuana, and cocaine. Ann Epidemiol. 1993;3(6):592–4.
135. Sadeu JC, Hughes CL, Agarwal S, Foster WG. Alcohol, drugs, caffeine, tobacco, and environmental contaminant exposure: reproductive health consequences and clinical implications. Crit Rev Toxicol. 2010;40(7):633–52.
136. Sadeu JC, Foster WG. Cigarette smoke condensate exposure delays follicular development and function in a stage-dependent manner. Fertil Steril. 2011;95(7):2410–7.
137. Dechanet C, Anahory T, Mathieu Daude JC, Quantin X, Reyftmann L, Hamamah S, Hedon B, Dechaud H. Effects of cigarette smoking on reproduction. Hum Reprod Update. 2011;17:76–95.
138. Gannon AM, Stämpfli MR, Foster WG. Cigarette smoke exposure leads to follicle loss via an alternative ovarian cell death pathway in a mouse model. Toxicol Sci. 2012;125(1):274–84.
139. Gaur DS, Talekar MS, Pathak V. Alcohol intake and cigarette smoking: impact of two major lifestyle factors on male fertility. Indian J Pathol Microbiol. 2010;53(1):35.
140. Mueller BA, Daling JR, Weiss NS, Moore DE. Recreational drug use and the risk of primary infertility. Epidemiology. 1990;1(3):195–200.
141. Fronczak CM, Kim ED, Barqawi AB. The insults of illicit drug use on male fertility. J Androl. 2012;33(4):515–28.
142. Mendelson JH, Mello NK, Ellingboe J. Acute effects of marihuana smoking on prolactin levels in human females. J Pharmacol Exp Ther. 1985;232(1):220–2.
143. Park B, McPartland JM, Glass M. Cannabis, cannabinoids and reproduction. Prostaglandins Leukot Essent Fatty Acids. 2004;11:189–97.
144. Battista N, Pasquariello N, Tommaso M D, Maccarrone M. Interplay between endocannabinoids, steroids and cytokines in the control of human reproduction. J Neuroendocrinol. 2008;11(Suppl 1):82–9.
145. Gold MS, Jacobs WS. Cocaine (and crack): clinical aspects. In: Lowinson JH, editor. Substance abuse: a comprehensive textbook. 3rd edn. Baltimore: Williams & Wilkins; 1997. pp. 181–199.
146. George VK, Li H, Teloken C, Grignon DJ, Lawrence WD, Dhabuwala CB. Effects of long-term cocaine exposure on spermatogenesis and fertility in peripubertal male rats. J Urol. 1996;11:327.
147. Gold MS, Miller NS. Cocaine and crack. In: Lowinson JH, editor. Substance abuse: a comprehensive textbook. 3rd edn. Baltimore: Williams & Wilkins; 1997. pp. 195–218 (Neurobiology).
148. Wang C, Chan V, Yeung RT. The effect of heroin addiction on pituitary-testicular function. Clin Endocrinol (Oxf). 1978;11:455–61. doi:10.1111/j.1365–2265.1978.
149. Ragni G, De Lauretis L, Gambaro V, Pietro R D, Bestetti O, Recalcati F, Papetti C. Semen evaluation in heroin and methadone addicts. Acta Eur Fertil. 1985;11:245–9.
150. Anderson K, Niesenblat V, Norman R. Lifestyle factors in people seeking infertility treatment—a review. Aust N Z J Obstet Gynaecol. 2010;11:8–20.
151. Eggert J, Theobald H, Engfeldt P. Effects of alcohol consumption on female fertility during an 18-year period. Fertil Steril. 2004;81(2):379–83.
152. Jensen TK, Hjollund NHI, Henriksen TB, Scheike T, Kolstad H, Giwercman A, Ernst E, Bonde JP, Skakkebaek NE, Olsen J. Does moderate alcohol consumption affect fertility? Follow up study among couples planning first pregnancy. BMJ. 1998;317(7157):505–10.
153. Van der Colf AP, Kruger TF, Menkveld R, Seier JV, Finch Am JE, Swart Y. Effect of ethanol on semen characteristics of vervet monkeys. Syst Biol Reprod Med. 1991;26(1):25–9.
154. Pajarinen J, Karhunen PJ, Savolainen V, Lalu K, Penttilä A, Laippala P. Moderate alcohol consumption and disorders of human spermatogenesis. Alcohol Clin Exp Res. 1996;20(2):332–7.

Erratum to: Exercise and Human Reproduction: Induced Fertility Disorders and Possible Therapies

21

Diana Vaamonde, Stefan S. du Plessis and Ashok Agarwal

Erratum to:
D. Vaamonde et al. (eds.), *Exercise and Human Reproduction*,
DOI 10.1007/978-1-4939-3402-7

The publisher regrets to inform that the below mentioned corrections were missed out or incorrectly carried out in the print and online files:

1) The correct affiliation of corresponding book editor, "Diana Vaamonde" is as mentioned below and needs to be changed globally.

Diana Vaamonde, MS, PhD
Department of Morphological Sciences
School of Medicine
University of Cordoba
International Network on Physical Exercise and Fertility (INPEF)
Cordoba, Spain

2) In the Contributors List, the below mentioned authors have to be listed with their correct degrees:
   a) Ignacio Jimena-Medina, MD, PhD
   b) Luis Jiménez-Reina, MD, PhD
   c) Diana Vaamonde, MS, PhD
   d) Ricardo Vaamonde-Lemos, MD, PhD

3) In About the Authors, please edit the following:
   a) Write the corresponding book editor's name as "Diana Vaamonde MS, PhD (Diana Maria Vaamonde Martin)".
   b) In the second paragraph, first line, remove the word "the".
   c) In the second paragraph, third line, insert "human" before reproduction.
   d) In the third paragraph, change the sentence starting with "She is also…" to "She has also been the…".

The online version of the updated original book can be found under DOI 10.1007/978-1-4939-3402-7

D. Vaamonde (✉)
Department of Morphological Sciences, School of Medicine, University of Cordoba, International Network on Physical Exercise and Fertility (INPEF), Cordoba, Spain
e-mail: fivresearch@yahoo.com

S. S. du Plessis
Division of Medical Physiology, Department of Biomedical Sciences, Stellenbosch University, P.O. Box 19063, 7505 Tygerberg, Cape Town, South Africa
e-mail: ssdp@sun.ac.za

A. Agarwal
American Center for Reproductive Medicine, Cleveland Clinic Foundation, Cleveland, OH, USA

© Springer Science+Business Media New York 2016

D. Vaamonde et al. (eds.), *Exercise and Human Reproduction*, DOI 10.1007/978-1-4939-3402-7_21

Index

© Springer Science+Business Media New York 2016
D. Vaamonde et al. (eds.), *Exercise and Human Reproduction*, DOI 10.1007/978-1-4939-3402-7